Evaluation and Surgical Management of the Ankle

Dolfi Herscovici Jr. • Jeffrey O. Anglen
John S. Early

Editors

Evaluation and Surgical Management of the Ankle

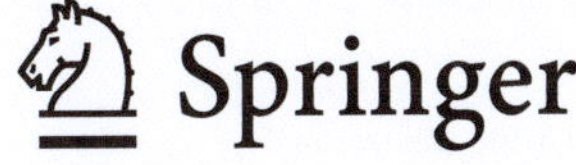

Springer

Editors
Dolfi Herscovici Jr.
Center for Bone and Joint Disease
Hudson, FL, USA

Jeffrey O. Anglen
Hughston Orthopedic Trauma
Indianapolis, IN, USA

John S. Early
Texas Orthopaedic Associates
Dallas, TX, USA

ISBN 978-3-031-33539-6   ISBN 978-3-031-33537-2   (eBook)
https://doi.org/10.1007/978-3-031-33537-2

This Springer imprint is published by the registered company Springer Nature Switzerland AG
The registered company address is: Gewerbestrasse 11, 6330 Cham, Switzerland

Preface

To learn is to change. Education is the process that changes the learner.
George B. Leonard, *Education and Ecstasy*, 1968

The junction between the lower leg and the foot is a unique articulation. The three bones that make up the ankle joint are the tibia above and medially, the fibula laterally, and the talus below. Here the vertical weight-bearing forces of the leg are dynamically transferred to the more horizontal support system of the foot. The muscular forces that result in bipedal ambulation are transferred around this corner by muscles and tendons acting upon the foot, constrained by the anatomy and structure of the ankle joint, the subtalar joint and their ligaments. It is a complex and beautiful machine that allows human gait while simultaneously maintaining stability on a variety of surfaces, allowing an individual the ability to walk, run, climb, kick a football, and dance.

Human gait is a pattern of repetitive muscular actions that can be analyzed using the term "stride." A single stride begins the moment that the heel strikes the ground and continues until the same heel strikes the ground again. Stride length is the distance between these two consecutive heel strikes and a "step" is defined as the distance between the heel strike of one foot and heel strike of the opposite foot. Normal gait is extremely efficient for both energy and oxygen consumption while a dysfunctional gait leads to increases in both energy and oxygen consumption. The many potential causes of a dysfunctional gait include pain, fractures, ligament instability, muscle or tendon problems, developmental abnormalities, and nerve damage.

Ankle disorders may result in changes in gait and can produce serious long-term complications that may be disruptive to the enjoyment of life. While many ankle injuries or conditions are self-limited and respond to conservative care, others may be best treated with surgical procedures. Some surgical conditions involving the ankle are among the most common problems that orthopedic surgeons encounter. Others are more complex and challenging. All deserve careful and thorough evaluation, consideration of alternatives, and a skillful application of evidence-based treatments. Too often, patients who present with significant problems may only be offered conservative care or an amputation as their only options due to physician inexperience, or concerns about arduous treatment courses, complications, or liability. Our goal with this textbook is to help physicians treating ankle problems with diagnosis, treatment strategy, and management for optimal outcomes.

As editors, we have assembled this textbook as a reference guide, with up-to-date chapter references, to help people tasked with managing patients with ankle problems. It is also intended as a primer with current concepts for the management of soft tissue disorders, fractures, diabetes chronic ankle problems, wound management, and osteochondral disorders. We have assembled a group of authors who are experienced and recognized as leading authorities in the management of ankle disorders. We have asked them to provide their practical, step-by-step approach to managing complex ankle problems along with tips and tricks and hazards to avoid. In addition, we have provided chapters discussing the anatomy, physiology, and biomechanics of the ankle along with radiographic approaches for the evaluation of these patients and a chapter outlining a differential to be considered when evaluating patients with ankle pain. By providing a better understanding, we can hopefully help patients maintain or return to productive and rewarding activity, and thereby produce happier patients and families. To the mid-level providers, students, residents, fellows, and physicians tasked with evaluating patients with ankle problems, we hope that the information provided in this textbook will better help guide your decisions when evaluating patients with ankle problems.

Hudson, FL, USA
Indianapolis, IN, USA
Dallas, TX, USA

Dolfi Herscovici Jr
Jeffrey O. Anglen
John S. Early

Acknowledgments

First, I would like to thank all the authors for their contributions. Your knowledge on the subject matter you were asked to write about is incredible. Thank you for putting up with all of our requests and helping to put together what we feel is an outstanding book. Second, I would like to thank my co-editors, Jeff Anglen and John Early; this project could not have been completed without both of you. Lastly, I would like to thank my beautiful wife, Lisa, for her support as my confidante and my de facto editor, for allowing me to sequester myself in my office to edit the manuscripts and for telling me when it was time to take a break and rejoin the real world.

—Dolfi Herscovici, Jr, DO, FAAOS

This book is the brainchild and labor of love of my friend Dolfi, who has spent his career studying orthopedic trauma with a specific focus on foot and ankle conditions. I am grateful to him for including me in the project. I, too, thank the authors for their hard work and willingness to spend a great deal of time producing this book. They are all busy people, and they have done this out of love of the topic and of teaching, because Lord knows no one is making any money off medical texts these days. I owe a great debt to my teachers, too many to mention, but hopefully this work will honor them and help pay it forward. Thanks also to Amy, for putting up with me most of the time.

—Jeff Anglen, MD, FIOTA

First and foremost, the concept and content of this work is the direct result of Dr. Herscovici's inspiration and perspiration. He was the driving force in this project. Thank you for allowing me to participate. Thanks also to my other co-editor, Jeff Anglen, for his valued efforts and contributions to making this a reality. To the authors, this is really your work. Without your expertise and ability to put your vast experience into words none of this would be possible. Thanks for working with us. Finally, thanks to my wife, CJ, for giving me the time and space to help with this project.

—John S. Early, MD, FAAOS

Contents

Part I

General Considerations

Embryology, Anatomy, and Physiology of the Ankle

Kristin A. Toy and Joshua N. Tennant

1 Introduction

In its development and form, the human ankle is an anatomical structure comprised of three bones with soft tissue structures, muscles, and neurovascular structures that allow for its unique function. Within the field of orthopaedics, knowledge of prenatal development of the lower extremity can aid in the understanding and treatment of congenital and acquired foot and ankle deformities. An understanding of anatomy and physiology further contributes to the foundational knowledge of clinical treatment of the ankle. This chapter will give a brief overview of the embryonic development and morphology, adult anatomy, and physiology of the ankle.

2 Embryology

Human embryologic development is a complex process that transforms a single cell into a multicellular organism composed of complex systems of specialized tissues. Driven by the integration of gene expression, cellular signaling, and structural elements, organogenesis is an intricate and delicately timed stage of development.

2.1 Ankle and Foot Formation in the Human Embryo and Fetus

The lower extremity will undergo many developmental and morphological changes during various stages of gestation. In 1929, Bohm classically described the embryonic foot development as four morphologic stages with distinct characteristics [1]. The majority of these changes occur between the second month and fourth month of development, with nearly all rudimentary structures of the foot formed by week 8 [2].

At 3 weeks post fertilization, the first sign of lower extremity formation occurs as a swelling along the lumbar and sacral myotomes. At week 4, this swelling gives rise to the lower limb bud parallel to the trunk. During this week, the limb bud grows and extends in the coronal plane, with separate identifiable regions of the thigh, leg, and foot. Internally, the neurovascular and myogenic

K. A. Toy
Department of Orthopaedic Surgery, University of North Carolina Hospitals, Chapel Hill, NC, USA
e-mail: Kristin.Toy@unchealth.unc.edu

J. N. Tennant (✉)
Foot and Ankle Service, Department of Orthopaedic Surgery, University of North Carolina Medical School, University of North Carolina Hospitals, Chapel Hill, NC, USA
e-mail: josh_tennant@med.unc.edu

© The Author(s), under exclusive license to Springer Nature Switzerland AG 2023
D. Herscovici Jr. et al. (eds.), *Evaluation and Surgical Management of the Ankle*,
https://doi.org/10.1007/978-3-031-33537-2_1

precursors begin to migrate into the growing limb buds [2, 3]. A foot disk is first visible at week 5, with the future plantar foot facing towards the head of the embryo. Digital rays become apparent at the end of the fifth week, but with digital notching present only at the hallux (great toe) [4]. By week 6, the limb will internally rotate 90-degrees along its longitudinal axis which brings the limb into the transverse plane. The preaxial (tibial) border of the foot is now cephalad and postaxial (fibular) border caudal. The foot plate is now in line with the long axis of the leg, resulting in an equinus position [1, 2]. Internally, previously dispersed mesenchymal cells gather into a tightly packed cell mass, known as mesenchymal condensations, and allow skeletal development to undergo chondrification (cartilage formation). During this period of development, the gastrocsoleus complex (gastrocnemius and soleus muscles) is distinct in form [2].

By week 7, the plantar surfaces of the feet are in the sagittal plane facing midline and the plantar pads are visible. The digits are distinct structures with well-defined interdigital spaces and the malleoli are of equal lengths. By week 8, the lower extremity remains in an externally rotated position in the transverse plane with the anterior surface of the knees laterally, and the soles of the feet touching at midline ("praying position"). Once cell differentiation has occurred the embryo enters the next stage known as the fetal stage. This period of development begins during the nineth week and lasts until birth. During fetal stage, the ankle joint begins to form, moving the foot out of equinus. During the fourth month, gradual pronation and dorsiflexion begins and continues for the remaining time in gestation [1].

Ligament development occurs prior to formation of the joint interzone and cavity formation and in general is complete by the second half of the fourth month. The syndesmosis ligaments and the deep layer of the deltoid ligament are the first to develop with the posterior tibiofibular ligament appearing during the eighth week. The inferior transverse and anterior tibiofibular ligaments appear next, along with the deep layer of the deltoid ligament and the superior retinaculum. Formed in a proximal to distal direction, the superior retinaculum will form a tunnel over the developing extensor tendons. During the nineth week, the superficial layer of the deltoid ligament, subtalar ligaments, and inferior retinaculum appear [5].

2.2　Morphological Changes Seen in Skeletal Structures

The four external morphological stages described by Böhm can be attributed to the individual changes and growth that occur as the skeletal elements develop (see Table 1). Like the foot, the ankle is also divided into preaxial (tibia) and postaxial (fibula) regions. Initially the preaxial border is more lateral with the plantar surface in the transverse plane facing cranially, and the medial malleolus is more distal than the lateral malleolus [6]. In week 6, the talus will form with a low dome of the talar body, in an oblique/adducted and wedged position angled 90° between the malleoli [5–7] (see Fig. 1).

Table 1 Böhm's developmental stages of the foot and ankle [1]

Stage	Gestation	Changes	Morphologic features
1	Month 2 (week 6)		• Leg/thigh in marked external rotation • Foot is adducted and in equinus
2	Month 3 (week 9)	• Internal rotation of leg, 90-degree rotation of foot along axis of the leg	• Foot is in equinus, adduction, with significant supination
3	Month 3 (week 10)	• Resolution of equinus and adduction with growth of talus	• Dorsiflexion of the ankle with mild equinus • Adduction of first metatarsal and significant supination of foot
4	Month 4 (week 12)	• Gradual pronation of the foot	• Dorsiflexion of the ankle with resolution of equinus • Pronation of the foot

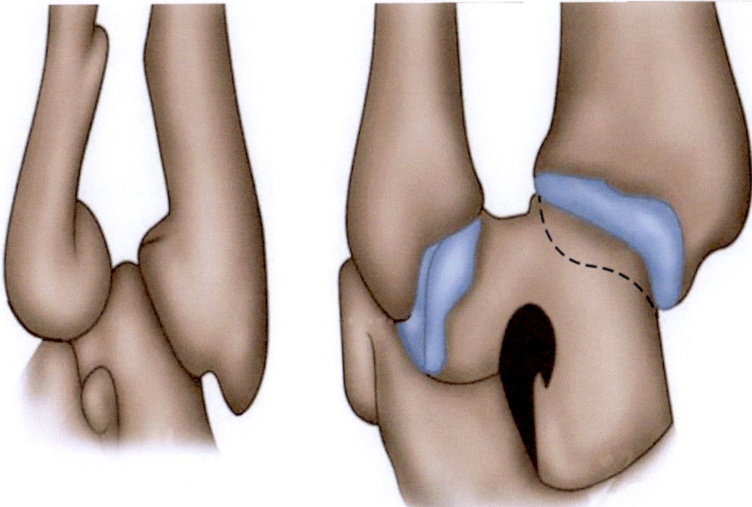

Fig. 1 Week 6 and 7 embryonic ankle. Appearance of the ankle during week 6 of development. The talus is obliquely wedged between the malleoli which are of equivalently distal. The talar dome is low compared to the adult and the future trochlea is adjacent to the distal tibia. (Adapted and modified from Sarrafian SK. *Anatomy of the Foot and Ankle: Descriptive, Topographic, Functional.* Third ed. Philadelphia: Lippincott; 2011. Original source; Olivier G. *Formation du Squelette des Membres chez l'Homme.* Vigot frères; 1962)

Internal rotation of the leg brings the footplate with the preaxial border cephalad and plantar surface facing midline. The position of the talus influences the position of the remaining tarsal bones and overall morphological features seen in Bohm's stage 1. The calcaneus lies lateral to the talus and is covered by the lateral third of the talus, while the navicular is displaced medially towards the tibia resulting in adduction of the metatarsal heads [1]. Secondary to the wedged position of the talus, the distal tibia is oblique and concave and the foot is in equinus at 90° of plantarflexion.

The malleoli become equivalently distal in week 7, with the lateral malleolus becoming more distal towards the end of the seventh week. At the end of the embryonic period, the distal tibiofibular joint is formed while the foot remains in equinus and adduction. The talus will elongate and extend over the calcaneus onto the newly formed sustentaculum tali, while the trochlea of the talus remains considerably flattened with a posterior declination of the ankle [5, 7]. Equinus persists due to the plantigrade position of the talar head and neck and posterior declination angle of the distal tibia. A difference in medial and lateral talus height causes a lateral tilting of the tibiotalar joint and a calcaneovarus position at the talocalcaneal joint [8]. These positions persist until the first 2 months of the fetal period where unequal growth along the distal tibia and trochlea brings the ankle out of equinus and varus.

At the beginning of week 9 the posterior declination angle decreases, bringing the distal tibia to 90° perpendicular to the shaft. In later weeks, the tibia will acquire an anterior inclination, which persists in adults with the articular surface at 93.3 ± 3.2° to the shaft [5, 9]. As the trochlea becomes elevated and rounded, there is increased growth in overall talus height and width. This decreases the calcaneal varus and moves the talar head laterally to increase the angle of torsion. At the mortise joint, there is increased growth along the medial side of the trochlea and lateral side of the plafond which resolves the lateral tilt of the tibiotalar joint [6, 8, 10]. By the end of the fourth month, these changes result in the feet acquiring a position of dorsiflexion and pronation [1, 10]. The secondary ossification center of the talus appears during the eighth month of gestation, while the secondary ossification centers of the distal tibia and fibula appear after birth.

Dorsiflexion and pronation continue to increase until birth, at which time additional morphological changes occur until the adult form of the ankle is reached.

2.3 Postnatal Development of the Ankle

Postnatal skeletal development of the ankle occurs in females earlier than in males. In females the secondary ossification centers appear during the fourth (distal tibia) and nineth month (distal fibula) and close around 14 years of age. In males, secondary ossification begins during the fourth (distal tibia) and 13th month (distal fibula) and close around 16 years of age. During this period, the talar head and neck continue to lateralize which decreases the neck-trochlear angle while increasing the torsional angle of the talus neck and head [10]. The distal tibia will externally rotate until age 5 with the most significant changes occurring during the first 3 months of life and between the fourth and fifth year of life [5, 11].

3 Anatomy

3.1 Osteology

The osseous anatomy of the ankle joint is comprised of three bones: the distal fibula, distal tibia, and talus. The bimalleolar form of the mortise of the ankle is rigid medially, and mobile laterally.

3.1.1 Tibia

The tibia is the primary weight bearing bone found in the leg and articulates with the talus to form the ankle joint. Distally, the logintudinal axis of the tibia is externally rotated relative to the axis of the tibia plateau approximately 30° (tibia torsion). The distal end of the tibia has five distinct surfaces; inferior, anterior, posterior, lateral, and medial.

The inferior surface, also known as the plafond, is composed of articular cartilage and artic-

ulates with the trochlea of the talus. Quadrangular in shape, the lateral and anterior borders are larger than the medial and posterior borders, respectively. The surface is concave from anterior to posterior, and transversely it is slightly convex, with a slightly elevated ridge seperating the lateral and medial segments. Described as the frustum of a cone (base of a cone after being cut into two pieces horizontally) with a mean medial apical angle of 22 ± 4°. The radius of curvature is smaller on the medial than lateral side [10] (see Fig. 7).

The anterior surface of the plafond is a continuation of the lateral surface of the tibial shaft, found between the borders of the interosseous membrane and the anterior crest. At the distal tibia, the tibia is externally rotated and brings the lateral surface anterior. A transverse ridge is located 0.5–1 cm proximal to the anterior plafond, and serves as the attachment site for the joint capsule [5]. Posteriorly, the tibial shaft is continuous with the posterior surface of the plafond which is smooth and slightly convex. On the medial aspect of the posterior surface there is vertical groove traveling towards the posterior malleolus which holds the posterior tibialis tendon. The neurovascular bundle travels lateral to the vertical groove along the posterior surface.

The lateral surface of the distal tibia forms the triangular shaped fibular notch, or incisura fibularis. Proximally, there is a roughened area of bone known as the interosseous crest, that is contiguous with the anterior and posterior borders of the incisura. These two areas diverge from the crest and terminate distally as forming the larger anterior and smaller posterior tubercles. These tubercles allow for the attachment of the respective anterior and posterior tibiofibular ligaments. The incisura holds the distal fibula and interosseous ligament proximally, which contributes to the stability of the syndesmosis joint. The medial surface of the distal tibia is found between the medial tibial shaft and malleolus. Bordered by the anterior and posterior surfaces of the tibial shaft, it is broad proximally and narrow distally. It serves as the attachment site for both the flexor and extensor retinaculum and is superficial and easily palpable on physical exam. This surface may extend towards the malleolus, serving as squatting facets which articulate with the talus during extreme dorsiflexion [12].

Distal to the medial surface of the distal tibia is the medial malleolus, which serves as a constraint on the medial side of the ankle mortise. The medial malleolus is pyramidal in shape and larger in the anteroposterior direction and narrow transversely. It does not extend as far distally as the lateral malleolus. The lateral aspect is concave and consists of articular cartilage to form the medial wall of the mortise. It is formed by two segments or colliculi, the anterior and posterior colliculus, separated by an intercollicular groove. This groove serves as the attachment site for the deep talotibial component of the deltoid ligament. The anterior colliculus also serves as an attachment for the superficial component of the deltoid ligament. Posteriorly, the malleolus serves as an attachment site for the flexor retinaculum and has a groove that holds the posterior tibialis tendon tunnel [5].

3.1.2 Fibula

The portion of the distal fibula that contributes to the tibiotalar joint includes the distal ¼ of the shaft and the lateral malleolus. The distal fibular shaft is quadrilateral in shape along the axial plane and can be divided into two surfaces, medial and lateral, that are separated by an anterior and posterior border. The anterior border of the fibula is divided by the interosseous crest into anteromedial and anterolateral segments [13]. On the anteromedial surface lies the origin of peroneus tertius while on the posteriomedial border lies the flexor hallucis longus muscle. Near the syndesmosis, on the lateral surface of the distal fibula, the anterior border of the distal fibula divides into two branches, anterior and posterior. The anterior branch merges with the interosseous crest, and continues distally to become the anterior border of the lateral malleolus. The point of convergence, of the anterior border and interosseous crest, marks the distal end of the anteromedial segment and interosseous membrane, and the beginning of syndesmosis ligament attachment sites [14].

The posterior branch of the anterior border, also called the oblique crest, travels posteriorly before becoming the posterior border of the lateral malleolus. The oblique crest demarcates two surfaces, anteroinferior and posterosuperior [13]. The anteroinferior surface is oriented laterally, is flat in shape and is subcutaneous. The posterosuperior surface twists and becomes continuous with the posterior aspect of the lateral malleolus. Near the tibiotalar joint, the fibula is externally rotated, which positions the peroneal tendons posterior to the lateral malleolus. Here the tendon of the peroneal brevis lies deep to the peroneal longus. Distally the fibula becomes triangular in the axial plane with both surfaces, as previously stated, becoming contiguous with the lateral malleolus [5].

The lateral malleolus is composed of the lateral, medial, and posterior surfaces, which gives it a pyramidal shape. It extends approximately 1 cm distal to the medial malleolus and is inverted with the apex of the pyramid directed inferoposterior. The lateral and medial surfaces converge towards the anterior border. The medial surface is limited to the level of the fibularis incisura. The anterior and posterior borders of the medial surface meet anteroinferiorly, and form a convex articular surface, along its long axis, to articulate with the lateral articular surface of the talus. Inferior and anterior to the articular surface are the attachment sites for the anterior talofibular, anterior tibiofibular, and calcaneofibular ligaments [5, 12]. Posterior to the articular surface are the attachment sites for the posterior talofibular and posterior tibiofibular ligaments. On the posterior surface lies the peroneal sulcus. This is a shallow groove, usually concave in shape, which houses the peroneal tendons. Also along the posterior surface are the posterior fibular tubercle and malleolar fossa which serve as the attachment site for the posterior tibiofibular ligament [5]. The lateral surface lies anteriorly and is smooth and convex and can be easily palpated on physical exam.

3.1.3 Talus

The talus is located between the bimalleolar plafond of the ankle and the tarsus. It is formed by three parts: the head, neck, and body. It has strong ligamentous but no tendinous attachments. The head articulates with the navicular, the calcaneus, and the calcaneonavicular ligaments and is rotated clockwise on the right and counterclockwise on the left.

The neck lies between the head and body. Its axis is angled inferiorly and medially, both at an average of 24° relative to the axis of the body of the talus, and has an average length of 17 mm. The neck has been divided into four surfaces: medial, lateral, inferior, and superior [5].

The body of the talus has five surfaces: medial, lateral posterior, inferior, and superior. When viewed in the coronal plane, it is wider anteriorly and narrower posteriorly, due to the shorter oblique lateral border of the talus. The *superior* surface is pulley shaped, and articulates with the articular surface of the tibia. The groove of the pulley lies more medial, making the lateral superior surface wider than the medial superior surface. The *lateral* surface is concave vertically and convex transversely and articulates with the fibula. On the apex the lateral talocalcaneal ligament inserts while the anterior talofibular ligament inserts along the anterior border of the lateral surface. The *medial* surface projects medially and inferiorly to articulate with the medial malleolus. Inferior to the articular segment lies a large oval surface which contains the insertion of the deep deltoid ligament. The *posterior* surface superiorly is non-articular. It has two projecting bony tubercles, posteromedial and posterolateral, with a sulcus running between them. The tubercles give insertion to the posterior talofibular ligament and the talar component of the fibulotalocalcaneal ligament of Rouvière and Canela Lazaro. The latter ligament inserts on the lateral aspect of the posterolateral tubercle. The flexor retinaculum inserts on the medial aspect of the surface while the posterior talocalcaneal ligament inserts on the inferior surface [5, 15].

3.2 Ligaments of the Ankle

3.2.1 Syndesmosis

The syndesmosis is the group of three ligaments which bind the distal fibula to the distal tibia, creating stability between the two bones. It consists of the anterior tibiofibular ligament, the posterior tibiofibular ligament, and the interosseous ligament. The anterior tibiofibular ligament originates on the anterior border of the distal fibula, inserting on the anterolateral and anterior distal tibia, the area known as Wagstaffe's tubercle. The fibers increase in length distally, with the most distal fibers being as long as 25 mm. The most distal fibers may overlay the superior fibers of the anterior talofibular ligament.

The posterior tibiofibular ligament has both deep and superficial components, originating on the posterior fibular tubercle. The superficial component, has fibers sweeping upward and medially to insert on the posterolateral tibial tubercle. The deep component is transverse and stout, and it has a twist of its fibers. Its insertion goes as far as the medial malleolus, effectively deepening the posterior tibial articular surface. The deep component of the ligament also articulates with the posterolateral superior talar dome, which has a corresponding facet at the ligament's contact point.

The interosseous ligament originates from the medial aspect of the distal fibular shaft, from an anterior-superior to posterior-distal footprint, that inserts on a similar footprint on the lateral border of the tibia. Proximally the interosseous ligament is in continuity with the interosseous membrane.

The superior extensor retinaculum is a thickening of the distal anterior compartment fascia of the leg, lacking distinct proximal and distal borders. It contains the anterior tibialis, extensor digitorum longus, extensor hallucis longus, and peroneus tertius tendons. Medially and laterally it inserts on the respective malleoli of the ankle, and is in continuity with the flexor retinaculum and the superior peroneal retinaculum, respectively.

3.2.2 Lateral Ankle Ligaments

The lateral ankle ligaments consist of the anterior talofibular ligament, the calcaneofibular ligament, and the posterior talofibular ligament.

The *anterior talofibular ligament* (ATFL) is a flat, rectangular structure that originates from the anterior fibula and inserts on the talar body just anterior to the articulation with the fibula. The upper and lower extents may be confluent with the anterior tibiofibular ligament and calcaneofibular ligament, respectively. In plantarflexion, the ligament is in its tightest position as it is stretched over the anterolateral corner of the talar body.

The *calcaneofibular ligament* (CFL) originates from the anterior distal lateral malleolus, just distal to the origin of the inferior band of the ATFL. The CFL lies deep to the peroneal tendon sheath as the tendons course under the distal fibula. The orientation of the CFL relative to the long axis of the fibula is variable, but it typically courses posteriorly at approximately 30° and inserts on the lateral surface of the posterior calcaneus. In this orientation, the ligament is taut in dorsiflexion and relaxed in plantarflexion. The average angle between the anterior talofibular ligament and the calcaneofibular ligament is $105 \pm 24°$ in the sagittal plane, allowing a synergistic and more efficient support of lateral ankle stability through the normal ankle range of motion [9] (Fig. 2).

The *posterior talofibular ligament* (PTFL) originates from the medial border of the posterior fibula, and courses in a horizontal plane to insert on the posterior talus, including the posterolateral tubercle or trigonal process. It forms the distal aspect of the flexor hallucis longus sheath at the level of the subtalar joint. It has increased tension in dorsiflexion, when it provides increased stability to the ankle joint, and decreased tension in plantarflexion.

3.2.3 Deltoid Ligament

The deltoid ligament is a complex confluence of multiple non-distinct fibers that stabilize the medial talus, navicular, and calcaneus, composed of superficial and deep layers. The ligament is in continuity anteriorly with the anterior ankle capsule, and the deep crural fascia, including the flexor retinaculum posteriorly. The deep talotibial fibers make up the only distinct component; the remaining divisions are surgically created, and named by their origins and insertions. The tendon sheaths of the posterior tibialis and flexor digitorum longus tendons are also confluent with the deltoid ligament.

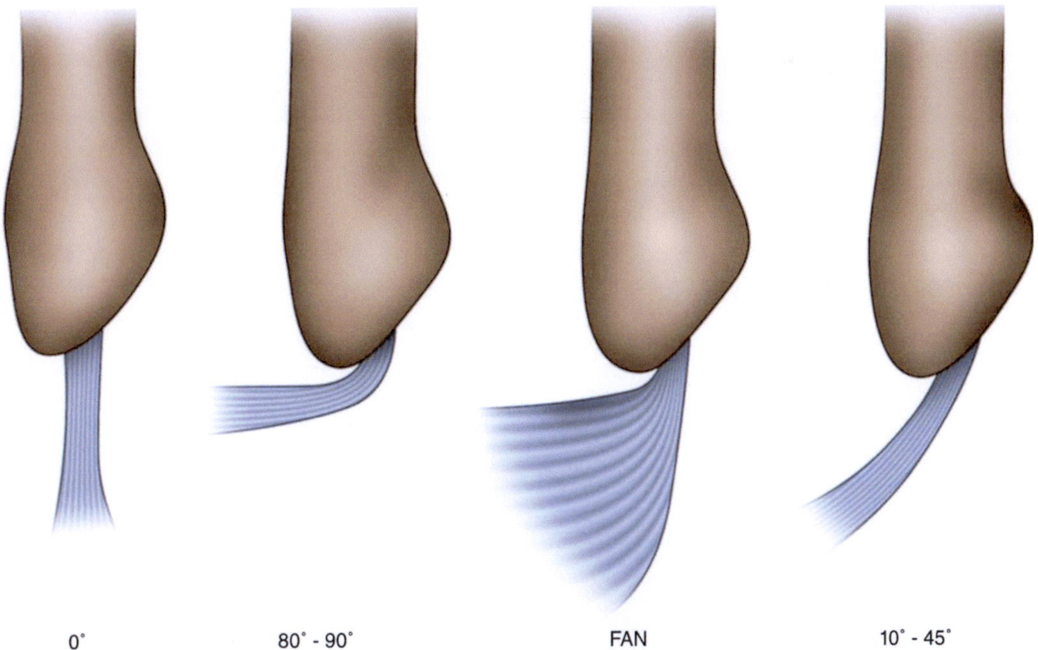

Fig. 2 The calcaneofibular ligament with various morphological appearance. (Adapted and modified from Ruth CJ. The surgical treatment of injuries of the fibular collateral ligaments of the ankle. *JBJS*. 1961;43(2):229–239)

The superficial layer of the deltoid ligament is triangular in shape, and originates from the anterior colliculus of the medial malleolus. The superficial layer consists of the anterior superficial tibiotalar fascicle, the tibionavicular fascicle, the tibioligamentous fascicle, the tibiocalcaneal ligament (the strongest portion of the superficial ligament), and the superficial posterior tbiotalar ligament.

The deep deltoid ligament is comprised of an anterior and posterior components. The deep anterior deltoid arises from the anterior colliculus and inserts on the medial wall of the talus; but is not always present [16]. The strongest portion of the entire deltoid ligament is the deep posterior tibiotalar ligament. The deep posterior ligament originates from the entire posterior colliculus, the intermolecular fossa between the two colliculi, and the upper posterior portion of the anterior colliculus. Its insertion is on the medial wall of the talar body. The deep posterior tibiotalar ligament resists external rotation and lateral displacement of the talus relative to the tibia (Fig. 3).

3.3 Myology

3.3.1 Anterior

Passing across the anterior aspect of the ankle are the tendons of (from medial to lateral); tibialis anterior (TA), extensor hallucis longus (EHL), extensor digitorum longus (EDL), and peroneus tertius (PT). These muscles originate along either the distal femur or tibial shaft and travel across the ankle and foot joints to allow for extension of the foot and ankle. The primary extensor of the ankle is the tibialis anterior (TA) muscle. Innervated by the deep peroneal nerve, the tibialis anterior muscle has a predominance of the L4 and L5 nerve roots [12]. The tibialis anterior muscle originates from the lateral condyle of the femur, lateral edge of the proximal half of the tibia and interosseous membrane. It is supplied by the branches of the anterior tibial artery and crosses the ankle joint anteriorly before inserting, with some variations, on medial plantar surface of the first cuneiform bone of the midfoot and base of the first metatarsal [17].

Fig. 3 Medial view of the ankle demonstrating the deltoid ligament

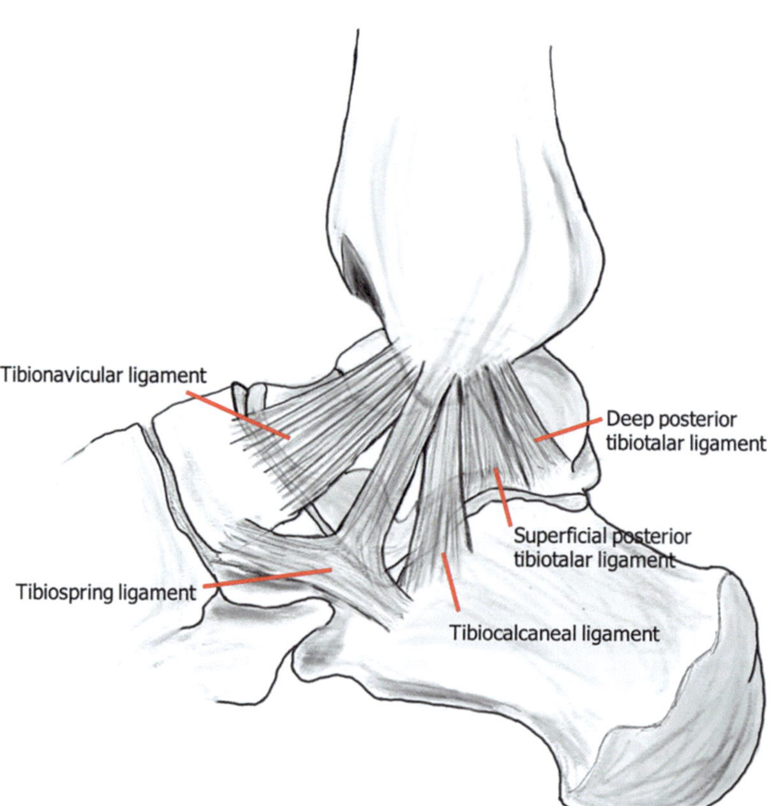

EHL originates along the anterior surface of the interosseous membrane and medial surface of the midshaft of the fibula and is innervated by the deep peroneal nerve with predominance for L5 nerve root. The EDL muscle originates along the anterior surface of interosseous membrane and medial surface of fibula and inferior surface of tibial lateral condyle, and is innervated by nerve roots L5, S1 of the deep peroneal nerve. Both EHL and EDL allow for dorsiflexion of the ankle and extension of the great toe and digits 2–5, respectively [12]. The peroneal tertius muscle originates along the medial border of distal fibula and inserts on the dorsal surface of the base of the fifth metatarsal. Also innervated by the deep peroneal nerve, it contributes to dorsiflexion and eversion during the gait cycle.

Near the distal tibia there is a thicking and reinforcement of the aponeurosis of the leg, which forms the superior and inferior extensor retinaculum (discussed in more detail in Sect. 3.3.5). Deep to the retinaculum, the tendons cross the anterior aspect of the ankle and are housed in synovial tendon sheaths.

There are three synovial sheaths that house the tendons of four anterior muscles, which begin and end at different locations along the foot and ankle. The tendon of TA is the only extensor tendon with a sheath beginning proximal to the superior extensor retinaculum, and extends to the talonavicular joint. The sheath is unique in containing a mesotenon layer that extends its entire length. The tendon sheath of EDL begins 2–3 cm proximal to the ankle joint and courses deep to the undivided inferior extensor retinaculum. This sheath also houses the peroneus tertius. Approximately 1 cm distal to the EDL sheath origin, the tendon sheath of EHL begins before traveling deep to the proximal limb of the inferior extensor retinaculum and continuing to the midfoot.

3.3.2 Lateral

The tendons of the peroneal longus and brevis pass along the lateral aspect of the ankle, posterior to the lateral malleolus before inserting in the foot. Both muscles originate in the lateral compartment of the leg, and insert within the foot.

The peroneal longus originates from the proximal 2/3 of the fibula and surrounding structures and forms a long tendon around the distal 1/3 of the leg. The tendon runs deep to the inferior peroneal retinaculum (the continuation of inferior extensor retinaculum), before traveling along the plantar surface of the foot where it inserts on the base of the first metatarsal and lateral edge of the medial cuneiform. The peroneal brevis muscle belly lies anterior to the peroneal longus and originates along the distal 2/3 of the lateral surface of the fibula. Its tendon is shorter than the peroneal longus, but similarly begins in the distal 1/3 of the leg before passing posterior to the lateral malleolus [12]. The peroneal brevis will insert on the lateral side of the base of the fifth metatarsal once it emerges from the inferior peroneal retinaculum. Both of these muscles are innervated by the superficial peroneal nerve, and are the primary evertors the foot.

3.3.3 Posterior

The posterior compartment of the leg is subdivided into superficial and deep compartments by the transverse intermuscular septum. Residing within the deep compartment are the flexor digitorum longus (FDL), flexor hallucis longus (FHL), and posterior tibialis muscles, which cross along the medial aspect of the ankle and insert on the foot. These muscles will be discussed in further detail in Sect. 3.3.4.

The superficial compartment contains the gastrocnemius and soleus muscles serve as the primary flexors of the foot and ankle. The tendons of these muscles pass along the posterior aspect of the ankle and share a common tendinous insertion on the calcaneal tuberosity. Together these two muscles are known as the gastrocsoleus complex or triceps surae and serve as the main antagonist to the tibialis anterior muscle. The gastrocnemius is located most superficially and originates as two heads (lateral and medial) from the posterior surface of the lateral and medial femoral condyles, respectively. The fibers of the two heads unite at midline as they insert onto a broad aponeurosis which forms the posterior fibers of the conjoint calcaneal (Achilles) tendon. The soleus is deep to the gastrocnemius and originates along the posterior proximal 1/3 of the fibula and tibia. The oblique muscle fibers insert on the posterior aponeurosis to form the anterior aspect of the conjoint calcaneal tendon (Achilles tendon) [12]. At 12–15 cm proximal to the calcaneal tubersity, the conjoint tendon will begin a progressive internal rotation that continues until 2–5 cm from insertion [5, 18]. This brings the gastrocnemius fibers anterolaterally and soleus fibers posteromedially, with both fiber types contributing to the conjoint tendon. Due to variation within the degree of rotation, it was originally estimated that composition of conjoint tendons was 50–66% soleus fibers, however recent studies have indicated that this range may be higher [19, 20]. The clinical implications of these findings continues to remain unknown and necessitates future further investigation.

3.3.4 Medial

Along the medial aspect of the ankle, the tendons of FHL, FDL, and posterior tibialis muscles and posterior tibial artery and nerve travel behind the medial malleolus and through the tarsal tunnel before inserting in the foot. The borders of tarsal tunnel are formed from the flexor retinaculum (roof), posterior medial malleolus (anterior aspect of the tunnel), and medial wall of the talus/calcaneus (floor). The structures within the tarsal tunnel are arranged in the following order from anterior medial to posterior lateral; posterior tibialis, FDL, neurovascular bundle, and FHL. After emerging from the tarsal tunnel, these structures travel distally to the foot to their insertion points.

These muscles all originate within the deep posterior compartment of the leg and are innervated by the deep peroneal nerve. FHL originate along the posterior surface of the middle 1/3 of the tibia and inserts along the plantar surface of the base of the distal phalanges to allow for flexion of toes. FDL originates along the distal 2/3 of the posterior surface of the fibula and surrounding structures and will travel obliquely in the leg towards the medial malleolus, before entering the foot. Ultimately, FHL inserts on the plantar surface of the base of the first distal phalanx to allow for flexion of the MTP and IP joints. The posterior tibialis muscle originates along the posterior surface of the interosseous membrane, middle 1/3 of the posterior tibia and proximal half of posterior fibula between FHL and FDL. It is the deepest muscle found within the posterior leg and inserts on the plantar surface of the navicular, cuneiforms, cuboid, and base of second to fourth metatarsal bones. Acting as the primary inverted of the foot, the posterior tibialis also has a weak contribution to plantarflexion.

3.3.5 Tendon Sheaths

The tendon sheaths of the foot and ankle muscles have a close anatomic relationship with the superior and inferior extensor retinaculum and flexor retinaculum as they pass the ankle joint. The retinaculum are aponeurotic bands that serve as reinforcement and retaining systems for tendons as they cross over the foot and ankle joints. Forming fibrous tunnels for tendons to pass through, the retinaculum will also act as pulleys. As tendons traverse under the retinaculum, they are covered and protected by synovial sheaths which is composed of three layers (parietal, visceral, and mesotenon) [5]. These sheaths provide nutrients for the tendons and are essential for maintaining the health and function of tendons. Synovial fluid is produced to facilitate gliding of the tendon and inflammation can result in tenosynovitis. Surgically, it is important to repair these structures to allow for proper healing and to prevent adhesions from forming.

3.4 Vascular Anatomy

The arterial supply of the ankle forms from an arterial network of anastomoses consisting of branches from the anterior tibial, posterior tibial, and peroneal arteries. The anterior and posterior tibial arteries are the terminal branches of the popliteal artery, while the peroneal artery branches from the proximal aspect of the anterior tibial artery. The two tibial arteries usually provide the majority of arterial supply to the foot and ankle. However, due to various anastomosing networks, and due to an absence or attenuation, the peroneal artery can become the dominant supply and provide collateral flow [5].

The *anterior tibial artery* travels alongside the deep peroneal nerve, within the anterior compartment of the leg. It provides blood supply to the anterior aspect of the ankle and contributes to both the lateral and medial malleolar anastomoses before traveling distally to the foot as the dorsalis pedis artery. Proximal to the ankle, the anterior tibial artery will give rise to a number of terminal branches including; the artery to sinus tarsi, the anterolateral and anteromedial malleolar arteries, and the lateral and medial tarsal arteries. These arteries will contribute to the lateral and medial malleolar anastomoses at the ankle.

The *posterior tibial artery* travels with the tibial nerve in the posterior compartment of the leg and supplies the tibia via nutrient and perforating arteries. Proximally it gives rise to the peroneal artery before traveling distally along the posterior side of the interosseous membrane. At 5 cm proximal to the distal tibia, the posterior tibial artery gives rise to the communicating branch which forms an anastomosis with transverse communicating branch of the peroneal artery. At the level of the ankle, the posterior

medial malleolar artery and medial calcaneal branch and join their respective anastomosis networks. Distally, the posterior tibial artery will traverse through the tarsal tunnel before bifurcating into the medial and lateral plantar arteries to supply the distal foot.

The *peroneal artery* is also in the posterior compartment of the leg and serves as the main arterial supply for the fibula. As it approaches the ankle, the peroneal artery gives off a number of branches that contribute to the anastomosis networks of the ankle, before terminating as the lateral calcaneal branch to supply the calcaneus. These branches and anastomoses connections include: the main perforating branch (anterior lateral malleolar artery), the transverse communicating branch of the peroneal artery (communicating branch of the posterior tibial artery), and posterior lateral malleolar branch (lateral malleolar anastomosis) before terminating as the lateral calcaneal branch. Each of these branches and their arborizations will participate in the anastomotic networks around the ankle (Fig. 4).

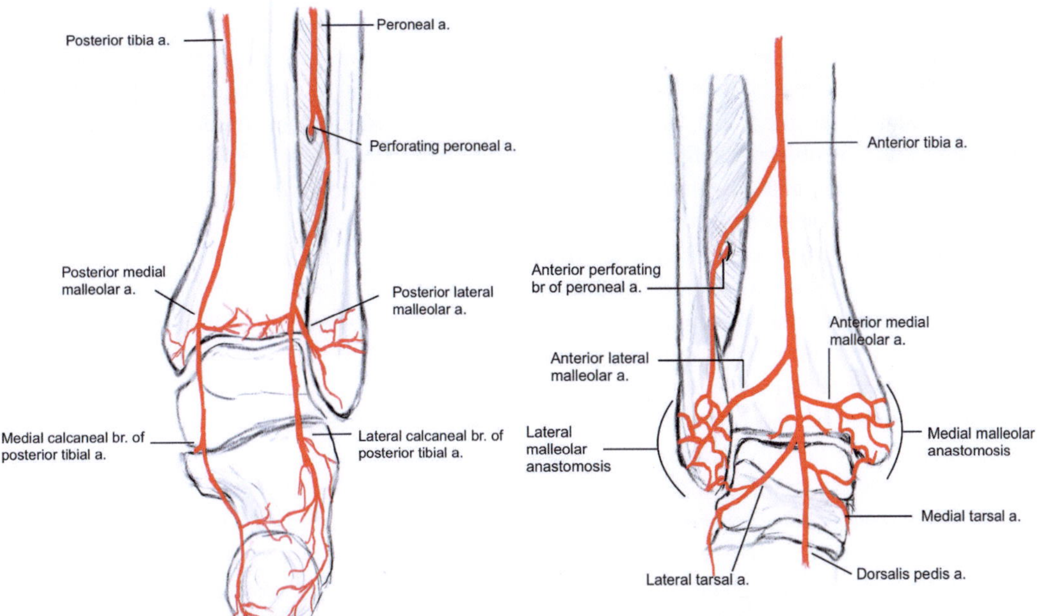

Fig. 4 Arterial supply of the ankle joint. This image illustrates the anterior and posterior vascular supply of the ankle. The left image demonstrates the posterior anastomosis formed from the branches from the posterior tibial artery and peroneal artery. The right image shows an anterior view of the ankle, demonstrating the lateral and medial anastomosis

3.4.1 Anastomosis Network and Arterial Supply to Distal Tibia and Fibula

There are three main anastomosis networks that supply the distal tibia and fibula: a proximal anastomosis, and an interconnected medial malleolar anastomosis and lateral malleolar anastomosis. The first anastomosis network occurs 5 cm proximal to the medial malleolus at the distal tibia. The main perforating branch (peroneal artery) will pierce the interosseous membrane to anastomose with lateral anterior malleolar artery (a branch of the anterior tibial artery). While the transverse communicating artery (peroneal artery) will anastomose with the posterior tibial artery communicating branch. Together these two anastomoses allow for complete collateral flow distally to the foot and ankle, which as previously stated, may occur in the event of a simultaneous anterior and posterior tibial artery absence or occlusion [12]. The medial and lateral malleolar anastomoses are connected by the transverse perimalleolar and lateral malleolar sagittal arterial anastomotic loops and consist of branches from the anterior tibial, posterior tibial, and peroneal branches.

The blood supply on the medial side of the ankle is provided by branches from the anterior tibial or dorsalis pedis artery and medial malleolar anastomosis. The tibial metaphysis and epiphysis plate or remnant, and articular cartilage are all supplied by the lateral and medial metaphyseal arteries and their branches. Branching from the posterior tibial artery, an average of 3.7 cm proximal to the ankle joint (talocrural), the lateral metaphyseal artery will provide nutrient vessels to the dorsolateral tibial metaphysis before joining the perforating peroneal artery. The medial metaphyseal artery usually originates 3.1 cm proximal to the ankle joint and contributes to the posterior and medial anastomoses. While it typically gives rise to three branches, it can also serve as the origin of the lateral metaphyseal artery.

The perforating peroneal artery will supply the distal fibula via the peroneal metaphyseal artery and lateral malleolar anastomosis in 60% of ankles. The fibular metaphyseal artery will then branch near the tibiofibular syndesmosis before anastomosing with the anterior lateral malleolar artery. Composed of the anterior lateral malleolar, lateral tarsal, posterior lateral malleolar artery, and lateral calcaneal arteries, the lateral malleolar anastomosis includes branches from each of three main arteries [12, 17].

3.4.2 Arterial Supply to Talus

The anterior tibial or dorsalis pedis, posterior tibial, and peroneal arteries and their branches contribute to the extraosseous and interosseous vascularity of the talus. The majority of the blood supply to the talar body is provided by the artery of the tarsal canal, with minor supplies from the artery of the tarsal sinus and deltoid branch, while the lateral talus is supplied mainly by the first perforating branch of the peroneal artery. With 70% of the talus covered by articular cartilage, extraosseous supply occurs by penetrating a limited number of non-articulating areas. Intraosseous sources include the arteries of the tarsal sinus and tarsal canal, superior neck and posterior tubercle vessels, and the deltoid branches. Anatomic studies have demonstrated that some anastomoses occur between intraosseous vessels, but these anastomoses are not thought to be significant enough for ankle vascularity [12]. Gelberman and Mortensen demonstrated that the contribution from the dorsalis pedis, superior neck, and posterior tubercle vessels are minor [21]. The limited and tenuous vascular supply makes the talus highly sensitive to insults that compromise arterial supply, which can have important surgical and prognostic implications following an injury [5].

3.4.3 Venous Supply

Venous drainage is essential for maintaining vascular homeostasis and carries away deoxygenated blood and metabolic waste. There are both superficial (cutaneous) and deep venous systems that are interconnected and supply the foot and ankle.

The superficial venous system of the lower extremity begins with the confluence of the digital veins which forms the dorsal venous arch of the foot. Formation of the great saphenous

(saphenous magna, or long saphenous) and small saphenous (lesser or short saphenous) veins occurs as additional venous tributaries contribute to the dorsal venous arch [12, 17]. On the medial aspect of the arch, the great saphenous vein is formed from the confluence of the medial marginal vein and medial dorsal venous arch. As it travels anterior to the medial malleolus, it obtains superficial tributaries from the medial malleolar and posterior tibial veins. The medial malleolar coronal network of veins will also connect to the deep venous system by draining into the posterior tibial vein at the three different points between the mid-calf and ankle [12]. The deep venous system (dorsalis pedis and anterior tibial veins) begins with the confluence of digital veins from the toes and run alongside their corresponding arteries. Before traveling posterior to the medial malleolus, this system will communicate with the greater saphenous vein via the anteromedial malleolar vein.

The short saphenous vein is also superficial and resides on the lateral side of the foot and ankle. Forming at the confluence between the lateral dorsal venous arch and lateral marginal vein, it lies posterior to the lateral malleolus. The lateral marginal vein will indirectly connect to the greater saphenous vein through the dorsal venous system. Similar to the great saphenous vein, the small saphenous is connected to the deep venous system. Two anterolateral malleolar veins serve as tributaries from the lateral malleolar venous system and dorsalis pedis vein (deep venous system). The small saphenous vein travels near the sural nerve as it moves proximally towards the heart. The final confluence of the vein is variable and can become a tributary to the popliteal, great saphenous, or sural veins [17].

3.5 Nerves

Within the lower extremity there are four nerves that provide sensory and motor innervation to the ankle joint and surrounding muscles. This includes the deep peroneal nerve, superficial peroneal nerve, sural nerve, and tibial nerve.

3.5.1 Deep Peroneal Nerve

The deep peroneal nerve (also known as the anterior tibial nerve) is a mixed sensory and motor nerve composed of L4-S1 nerve roots. As one of the terminal branches of the common peroneal nerve, it originates in the lateral compartment of the leg just distal to the fibular head. It will pass obliquely through the lateral compartment of the leg to enter the anterior compartment. It pierces the extensor hallus longus muscle to begin its distal descent, anterior to the interosseous membrane. In the distal half of the leg, the deep peroneal nerve is joined by the anterior tibial artery. Within the anterior compartment of the leg, the deep peroneal nerve supplies motor branches to the anterior compartment muscles and a sensory articular branch for the ankle joint [13]. At approximately 1.3 cm proximal to the ankle joint the deep peroneal nerve is deep to the inferior extensor retinaculum and divides into medial and lateral terminal branches [22]. The medial branch lies medial to the dorsalis pedius, between the extensor hallicus longus tendon and extensor hallicus brevis muscle. Distally, this medial branch (cutaneous branch only) provides sensory innervation of the great and second toes and to the dorsum of the first webspace. The lateral (mixed) branch travels lateral to the dorsalis pedius beneath the extensor digitorum brevis and provides motor innervation to the extensor digitorium brevis muscle and sensory innervation to the tarsal and metatarsal joints.

3.5.2 Superficial Peroneal Nerve

The superficial peroneal nerve is a mixed nerve composed of L5-S2 nerve roots and the other terminal branch of the common peroneal nerve. Providing innervation to the lateral compartment of the leg, it travels between the peroneus longus and brevis muscles. Distally, it will pierce the deep fascia of the leg (covering the peroneal longus and brevis muscles) to emerge superficially along the anterior border of the lateral fibula.

The distance at which the nerve becomes superficial has been shown to be variable and range from 5 cm to above 12.5 cm from the distal lateral malleolus in anatomic studies. However, these studies indicate that in over 98% of legs, the superficial peroneal nerve will pierce the deep fascia between 10 and 12.5 cm proximal to the tip of the lateral malleolus [23, 24]. Within 1–3 cm of piercing the deep fascia of the anterolateral leg, the nerve will divide into two terminal branches, the medial and intermediate dorsal cutaneous nerves, which provide sensory innervation over the anterior ankle and dorsum of the foot. The medial dorsal cutaneous nerve is the largest branch and travels parallel to the extensor hallucis longus tendon while the intermediate dorsal cutaneous nerve travels along the lateral aspect of the dorsal foot. Once over the dorsum of the foot, these cutaneous nerves will continue to arborize and ultimately provide cutaneous innervation over the dorsal distal foot and toes. Often these terminal branches will anastomose with terminal branches of other sensory nerves.

3.5.3 Sural Nerve

The sural nerve is composed of S1-S2 nerve roots and is a terminal branch of the tibial nerve, formed from the medial and lateral sural nerves. It will provide cutaneous innervation over the posterolateral aspect of the leg and foot and is purely a sensory nerve. Branching from the tibial nerve in the popliteal fossa, the medial sural nerve travels between the two heads of the gastrocnemius, before piercing the deep fascia to travel superficially in the cutaneous tissues of the leg towards the foot [12]. The lateral sural nerve branches from the common peroneal nerve, near the head of the fibula and travels in the cutaneous tissue of the leg before joining the medial sural nerve to form the (median) sural nerve [17]. This anastomosis typically occurs around midleg, but anatomic variation has been seen with the anatomosis occurring in both the proximal and distal directions [24].

The sural nerve will travel distally along the lateral border of the Achilles tendon, along with the short saphenous vein, until it reaches the posterior border of the lateral malleolus. It turns to travel towards the dorsolateral surface of the foot, passing 1–1.5 cm distal and plantar to the lateral malleolus. At approximately 2–3 cm distal to the lateral malleolus, it will arborize to supply articular tissues (inferior tibiofibular, ankle, and talo-

calcaneus joints), and cutaneous tissue overlying the lateral malleolus, calcaneus, and dorsum of the foot. A number of anatomic studies have confirmed the course of the main trunk of the sural nerve, which has important surgical implications. Eastwood et al. identified the mean distance, within a 95% confidence interval, between the main trunk of the sural nerve and the distal fibula and lateral malleolus. Measuring the distance from the distal tip of the lateral malleolus, at 10 cm proximal, 5 cm proximal, directly posterior and directly inferior to the tip, the sural nerve was identified at the mean distances of 2.5 cm, 2.1 cm, 1.4 cm, and 2.3 cm, respectively (seen in Table 1) [25]. Later studies confirmed these findings with all of the subsequent measurements falling within the 95% confidence intervals [26, 27]. Surgical incisions over the distal fibula and malleolus should thus be placed outside of the ranges defined by Eastwood et al., in order to prevent itrogenic injury to the sural nerve (Fig. 5, Table 2).

3.5.4 Tibial Nerve

The tibial nerve is a mixed nerve composed of L4-S3 nerve roots that is a terminal branch of the sciatic nerve in the popliteal fossa. Traveling distally with the posterior tibial artery, and deep to the triceps surae, the tibial nerve will provide innervation to the muscles of the posterior leg [13]. Near the tarsal tunnel the tibial nerve bifurcates into two terminal branches; the medial and plantar nerves. The tibial nerve will give rise to articular and cutaneous branches that innervate the medial ankle joint capsule and medial malleolus cutaneous skin, respectively. While these articular and cutaneous branches typically originate near the bifurcation of the medial or plantar nerves, they can also arise from the plantar nerves if the tibial nerve bifurcation is proximal to the malleolus [5, 29].

Following the bifurcation, the medial plantar nerve (mixed) will travel deep to the abductor hallucis where it innervates the abductor hallucis, flexor digitorum brevis (FDB) before dividing into three terminal branches (common digital nerves 1 through 3). Distally, these nerves supply the lumbrical 1 and 2 before providing sensory

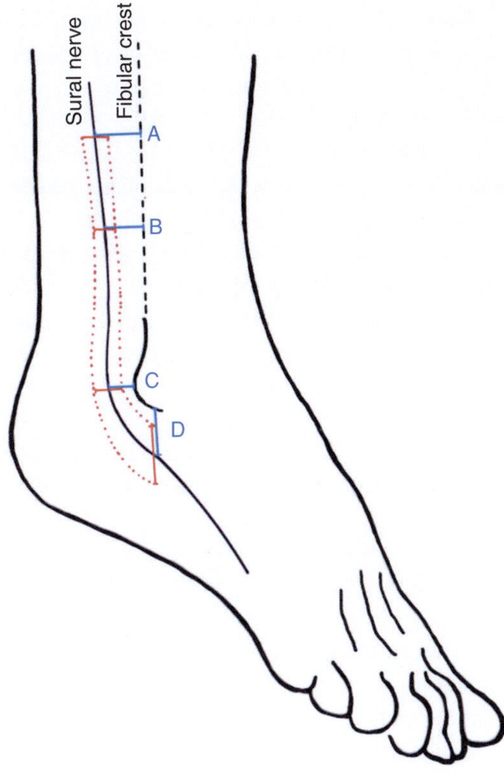

Fig. 5 Anatomical path of the sural nerve. Dotted black line demarcates fibular crest, Dark blue line represent Sural nerve. Light blue lines A–D represent distance of sural nerve from anatomical landmarks seen in Table 1. Solid red lines represents 95% confidence interval of anterior and posterior limits of main trunk seen in Table 1. Red dotted lines represents extrapolated danger zone border of sural nerve path based on calculated 95% confidence interval. (Based on findings from Eastwood et al. [28])

Table 2 Distances of sural nerve

Position	Mean distance ± SE (cm)	95% Confidence interval (± 1.96 SD) (cm)
A	2.5 ± 0.1	1.7–3.2
B	2.1 ± 0.1	1.5–2.7
C	1.4 ± 0.1	0.6–2.2
D	2.3 ± 0.2	0.7–3.9

Anatomical landmarks (position A–D) are based upon relative to the tip of the lateral malleolus. A; 10 cm proximal, B; 5 cm proximal, C; directly posterior, D; directly inferior. Based on findings from Eastwood et al. [28]

innervation for digits 1 through 3 and half of digit 4. The lateral plantar nerve (mixed) will travel with the lateral plantar artery between flexor digitorium brevis (FDB) and quadratus planae (QP)

before dividing into a deep and superficial branch. The deep branch (motor only) supplies the first and second interossei muscles, lumbricals 2–4, and adductor hallicus. The superficial branch (mixed) will continue to bifurcate and provide motor innervation to the FDB, FDM, and third and fourth interossei muscles and before supplying cutaneous innervation to digits 4 and 5.

3.5.5 Capsular and Ligament Innervation

Innervation of the ankle joint has significant anatomic variation in both number of articular branches and location of innervation, with contributions from the deep and superficial peroneal, tibial, sural, and saphenous nerves [5, 22, 30]. The lateral capsule is supplied predominantly by articular branches of the sural nerve, while the medial capsule is predominantly innervated by the tibial nerve. Innervation of the anterior and posterior capsule tends to be more variable. The anterior capsule may have contribution branches from the saphenous, sural, superficial, and deep peroneal nerves, while the posterior capsule may be supplied by the tibial, saphenous, and sural nerves [22]. In addition to supplying the lateral capsule, the sural nerve will also innervate the surrounding capsuloligamentous structures including posterior inferior tibiofibular and talocalcaneal ligaments. The tibial nerve supplies the deltoid, anterior inferior tibiofibular, and anterior talofibular ligaments along with the capsule [30].

4 Physiology

The axis of motion of the ankle joint is formed by a line drawn between the distal tips of the medial and lateral malleoli, giving the axis of the ankle joint a laterally tilted and externally rotated position. In the coronal plane, a line drawn vertically down the anatomic axis of the tibia that intersects the axis forms an 83° angle. This is known as the talocrural angle (Fig. 6).

Due to the position of the axis of external rotation for the ankle in the axial plane, there is 20–30° more external rotation of the ankle than the knee [9].

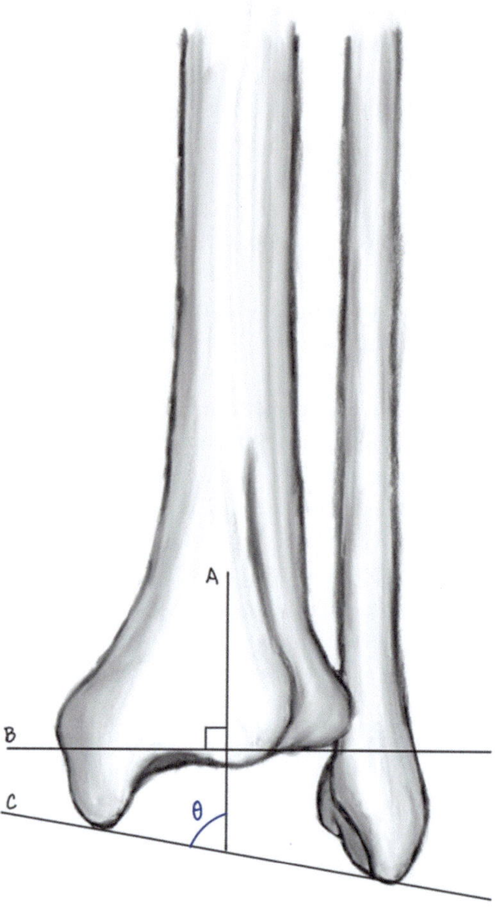

Fig. 6 Talocrural angle. Line A is parallel to the shaft of the tibia and perpendicular to Line B which is parallel to the tibial plafond. Line C runs between the distal most portion of the medial and lateral malleolus. The Talocrural angle (theta, *θ*) is formed from the intersection of Line A and Line C

Range of motion of the ankle has been variably reported in studies, as consisting of between 10° and 30° dorsiflexion, and 23–56° of plantarflexion [28, 31, 32]. The talus externally rotates within the mortise with ankle dorsiflexion and internally rotates with ankle plantarflexion, with a 6° range of rotation. Regular instability of the talus within the mortise is not seen, despite the fact that the talus is on average 4.2 mm wider anteriorly than posteriorly. Although the medial dome of talar trochlea is anatomically narrower and shorter than the lateral dome, the talus itself acts like rolling an ice cream cone (frustum) rather than a cylinder (see Fig. 7). This prevents instability with rotational motion of the ankle [33].

The motion of the tibiofibular syndesmosis is also critical to the stability of the tibiotalar joint. Elasticity of the syndesmosis allows the mortise to widen and narrow with dorsiflexion and plantarflexion, respectively [5, 34]. Under weight-bearing loads and external rotation, Beumer et al. measured the in vivo motion of the distal syndesmosis with implanted radiostereometry markers. From a neutral ankle position, external rotation of the fibula was measured between 2° and 5°, with posterior translation of up to 3 mm [35].

The load bearing surface characteristics of the tibiotalar joint are sensitive to change due to the constrained anatomy. Ramsey and Hamilton demonstrated, using a carbon transference technique, that a 1 mm shift of lateral talar displacement decreased by 42% the contact surface of the

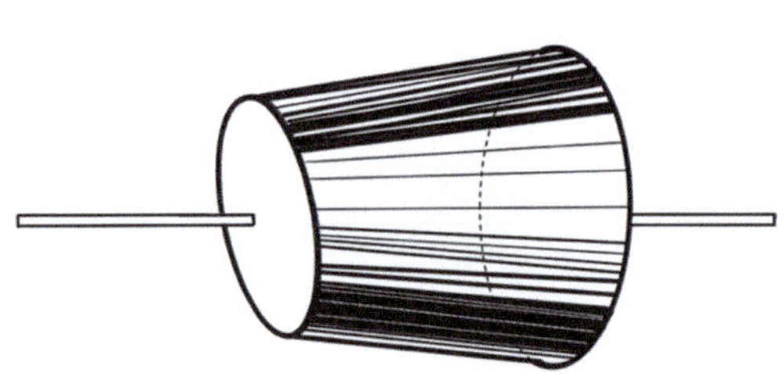

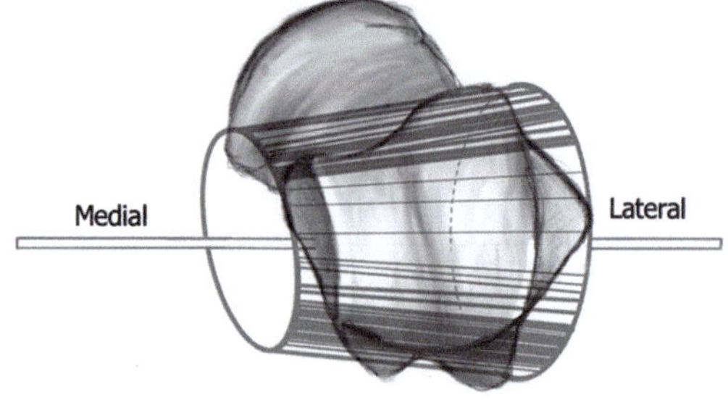

Fig. 7 The talus as a frustum of a cone. The radius of curvature of the talus is smaller on the medial side compared to the lateral side. The face of the medial facet is elliptical and closer to the apex of the cone. As a result, the trochlear surface is a frustum which influences ankle stability during motion and the axes of rotation. (Adapted and modified from Close JR, Inman VT. *The action of the ankle joint. Report to the Advisory Committee on Artificial Limbs, National Research Council.* Vol 22. Berkeley, CA: Prosthetic Devices Research Project, Institute of Engineering Research, University of California; 1951)

tibial plafond and talar dome [36]. Ankle stability is therefore dependent on the articular anatomy, medial/lateral collateral ligaments, and distal tibiofibular ligaments for passive stability. Gravity, muscle forces, and ground reaction forces by the foot provide active stability [37].

5 Conclusion

The development of the ankle is a complex process that begins within weeks of conception and continues until early adolescence. The various developmental, morphological and functional changes are carefully timed events that allow for the unique anatomy and function of the ankle joint. Knowledge of the stages of prenatal development, anatomy, and physiology can aid in the understanding of various foot and ankle deformities and contribute to the foundational knowledge. This chapter covered a brief overview of ankle embryonic development and morphology, adult anatomy and physiology necessary for orthopaedic practice and clinical treatment of the ankle.

References

1. Böhm M. The embryolgic origins of club-foot: the Krüppelfürsorgestelle of the city of Berlin in St. Hildegard's Hospital. JBJS. 1929;11(2):229–59.
2. O'Rahilly R, Gardner E. The timing and sequence of events in the development of the limbs in the human embryo. Anat Embryol (Berl). 1975;148(1):1–23.
3. Bardeen CR, Lewis WH. Development of the limbs, body-wall and back in man. Am J Anat. 1901;1(1):1–35.
4. Bernhardt DB. Prenatal and postnatal growth and development of the foot and ankle. Phys Ther. 1988;68(12):1831–9.
5. Sarrafian SK. Anatomy of the foot and ankle: descriptive, topographic, functional. 3rd ed. Philadelphia, PA: Lippincott; 2011.
6. Bardeen CR. Studies of the development of the human skeleton. Am J Anat. 1905;4:265–302.
7. Olivier G. Formation du Squelette des Membres chez l'Homme. Paris: Vigot frères; 1962.
8. Kawashima T, Uhthoff HK. Development of the foot in prenatal life in relation to idiopathic club foot. J Pediatr Orthop. 1990;10(2):232–7.
9. Stiehl JB. Inman's joints of the ankle. Baltimore, MD: Williams & Wilkins; 1991.
10. Straus WL. The growth of the human foot and its evolutionary significance. Contrib Embryol. 1927;101:93–134.
11. Le D. La torsion du tibia, normeale, pathologique, experimentale. J Anat Paris. 1909;45:598–615.
12. Standring S. Gray's anatomy: the anatomical basis of clinical practice. Philadelphia, PA: Elsevier; 2016.
13. White TD, Black MT, Folkens PA. Human osteology. London: Academic Press; 2011.
14. Cunningham C, Scheuer L, Black S. Developmental juvenile osteology. London: Academic Press; 2016.
15. Rouvière H, Canela Lazaro M. Le ligament peroneo-astragalo-calcaneen. Paper presented at: Annales d'anatomie Pathologique;1932.
16. Bremer S. The unstable ankle mortise-functional ankle varus. J Foot Surg. 1985;24(5):313–7.
17. Gray H. Anatomy of the human body. 20th ed. Philadelphia, PA: Lea & Febige; 1918.
18. Testut L. Traité d'anatomie humaine. Paris: Doin; 1921.
19. Cummins EJ, Anson BJ. The structure of the calcaneal tendon (of Achilles) in relation to orthopedic surgery, with additional observations on the plantaris muscle. Surg Gynecol Obstet. 1946;83:107–16.
20. Edama M, Kubo M, Onishi H, et al. The twisted structure of the human Achilles tendon. Scand J Med Sci Sports. 2015;25(5):e497–503.
21. Gelberman RH, Mortensen WW. The arterial anatomy of the talus. Foot Ankle. 1983;4(2):64–72.
22. Han JR, Tran J, Agur AMR. Overview of the innervation of ankle joint. Phys Med Rehabil Clin N Am. 2021;32(4):791–801.
23. Horwitz MT. Normal anatomy and variations of the peripheral nerves of the leg and foot: application in operations for vascular diseases: study of one hundred specimens. Arch Surg. 1938;36(4):626–36.
24. Kosinski C. The course, mutual relations and distribution of the cutaneous nerves of the metazonal region of leg and foot. J Anat. 1926;60(Pt 3):274–97.
25. Eastwood DM, Irgau I, Atkins RM. The distal course of the sural nerve and its significance for incisions around the lateral hindfoot. Foot Ankle. 1992;13(4):199–202.
26. Lawrence SJ, Botte MJ. The sural nerve in the foot and ankle: an anatomic study with clinical and surgical implications. Foot Ankle Int. 1994;15(9):490–4.
27. Ikiz ZAA, Üçerler H, Bilge O. The anatomic features of the sural nerve with an emphasis on its clinical importance. Foot Ankle Int. 2005;26(7):560–7.
28. Boone DC, Azen SP. Normal range of motion of joints in male subjects. J Bone Joint Surg Am. 1979;61(5):756–9.
29. Rüdinger N. Die Gelenknerven des menschlichen Körpers. Erlangen: Enke; 1857.
30. Gardner E, Gray DJ. The innervation of the joints of the foot. Anat Rec. 1968;161(2):141–8.
31. Bonnin JG. Injury to the ligaments of the ankle. J Bone Joint Surg (Br). 1965;47(4):609–11.

32. Sammarco GJ, Burstein AH, Frankel VH. Biomechanics of the ankle: a kinematic study. Orthop Clin North Am. 1973;4(1):75–96.
33. Close JR, Inman VT. The action of the ankle joint. Report to the Advisory Committee on Artificial Limbs, National Research Council. Vol 22. Berkeley, CA: Prosthetic Devices Research Project, Institute of Engineering Research, University of California; 1951.
34. Poirier P, Charpy A. Traité d'anatomie humaine, vol. 2. Paris: Bataille; 1901. p. 67.
35. Beumer A, Valstar ER, Garling EH, et al. Kinematics of the distal tibiofibular syndesmosis: radiostereometry in 11 normal ankles. Acta Orthop Scand. 2003;74(3):337–43.
36. Ramsey P, Hamiiton W. Changes in tibiotalar area of contact caused by lateral talar shift. J Bone Joint Surg. 1976;58(3):356–7.
37. McCullough C, Burge P. Rotatory stability of the load-bearing ankle. An experimental study. J Bone Joint Surg (Br). 1980;62(4):460–4.

Biomechanics of the Ankle

Patricia K. Wellborn, Joshua N. Tennant,
and Trapper A. J. Lalli

1   Introduction

The biomechanics and function of the human foot and ankle are the product of its unique anatomy and structure. The ankle joint complex consists of three primary joints: tibiotalar (or talocrural), subtalar (or talocalcaneal), and the transverse tarsal joint. These joints work synergistically to conduct ankle motion and provide stability to the complex, which is fundamental in the ability to ambulate and efficiently manage weight-bearing forces. This chapter will explore the biomechanical properties of the ankle joint complex and its role in ambulation, as well as some examples of abnormal gait and force distribution.

2   Anatomical Contributions to Biomechanics

2.1   Tibiotalar Joint

The tibiotalar joint is the articulation between the distal tibia and the talar body. It is less commonly referred to as the talocrural joint, but the two terminologies are interchangeable. This joint serves as the primary dorsiflexor and plantarflexor of the ankle joint complex. It is also the primary weight-bearing joint of the ankle joint complex.

The tibiotalar joint is most stable in dorsiflexion [1, 2]. In dorsiflexion, as well as the stance phase of gait, the primary contributor to stability is the bony anatomy [1]. As the tibiotalar joint plantarflexes, the joint becomes more heavily reliant on the surrounding soft tissues for stability [1]. Three ligamentous groups are key for stabilization of the tibiotalar joint. From medial to lateral, these consist of the medial deltoid ligaments, the syndesmosis, and the lateral ankle ligaments. The deltoid ligament stabilizes the medial portion of the joint and resists eversion and valgus stress. The deltoid ligament is composed of a combination of six individual ligaments that are variably present amongst individuals. The tibionavicular, tibiospring, and deep posterior tibiotalar ligaments are present in all individuals. The tibiocalcaneal, superficial posterior tibiotalar, and deep anterior tibiotalar ligaments have a variable presence [3].

The syndesmotic ligaments lie between the tibia and the fibula. The syndesmosis consists of the anterior inferior tibiofibular ligament (AITFL), the posterior tibiofibular ligament (PTFL), and the interosseous tibiofibular ligament. These syndesmotic ligaments help stabilize the distal part of the fibula. The lateral ligamentous complex consists of the anterior talofibular, posterior talofibular, and calcaneofib-

P. K. Wellborn (✉) · J. N. Tennant · T. A. J. Lalli
Department of Orthopaedics, University of North Carolina, Chapel Hill, NC, USA
e-mail: Patricia.Wellborn@unchealth.unc.edu;
josh_tennant@med.unc.edu; trapper_lalli@med.unc.edu

ular ligaments. These lateral ligaments resist inversion and varus stress [1].

As the tibiotalar joint progresses from plantarflexion to dorsiflexion, there is both rotational and translational motion. Leardini et al. defined the articular contact point as the area of maximal contact and greatest pressure on the articular surface of either the distal tibia or talus. They discovered that that the articular contact point in the distal tibia shifts in relation to the amount of ankle dorsiflexion. At maximum plantarflexion, the articular contact point is on the posterior half of the tibial articular surface. As the ankle dorsiflexes, this contact point shifts to the anterior half of the tibial articular surface [4]. The center of contact behaves similarly in the talus. As the tibiotalar joint moves from dorsiflexion to plantarflexion, the center of contact on the talus moves from anterior to posterior [5]. In dorsiflexion, the talus is translated posteriorly and flexes forward. Conversely, in plantarflexion, the talus is translated anteriorly and extends backward [4].

In addition to the articular contact point shifting on the distal tibia and talus, there are varying degrees of contact area depending on ankle position. Numerous studies have attempted to identify the contact area between the tibia and the talus and the degree to which the area changes with tibiotalar motion [5–7]. Castro reported the contact area at the tibiotalar joint varies between 1.5 and 9.4 cm². In his meta-analysis, it was inconclusive whether contact area increases with dorsiflexion or whether the variations seen in studies were due more to differences in technique amongst the studies themselves [6]. Kimizuka et al. performed a cadaveric study and found that the weight-bearing contact area is localized to the anterior and lateral portion of the joint (Fig. 1). They found that the average articular contact area between the tibia and talus was 4.8 cm² with a maximal intra-articular pressure of 9.9 MPa. Intra-articular pressure is defined as the pressure within the tibiotalar joint. With increasing force applied to the joint, the articular contact area increased in size. With traction applied to the tibiotalar joint (diastasis), contact area decreased and intra-articular peak pressures increased [7]. Similar to Kimizuka et al., Calhoun et al. [5] per-

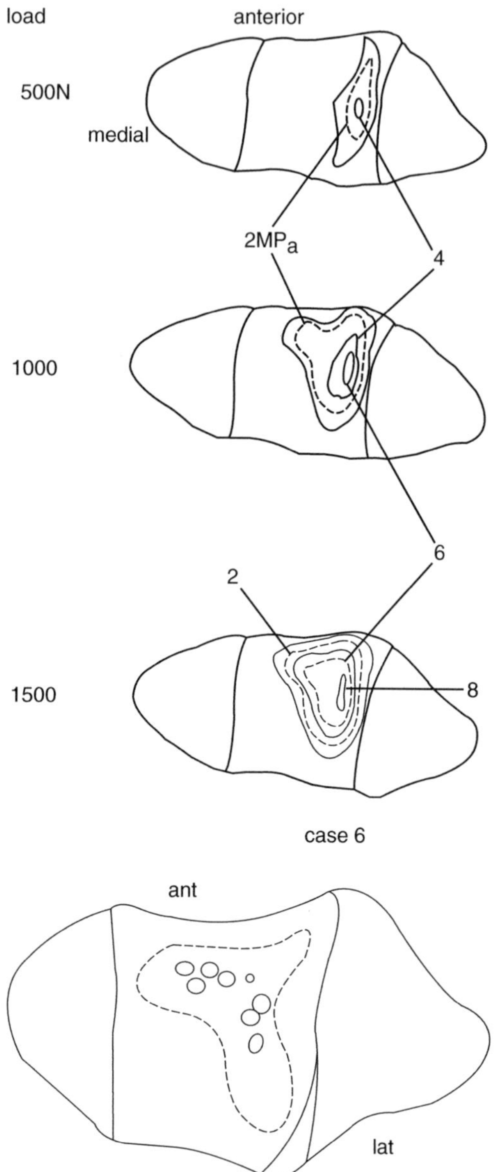

Fig. 1 The results of the force study are shown. Contact was localized to antero-lateral portion of joint, and contact area increased with increasing forces. (Reproduced from Kimizuka with permission [7])

formed a cadaveric study exploring the relationship between motion, contact area, and pressure. They found that contact surface area increased from a plantarflexed to dorsiflexed position. They also found that force per unit area (amount of force in a given articular area) decreased proportionately. Similar findings were found with both inversion and eversion in both neutral and dorsiflexed positions. This study also explored the impact of increasing forces across the tibiotalar joint. As applied force increased, contact area increased but articular pressure remained relatively the same [5, 6].

2.2 Talofibular/Distal Tibiofibular Joint

The talofibular and distal tibiofibular joints are the articulation between the distal fibula (lateral malleolus) and the distal tibia and talus. The fibula plays an important role in bony stability for the tibiotalar joint during weight-bearing. It is estimated that the fibula supports around 15–20% of the weight-bearing forces [6]. As the tibiotalar joint dorsiflexes, the fibula translates laterally and distally as well as externally rotates [6]. Conversely, the fibula translates medially and proximally, and internally rotates, as the tibiotalar joint plantarflexes. This complex three dimensional movement contributes to both static and dynamic stability of the ankle joint complex.

2.3 Subtalar Joint

The subtalar joint is the articulation between the talus and the calcaneus. It is less commonly referred to as the talocalcaneal joint. It is a triplanar, uniaxial joint and serves as the primary inverter and evertor of the ankle joint complex. Its complicated motion is a manifestation of its complex anatomy. At the anterior portion of the joint, the inferior talus is convex and the superior calcaneus is concave. Conversely, in the posterior portion of the joint, the inferior talus is concave and the superior calcaneus is convex. The subtalar ligamentous complex includes the interosseous talocalcaneal, lateral talocalcaneal, and anterior talocalcaneal ligaments as well as the calcaneofibular portion of the lateral ligamentous complex and the tibiocalcaneal portion of the deltoid ligament [1]. When the foot is dorsiflexed, the subtalar joint extends (dorsiflexes), abducts, and pronates [8]. This places the heel in valgus.

As the foot is plantarflexed, the subtalar joint flexes (plantarflexes), adducts, and supinates which places the heel in varus [8].

2.4 Transverse Tarsal Joint

The transverse tarsal joint is the articulation between the talus, calcaneus, cuboid, and navicular bones. It is also commonly referred to as the Chopart joint. This joint contributes to inversion and eversion but serves its greatest role in gait biomechanics. It can be "locked" and "unlocked" throughout gait. This allows for control of either a rigid or flexible foot. This concept will be expanded on later in the chapter in Sect. 5.

3 Motion of the Ankle Joint Complex

The motion of the ankle joint complex involves various joints with different axes. It is the combination of motion in multiple joints that create familiar ankle movements.

3.1 Range of Motion

Sagittal ankle motion (plantarflexion and dorsiflexion) is the principal movement of the ankle joint complex. The vast majority of this motion occurs at the tibiotalar joint, with an average 60° of sagittal motion [9]. This is comprised of approximately 10–30° of dorsiflexion and 40–55° of plantarflexion [1, 6]. Range of motion of the ankle is best measured in a weight-bearing stance rather than passively, as this is the most accurate representation of functional range of motion [6]. The required range of sagittal motion for walking is around 30° [1, 10], around 37° is needed for ascending stairs, and around 56° is needed for descending stairs [1]. With increasing age, there is a loss of sagittal motion, primarily plantarflexion [6].

Coronal motion refers to inversion and eversion of the ankle joint complex. The average motion is 23° of inversion and 12° of eversion [1,

9]. It is controversial what percentage of this motion originates in the subtalar joint versus the tibiotalar joint [1, 9]. There is likely variation among individuals regarding the contribution from each joint [9].

Translational motion of the tibiotalar joint describes anterior or posterior motion of the talus relative to the plafond. This motion is most relevant when the tibiotalar joint undergoes destabilizing forces, such as ligamentous instability or fractures. The greatest amount of translational motion (and therefore, laxity of the ankle joint) is seen at a neutral position of the tibiotalar joint. As the tibiotalar joint approaches the extremes of both plantarflexion and dorsiflexion, translational motion is decreased. Flexion angle of the tibiotalar joint remains the most important parameter in determining laxity [4].

multiaxial, or whether the axis moves with different positions. Lundberg et al. studied the tibiotalar rotational axis and found that the axis shifts throughout the course of motion from plantarflexion to dorsiflexion. In plantarflexion, the axis is angled from inferomedial to superolateral. In dorsiflexion, the axis is angled from inferolateral to superomedial (Fig. 2). The transition of the axis was found to be abrupt in some subjects and a more gradual transition in others [11]. Throughout motion, the midpoint of the axis remained near the midpoint of a line between the tips of the two malleoli at a central point in the talus, suggesting that this point represents a center of rotation and movement of the tibiotalar joint [2, 10]. Overall, this continues to be explored and further studies are needed to fully understand the axis of rotation [6].

3.2 Tibiotalar Axis of Rotation

The tibiotalar joint has the greatest motion of the joints within the ankle joint complex. It is controversial whether the tibiotalar joint is uniaxial or

3.3 Subtalar Motion

Subtalar motion is crucial for inversion and eversion of the ankle joint complex. It also contributes to motion in the sagittal plane as well as

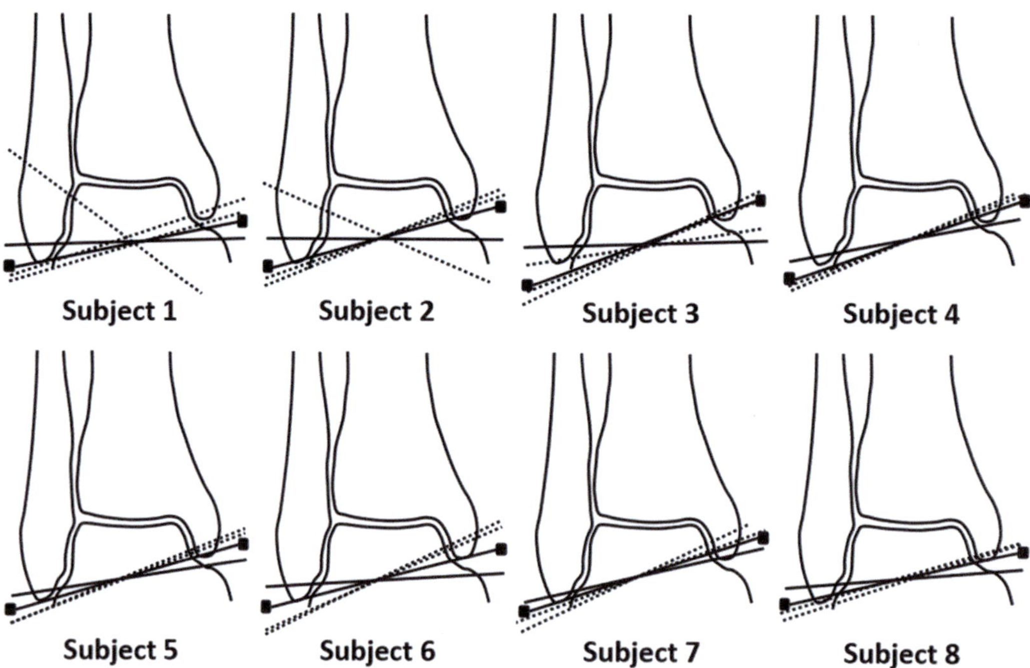

Fig. 2 Results from Lundberg's study demonstrating the tibiotalar axis of rotation. Lines represent the variation in the axis with varying degrees of dorsiflexion. (Reproduced from Lundberg with permission [11])

some rotation. During ambulation, there is approximately 10° of combined sagittal and rotational motion produced at the subtalar joint [10]. This motion is often described as triplanar. The subtalar joint has two different centers of rotation, due to having both an anterior and a posterior aspect to the joint. Contributing to the complexity of subtalar motion is the rotational nature of the calcaneus. Both the talus and calcaneus can rotate and translate during motion, which produces a screw-like motion of the joint [2, 10]. Even small degrees of motion in the subtalar joint create powerful movements in the ankle joint complex.

3.4 Four-Bar Linkage Model

The four-bar linkage model is a popular method for describing the motion of the ankle joint complex. In this model, there are four bars connecting the tibia, fibula, talus, and calcaneus (Fig. 3, line segments representing the calcaneofibular and

tibiocalcaneal ligaments). The talus-calcaneus and tibia-fibula then rotate around each other on these line segments. The talus has two radii representing the varying center of rotation. The advantage of this model is its ability to account for the irregular shape of the talus, as well as the translational motion of the talus under the tibia. Using this model accounts for the combination of the "rolling" and "sliding" motions of the ankle joint complex [4, 6, 12, 13].

3.5 Pronation/Supination

A combination of all aspects of motion described above creates the motions of pronation and supination. Pronation and supination are described relative to the plantar aspect of the foot. Pronation results in the plantar foot pointing laterally, while supination results in the plantar foot pointing medially. Pronation is a combination of ankle joint complex dorsiflexion, eversion, and abduction. Conversely, supination is a combination of

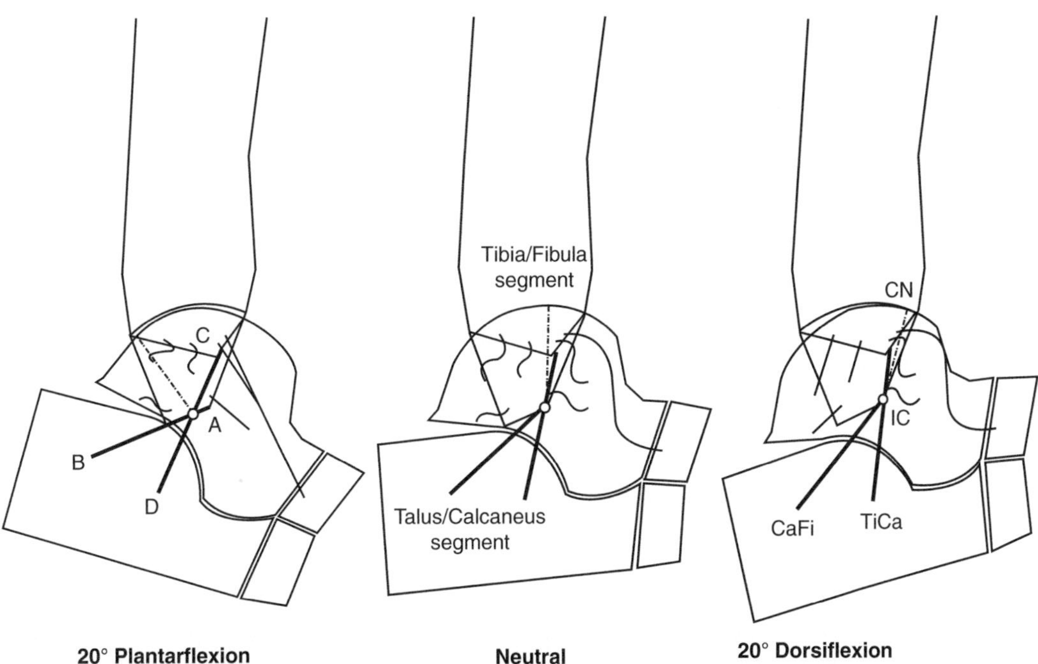

Fig. 3 The four-bar linkage model. The solid lines represent the calcaneofibular (CaFi) and tibiocalcaneal (TiCa) ligaments. The center of rotation (IC) is the location where the two ligament fibers cross. CN represents the common normal articular contact point. (Reproduced from Leardini with permission [4])

plantarflexion, inversion, and adduction, combining motions of multiple ankle and hindfoot joints [1, 14]. Five triplane joints contribute to the motion: the tibiotalar joint, subtalar joint, Chopart joint, first metatarsal-cuneiform joint, and the fifth metatarsal-navicular joint [14]. The complex motions of pronation and supination are critical to the ankle joint complex's ability to handle uneven ground and other varying forces.

4 Static and Dynamic Stabilizers of the Ankle

The ankle joint complex requires stability from both static and dynamic forces to manage the significant ground reaction forces and uneven ground surfaces during ambulation. Static stabilizers include: the tibia, talus, fibula, calcaneus, along with their joint congruity and associated ligaments and fascia. Dynamic stabilizers include: the surrounding muscles, tendons, and the dynamic nature of tarsal bone motion. At different stages of ambulation, there is a variable impact between the static and dynamic stabilizers.

4.1 Static Stabilizers

A vast majority of the stability of the ankle joint complex is attributed to the bony structures and their articular congruity. Calhoun et al. found articular congruity to be responsible for 70% of the anterior to posterior stability, 50% of stability in inversion/eversion, and 30% of internal/external rotational stability [13]. In weight-bearing conditions, articular congruity provides 100% of the stability in eversion and inversion [2, 6, 9]. However, this only provides around 30% of rotational stability [2, 6, 9]. When the ability for bony structures to provide stability has been maximized, the ankle joint complex relies on ligamentous structures for the remainder of stability.

The ankle joint complex has numerous ligaments on both the medial and lateral aspects. These ligaments tend to be relaxed during functional range of motion, i.e., the motion needed to

perform routine daily tasks. However, the ligaments are tensioned as the ankle increases towards the maximal range of motion [9]. The ligamentous structures are the primary determinant of the maximal range of motion [9].

The lateral ligament complex consists of the anterior talofibular (ATFL), calcaneofibular (CFL), and posterior talofibular (PTFL) ligaments. The ATFL prevents internal rotation and anterior translation of the talus. The CFL provides subtalar stability and prevents adduction. The PTFL prevents external rotation of the talus [2, 9]. These three ligaments play a key role in resisting inversion of the ankle joint complex and are also the primary restraint to anterior translation of the talus [6]. Anatomically, the CFL is parallel to the axis of motion of the subtalar joint, which allows it to stabilize the subtalar joint while not restricting motion [6]. The ATFL and CFL are in 90-degree orientation to each other and work in perpendicular planes [6]. The ATFL is the primary restraint in plantarflexion while the CFL is primary in dorsiflexion [6].

Hinterman et al. performed a cadaveric study examining the role of the lateral ligamentous complex. The lateral ligaments were sequentially transected under varying loads. Under a true axial load, there was stable internal tibial rotation and calcaneal eversion regardless of the competency of lateral or medial ligaments. This further demonstrated the role of articular congruity in the ankle joint complex. When the ATFL was released, there was a significant increase in tibial internal rotation. However, there was no further change in rotation with the transection of the remaining ligaments. On the other hand, a release of the final subtalar interosseous ligaments significantly increased the internal rotation of the tibia. There was a greater loss of stability in plantarflexion than dorsiflexion with the release of all ligaments. Although there were similar findings for calcaneal eversion, the calcaneus was always stable in dorsiflexion regardless of ligamentous integrity [15]. This study demonstrated key findings of the importance of articular congruity, greater ankle stability in dorsiflexion, and that the ATFL is the most important component of the lateral ligamentous complex.

The medial ligamentous structures are collectively known as the deltoid ligament. The deltoid ligament resists valgus tilt of the talus, anterior translation, lateral translation, and eversion of the ankle [2, 9]. It has both superficial and deep components [3, 6] and, as previously discussed, can be composed of up to six ligamentous bands [3]. An anatomic study by Campbell et al. identified the tibionavicular, tibiospring, and deep posterior tibiotalar ligaments to be present in all cadaveric specimens with the deep posterior tibiotalar ligament being the largest [3]. The other three bands (tibiocalcaneal, superficial posterior tibiotalar, and deep anterior tibiotalar) were variably present amongst specimens [3]. In the cadaveric study by Harper et al., they identified the deltoid ligament to be the primary restraint against valgus tilt with both the superficial and deep components contributing equally. They also found that the deep deltoid ligament is a secondary restraint to both anterior and lateral translation of the talus (lateral malleolus and lateral ligamentous complex are primary restraints) [6, 16]. When the deltoid ligament was transected, the articular contact area of the tibiotalar joint decreased and intra-articular pressure increased [13].

Additional static stabilizers of the ankle joint complex include the plantar aponeurosis and the stabilizers of the arch. The plantar aponeurosis bears up to 60% of the stress forces during weight-bearing [14]. With toe extension, the aponeurosis becomes tighter, and therefore, is able to handle more force. This is known as the "windlass effect" [14] (Fig. 4). Other static stabilizers of the arch include the short and long plantar ligaments and the calcaneonavicular ligament (spring ligament) [6].

4.2 Dynamic Stabilizers

The dynamic stabilizers of the ankle joint complex are the surrounding muscles and tendons that pass around the ankle joint complex. This includes the peroneus brevis, peroneus longus, peroneus tertius (if present), tibialis anterior, posterior tibialis, extensor digitorum, extensor hallucis longus, flexor hallucis longus, flexor

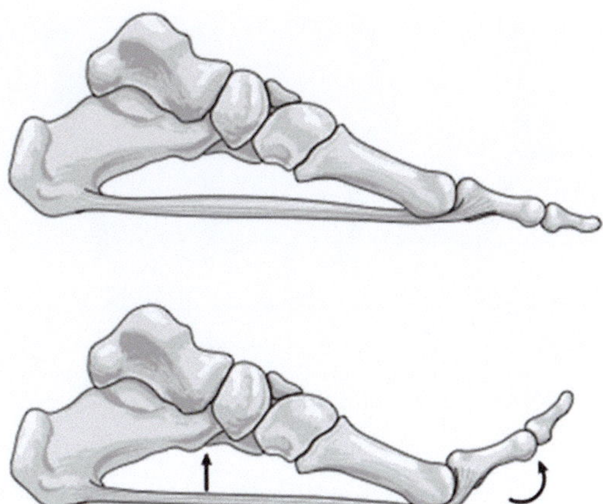

Fig. 4 The windlass effect. Extension of the toes tightens the plantar fascia. (Reproduced from Rosenbaum with permission [17])

digitorum, and the gastrocnemius/soleus complex [8]. The role of dynamic stabilizers will be expanded upon in Sect. 5.

5 Gait

The ankle joint complex's primary purpose is to provide a stable weight-bearing platform that supports the forces of ambulation in an energy-efficient manner. Weight-bearing forces reach as high as 5.5 times body weight during normal ambulation [6]. This is in addition to the destabilizing stresses that occur when walking on uneven ground or making lateral movements.

5.1 Phases of Gait

In normal gait, there are two distinct phases: stance and swing (Fig. 5). Stance phase occurs when any portion of the foot is in contact with the ground. Swing phase occurs when that foot is not in contact with the ground. A complete cycle occurs when the ipsilateral foot makes contact with the ground again after a full cycle of gait. A "double support period" occurs when both feet are in contact with the ground simultaneously. This occurs at two separate instances during the gait cycle, with each instance comprising around 10% of the total

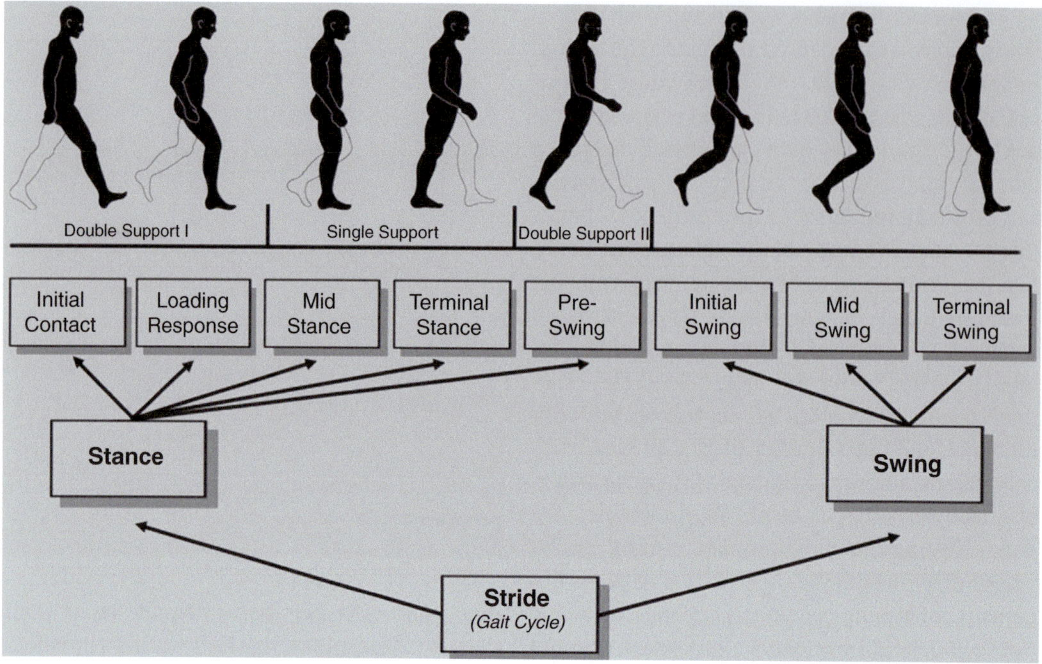

Fig. 5 This depicts normal gait. One cycle is composed of both stance and swing phases. These are further subdivided as shown. One complete cycle is referred to as a stride. (Reproduced from Shah with permission [18])

gait cycle (total 20%). These double support periods are replaced in running with "floating periods", which are defined as times when neither foot is touching the ground [18].

5.1.1 Stance Phase

During normal ambulation, approximately 60% of the gait cycle is spent in the stance phase [14, 18, 19]. The stance phase is further subdivided into five subphases [18].

Initial Contact

Initial contact occurs when the heel of the first foot makes initial contact with the ground. This also initiates the first double support period [18]. At this subphase, around 80% of the body weight is directly over the ipsilateral calcaneus. Body weight provides for a vertical compressive force and is the first period of increased forces [14].

Loading Response

The loading response subphase occurs when the entire first foot is in contact with the ground [18].

This is a period of controlled plantarflexion of the ankle and foot through eccentric contraction (lengthening of a muscle during contraction) of tibialis anterior (TA), extensor hallucis longus (EHL), and extensor digitorum longus (EDL). The knee passively flexes to maintain a center of gravity directly over the ankle [20]. This subphase is a shock absorption period and to accommodate the encountered forces, the foot pronates [14]. The hindfoot swings into valgus, the talus plantarflexes and adducts, and there is eccentric contraction of the supinators (TA, EHL, EDL). This is referred to as the "torque converter of the lower limb" [14]. During this subphase, the contralateral foot leaves the ground and enters its own swing phase, which ends the double support period [18].

Mid-Stance

The mid-stance subphase occurs as the body continues to move forward due to momentum. The entire foot remains in contact with the ground. There is passive dorsiflexion of the ankle and the knee becomes locked in extension. Minimal energy is needed in this phase as momentum provides forward movement. Ground reaction forces are anterior to the knee and ankle joint complex at this subphase [18].

Terminal Stance

The terminal stance subphase starts as the heel begins to lift off of the floor. Body weight shifts towards the metatarsal heads. The gastrocnemius/soleus complex fires concentrically to generate the power needed for propulsion [18]. As the weight continues to shift towards the metatarsal heads, the foot begins to supinate [14]. There is contraction of the gastrocnemius/soleus as well as posterior tibialis, flexor digitorum longus, and flexor hallucis longus. The intrinsic foot muscles also contract to allow for stabilization of the midtarsal joint. With supination of the subtalar joint and intrinsic muscle contraction, the midtarsal joint becomes locked. This creates the rigid lever needed to generate the force for foot push off in the next subphase [14].

Pre-swing

The pre-swing subphase begins at the "toe off" period as the foot begins to leave the ground. There is concentric tibialis anterior contraction and EHL contraction producing dorsiflexion of the ankle, foot, and hallux [18, 21]. During this subphase, the knee and hip also flex to prepare for foot clearance in the swing phase [18].

5.1.2 Swing Phase

The swing phase of the gait cycle occurs when the foot is no longer in contact with the ground. It is subdivided into the initial, mid, and terminal subphases. Minimal energy is needed for the foot in swing phase as it is being driven forward by momentum. Adequate dorsiflexion of the foot is critical to a successful swing phase in order to clear the ground. The tibialis anterior continues to contract concentrically throughout the swing phase. In addition, there is hip and knee flexion, which assist with clearing the foot from the ground [18].

5.2 Three Rocker Model

The "three rocker model" is another model for describing the subphases of the stance phase (Fig. 6). It was developed to describe the shifting of the fulcrum as the stance phase progressed. Each rocker (or point of rotation) has a primary purpose of either stiffening the foot to allow for propulsion and power or flexing the foot to allow for force absorption [4, 18, 19].

5.2.1 First Rocker

The first rocker begins with the foot's initial contact with the floor and comprises 10% of the gait cycle [22]. As the heel makes contact, there is a controlled lowering of the foot to the floor through eccentric tibialis anterior contraction. The heel is the fulcrum in this stage which produces ankle plantarflexion and knee flexion. As the heel makes contact with the ground, the ankle is pushed into valgus. This unlocks the Chopart joint which causes the foot to become flexible and allows it to act as a shock absorber for the increasing forces generated in this phase of gait [4, 18, 19].

5.2.2 Second Rocker

The second rocker occurs during midstance and comprises 20% of the gait cycle [22]. In this subphase, the foot is entirely in contact with the ground. The ankle is now the fulcrum. The goal of this subphase is to control forward motion. This is achieved through passive dorsiflexion of the ankle with eccentric contraction of the gastrocnemius/soleus complex [4, 18, 19].

5.2.3 Third Rocker

The third rocker is the final stance subphase and comprises 30% of the gait cycle [22]. As momentum continues to shift forward, the ankle reaches its limit of passive dorsiflexion. The gastrocnemius/soleus complex then starts to concentrically contract. This shifts the fulcrum to the metatarsal heads. As this occurs, concentric contraction of the posterior tibialis shifts the hindfoot into varus [4, 18, 19]. As the metatarsophalangeal joints dorsiflex during toe off, the plantar fascia is ten-

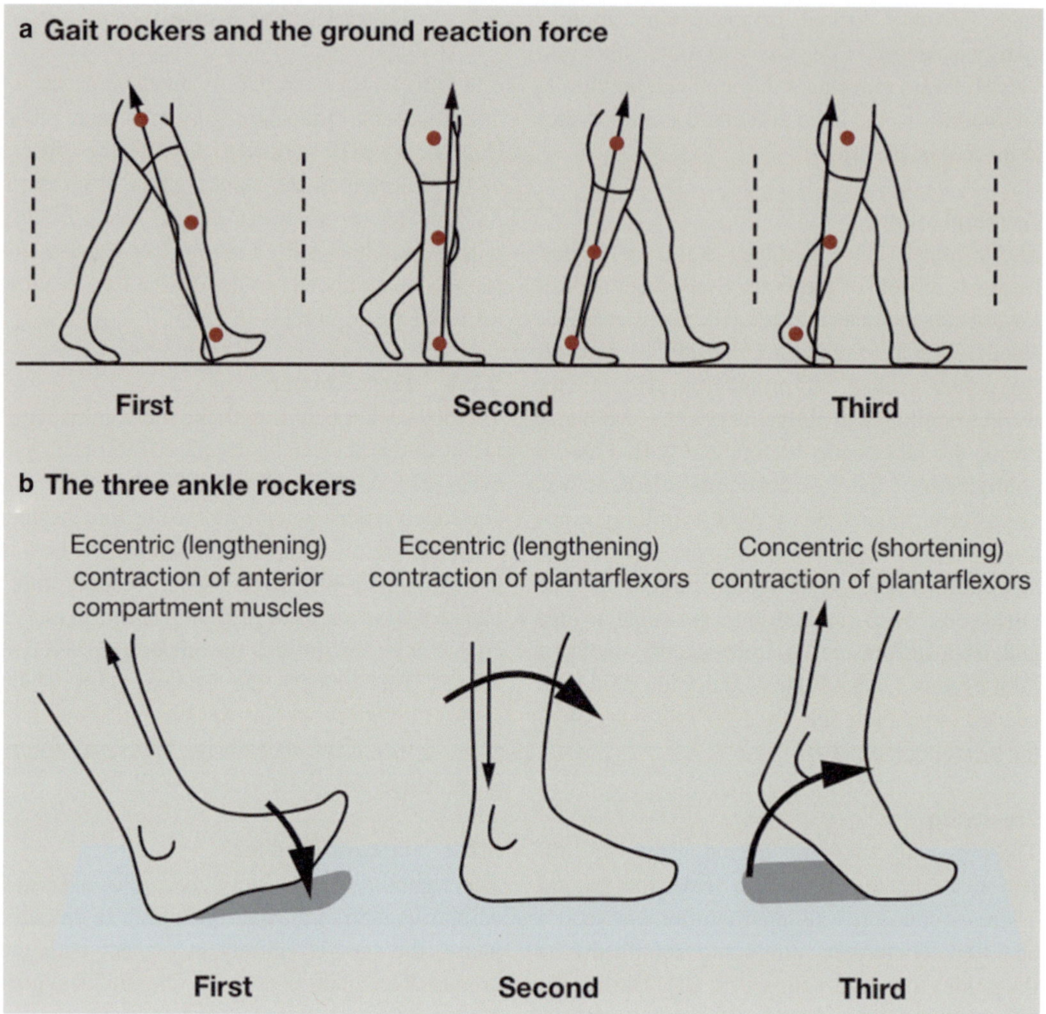

Fig. 6 The three rocker model. (**a**) Red dots represent the center of rotation at each joint. The line represents the ground reaction force direction. (**b**) The three rocker model with respect to foot position and the necessary muscle contractions. (Reproduced from Shah with permission [18])

sioned through the windlass effect. This creates the rigid lever arm that allows for the production of power needed for push off [4, 18, 19].

5.3 Pre-requisites for Normal Gait

Perry originally described the five prerequisites for normal gait [19]. First, there must be stability during the stance phase. This requires a stable foot position. Second, there must be adequate clearance during the swing phase, i.e., the foot needs to be able to clear the ground. Third, there must be adequate step length. This requires balance, a stable stance side, and sufficient hip and knee flexion on the swing side. Fourth, there must be appropriate pre-positioning during swing phase. Lastly, normal gait requires energy conservation and efficient use of energy in the gait cycle [18, 19].

5.4 Motion During Gait

Normal, energy-efficient gait requires around 30° of sagittal motion in the tibiotalar joint [4]. Typically, around 20° of plantarflexion is needed at toe off phase [21]. Ankle dorsiflexion needs are more variable but the typical motion is around 10–30° of dorsiflexion during ambulation [21]. In addition to sagittal motion, the triplanar motion of normal gait also includes approximately 14° of coronal motion and 22° of axial motion [4].

5.5 Energy Needs During Gait

Normal gait is an energy-efficient process. The body maximizes passive movements and utilizes forward momentum to achieve extreme efficiency. Normal gait requires around 2.5 kcal/min. These energy needs are just slightly greater than those required for sitting and standing (both around 1.5 kcal/min) [19]. Any modification to gait that affects the normal gait cycle will increase energy needs. The most common needs for increased energy are due to faster pace, antalgic gait, or use of an assistive device. Additionally, energy needs may increase with a lower leg amputation at any level, the use of a brace, or the presence of a knee flexion contracture [19]. As discussed above, the body frequently relies on eccentric contraction of various muscles for control during the gait cycle. Eccentric muscle contraction is the most energy-efficient form of muscle contraction [20]. Disruptions to this process have a profound effect on biomechanics and function.

5.6 Forces During Gait

The ankle joint complex and foot experience tremendous forces throughout normal gait which increase even more during running and destabilizing activities. There is substantial variability in different studies about the amount of force seen in gait. It is estimated that these forces are around 120% of body weight at heel strike [2]. During stance phase, the tibiotalar joint endures forces around 4 times body weight (BW), with averages between 3 and 5 × BW [1, 9]. The subtalar joint experiences forces around 2.4 × BW and the Chopart joint around 2.8 × BW [9]. At heel rise, tibiotalar forces increase to around 4.5–5.5 × BW [6]. These forces may increase up to 13 × BW during running [1].

5.7 Dynamic Changes in Intra-articular Pressure

During normal gait, there are significant changes that occur to the intra-articular pressure of the tibiotalar joint. This is important due to the potential for accelerated wear and arthritis formation with variable loading. Suckel et al. performed a cadaveric study and found that the major area of stress and greatest torque changes were seen in the anterolateral portion of the tibiotalar joint [23]. The medial talus had significantly lower pressures compared to the lateral aspect of the talus. This is consistent with the typical anterior tibial osteophytes seen in tibiotalar osteoarthritis. During heel strike, there was a rapid increase in intra-articular pressure throughout the tibiotalar joint. This reached a plateau after around 20% of stance phase occurred. During push off, the intra-articular pressure continued to increase. Intra-articular pressure reached a maximum at around 70% through the push off phase [23].

5.8 Running/Sprinting

The body makes several changes to the gait cycle when running, and even more when sprinting. The primary difference is the change from double support periods to floating periods, where neither foot is in contact with the ground. The time spent in stance phase also decreases significantly. As speed increases, stance time decreases from around 60% when walking, to 31% while running, to 22% while sprinting [24]. As speed increases, sagittal plane motion of the ankle increases. This enables a lower center of gravity. Similarly, hip and knee flexion also increase. To achieve greater dorsiflexion, tibialis anterior contraction changes from eccentric while walking to concentric during running and sprinting [24]. It is important to note that while this allows greater speed, the change to concentric contraction comes at the cost of increased energy expenditure.

6 Abnormal/Altered Biomechanics

Given the complexity of gait and normal ambulation, the process is easily altered by ankle joint complex pathology. Any alteration to the typical gait cycle results in a less efficient process and, therefore, requires increased energy. Various accommodative strategies occur either consciously or, more typically, subconsciously.

6.1 Antalgic Gait

An antalgic gait, or limp, occurs as a result of increased pain or other symptoms in one affected leg. This may arise from several sources of pain ranging from the hip/pelvis down to the toes. An antalgic gait arises to limit the amount of weight-bearing time spent on the affected side. This results in increased stance time on the contralateral side and greater total time spent in double support periods [18].

6.2 Planovalgus Foot

A planovalgus foot, or flatfoot, is defined as the hindfoot in increased valgus and a loss of the normal arch of the midfoot. This produces an increase in ankle plantarflexion, a contracture of the triceps surae, and an overall reduction in the normal ankle range of motion. The loss of ankle motion is accommodated by increased dorsiflexion and flexibility through the transverse tarsal (Chopart) joint. With increased motion at the transverse tarsal joint, the hindfoot is driven into more valgus through the subtalar joint. In sum, these changes lead to a shift towards pronation of the foot during all phases of gait [25].

6.3 Foot Drop

Foot drop results from either a weakness or a complete loss of ankle dorsiflexion. This may have several different etiologies including peripheral neuropathy, peroneal nerve injury, tibialis anterior muscle/tendon injury, or lumbar pathology. Ultimately, this results in an equinus (plantarflexed) position of the ankle and an inability to fully dorsiflex the ankle. Using the rocker model to describe foot drop, during the first rocker phase, there is loss of the controlled plantarflexion, and instead, there is a "slap" type impact of the foot [18]. There are several accommodative strategies for gait that patients with foot drop may do either consciously or subconsciously. Since the ankle is plantarflexed, the affected extremity is functionally longer than it should be. To compensate, the body enacts strategies to "shorten" this limb [20]. In order for the foot to clear the ground, the ipsilateral hip and knee will increase the amount of flexion [18, 20]. Similarly, pelvic obliquity may develop to accommodate foot clearance [18, 20]. A steppage (or marching) type gait, circumduction of the affected limb, and abduction of the affected limb are other maneuvers to help shorten the functionally long leg [20].

6.4 Ankle Joint Complex Osteoarthritis

One of the most common sources of altered biomechanics is the development of ankle osteoarthritis. This may be present in any of the three joints of the ankle joint complex independently or in combination. In contrast with the hip and knee, ankle osteoarthritis is primarily post-traumatic rather than idiopathic [21, 26]. Therefore, it is much easier to identify those patients at risk of developing arthritis in the future. As arthritis progresses, there is loss of both active and passive sagittal motion of around $10°$ [21]. With the loss of plantarflexion, there is also a decrease in peak plantarflexion moment and ankle power [4, 21]. Similarly, there is a loss of the standard motion coupling between the tibiotalar and subtalar joints [21]. To accommodate for these motion losses, the body spends less time in stance phase on the affected leg [21]. This also limits the maximum force that can be loaded on the affected leg [21]. These changes result in a shorter stride length and slower walking speed [4, 18, 21].

There are several conservative and surgical treatment options utilized in the management of ankle osteoarthritis and these will be discussed in other chapters.

7 Conclusion

The ankle joint complex is a uniquely formed structure where the combination of articular anatomy, ligamentous support, and muscular force through tendon attachments is essential for gait and managing weight-bearing forces. An energy-efficient gait cycle requires coordination from the hip through the ankle, with the ankle joint complex serving the greatest role. Biomechanics of the foot and ankle thus form a foundation from which to build our understanding of diagnosis and treatment of foot and ankle pathology.

References

1. Brockett CL, Chapman GJ. Biomechanics of the ankle. Orthop Trauma. 2016;30(3):232–8.
2. Snedeker JG, Wirth SH, Espinosa N. Biomechanics of the normal and arthritic ankle joint. Foot Ankle Clin. 2012;17:517–28.
3. Campbell KJ, Michalski MP, Wilson KJ, Goldsmith MT, Wijdicks CA, LaPrade RF, Clanton TO. The ligament anatomy of the deltoid complex of the ankle: a qualitative and quantitative anatomical study. J Bone Joint Surg. 2014;96(8):e62.
4. Leardini A, O'connor JJ, Giannini S. Biomechanics of the natural, arthritic, and replaced human ankle joint. J Foot Ankle Res. 2014;7:8.
5. Calhoun JH, Eng M, Li F, Ledbetter BR, Viegas SF. A comprehensive study of pressure distribution in the ankle joint with inversion and eversion. Foot Ankle Int. 1994;15(3):125–33.
6. Castro MD. Ankle biomechanics. Foot Ankle Clin. 2002;7:679–93.
7. Kimizuka M, Kurosawa H, Fukubayashi T. Load-bearing pattern of the ankle joint: contact area and pressure distribution, vol. 96. Arch Orthop Traumat Surg; 1980. p. 45–9.
8. Sarrafian SK. Sarrafian's anatomy of the foot and ankle. 2nd ed. Philadelphia, PA: Lippincott; 1993. p. 544.
9. Kleipool RP, Blankevoort L. The relation between geometry and function of the ankle joint complex: a biomechanical review. Knee Surg Sports Traumatol Arthrosc. 2010;18:618–27.
10. Procter P, Paul JP. Ankle joint biomechanics. J Biomech. 1982;15(9):627–34.
11. Lundberg A, Svensson OK, Nemeth G, Selvik G. The axis of rotation of the ankle joint. J Bone Joint Surg (Br). 1989;71(1):94–9.
12. Leardini A, O'connor JJ, Catani F, Giannini S. A geometric model of the human ankle joint. J Biomech. 1999;32:585–91.
13. Kakkar R, Siddique MS. Stresses in the ankle joint and total ankle replacement design. Foot Ankle Surg. 2011;17:58–63.
14. Donatelli R. Normal biomechanics of the foot and ankle. J Orthop Sports Phys Ther. 1985;7:91.
15. Hintermann B, Sommer C, Nigg BMN. Influence of Ligament transection on tibial and calcaneal rotation with loading and dorsi-plantarflexion. Foot Ankle Int. 1995;16(9):567–71.
16. Harper MC. Deltoid ligament: an anatomical evaluation of function. Foot Ankle Int. 1987;8(1):19–22.
17. Rosenbaum AJ, DiPreta JA, Misener D. Plantar heel pain. Med Clin N Am. 2014;98(2):339–52.
18. Shah K, Solan M, Dawe E. The gait cycle and its variations with disease and injury. Orthop Trauma. 2020;34(3):153–60.
19. Gage JR, Deluca PA, Renshaw TS. Gait analysis: principles and applications. Instr Course Lect. 1995;77-A(10):1607–23.
20. Gait DA. The role of the ankle and foot in walking, vol. 98. Medical Clinics of North America; 2014. p. 205–11.
21. Nüesch C, Barg A, Pagenstert GI, Valderrabano V. Biomechanics of asymmetric ankle osteoarthritis and its joint-preserving surgery. Foot Ankle Clin. 2013;18:427–36.
22. Espinosa N, Maceira E, Myerson M. Current concept review: metatarsalgia. Foot Ankle Int. 2008;29(8):871–9.
23. Suckel A, Muller O, Wachter N, Kluba T. In vitro measurement of intraarticular pressure in the ankle joint. Knee Surg Sports Traumatol Arthrosc. 2010;18(5):664–8.
24. Mann RA, Hagy J. Biomechanics of walking, running, and sprinting. Am J Sports Med. 1980;8(5):345–50.
25. Saraswat P, MacWilliams BA, Davis RB, D'Astous JL. Kinematics and kinetics of normal and planovalgus feet during walking. Gait Posture. 2014;39(1):339–45.
26. Singer S, Klejman S, Pinsker E, Houck J, Daniels T. Ankle arthroplasty and ankle arthrodesis: gait analysis compared with normal controls. J Bone Joint Surg. 2013;95(24):e191.1.

Radiologic Imaging of the Ankle

Alexander B. Peterson and Eric W. Tan

When evaluating the ankle, the proper use of diagnostic imaging is critical for accurate diagnosis and guiding the appropriate treatment. This chapter will discuss imaging techniques that are commonly used to assess the ankle. This encompasses traditional modalities, such as radiography, magnetic resonance imaging (MRI), and computed tomography (CT), as well as more specialized techniques including weight bearing CT (WBCT) and single photon emission computed tomography (SPECT) scans.

1 Radiography

Radiographs, colloquially known as X-rays, are the most utilized form of imaging in the foot and ankle. Image acquisition is rapid, cost is relatively inexpensive, and the required equipment can be readily installed in the office setting. In the modern era, digital radiography has replaced conventional film-based radiographs. At its core, radiographs are produced by passing ionizing radiation, such as X-rays, through a patient. The penetration of the radiation is variable based on the density of the tissue, with bone and metallic implants generally being the densest. The penetrating radiation effectively produces a shadow of the anatomy, which is captured on the detector. Detectors were traditionally photographic film but are now commonly digital. The digital detector then produces the radiographic image for diagnostic interpretation [1, 2].

A thorough history and physical examination is critical for guiding the decision to obtain radiographic imaging. Beyond standard radiographs of the ankle, the history and exam may guide the practitioner to order special views, stress views, or images of adjacent anatomy, such as the foot, tibia and fibula, or full-length films of the limb. In general, radiographs provide a good initial evaluation of the ankle joint and can direct the need for more advanced imaging studies, as needed.

Due to a concern that radiographs were being overutilized to evaluate ankle injuries, the Ottawa rules were developed to guide practitioners on the proper use of radiographic examination in the setting of an acute ankle injury [3]. As most ankle injuries are sprains that do not involve fractures of the bones, unnecessary X-rays may be avoided by following restrictions laid forth by the Ottawa guidelines. These rules are defined as bony tenderness at the malleoli or the inability to bear weight; if any of these are present, radiographic assessment is warranted. Sensitivity of this decision-making tool has been shown to be 100% for fractures, with moderate specificity. When implemented in clinical practice, the rate of ankle radiographs is reduced by up to 40% [4–6].

A. B. Peterson · E. W. Tan (✉)
Department of Orthopaedic Surgery, Keck School of Medicine of USC, Los Angeles, CA, USA
e-mail: Alexander.Peterson@med.usc.edu; Eric.Tan@med.usc.edu

© The Author(s), under exclusive license to Springer Nature Switzerland AG 2023
D. Herscovici Jr. et al. (eds.), *Evaluation and Surgical Management of the Ankle*,
https://doi.org/10.1007/978-3-031-33537-2_3

Ottawa ankle rules are effective for ruling out unstable ankle fractures in the acute setting, arguably making them appropriate in the emergency department, but radiographs are useful for more than detecting fractures. As such, the authors have a low threshold to obtain ankle radiographs, which can provide information about potential arthritis, focal articular lesions, anatomic alignment, tumors, infection, and certain soft tissue conditions, among others. It is also important to point out that patients may present with ankle pain in the absence of trauma.

If imaging is warranted, standard views of the ankle are obtained. These include anteroposterior (AP), lateral, and internal oblique (mortise) views (Fig. 1). Whenever possible, standing (i.e., weight-bearing) radiographs are obtained in lieu of non-weight-bearing films. Weight-bearing radiographs provide important information about the overall structural alignment of the ankle as it exists in daily life. In most cases, it is when the patient is using and loading the ankle that they experience pain or discomfort. Therefore, the weight-bearing images create the physiologic stresses on the ankle joint and surrounding ligaments that illustrate key findings like joint space narrowing, bony impingement, and joint subluxation that would go unappreciated in a non-weight-bearing radiograph. Non-weight-bearing films should only be obtained when the patient is unable to stand on the limb, either due to pain or other physical restriction.

The *AP view*, with the knee and the axis of the first ray of the foot pointing forward, allows evaluation of the tibiotalar joint, distal tibia and fibula, peripheral borders of the tarsals, talar dome, and the syndesmosis (Fig. 2) [7, 8]. The lateral gutter is poorly visualized due to overlap between the fibula and the lateral aspect of the talus.

The *mortise view*, or internal oblique, is obtained with the leg internally rotated 15–20° relative to the AP position. There should be no overlap of the malleoli with the talus [9]. It provides additional information about the ankle mortise and syndesmotic alignment, talar dome integrity, different views of the malleoli, and allows for inspection of the lateral talar process. The mortise view produces the optimal assessment of tibiotalar and talofibular congruity.

The *lateral view* is obtained with the medial border of the foot against the cassette and the beam perpendicular. A true lateral has perfect overlap of the medial and lateral talar dome, and no overlap between the tibial plafond and the talar dome. The fibula will be superimposed on the tibia. It allows for assessment of the ankle for effusion, hindfoot integrity and talocalcaneal relationship, tibiofibular integrity and syndesmosis, and tibiotalar congruity. In the case of fracture, particular attention should be paid to the posterior malleolus. The fifth metatarsal base, often fractured from inversion injuries, may also be well-visualized on a lateral radiograph.

At some institutions, an *external oblique radiograph* is included in the standard trauma series. To obtain this view, the leg is rotated externally 45°, relative to a true AP [7]. This allows for improved assessment of the posterior colliculus of the medial malleolus, which can otherwise be difficult to visualize [10].

If an isolated medial or posterior malleolar ankle fracture or isolated medial clear space widening is identified, it is critical that the practitioner examines the entire lower leg and obtains films of the complete tibia and fibula to rule out a Maisonneuve injury-pattern with a more proximal fibula fracture (Fig. 3).

When obtaining a non-weight-bearing image, the ankle should be dorsiflexed to neutral, with some pronation through the foot to create a more physiologic view [7]. Due to the normal anatomy of the talus, it is broader anteriorly than posteriorly, so if the talus is plantarflexed during the AP or mortise radiographs, the medial clear space measurements may be distorted. Stress views of the ankle are also important diagnostic tools in cases when the patient is unable to bear weight.

1.1 Radiographic Evaluation

It is important to understand the measurements commonly applied to the standard ankle series, particularly in the setting of trauma, with most establishing the stability status of the ankle

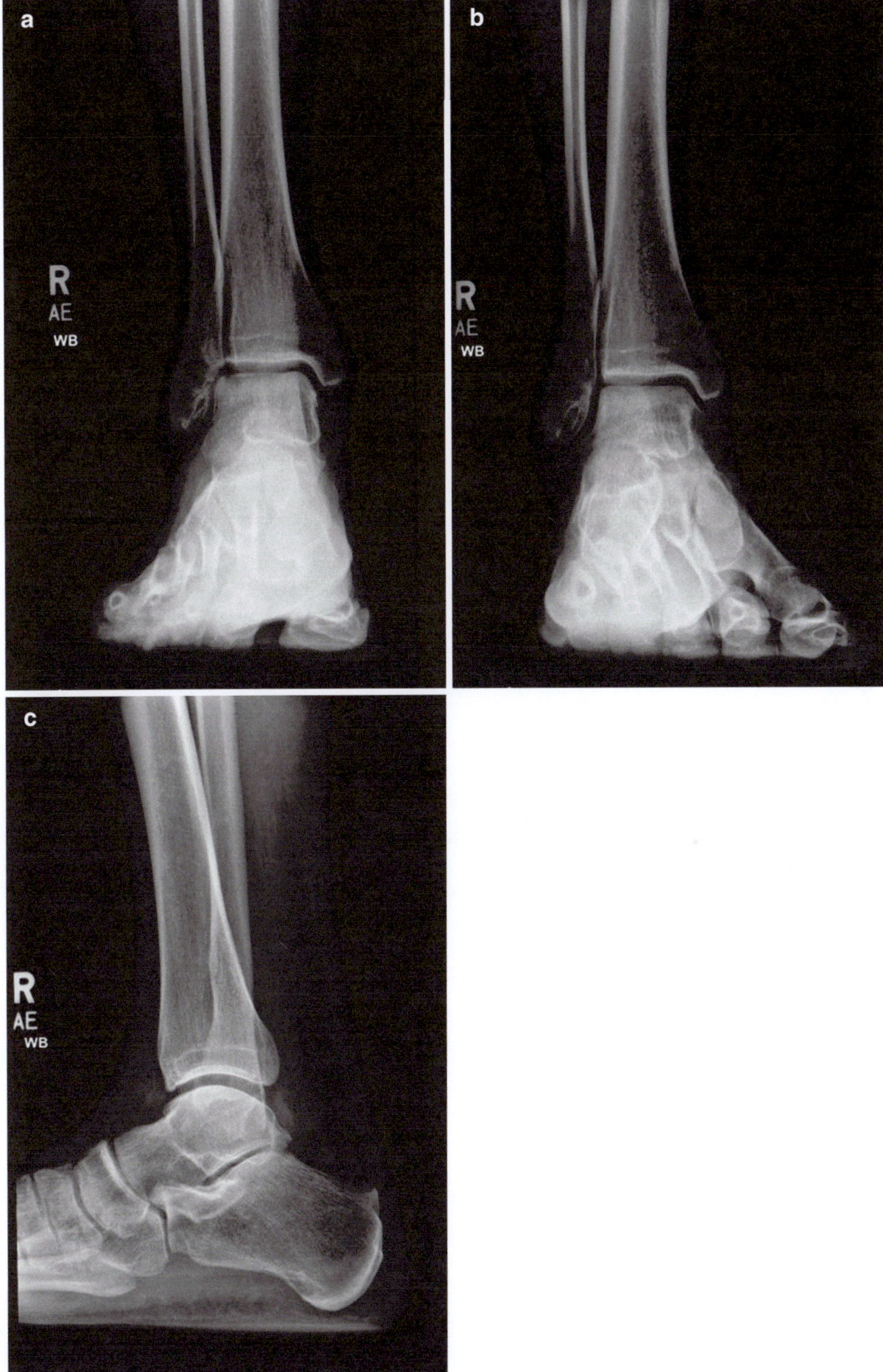

Fig. 1 Standard radiographic weight-bearing views of the ankle. (**a**) Anteroposterior. (**b**) Mortise. (**c**) Lateral

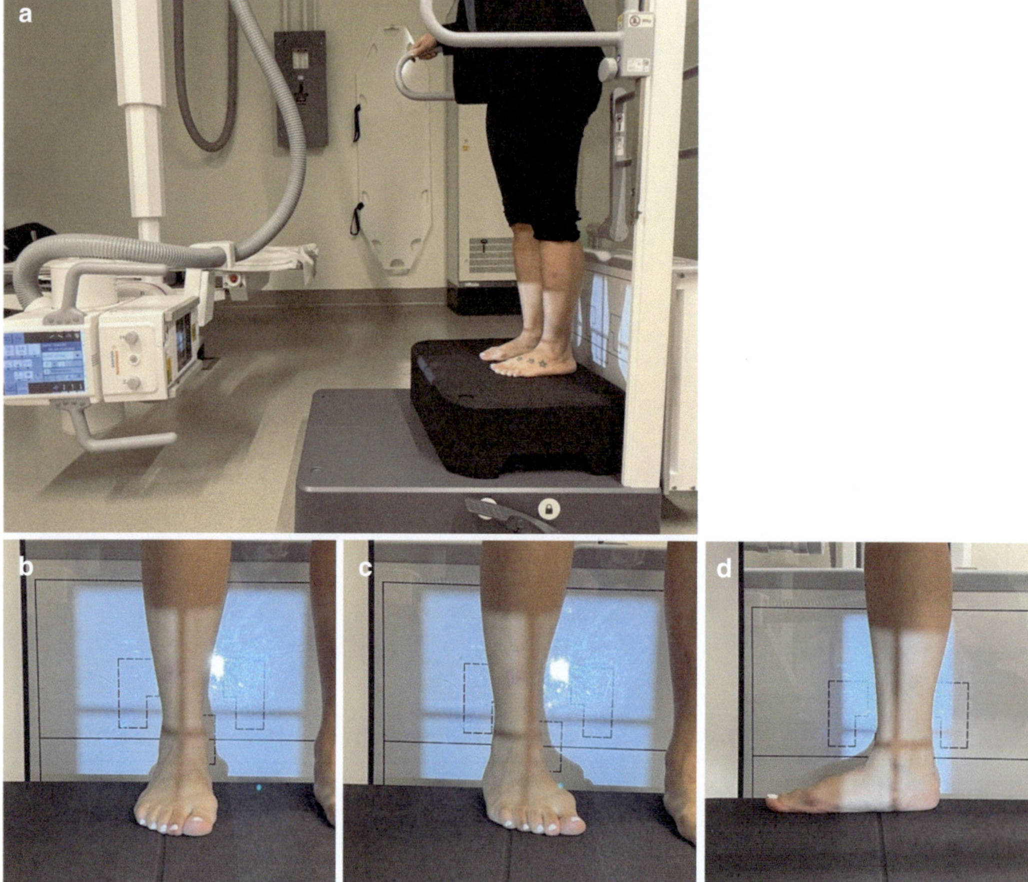

Fig. 2 Techniques for the acquisition of standard weight-bearing radiographs of the ankle. (**a**) The patient stands on an elevated platform between the beam and the cassette. The beam is angled parallel to the floor. (**b**) Anteroposterior view: The first ray and patella are pointed forward, parallel to the beam. (**c**) Mortise view: The leg is internally rotated 15–20°. (**d**) Lateral view: the first ray is oriented perpendicular to the beam

following fracture or ligamentous disruption. The *medial clear space* gives information about the integrity of the deltoid ligament. Measured on a weight-bearing or stress mortise view, it is defined as the distance between the medial border of the talus and the lateral border of the medial malleolus (Fig. 4) [9, 11]. Specifically, the measurement should be made 5 mm distal to the dome of the talus [12]. Values >5 mm or >1 mm greater than the tibiotalar distance (between the tibial plafond and talar dome) have been proposed at cutoffs for clinically significant deltoid injury [13, 14]. Practically, this could lead a surgeon to fixation of the fibula in an unstable isolated lateral malleolus fracture. The *tibiofibular clear space* and the *tibiofibular overlap* assess the ligaments, integrity and alignment of the syndesmosis and can also be measured on weight-bearing or stress views. The *tibiofibular clear space* is measured from the medial border of the fibula to the incisura fibularis (tibial concavity at the distal tibiofibular articulation) [15]. It is measured 1 cm proximal to the tibial plafond [16]. Widening represents potential disruption of the ankle syndesmosis, either through fracture or frank ligamentous injury (such as a "high ankle sprain"). Traditionally, normal values were considered normal if they were less than 6 mm on AP and mortise views. *Tibiofibular overlap* measures the radiographic overlay of the fibula and the anterolateral fibula on AP and mortise views. Again, it is measured 1 cm proximal to the tibial

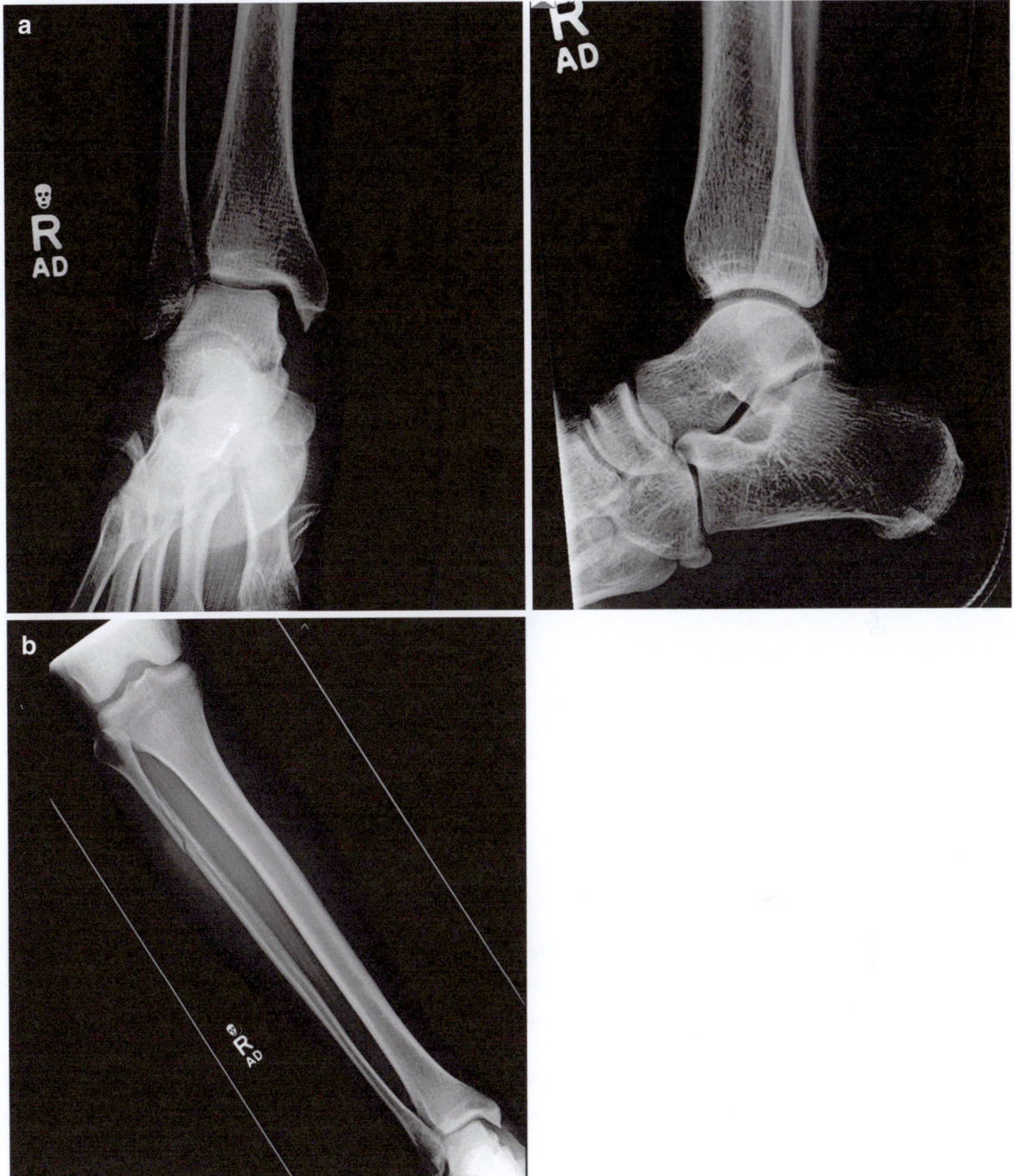

Fig. 3 Maisonneuve injury pattern. (**a**) Isolated medial clear space widening is seen on the initial radiographs. (**b**) Tibia fibula films demonstrate a fracture of the proximal fibula, consistent with a Maisonneuve injury with syndesmotic disruption

plafond. Normal values are traditionally >6 mm on the AP view and >1 mm on the mortise view. Though helpful for guiding evaluation, these values for tibiofibular clear space and overlap have been challenged, as significant variation has been found in normal controls [15]. The *anterior to posterior fibular gap* is specific to rotational ankle fractures and is measured on the lateral view. The orthogonal distance between the proximal and distal fibula fragments is measured, immediately anterior to the disruption in the posterior cortex [14]. Values greater than 1 mm on initial injury radiographs are associated with medial tibiotalar instability.

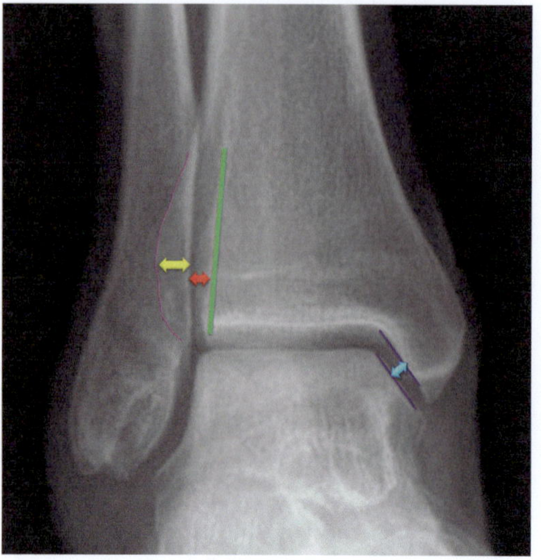

Fig. 4 Common radiographic measurements of the ankle. *Medial clear space* (cyan arrow) is measured 5 mm below the level of the talar dome, between the medial aspect of the talus and the lateral aspect of the medial malleolus. *Tibiofibular clear space* (red arrow) is measured 1 cm proximal to tibial plafond, between the medial border of the fibula and the medial shadow of the incisura fibularis (green line). *Tibiofibular overlap* (yellow arrow) is measured 1 cm proximal to the tibial plafond, between the lateral border of the tibia (magenta line) and the medial border of the fibula

1.2 Stress Radiographs

Plain radiographs may not adequately identify the presence of any associated soft tissue injuries. To evaluate these injuries, stress radiographs have been described. Stress radiographs assess ligamentous instability and may be considered for acute or chronic ankle injuries. To evaluate distal syndesmotic or medial ankle deltoid ligament tears, especially in setting of a fibula fracture, the use of *gravity stress* or *manual external rotation stress* radiographs have been described [11, 17]. The purpose of these two stress radiographs is to guide the practitioner in determining both the optimal treatment (operative versus nonoperative care) and the recommended weight-bearing status. When positive, the images will demonstrate relative widening of the medial clear space, indicative of a deltoid injury, and/or widening of the tibiofibular joint, indicative of a syndesmotic injury. It is not uncommon for a distal fibula fracture to have a stable appearance on a non-weight-

bearing mortise view, only to have significant subluxation on a stress exam. Gravity stress radiographs are performed with the patient in the lateral decubitus position, injured side down. The limb's rotation and the beam are adjusted to obtain a mortise view of the ankle (Fig. 5). It is imperative that the medial malleolus is closer to the ceiling and the lateral malleolus closer to the ground. This allows the foot and talus, under their own weight (gravity), to "fall down" away from the medial malleolus. The *manual external rotation stress* is obtained by stabilizing the tibia with one hand, while applying a steady external rotational

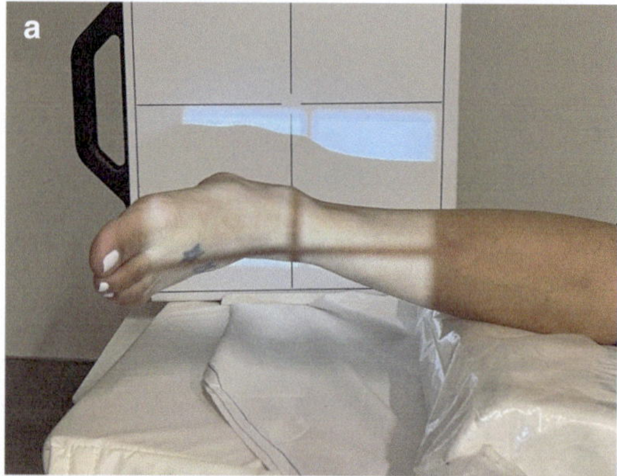

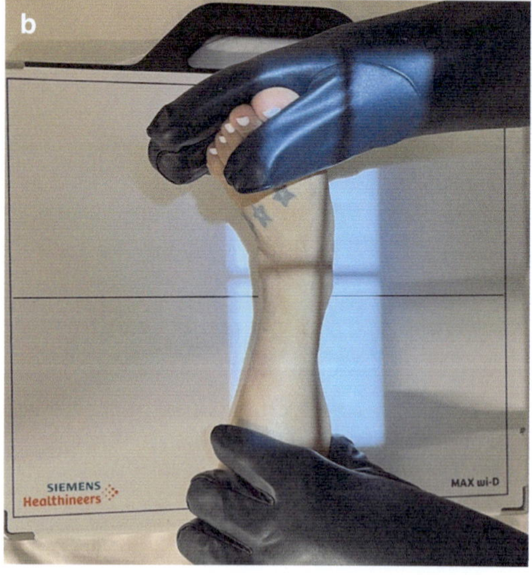

Fig. 5 Ankle stress tests are used to diagnose joint instability. (**a**) Gravity stress view: The affected ankle is suspended, with the medial side toward the ceiling. A mortise view is obtained. (**b**) Manual external rotation stress: Utilizing lead gloves to avoid unnecessary radiation exposure, the provider stabilizes the leg while applying an external rotation force through the foot

force through the foot, preferably in neutral to slight dorsiflexion during a mortise radiograph [18, 19]. It is best practice for the practitioner applying the stress to utilize lead-lined gloves to limit radiation exposure. A weight-bearing ankle radiograph is also a stress view, as it applies a physiologic load to the joint. Recent studies have shown that weight-bearing films alone are adequate for determining the stability of ankle fractures, and that positive gravity stress radiographs may result in unnecessary surgical intervention [11, 17]. It is the authors' practice to only use gravity and manual stress radiographs when the patient is unable to receive a weight-bearing film, either due to pain or other disability, or when the weight-bearing radiographs are inconclusive (Fig. 6). From a practical perspective, these stress views can be obtained in the office, urgent care, or emergency department. When assessing ankle stability in the operating room, often the manual external rotation stress test is performed under fluoroscopic imaging, given the limits of patient positioning and participation.

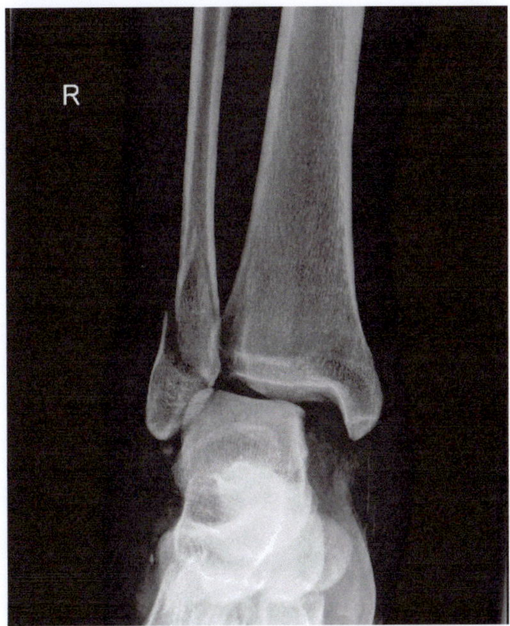

Fig. 6 Due to polytrauma, this patient was unable to stand for a weight-bearing film. A manual external rotation stress demonstrated significant widening of the medial clear space via rotation and lateral translation of the unstable talus

Additional stress views also exist and are helpful for evaluating the ankle ligaments. The *anterior drawer stress* radiograph primarily evaluates the competency of the anterior talofibular ligament (ATFL) [7]. The ATFL is an important restraint to anterior subluxation of the talus, relative to the tibial plafond and is best evaluated using a lateral ankle radiograph. This can be obtained using specialized mechanical devices for applying the anterior drawer force, in a reproducible manner with a standardized force typically 15 kPa, or can be performed manually. When performed manually, the patient is positioned supine with the heel elevated on a firm bolster. Utilizing one hand to stabilize the tibia with a downward force, the second hand is placed behind the heel and pulls the foot forward [8]. A positive test will demonstrate anterior subluxation of the talus, with either 10 mm of absolute subluxation, or 3–5 mm of relative subluxation, compared to the contralateral side [20, 21]. The *talar tilt test*, or varus stress, primarily evaluates the integrity of the calcaneofibular ligament (CFL) by assessing the ankle's ability to resist a varus directed force. This is performed using an AP radiograph. While the patient is in the supine position, a varus force is manually applied through the ankle. The relative coronal plane angulation of the talus and the tibial plafond (talar tilt) is measured. Laxity of the lateral ankle ligaments will lead to greater talar tilt. The stress test is positive if there is 10° of talar tilt, or 3–5° of tilt relative to the contralateral ankle [20, 21]. The anterior drawer and talar tilt stress radiographs are certainly not a mandatory study for evaluating lateral ankle instability, as the diagnosis can be made based on history and physical examination. Studies have shown that these two stress views may underestimate the true severity of instability [20]. The images can, however, provide additional objective information to support the diagnosis and decision for treatment. Similarly, an ankle *valgus stress test* can be performed in an identical manner, providing information about the integrity of the deltoid ligament. This can be valuable in the setting of medial ankle instability or flatfoot reconstruction [22].

1.3   Specialized Radiographic Evaluations

Additional views, beyond the routine ankle series, can be helpful, and in some cases imperative for an adequate clinical assessment. Suggestion of injuries to the foot should certainly receive standard foot radiographs (AP, lateral, and external oblique). If one suspects a fracture to the calcaneus, two additional radiographs can be obtained to assess the fracture. The first is a *Harris (axial) heel* view, allowing one to visualize a longitudinal axial view of the calcaneus and the second is a *Broden* view, which provides further information about the subtalar joint integrity [8].

Suspected fractures of the talar neck can be evaluated with a *Canale view* radiograph. The *Canale* view is obtained by maximally plantarflexing the ankle and pronating the foot 15°. This allows for less obstructed visualization of the talar neck by reducing the overlap of the calcaneus on the talus. The *Canale* view is also useful for preoperative planning as well as postoperative assessment of reduction [23, 24].

Understanding the relationship between the hindfoot, ankle, and tibia is critical when planning for a deformity correction. A specialized radiograph that is helpful evaluating the ankle/hindfoot alignment and the presence of any coronal plane deformity is the *Saltzman hindfoot alignment view* (Fig. 7). Although visualization of the tibiotalar alignment is clear on the standard AP and lateral ankle radiographs, it does not provide a full assessment of the axial heel position

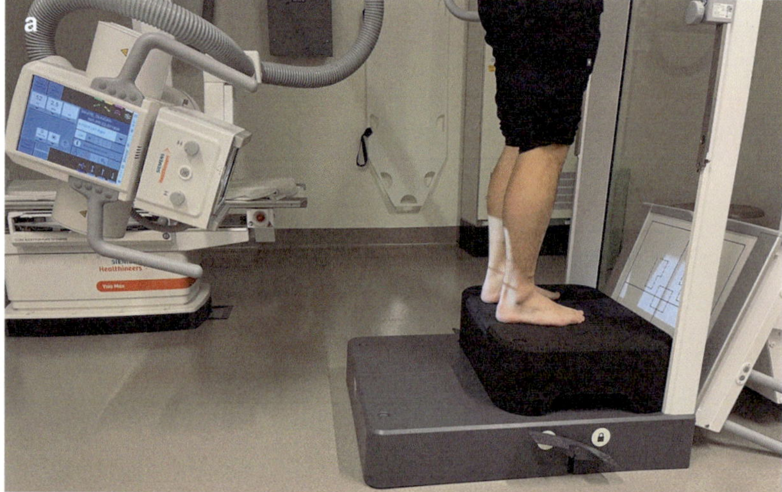

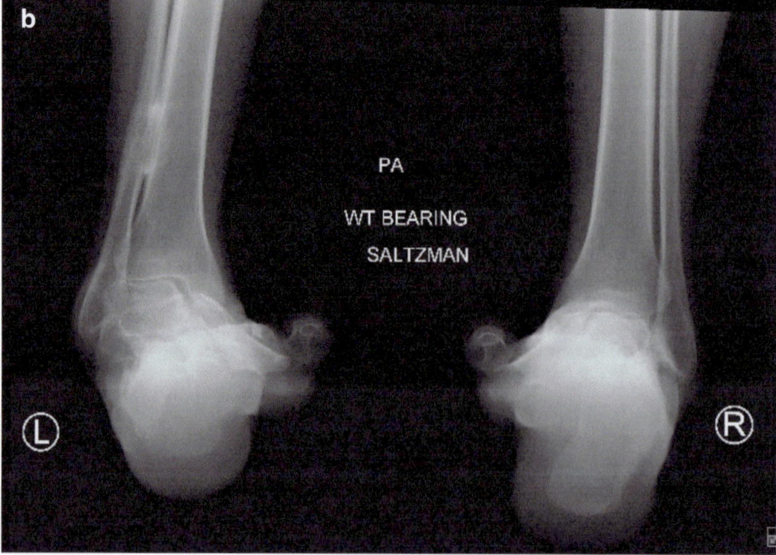

Fig. 7 Saltzman hindfoot alignment view: (**a**) The patient stands on a radiolucent platform. The cassette is angled 20° off the vertical, with the beam perpendicular to the cassette. (**b**) The Saltzman hindfoot alignment view shows significant hindfoot varus deformity in this patient

relative to the ankle and distal tibia. Multi-level deformity is not uncommon, and the Saltzman hindfoot alignment view provides a method for radiographically imaging the coronal plane alignment of the hindfoot in relation to the weight-bearing line of the tibia. With the patient standing, the beam is oriented in a posteroanterior direction and slightly plantar, 20° from the horizontal, with a detector cassette oriented 20° from the vertical [25, 26].

Lastly, *full-length extremity films*, also known as hip-to-calcaneus radiographs, are useful for evaluation of multilevel deformity as well as limb length discrepancies (Fig. 8) [27, 28]. They

simultaneously provide information about coronal plane deformity at the femur, knee, tibia, ankle, and hindfoot. To obtain this radiograph, the patient stands on a radiolucent box while facing away from the beam with the patella centered. The beam is angled level to the horizontal at the level of the knee. The radiograph should project an image from the lower part of the pelvis through the calcaneus [27]. Mechanical and anatomic axis measurements can then be made to determine the necessary level(s) of correction. If both limbs are captured, leg length discrepancies can be measured. It has been shown surgical management of a deformity at the knee can have a direct impact on the improvement or exacerbation of deformity at the hindfoot and ankle [29].

2 Magnetic Resonance Imaging

Magnetic resonance imaging (MRI) is an advanced imaging modality that is commonly used in the diagnosis of pathology around the foot and ankle. MRI technology uses magnetic fields and radio waves to collect data on a range of tissue characteristics, which is subsequently processed to produce a variety of different cross-sectional images [30]. MRI takes advantage of the magnetic properties of unpaired hydrogen protons in the targeted tissues. The magnet of the MRI produces a strong electromagnetic (EM) field, which causes the unpaired hydrogen atoms to align in a particular orientation [31]. Subsequently, a radiofrequency (RF) pulse is directed at the tissue, which causes the protons to enter a higher energy state. When the RF pulse ceases, the protons undergo relaxation, returning to their original energy state. In the process, they emit that energy differential in the form of RF energy, which maintains information about its source tissue. The MRI system detects the emitted RF energy and subsequently processes the data to produce images reflecting the unique biochemical tissue properties. The protons of muscle, fat, tendon, ligaments, bone, cartilage, and synovial fluid respond in different, but consistent ways to the MRI scanning process. This leads to

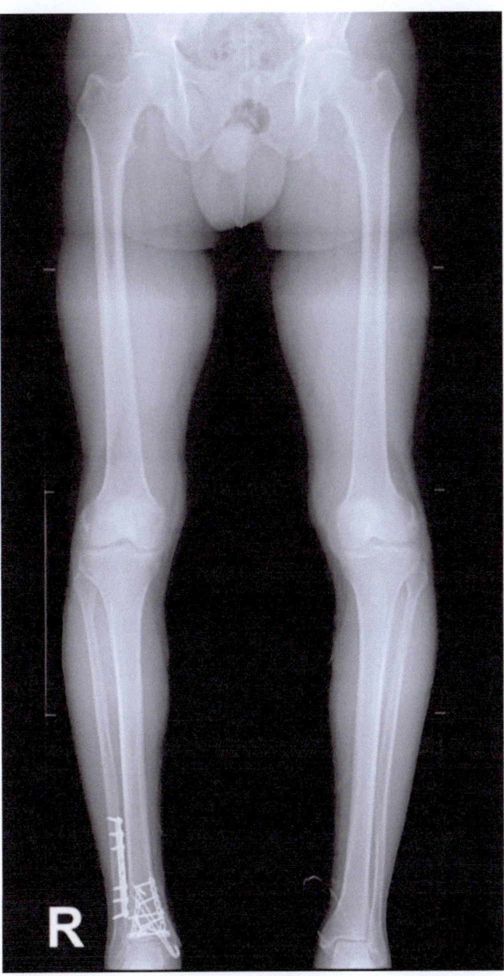

Fig. 8 Full length alignment radiographs. Full length films are useful for assessing multiple levels of deformity, as well as for measuring leg length discrepancies

images with good differentiation between the various tissues, and potential for excellent definition of anatomic structures.

The way the MRI machine pulses RF energy affects the response of the unpaired protons in the imaged tissue. By controlling the variables around the pulsed RF energy, different MRI "sequences" can be obtained. Each sequence has unique characteristics that highlight different types of tissue (Fig. 9). Common examples include T1, T2, short tau inversion recovery (STIR), and proton density-weighted fast spin-echo (PD FSE) sequences [32]. The T1-weighted sequences display fat, subacute hemorrhage, and proteinaceous fluid as high signal, or bright, whereas edema and other fluid appears low signal, or dark [30]. A T1 image provides high anatomic detail and is useful for assessing findings like fracture lines, but is poor for evaluating cartilage. T2-weighted sequences display fluid as high signal and fat as low signal. They are important for looking for sites of edema. The PD-weighted FSE sequences provide high anatomic detail and, unlike T1 sequences, provide

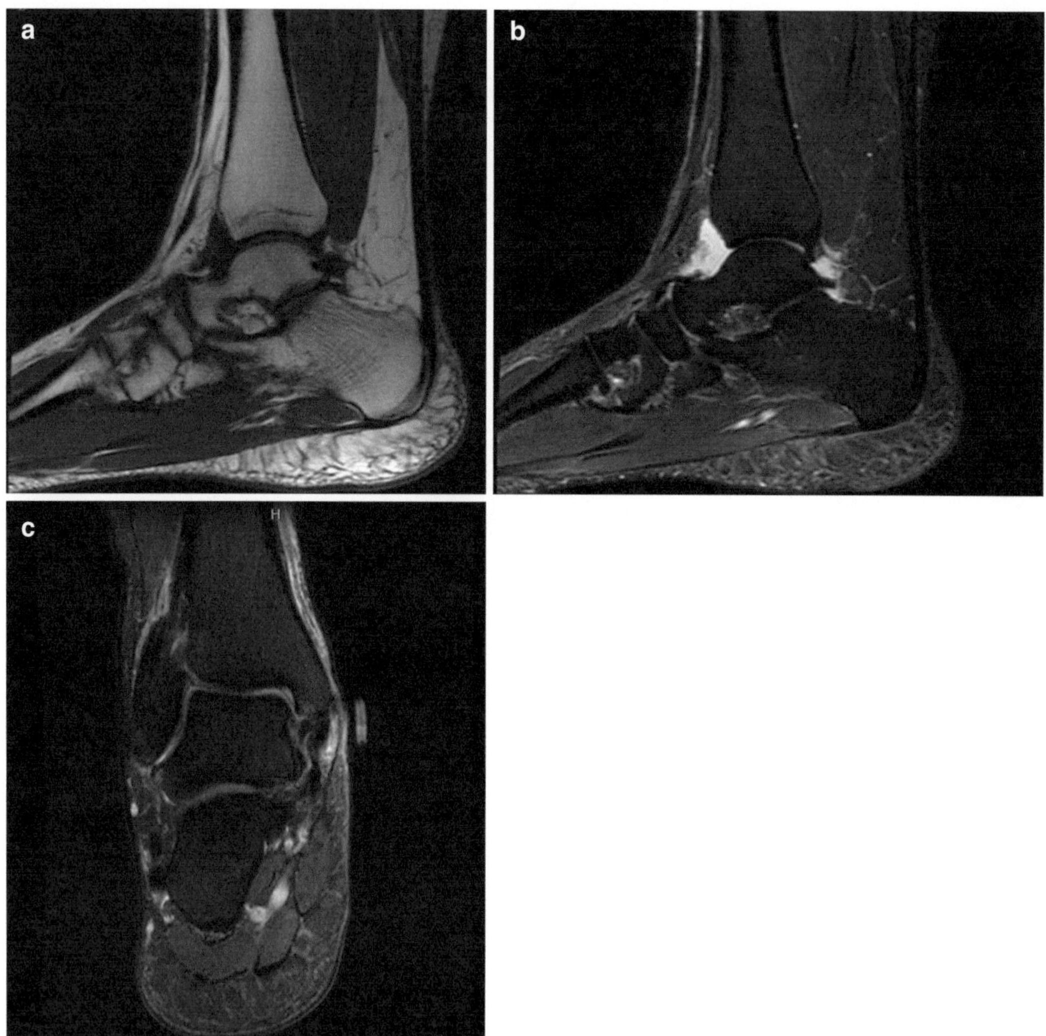

Fig. 9 Different MRI sequences highlight unique elements of patient anatomy and pathology. (**a**) T1 MRI image sagittal view of the ankle. (**b**) STIR MRI image sagittal view of the ankle. (**c**) PD MRI image coronal view of the ankle

excellent evaluation of articular cartilage. The STIR sequences highlight fluid, while suppressing fat, which is excellent for identifying edematous sites of pathology. Their long sequencing times, however, lead to worse resolution.

MRI is an important tool used in the evaluation of acute and chronic soft tissue, chondral, and osseous injuries. Often, given the close proximity of anatomic structures in the ankle and hindfoot, it can be difficult to definitively diagnose the exact source of a patient's symptoms on examination alone. For example, following inversion injuries (ankle sprains), an MRI can be useful for evaluating multiple adjacent structures simultaneously. MRI can assess the lateral ankle ligaments, the ATFL and CFL, as well as the syndesmosis for disruption. The peroneal tendons can be evaluated for tears, degeneration, or dislocation. Looking deeper, the tibiotalar joint may display osteochondral lesions of the talus and tibia, or synovitis with an associated ankle joint effusion. The adjacent hindfoot joints can also be assessed for chondral injury and potential coalitions. Similarly, medial sided pain can be assessed simultaneously for pathology of the deltoid ligament, posterior tibial tendon, tarsal tunnel, osteochondral lesions, medial malleolar stress fractures, among other possibilities. Thus, MRI can provide critical information to guide treatment.

In addition, MRI can aid in the diagnosis of an array of bony pathologies that may go unnoticed on plain radiographs. This includes bone marrow edema syndrome, stress fractures, as well as avascular necrosis (AVN) of the talus [33]. Furthermore, MRI, alongside radiographs and CT, is used to stage the progression of AVN, which can help guide future treatment [34].

Of particular interest, when considering MRI of the ankle, is the imaging of osteochondral lesions of the talus (OLT). Most OLTs occur in the talar dome, specifically in the posteromedial and centromedial aspect [35, 36]. Due its radiographic properties, MRI can reveal elements of bone edema, cyst formation, subchondral bone compression, cartilage delamination, and unstable osteochrondral fragments. Knowledge of the lesion's exact location, size, and depth, among other characteristics, is critical for determining operative positioning, approach, and treatment (Fig. 10) [37].

In addition, tendons are well visualized on MRI. Following lacerations or ruptures, the degree of tendon disruption and potential level of retraction can be determined. Evaluation for chronic pain can demonstrate various degrees of tendinopathy, in the form of peritendinous fluid, tendon thickening, split tears, and rupture. Although Achilles ruptures may be diagnosed by

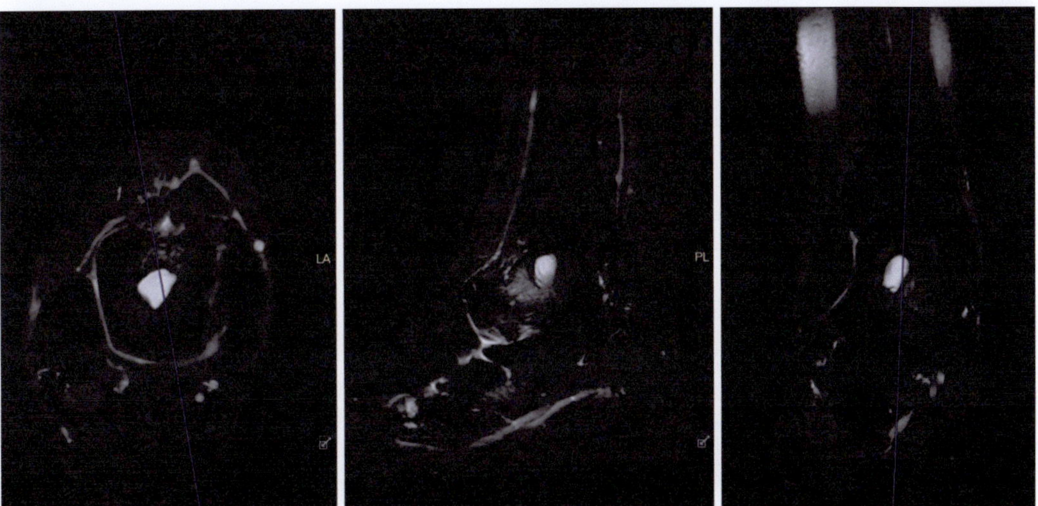

Fig. 10 MRI demonstrates a large talar subchondral cyst. Defining the location and size of the cyst is important for surgical planning

examination alone, an MRI with the ankle in plantarflexion can reveal the exact location of the rupture as well as evidence of tendon gapping, which may be important information when deciding on operative versus nonoperative management (Fig. 11) [38].

MRI is also an effective diagnostic modality for evaluating infection, as well as working up soft tissue and osseous masses. Though physical exam is a critical component of diagnosis, MRI can help define the extent and location of an infectious process. It can differentiate simple cellulitis from an abscess, or complex phlegmon. More importantly, MRI can provide evidence for underlying osteomyelitis, particularly when early or indolent, helping to guide operative management and antibiotic duration. When assessing masses about the foot and ankle, an MRI can define the structure, extent, and likely composition of soft tissue masses, to determine if the lesion is benign or malignant, and the need for excision versus staged biopsy versus observation. It can also provide further details about osseous lesions and reveal associated soft tissue components. When combined with an intravenous contrast, it is ideal for comprehensive assessment of tumors as well as lesion surveillance [39].

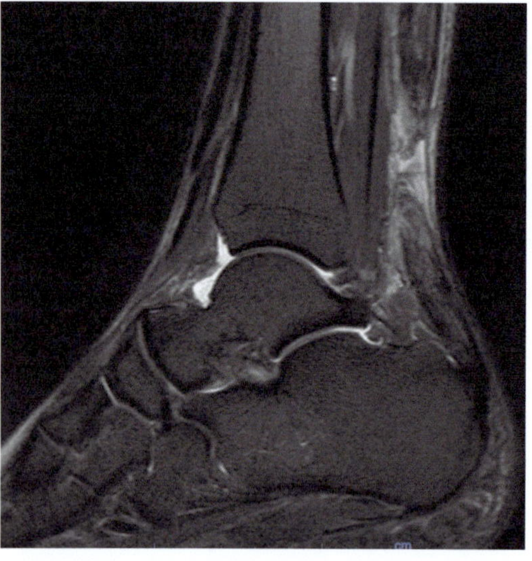

Fig. 11 MRI of the ankle demonstrates an acute Achilles rupture at its midsubstance. Gapping is noted between the tendon edges

3   Computed Tomography

Modern computed tomography (CT) allows for rapid acquisition of cross-sectional imaging. It can produce high resolution, thin-slice digital renderings of three-dimensional anatomic structures. At their core, CT scanners are composed of a gantry and a movable table [40]. The gantry is the frame that houses a rotating X-ray tube including collimators/filters, detectors, rotational components, angulation motors, and positioning laser lights. As the patient slides through the gantry aperture on the moving table, the rotating X-ray tube and detectors acquire image slices of the targeted anatomy. Modern helical or spiral CT scanner designs have multiple detectors, allowing the machine to acquire multiple slices with every rotation, effectively speeding up the required imaging time [41]. This process is termed "data acquisition." Three-dimensional CT images are broken up into small units of volume, or voxels. The amount of radiation that is absorbed, or attenuated, by each voxel of tissue dictates how it is displayed in the ultimate image rendering [30, 41]. The attenuation is then given a number based on a comparison with a similar voxel of water. For example, a voxel of bone will have higher attenuation than a voxel of gas in soft tissue. Each voxel in a CT slice is represented visually by a pixel on the two-dimensional slice renderings. The voxels are assigned values, known as Hounsfield units, based on their degree of X-ray attenuation. Hounsfield unit values represent the voxel's relative position on a visual gray scale [30]. At the extremes of the relative scale, dense bone will typically be white, while air will be black [41]. Through this process, the CT scanner can produce images with high resolution between different types of tissue. Due to the three-dimensional nature of the data acquisition, two-dimensional images can be reconstructed in multiple planes. Conventionally this is in the coronal, sagittal, and axial planes; however, the CT technologist can reformat slices in nearly any anatomic plane desired. The thinner the slices obtained, the higher the resolution in the various planes. The addition of picture archiving communication systems (PACS) has allowed higher-resolution scans to be obtained and stored.

A common concern with CT imaging is the inherent radiation exposure. Traditionally, a CT of the ankle delivered nearly fourfold the radiation of a chest radiograph [30]. Improvement in CT image resolution requires an increase in the density of voxels and number of slices. This, in turn, requires increased radiation exposure [41]. Fortunately, progress is being made to reduce radiation risks. Recent studies regarding radiation reduction protocols for the purpose of extremity trauma imaging have demonstrated tenfold reductions in exposure, relative to conventional protocols, without a significant sacrifice in resolution [42]. One study showed that their ankle fracture CT protocol exposed the subjects to less radiation than multiple views with conventional radiograph [43].

CT scans, which provide fine bony detail in multiple planes, and have become the standard of care for assessing a wide breadth of ankle pathology, from traumatic injury to tumors. Unlike a plain radiograph, which requires a fair amount of interpretation given the inherent bony overlap in the image, a CT can give definitive information about the three-dimensional status of the anatomy.

3.1 Fracture Management

CT imaging has proven to be highly advantageous in the evaluation of fractures about the ankle [44]. Injury patterns that often benefit from CT scanning include pilon fractures, malleolar ankle fractures, pediatric triplane and tillaux fractures, and talus fractures (Fig. 12) [30]. Providers can evaluate the size, location, and orientation of fragments involved, as well as the status of the joint surface, intra-articular fragments, and presence of bone loss. Another advantage of CT is the visualization of occult fractures that are otherwise not visible or very difficult to visualize on plain radiographs. They can also reveal soft tissue injuries, such as peroneal dislocation or soft tissue entrapment, helping with preoperative planning and having an important impact on sur-

gical decision making. Studies have found that surgeons altered their surgical plans, including patient positioning and operative approach, in 23–44% of cases after obtaining CT imaging for rotational ankle fractures [45, 46]. The primary driving force for altering the surgical plan was the additional information obtained about the posterior malleolus fracture (Fig. 13). The additional use of three-dimensional reconstructions provides an intuitive rendering of the injury, akin to a physical model. Additionally, CTs can evaluate the quality of reduction either postoperatively or intraoperatively. One of the more common applications is to assess syndesmotic reduction in ankle fractures. Malreduction of the syndesmosis may be indicated for a revision of the previous fixation (Fig. 14) [47].

3.2 Supplementary Management

Osteochondral lesions of the talus (OLT) can be evaluated with CT as well as MRI. Although MRI is an important tool for detection of OLTs, it can often overestimate the size of the lesion, as bony edema is prominently displayed. CT is more precise in defining the bony involvement of the OLT, its size, cystic quality, and for guiding potential fixation in the acute setting [37]. CT arthrography is an alternative to MRI for evaluation of the chondral surface in the setting of patients with contraindications to MRI, such as an incompatible implanted cardiac device [30].

Evaluating bony union in the setting of fracture and fusion may be difficult due to obscuring hardware or overlapping bony projections, especially in cases like ankle fusions, subtalar fusions, or comminuted pilon fractures (Fig. 15). A CT can reveal all aspects of the joint, the fracture, or the fusion site, and can help visualize the degree of healing (with the exception of metal artifact).

Using intravenous (IV) contrast is an important adjunctive element of CT scans in select scenarios. In the acute setting, CT with contrast can confirm the level of a potential vascular disruption. It can also provide additional information about the blood flow to musculoskeletal tumors.

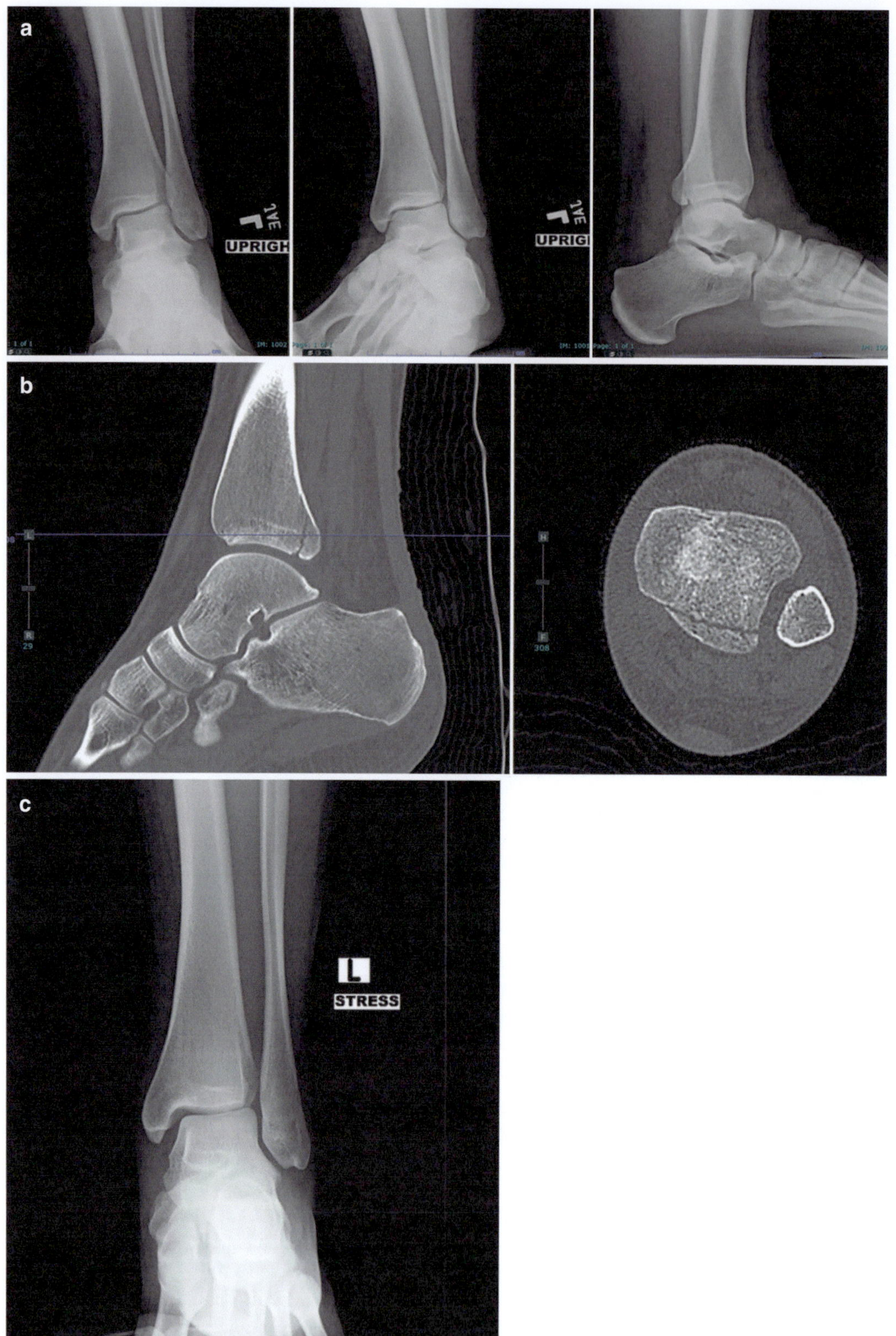

Fig. 12 CT scans are useful in assessing the size and morphology of malleolar fractures. (**a**) Radiographs demonstrate an isolated posterior malleolar fracture. (**b**) CT scan defines the size and orientation of the posterior malleolus fracture line. (**c**) Stress radiograph reveals medial clear space widening, suggestive of deltoid and syndesmotic instability

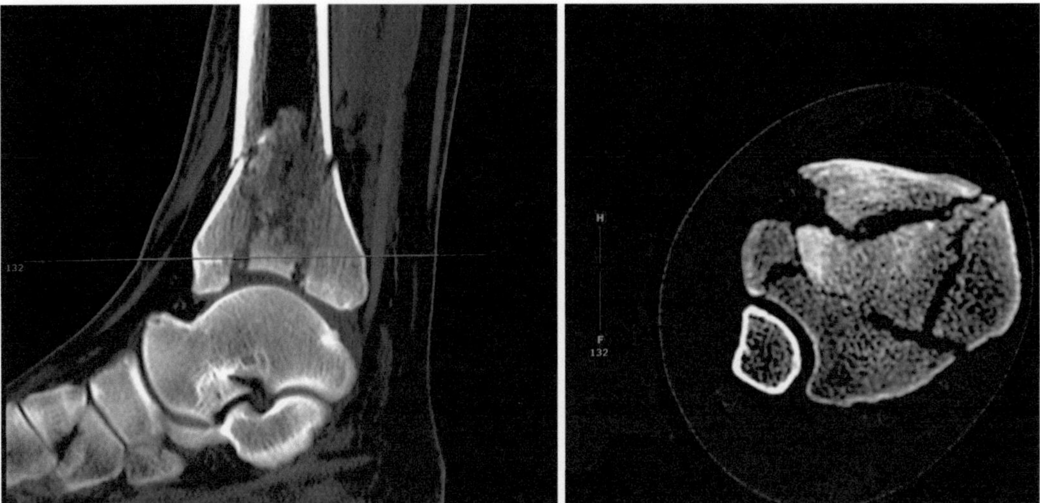

Fig. 13 CT of the ankle demonstrating a comminuted pilon fracture. Evaluation of the fracture in multiple planes is important for understanding the three-dimensional nature of the injury, particularly the location of fracture planes, independent fragments, and bone loss

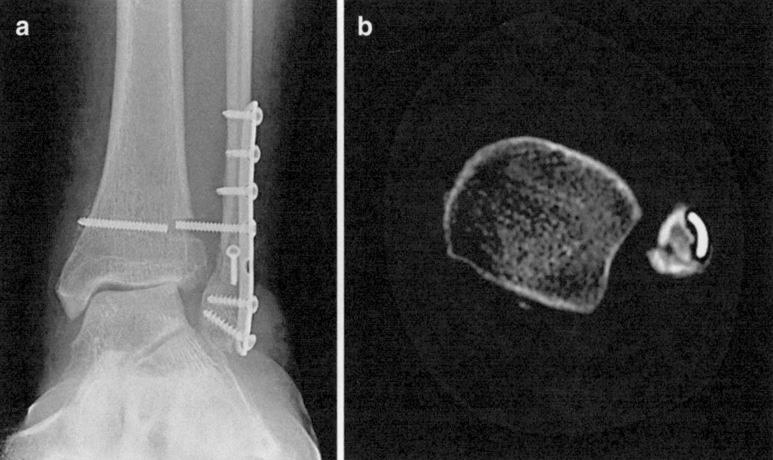

Fig. 14 CT imaging can demonstrate the presence of syndesmotic malreduction. (**a**) Mortise view radiograph suggesting syndesmotic disruption with failed hardware. (**b**) CT scan axial view demonstrates anterior translation of the fibula, with a malreduced syndesmosis

CT is an important adjunct in the diagnosis of ankle and hindfoot arthritis. It can reveal the extent of bone loss and the presence of bony cysts, which can affect surgical decision making, particularly when considering the use of a total ankle arthroplasty (TAA) [48]. Identifying significant bone loss in the talus, or the existence of large osteophytes can be used preoperatively as part of the surgical plan, while postoperatively it may detect peri-implant cysts (Fig. 16), compo-nent subsidence, loosening, a polyethylene fracture, or a malleolar fracture [49].

The advent of *weight bearing CT* (WBCT) technology has produced a paradigm shift in the evaluation of foot and ankle deformity. It effectively merges the valuable three-dimensional data of CT with the practical elements of a standing radiograph. One can view the bony anatomy, while also assessing the structural alignment of the foot and ankle under physiologic loading

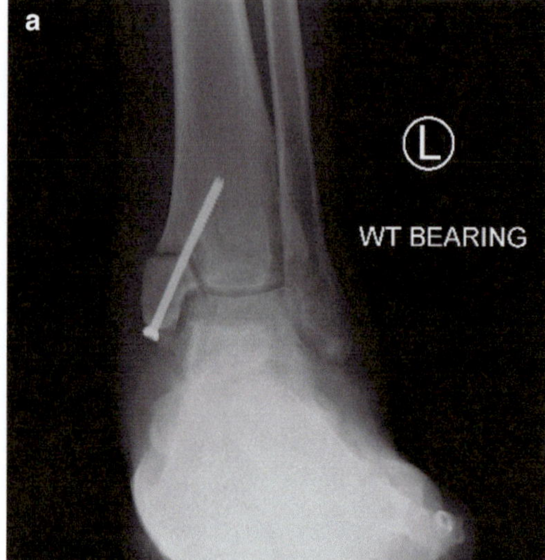
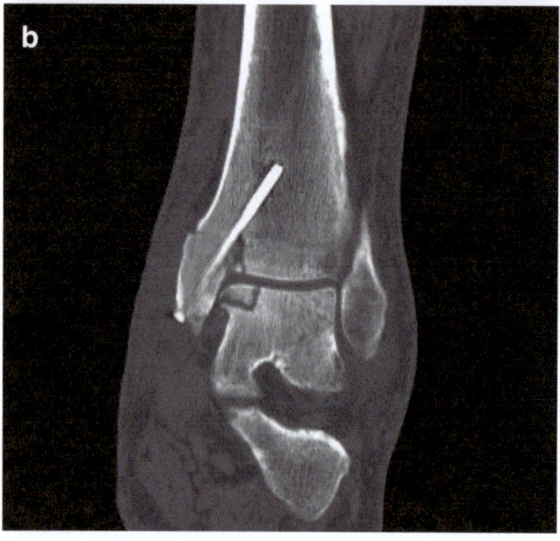

Fig. 15 Radiographs (**a**) demonstrate a nonunion of a prior medial malleolar osteotomy. A lucency is visible at the site of the medial talar osteochondral allograft, but it is unclear if it has united. (**b**) CT scan confirms nonunion of both the medial malleolus and the talar allograft

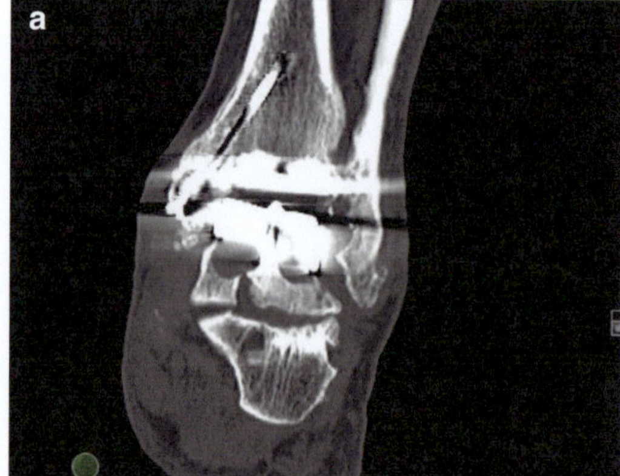
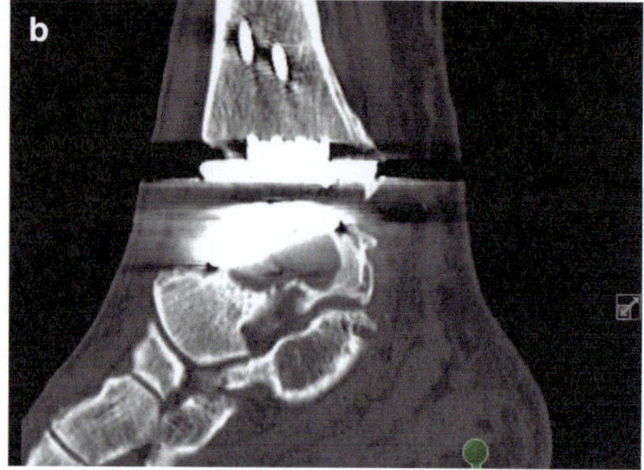

Fig. 16 CT demonstrating large talar cysts adjacent to the talar component of a total ankle replacement. (**a**) Coronal view. (**b**) Sagittal view

(Fig. 17). This has been particularly beneficial in evaluating the subtalar joint and subfibular impingement. This improves the physician's understanding of the relative position of the bones and joints in their weight-bearing state when patients experience pain or dysfunction. It is valuable for evaluating post-traumatic malunion, ankle and hindfoot arthritis with associated malalignment, as well as complex and potentially dynamic deformities such as progressive collapsing foot deformity, and conditions like Charcot Marie Tooth disease [50, 51]. This effectively raises the bar with regards to clinical diagnosis and preoperative planning and provides insights that would not be available using non-weight-bearing CT scans.

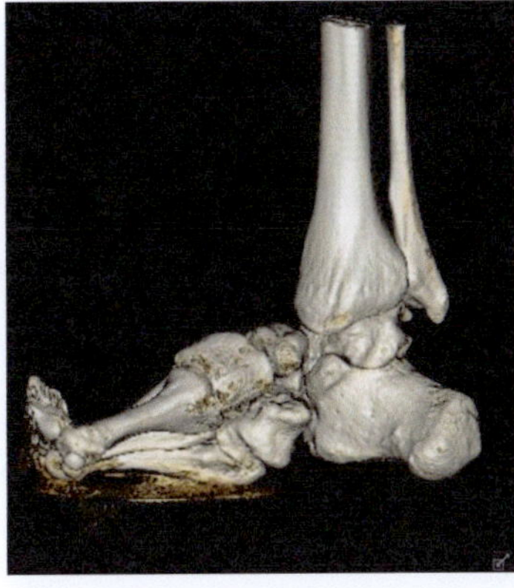 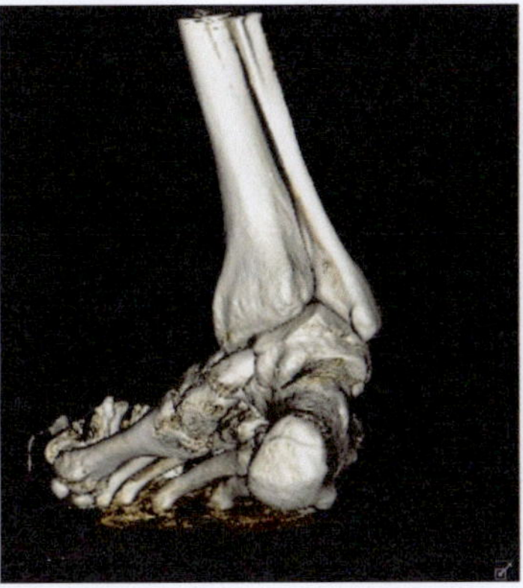 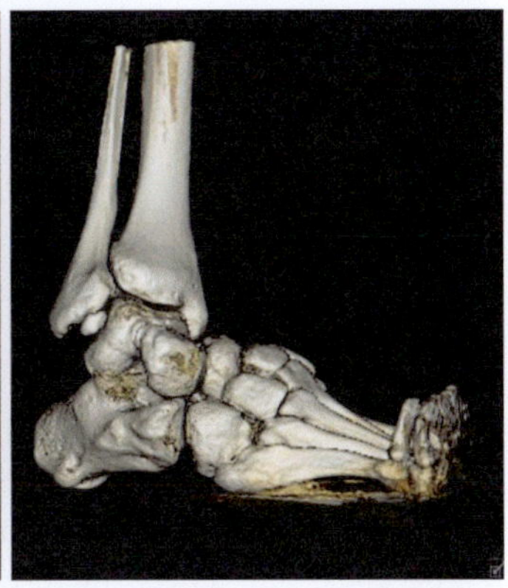

Fig. 17 Weight-bearing CT imaging allows for visualization of foot and ankle alignment under physiologic loading. This is valuable for understanding deformity and planning surgical correction. Furthermore, 3-dimensional reconstruction views give the provider a practical rendering of the patient's anatomy

4 Ultrasound

Ultrasound allows for real-time, dynamic imaging of the foot and ankle. It works in a manner similar to naval SONAR (sound navigation and ranging) systems, in which sound waves are emitted, reflected, and subsequently detected, providing information about the structures they encounter [30]. Ultrasound transducers produces high-frequency sound waves in the range of 5–18 MHz. As air can cause disturbances in image acquisition, ultrasound gel is placed between the probe and the patient's skin. Alternatively, the anatomy of interest can be submersed in liquid. Ultrasonic waves are passed from the probe into the tissue, reflecting at different acoustic interfaces. With these reflected echoes, the ultrasound system can produce a diagnostic image in real-time. In general, higher frequency probes produce high detail, but limited depth of imaging. Low frequency probes produce lower resolution but can detect structures at greater depths.

Ultrasound use has good musculoskeletal applications including the evaluations of tendons, nerves, and allowing guidance to ensure accurate targeted injections. When used for the evaluation of tendons, it can diagnose, in real-time, the pathology of the tendons. The peroneal tendons can be evaluated for split tears and tenosynovitis, with the patient actively moving, along with sub-luxation and dislocation. The Achilles tendon can also be reliably imaged, with some studies showing 96% accuracy for diagnosing a full rupture [38, 52]. Combining physical examination with real-time ultrasound improves diagnostic accuracy [53].

It can also evaluate a variety of nerve pathologies about the ankle and hindfoot by allowing direct visualization of the course of the nerve. Often, if there is a nerve entrapment, structural changes can be seen at typical compression sites, such as passing through fascial planes. Entrapment will create a typical appearance of swelling proximal to the compression site, with return of normal caliber distal to the site [52]. This is specifically helpful for the evaluation of tarsal tunnel syndrome. Not only can direct nerve changes be detected, but ultrasound can also show compressive lesions, like ganglions or enlarged vessels, as well as scar tissue formation.

In addition to identifying the musculoskeletal pathologies, many providers utilize ultrasound guidance when performing targeted injections to ensure accuracy, whether into the tibiotalar joint or around tendons. Similarly, cystic masses, like ganglions, can be visualized so that an accurate aspiration is performed [52]. Another use for ultrasound is assessing for and localizing the presence of a foreign body, especially those that are radiolucent, such as a splinter.

Lastly, although not an ankle injury, ultrasound is the most common modality used to confirm a deep venous thrombosis (DVT) of the leg [54].

5 Nuclear Medicine

Nuclear Medicine is a unique imaging modality that is utilized to diagnose pathology that would be otherwise undetectable on conventional radiographs, like stress fractures and osteomyelitis [30]. It has also gained value in the workup of painful total ankle replacements, to help localize the offending source of pain. Nuclear scans require the injection of radioactive agents into the patient prior to imaging. There are various radiopharmaceutical agents available for an array of diagnostic purposes. They are labeled with ligands, which are ions, molecules, or functional groups that bind to another chemical entity to form a larger complex, during specific physiologic processes. Once injected, the nuclear agents generally have preferential uptake in sites of elevated metabolic activity, leading to a localized concentration [55]. By their nature, the agents emit radioactive energy. A gamma camera detects the emission, and after converting the radioactive energy to photos, ultimately produces a visual representation of the localized radiopharmaceutical uptake in the body. Although relatively crude in appearance, these images are unique in their ability to represent a physiologic process.

Technetium-99m-methylene diphosphate *bone scans* are useful for detecting sites of increased osteoblastic activity, such as fractures, tumors, and growth plates. As such it can be utilized to detect stress fractures, bony tumors, and osteochondral injuries [30, 56]. Indium-111, as well as technetium-99m, can be utilized for white blood cell-tagged studies for evaluation of osteomyelitis (Fig. 18) [30]. When investigating for an infection, the radiopharmaceutical agent is incubated

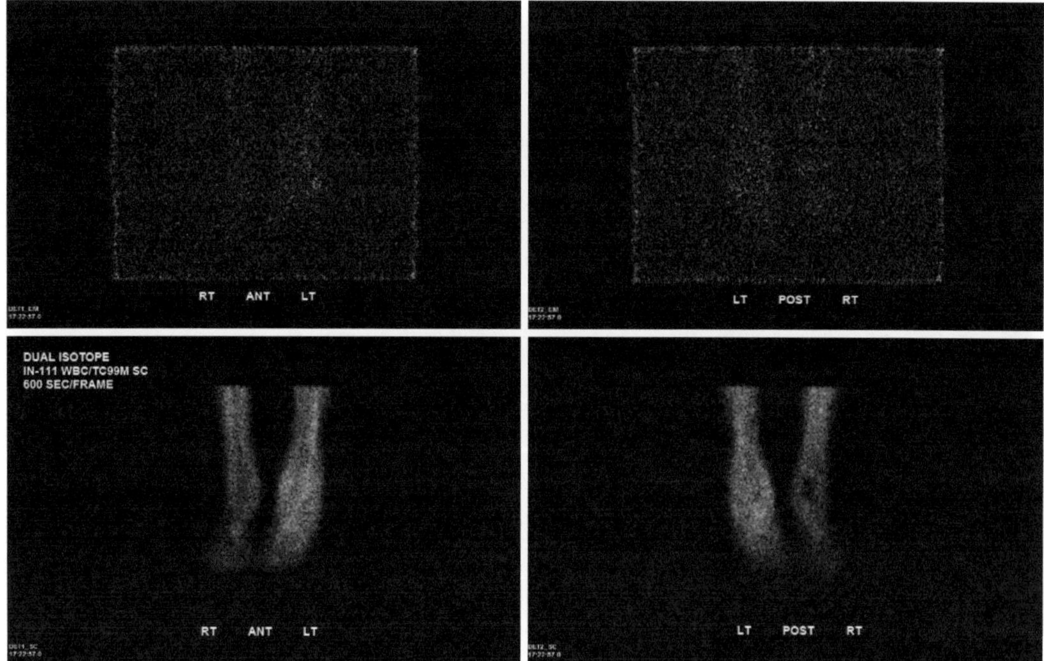

Fig. 18 Indium-111 white blood cell-tagged study performed to rule out osteomyelitis of the distal tibia. In this case, the lack of signal suggests no active infection

with isolated leukocytes with isolated leukocytes from the patient's blood draw. They are then reinjected, and the leukocytes will tend to concentrate in areas of active infection, such as an area of suspected osteomyelitis. The patient will undergo scanning at 4 and 24 h following the injection. The resultant images will demonstrate focal uptake in the event of infection. Charcot arthropathy can often be particularly difficult to differentiate from osteomyelitis with a high false positive rate with both MRI and routine bone scan. The advent of dual bone scans, utilizing Indium-111 labeled white blood cells alongside technetium-99 sulfur colloid has improved the specificity of nuclear scans for diagnosing osteomyelitis to differentiate from an acute Charcot arthropathy [57].

An increasingly valuable imaging modality is single photon emission computed tomography (SPECT). Unlike the crude images rendered in traditional bone scans, SPECT can blend the clarity of modern CT imaging with the functional data obtained from nuclear medicine. Its primary advantage is being able to pinpoint sites of increased metabolic activity. This is particularly helpful after patients have undergone complex surgery, where pain is diffuse, and there are many potential sources of pain. An important application is in the work up of painful total ankle arthroplasty [58, 59]. In these patients, their postoperative pain could be secondary to component subsidence, loosening, cyst formation (at multiple sites), impingement, stress fracture, and infection, among others (Fig. 19). SPECT can help the physician localize the most likely origin of symptoms.

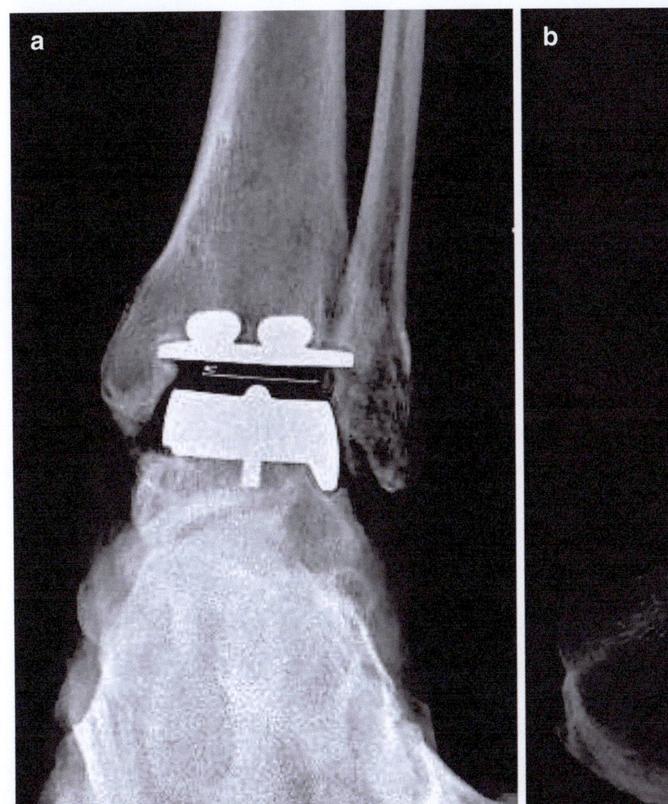
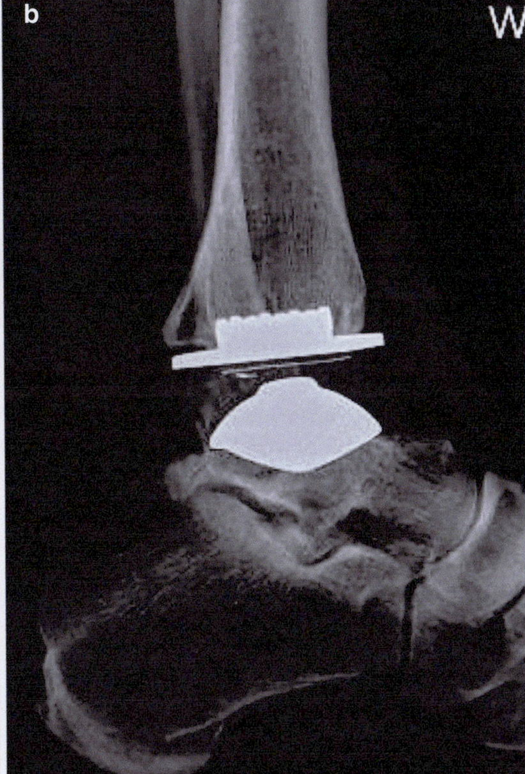
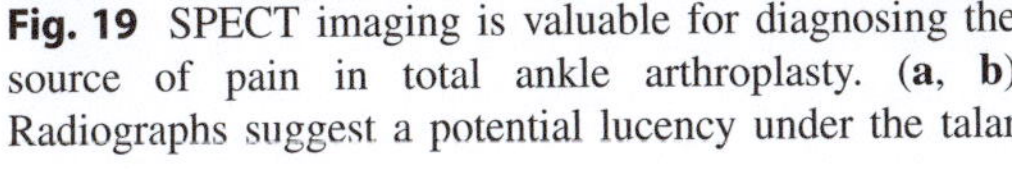

Fig. 19 SPECT imaging is valuable for diagnosing the source of pain in total ankle arthroplasty. (**a, b**) Radiographs suggest a potential lucency under the talar component but are inconclusive. (**c, d**) SPECT scan demonstrates increased signal under the talar component. The CT confirmed a large cyst

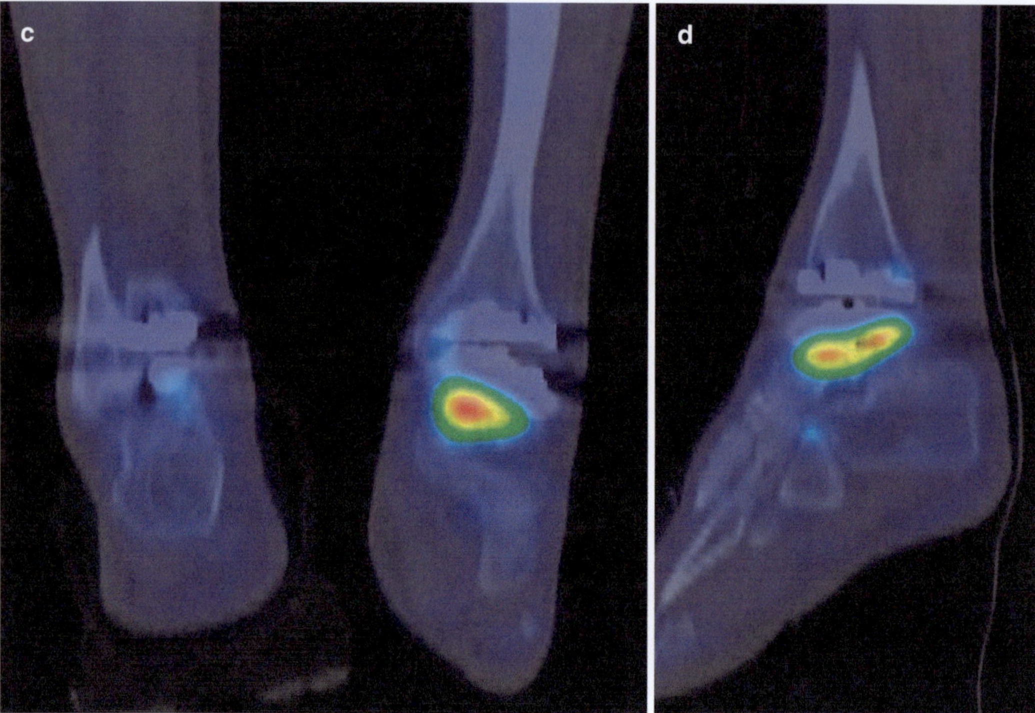

Fig. 19 (continued)

6 Conclusion

There are many options when it comes to imaging of the ankle. As such, the provider must be prudent with their diagnostic workups. Factors such as radiation exposure, patient burden, and cost should not be overlooked. As such, it is important to have clear indications for the various imaging modalities. When doing an initial evaluation of ankle pain or instability, it is the author's opinion that a routine weight-bearing ankle series is nearly always appropriate and can provide significant information about osseous injury and quality, joint degeneration, ligamentous stability, and overall alignment of the ankle and hindfoot. Synthesizing information from the patient's history, examination, and radiographs, the provider can then determine the need for further imaging. The judicious use of CT, MRI, nuclear scans, and ultrasound can provide unique data that can assist with diagnosis, treatment choice, and nuances of surgical planning.

References

1. Chotas HG, Dobbins JT III, Ravin CE. Principles of digital radiography with large-area, electronically readable detectors: a review of the basics. Radiology. 1999;210(3):595–9.
2. Bushberg JT. The essential physics of medical imaging. 3rd ed. Philadelphia, PA: Wolters Kluwer Health/Lippincott Williams & Wilkins; 2012.
3. Stiell IG, Greenberg GH, McKnight RD, Nair RC, McDowell I, Reardon M, et al. Decision rules for the use of radiography in acute ankle injuries. Refinement and prospective validation. JAMA. 1993;269(9):1127–32.
4. Bachmann LM, Kolb E, Koller MT, Steurer J, ter Riet G. Accuracy of Ottawa ankle rules to exclude fractures of the ankle and mid-foot: systematic review. BMJ. 2003;326(7386):417.
5. Morais B, Branquinho A, Barreira M, Correia J, Machado M, Marques N, et al. Validation of the Ottawa ankle rules: strategies for increasing specificity. Injury. 2021;52(4):1017–22.
6. Stiell IG, McKnight RD, Greenberg GH, McDowell I, Nair RC, Wells GA, et al. Implementation of the Ottawa ankle rules. JAMA. 1994;271(11):827–32.
7. Berquist TH. Imaging of the foot and ankle. 3rd ed. Philadelphia, PA: Wolters Kluwer/Lippincott Williams & Wilkins Health; 2011.

8. Degwert R, Gaulrapp H, Kessler S, Roeser A, Staebler A, Szeimies U, et al. Diagnostic imaging of the foot and ankle. Stuttgart: Thieme; 2015.

9. Lau BC, Allahabadi S, Palanca A, Oji DE. Understanding radiographic measurements used in foot and ankle surgery. J Am Acad Orthop Surg. 2022;30(2):e139–e54.

10. Ebraheim NA, Wong FY. External rotation views in the diagnosis of posterior colliculus fracture of the medial malleolus. Am J Orthop. 1996;25(5):380–2.

11. Gregersen MG, Molund M. Weightbearing radiographs reliably predict normal ankle congruence in weber B/SER2 and 4a fractures: a prospective case-control study. Foot Ankle Int. 2021;42(9):1097–105.

12. Murphy JM, Kadakia AR, Irwin TA. Variability in radiographic medial clear space measurement of the normal weight-bearing ankle. Foot Ankle Int. 2012;33(11):956–63.

13. Arthur D, Pyle C, Shymon SJ, Lee D, Harris T. Correlating arthroscopic and radiographic findings of deep deltoid ligament injuries in rotational ankle fractures. Foot Ankle Int. 2021;42(3):251–6.

14. Cavanaugh ZS, Gupta S, Sathe VM, Geaney LE. Initial fibular displacement as a predictor of medial clear space widening in weber B ankle fractures. Foot Ankle Int. 2018;39(2):166–71.

15. Shah AS, Kadakia AR, Tan GJ, Karadsheh MS, Wolter TD, Sabb B. Radiographic evaluation of the normal distal tibiofibular syndesmosis. Foot Ankle Int. 2012;33(10):870–6.

16. Harper MC, Keller TS. A radiographic evaluation of the tibiofibular syndesmosis. Foot Ankle. 1989;10(3):156–60.

17. Seidel A, Krause F, Weber M. Weightbearing vs gravity stress radiographs for stability evaluation of supination-external rotation fractures of the ankle. Foot Ankle Int. 2017;38(7):736–44.

18. McConnell T, Creevy W, Tornetta P. Stress examination of supination external rotation-type fibular fractures. J Bone Joint Surg Am. 2004;86(10):2171–8.

19. Park SS, Kubiak EN, Egol KA, Kummer F, Koval KJ. Stress radiographs after ankle fracture: the effect of ankle position and deltoid ligament status on medial clear space measurements. J Orthop Trauma. 2006;20(1):11–8.

20. Hoffman E, Paller D, Koruprolu S, Drakos M, Behrens SB, Crisco JJ, et al. Accuracy of plain radiographs versus 3D analysis of ankle stress test. Foot Ankle Int. 2011;32(10):994–9.

21. Jolman S, Robbins J, Lewis L, Wilkes M, Ryan P. Comparison of magnetic resonance imaging and stress radiographs in the evaluation of chronic lateral ankle instability. Foot Ankle Int. 2017;38(4):397–404.

22. Francisco R, Chiodo CP, Wilson MG. Management of the rigid adult acquired flatfoot deformity. Foot Ankle Clin. 2007;12(2):317–27, vii.

23. Thomas JL, Boyce BM. Radiographic analysis of the Canale view for displaced talar neck fractures. J Foot Ankle Surg. 2012;51(2):187–90.

24. Canale ST, Kelly FB. Fractures of the neck of the talus. Long-term evaluation of seventy-one cases. J Bone Joint Surg Am. 1978;60(2):143–56.

25. Saltzman CL, El-Khoury GY. The hindfoot alignment view. Foot Ankle Int. 1995;16(9):572–6.

26. Cobey J. Posterior roentgenogram of the foot. Clin Orthop Relat Res. 1976;118:202–7.

27. Haraguchi N. Analysis of whole limb alignment in ankle arthritis. Foot Ankle Clin. 2022;27(1):1–12.

28. Kim J, Rajan L, Kumar P, Kim JB, Lee WC. Lower limb alignment in patients with primary valgus ankle arthritis: a comparative analysis with patients with varus ankle arthritis and healthy controls. Foot Ankle Surg. 2022;29:72.

29. Mansur H, Rocha FA, Garcia PBL, de Alencar FHU, Guilme P, de Castro IM. Alteration of hindfoot axis after total knee arthroplasty. J Arthroplast. 2019;34(10):2376–82.

30. Coughlin M, Saltzman C, Anderson R. Mann's surgery of the foot and ankle, vol. 2. 9th ed. Amsterdam: Elsevier Health Sciences; 2014.

31. Anderson J, Read J. Atlas of imaging in sports medicine. Sydney, NSW: McGraw-Hill Education Australia; 2016.

32. Grover VP, Tognarelli JM, Crossey MM, Cox IJ, Taylor-Robinson SD, McPhail MJ. Magnetic resonance imaging: principles and techniques: lessons for clinicians. J Clin Exp Hepatol. 2015;5(3):246–55.

33. Orr JD, Sabesan V, Major N, Nunley J. Painful bone marrow edema syndrome of the foot and ankle. Foot Ankle Int. 2010;31(11):949–53.

34. Zhang H, Fletcher AN, Scott DJ, Nunley J. Avascular osteonecrosis of the talus: current treatment strategies. Foot Ankle Int. 2022;43(2):291–302.

35. Pedowitz R, Chung CB, Resnick D. Magnetic resonance imaging in orthopedic sports medicine. 1st ed. Berlin: Springer; 2008.

36. van Diepen PR, Dahmen J, Altink JN, Stufkens SAS, Kerkhoffs GMMJ. Location distribution of 2,087 osteochondral lesions of the talus. Cartilage. 2021;13(1 Suppl):1344S–53S.

37. Wodicka R, Ferkel E, Ferkel R. Osteochondral lesions of the ankle. Foot Ankle Int. 2016;37(9):1023–34.

38. Dams OC, Reininga IHF, Gielen JL, van den Akker-Scheek I, Zwerver J. Imaging modalities in the diagnosis and monitoring of Achilles tendon ruptures: a systematic review. Injury. 2017;48(11):2383–99.

39. Rammelt S, Fritzsche H, Hofbauer C, Schaser KD. Malignant tumours of the foot and ankle. Foot Ankle Surg. 2020;26(4):363–70.

40. Mazonakis M, Damilakis J. Computed tomography: what and how does it measure? Eur J Radiol. 2016;85(8):1499–504.

41. Seeram E. Computed tomography: a technical review. Radiol Technol. 2018;89(3):279CT–302CT.

42. Konda SR, Goch AM, Haglin J, Egol KA. Ultralow-dose CT (reduction protocol) for extremity fracture evaluation is as safe and effective as conventional CT: an evaluation of quality outcomes. J Orthop Trauma. 2018;32(5):216–22.

43. Tuncer K, Topal M, Tekin E, Sade R, Pirimoglu RB, Polat G. The new ultralow dose CT protocol for the diagnosis of fractures of the ankle: a prospective comparative study with conventional CT. J Orthop Surg. 2020;28(3):2309499020960238.

44. Rammelt S, Boszczyk A. Computed tomography in the diagnosis and treatment of ankle fractures: a critical analysis review. JBJS Rev. 2018;6(12):e7.

45. Donohoe S, Alluri RK, Hill JR, Fleming M, Tan E, Marecek G. Impact of computed tomography on operative planning for ankle fractures involving the posterior malleolus. Foot Ankle Int. 2017;38(12):1337–42.

46. Kumar A, Mishra P, Tandon A, Arora R, Chadha M. Effect of CT on management plan in malleolar ankle fractures. Foot Ankle Int. 2018;39(1):59–66.

47. Sagi HC, Shah AR, Sanders RW. The functional consequence of syndesmotic joint malreduction at a minimum 2-year follow-up. J Orthop Trauma. 2012;26(7):439–43.

48. Cody EA, Scott DJ, Easley ME. Total ankle arthroplasty: a critical analysis review. JBJS Rev. 2018;6(8):e8.

49. Lee GW, Lee KB. Periprosthetic osteolysis as a risk factor for revision after total ankle arthroplasty: a single-center experience of 250 consecutive cases. J Bone Joint Surg Am. 2022;104(15):1334–40.

50. Barg A, Bailey T, Richter M, de Cesar Netto C, Lintz F, Burssens A, et al. Weightbearing computed tomography of the foot and ankle: emerging technology topical review. Foot Ankle Int. 2018;39(3):376–86.

51. Michalski MP, An TW, Haupt ET, Yeshoua B, Salo J, Pfeffer G. Abnormal bone morphology in Charcot-Marie-tooth disease. Foot Ankle Int. 2022;43(4):576–81.

52. Beard NM, Gousse RP. Current ultrasound application in the foot and ankle. Orthop Clin North Am. 2018;49(1):109–21.

53. Griffin MJ, Olson K, Heckmann N, Charlton TP. Realtime Achilles ultrasound Thompson (RAUT) test for the evaluation and diagnosis of acute Achilles tendon ruptures. Foot Ankle Int. 2017;38(1):36–40.

54. Bright JM, Fields KB, Draper R. Ultrasound diagnosis of calf injuries. Sports Health. 2017;9(4):352–5.

55. Waller ML, Chowdhury FU. The basic science of nuclear medicine. Orthop Trauma. 2016;30(3):201–22.

56. Leumann A, Valderrabano V, Plaass C, Rasch H, Studler U, Hintermann B, et al. A novel imaging method for osteochondral lesions of the talus--comparison of SPECT-CT with MRI. Am J Sports Med. 2011;39(5):1095–101.

57. Womack J. Charcot arthropathy versus osteomyelitis: evaluation and management. Orthop Clin. 2017;48(2):241–7.

58. Mason LW, Wyatt J, Butcher C, Wieshmann H, Molloy AP. Single-photon-emission computed tomography in painful total ankle replacements. Foot Ankle Int. 2015;36(6):635–40.

59. Vulcano E, Myerson MS. The painful total ankle arthroplasty: a diagnostic and treatment algorithm. Bone Joint J. 2017;99B(1):5–11.

Evaluation of Ankle Pain

Joseph Jacobson, Rishin Kadakia,
and Jason Bariteau

1 Introduction

Injuries below the knee constitute a large volume of both primary care and specialty visits. The complexity of these injuries is complicated by the intricate anatomy between the 28 bones, 33 joints, and numerous tendons and ligaments—all of which bear upwards of 45 times the body weight based on the activity the patient is participating in. A thorough history and anatomic-focused physical examination can often help the practitioner concisely identify a specific diagnosis.

2 History of Present Illness

Examination of all patients with foot and ankle pathology should begin with a complete history. Special attention should be placed into obtaining pertinent past medical and surgical history, duration and quality of symptoms, attempted treatment modalities, and the length of treatment prior to current presentation.

2.1 Medical History

Evaluation of a patient's medical history should start with a detailed list of chronic medical problems and current medications. While this helps the practitioner understand the patient's overall health, it also assists in surgical planning by identifying what pre-operative clearance must be obtained and the setting in which a surgical patient can be cared for (i.e., ambulatory surgery center versus in-patient). Furthermore, certain medications must be modified or held prior to surgery, such as anticoagulation immunomodulatory (affecting the immune system) medications.

Special attention should be paid to those with diabetes mellitus and chronic kidney disease. Identifying patient with these co-morbidities is critical. Further, obtaining updated lab work, such as Hemoglobin A1C levels and creatinine is important for the co-medical management of these patients. For diabetic patients, it is important to understand what their day-to-day blood glucose levels are and if they are controlled or if there are wide fluctuations. For those on dialysis, it is important to determine when their dialysis schedule is and where their vascular access points are located. Multiple studies suggest an A1C level less than 8.0% prior to proceeding with elective procedures [1, 2]. As mentioned above, immune compromising conditions and current immune-modulating agents should be identified and coordination with the patient's rheumatologist surrounding discontinuation of disease

J. Jacobson · R. Kadakia · J. Bariteau (✉)
Department of Orthopedic Surgery – Foot & Ankle,
Emory University School of Medicine,
Atlanta, GA, USA
e-mail: joseph.jacobson@emory.edu;
rishin.j.kakadia@emory.edu

modifying agents surrounding surgical procedures should be done. Patients with diabetes, chronic kidney disease, and rheumatologic conditions are often high-risk surgical candidates. Therefore, it is important to identify these conditions when counseling patients about surgical risks.

Past surgical and/or trauma history is also important to obtain as this can often point to the etiology of a patient's pain. For example, a previous history of a calcaneus fracture, and the subsequent development of subtalar joint arthrosis, may provide information as to why the patient is complaining of hindfoot pain. If patients sustain complications after surgery, documenting these problems may also play a role when counseling patients about any potential surgeries. Additionally, social factors, such as the patient's smoking history and whom they live with at home, may indicate sources available for their post-operative care. The amount of social support and self-efficacy, as demonstrated by the LEAP study, directly predict outcomes and patient's abilities to maintain engaged with the recovery process [3]. Thus, social support following an injury or surgery is critical because some patients are required to be partial or non-weight bearing, with long periods of immobilization. This significantly limits their mobility and their independence, to such activities as driving, further stressing the patient's social support network. All these factors are crucial in the ultimate recovery of the patient.

2.2 Symptoms/Previous Treatments

Patients will often present with a chief complaint of pain, which may also be accompanied by swelling and a deformity. While diffuse swelling can be a sign of an underlying systemic problem, swelling confined to the foot and ankle often indicates where the problematic area is. Having the patient identify their exact source of pain, ideally with one finger, can help to focus the examination to a more anatomic region (e.g., anterolateral ankle, lateral border of the forefoot, etc.) Duration of symptoms and history of any inciting event can also give a clue to chronicity of the patient's complaint.

Additionally, details listing previous treatment modalities, including surgical and non-surgical treatments, should be noted. Many patients will have often undergone some attempted non-surgical care (e.g., physical therapy, orthotics, trial of anti-inflammatories), and it is important to document these specific interventions. For patients presenting for a second opinion, in the setting of previous surgical care, it is imperative that you obtain previous operative reports. Patients may not completely understand the surgeries that they have undergone. Having the operative report will allow you to review the procedure(s) previously performed, identify the type(s) of implant that was used, and identify the name of the company that provided the implants. This last information is important because if further surgery is necessary, having this knowledge preoperatively will allow the correct instrumentation to be available for removal of these implants.

Lastly, if patients present with or describe a deformity that has developed, it is important to know if the deformity is progressing or static. Other questions to ask about any deformity include, how or when it occurred? Whether it was the result of the initial trauma or injury? And, whether the deformity occurred because of any previous surgeries? This may also include any discussion about difficulty with shoe wear.

After a thorough history has been obtained, the physical examination is the next step in helping to obtain a diagnosis. This should be completed with the patient in appropriate clothing, ideally shorts, so that the entirety of the lower extremity can be visualized from the patella to the tips of the toes. The following section will detail the examination and specific tests of the foot and ankle that the authors recommend for all new patients presenting with complaints of ankle pain.

3 Physical Examination

3.1 Inspection

The first step in the examination of a patient is to place them comfortably into gowns or paper shorts that will allow the examiner to evaluate the patient from the patella to the tips of their toes. A thorough inspection should also include an examination of the contralateral, non-affected limb.

The skin should be assessed first. Any skin changes, including ulcerations, should be noted as these may warrant a work-up for infectious diseases. Special attention should also be paid to any redness to the skin, commonly referred to as erythema or rubor. Dependent rubor, a common sequela of peripheral vascular disease, can be distinguished from erythema secondary to cellulitis by elevating the affected extremity. Erythema that remains, despite elevation of the leg above the level of the heart, may be indicative of cellulitis, and may also warrant a further work-up for infection. Ecchymosis and swelling often follow specific anatomic patterns and these may help provide a differential diagnosis for the examiner. Special notation should also be made of any previous surgical scars, their proximity to one another, and the quality of the surrounding tissue. This is crucial for preoperative planning as it allows surgeons a chance to evaluate the soft tissue envelope and best decide where future incisions can safely be placed to avoid skin breakdowns, wound complications, and surgical site infections. Lastly, especially in the setting of trauma, inspection of the skin is important to determine when further surgery can safely be performed. When a patient has a splint that cannot be removed, due to instability, we recommend removing the anterior half of the splint to allow for inspection of the skin and to evaluate the extent of swelling. The ability of the examiner to wrinkle the skin indicates that the edema of the extremity has decreased enough to safely proceed with any further surgical intervention the patient may require, while decreasing the risk of wound healing issues post-operatively [4].

Next, the anatomic axis of both extremities should be evaluated, anteriorly and posteriorly, with special attention paid to the patient's hindfoot alignment. If possible, this should be done with the patient standing and bearing full weight in an unassisted manner. One should also inspect and palpate all the bones and joints of the lower extremity as a potential cause of pain. Lastly, the greater and lesser toes should be inspected, and

any abnormalities should be evaluated to determine if they are fixed or flexible deformities.

3.2 Palpation

Palpation for areas of tenderness should follow a methodical, anatomic-based approach. We recommend starting lateral and proximal and working distal and medial. Following a strict approach for each patient visit will ensure that no areas are missed on routine examinations. If the patient has sustained a recent trauma, working furthest away from injured area and finishing with injured area is also an option.

3.3 Evaluation of Motion

Evaluating a patient's preoperative motion is important prior to initiating any treatment. The Silverskiöld test is a specific test to evaluate shortening or contractures of the Achilles tendon, as it affects ankle joint motion. It is performed in two different ways, first with the knee in full extension and then flexed to 90°. With the patient in a sitting position, and the hindfoot held in the neutral (0° of inversion and eversion) position, dorsiflexion of the ankle is assessed with the knee in full extension. The knee is then flexed to 90°, which takes tension off the gastrocnemius muscle, and passive dorsiflexion of the ankle is reassessed. If the patient demonstrates an increase in passive dorsiflexion with the knee flexed, this indicates that the patient has an isolated gastrocnemius contracture. If there appears to be no difference with either extension or flexion of the knee, this will indicate a combined gastroc-soleus contracture. Differentiation of the location of the contracture (e.g., an equinus position) is important if one anticipates that the patient will need any adjunctive soft tissue releases, to help realign the position of the ankle.

Subtalar joint motion should again be measured with the patient in sitting position. The ankle should be held into a neutral (0° dorsi- and plantarflexion) position to avoid any compensatory movement through the tibiotalar joint.

Subtalar motion, consisting of inversion and eversion, is then evaluated. Understanding how to place the foot and ankle into a neutral position, prior to testing the motion of the ankle or subtalar joints, is critical for patients with ankle pain as the foot can often influence the etiology and treatment of ankle pathology. As an example, patients with chronic ankle instability can present with a cavus (high-arched) foot deformity. As the arch increases in height, it causes the foot to supinate which places a greater strain on the lateral structures of the foot and ankle. This can lead to chronic lateral ligamentous instability and should be assessed prior to any surgical intervention.

Midfoot motion is assessed by stabilizing the hindfoot with one hand while the other moves the forefoot laterally for abduction and medially for adduction. Special attention should be placed on the first tarsometatarsal articulation for hypermobility, especially in the setting of flatfoot and hallux valgus. Limitations in movement of the toes can be secondary to degenerative changes, primarily in the hallux but may also be due to contractures of the tendons. Both hallux metatarsophalangeal joint dorsiflexion and plantarflexion should be assessed, with special attention paid to pain elicited throughout the arc of motion and at which points that pain is present. It is also important to examine the motion on the contralateral extremity, which can help to set baseline motions for the patient.

3.4 Neurologic

Muscle strength should be evaluated for all major muscle groups consisting of posterior tibial, peroneals, gastrocnemius-soleus complex, flexor hallucis longus, flexors to the lesser toes, and extensor hallucis longus and extensors to the lesser toes. Sensation should also be assessed in the following distributions: superficial peroneal, deep peroneal, sural, saphenous, and tibial nerves. Again, examining the contralateral extremity is important to set the baseline for the patient. In the setting of peripheral neuropathy, Semmes-Weinstein monofilament testing should be completed. This simple exam is performed with the patient's eyes closed and has a sensitivity and specificity of 91% and 86%, respectively, which increases with a minimum testing of four plantar sites (great toe, first, third, and fifth metatarsal heads) [5]. An inability to detect a 5.07 filament (10-g) Semmes-Weinstein monofilament indicates the loss of protective sensation [6].

3.5 Vascular

Vascular evaluation of both the dorsalis pedis and posterior tibial pulses should be documented. There is a relatively low percentage of congenitally absent posterior tibial (0.18%) and dorsalis pedis (2.7%) pulses [7]. If neither pulse cannot be palpated, we recommend the use of doppler ultrasound and specific notation of anatomic location pulses are found for future reference. Any concern for peripheral vascular disease warrants evaluation with ankle/toe brachial index or toe pressures and referral to vascular surgery if necessary.

4 Special Tests

In patients presenting with a suspected Achilles rupture, it is important to first discern whether the patient had any pre-existing pain, since this may be indicative of an acute rupture in a patient with chronic tendinosis. To adequately assess for a ruptured tendon, the patient is placed into a prone position. Integrity of the Achilles tendon is performed using three different tests. The first is to palpate the entire tendon for any defects. The second, known as the Thompson test, is performed by squeezing the gastrocnemius-soleus complex. If no plantarflexion of the ankle is felt or observed, then an Achilles tendon rupture is presumed. Lastly, the patient flexes their knee to 90° and comparing the resting tension and plantar flexion against resistance is performed. Again, comparison of the contralateral extremity is recommended. Current AAOS clinical guidelines recommend at least two clinical exam findings to establish the diagnosis, with the Thompson test having the highest sensitivity (0.96) and specificity (0.93) [8].

4.1 Differential Diagnoses of Pain

Once the history and physical examinations are performed, the examiner should consider the cause of the pain, based on their anatomic location.

4.1.1 Lateral Ankle Pain

In patients who provide a history of an inversion injury or feelings of instability, the authors recommend documenting the cumulative lifetime injury occurrences. This is followed by formal testing of the lateral ankle and syndesmotic ligaments. While this is less useful, and often very painful in the acute setting, it can be especially helpful in patients with more chronic symptoms. Anterior drawer test of the ankle elicits pain in patients with an injury of the anterior talofibular ligament. It is performed with the patient sitting, knee bent with the leg hanging off the exam table. One hand stabilizes the midshaft of the tibia while the other cups the hindfoot and places an anteriorly directed force on the ankle. The presence of an anterior shift and an endpoint should be noted and compared to the contralateral ankle. An inversion stress of the calcaneus that produces pain may suggest a calcaneofibular injury.

Syndesmotic stability must also be assessed, especially when a high ankle sprain is suspected. Several tests have been described to evaluate for a syndesmotic sprain. The first is the *squeeze test and* is performed by squeezing the fibula and tibia together at the junction of the distal third of the tibia [9]. Pain is produced by tensioning the fibers at the distal tibiofibular complex. The second test is *the tibiofibular shuck or Cotton test* and is performed with the distal leg steadied with one hand while the opposite hand grasps the heel and moves it side to side. Excessive movement of the talus within the mortise, as compared to the contralateral ankle, suggests an unstable mortise [10]. The third test is the *abduction and external rotation test* [11]. This test is performed by stabilizing the leg, with the knee flexed to 90°, while the foot is abducted and externally rotated. Pain at the syndesmosis suggests a positive test. The last test is the *fibular translation test* [12]. This is performed with the patient sitting while an attempt is made to translate the fibula anteriorly and posteriorly. Any pain and excessive motion at the distal fibula, as compared to the contralateral side, may indicate a syndesmotic injury. While these tests can indeed elicit pain, the literature does not support any specific biomechanical test as being superior to the others, other than suggesting that there may be a syndesmotic injury [11, 13]. The authors support the use of radiographs and magnetic resonance imaging (MRI) studies and the anatomic location of pain around the syndesmosis as better indicators to identify a syndesmotic injury.

Lateral malleolar stress fractures, while rare, must be included in the differential diagnosis of lateral ankle pain. The patient will often complain of vague lateral ankle pain proximal to the ankle joint and will be tender along the bone on examination. Unlike their counter parts on the medial side, these are considered low-risk stress injuries and often heal with nonoperative treatment [14]. Pain slightly distal to the tip of the fibula, versus on the actual bone as seen with stress fractures, can be secondary to peroneal tendon pathology, with or without an os fibularis. Peroneal pathology is a spectrum of disease, ranging from tendonitis to fulminant tears and can include both the longus and brevis tendon. This pain can extend proximal up the posterior aspect of the fibula as the tendons course through the retromalleolar groove. Exclusion of peroneal tendon dislocations, via attempted manual tendon dislocation from behind the fibula while the patient everts their hindfoot, is crucial in diagnosing this problem.

Anterolateral ankle pain can also be secondary to an accessory anterior inferior tibiofibular ligament, located just distal to the native AITFL, known as Bassett's ligament [15]. Recurrent trauma, leading to attenuation and fibrosis of this ligament, leads to anterolateral impingement and ultimately becomes a source of pain for the patient.

4.1.2 Posterior Ankle Pain

The differential diagnosis for posterior ankle pain includes insertional and non-insertional Achilles tendonitis, posterior ankle impingement, and flexor hallucis longus (FHL) tenosynovitis. Patients with insertional Achilles tendonitis often complain of pain most commonly at the insertion into the calcaneus. A large deformity near the insertion of the Achilles tendon may be present in the patients. Those with an inflamed retrocalcaneal bursa, may also have some tenderness with palpation, anterior to the distal aspect of the tendon. This contrasts with patients who have non-insertional Achilles tendinosis as the pain is often more diffuse and located more proximal, often times in the watershed region of the Achilles tendon but may extend up into the musculotendinous junction.

Another source of posterior ankle pain may be due to posterior impingement, often caused by patients with a symptomatic os trigonum. These patients will complain of pain with hyper-plantarflexion of the ankle, often seen in ballet dancers. This pain is reproducible on examination with hyper-dorsiflexion of the ankle. Given the proximity of the FHL to the os trigonum, these patients may also have a component of FHL tenosynovitis that can be exacerbated by dorsi- and plantarflexion of the great toe.

4.1.3 Anterior Ankle Pain

In patients who present with anterior ankle pain it is important to understand the position of the ankle that elicits the pain. Patients with anterior impingement, and a history of trauma, can develop anterior distal tibia osteophytes, which will produce pain and decreased motion with dorsiflexion of the ankle. These patients will be diffusely tender to palpation along the entire anterior joint line. This differs from patients who have pain secondary to the development of an osteochondral defect (OCD) in the talus. Patients with an OCD often have more point tender at the anteromedial region of the ankle, and less frequently at the anterolateral joint line.

Pathology of the tibialis anterior tendon is also a contributor to anterior ankle pain. Like any other tendon in the body, it is subject to inflammatory changes leading to tendonitis. Tendon rupture must also be on the practitioner's differential. These may or may not be preceded by an episode of trauma as they can be attritional in nature. If a palpable tendon defect is present

(e.g., a rupture) swelling may make this portion of the examination difficult to assess. Ankle dorsiflexion may still be present, even in complete rupture, due to the competence and recruitment of the toe extensors. A simple test to asses for a rupture is to have the patient attempt to walk on their heels, as this is nearly impossible to due in the absence of a tibialis anterior tendon.

4.1.4 Medial Ankle Pain

A patient's complaint of medial ankle pain may occur because of problems with the posterior tibial tendon, especially in the setting of pes planovalgus (flatfoot). These patients will describe pain proximal to the medial malleolus or point to the insertion of the posterior tibial tendon on the navicular tuberosity, as the location of their pain. To differentiate this foot problem from ankle pain, it is important to assess the mid- and hindfoot. This is performed with the patient standing on the affected limb. While balancing themselves, an attempt is made to perform a single leg heel rise (SLHR). In normal patients, the SLHR produces a reconstitution of the arch and a varus positioning of the hindfoot. Patients with tendinosis of the posterior tibial tendon may be unable or have some difficulty performing a SLHR.

Another potential cause of medial sided ankle pain are medial malleolar stress fractures. These commonly occur in active, high-demand patients. These patients present without a history of trauma and often describe a gradual onset of pain and swelling of the medial ankle that is alleviated with cessation of activity. They will often be point tender directly over the bone and plain radiographs or MRI studies will help to confirm the diagnosis.

5 Conclusions

Ankle pain can occur in multiple locations. A thorough and systematic approach to evaluating the patient's complaint will help to differentiate the potential causes of their pain. At the conclusion of the examination, and once a presumed diagnosis has been made, a better discussion between the examiner and the patient, regarding treatments and outcomes, can be undertaken.

References

1. Tarabichi M, et al. Determining the threshold for HbA1c as a predictor for adverse outcomes after total joint arthroplasty: a multicenter, retrospective study. J Arthroplast. 2017;32(9S):S263–7.
2. Cancienne J, Werner B, Browne J. Is there a threshold value of hemoglobin A1c that predicts risk of infection following primary total hip arthroplasty? J Arthroplast. 2017;32(9S):S235–40.
3. Mackenzie E, Bosse MJ. Factors influencing outcomes following limb-threatening lower limb trauma: lessons learned from the lower extremity assessment project (LEAP). JAAOS. 2006;14(10):205–10.
4. Tull F, Borrelli J. Soft-tissue injury associated with closed fractures: evaluation and management. JAAOS. 2003;11(6):431–8.
5. Herbst SA, Jones KB, Saltzman CL. Pattern of diabetic neuropathic arthropathy associated with peripheral bone mineral density. J Bone Joint Surg (Br). 2004;86:378–83.
6. Smieja M, Hunt DL, Edelman D, Etchells E, Cornuz J, Simel DL. Clinical examination for the detection of protective sensation in the feet of diabetic patients. International Cooperative Group for Clinical Examination Research. J Gen Intern Med. 1999;14:418–24.
7. Robertson GS, Ristic CD, Bullen BR. The incidence of congenitally absent foot pulses. Ann R Coll Surg Engl. 1990;72(2):99–100.
8. Chiodo CP, et al. American Academy of Orthopaedic Surgeons Clinical Practice Guidelines on Treatment of Achilles tendon rupture. JBJS Am. 2010;92(14):2466–8.
9. Teitz CC, Harrington RM. A biomechanical analysis of the squeeze test for sprains of the syndesmotic ligaments of the ankle. Foot Ankle Int. 1998;19:489–92.
10. Cotton FJ. Fractures and joint dislocations. Philadelphia, PA: WB Saunders; 1910.
11. Alonso A, Khoury L, Adams R. Clinical test for ankle syndesmosis injury: reliability and prediction of return to function. J Ortho Sports Phys Ther. 1998;27:276–84.
12. Ogilve-Harris DJ, Reed SC. Disruption of the ankle syndesmosis: diagnosis and treatment by arthroscopic surgery. Arthroscopy. 1994;10:561–8.
13. Beumer A, van Hemert WL, Swierstra BA, Jasper LE, Belkoff SM. A biomechanical evaluation of clinical stress tests for syndesmotic ankle instability. Foot Ankle Int. 2003;24:358–63.
14. Mayer SW, et al. Stress fractures of the foot and ankle in athletes. AJSM. 2014;6(6):481–91.
15. Bassett FH, Gates HS, Billys JB, Morris HB, Nikolaou PK. Talar impingement by the anteroinferior tibiofibular ligament. A cause of chronic pain in the ankle after inversion sprain. J Bone Joint Surg Am. 1990;72(1):55–9.

Part II

Soft Tissue Disorders

Managing Tendon Pathology of the Ankle

Kevin A. Schafer, Zijun Zhang, and Lew C. Schon

1 Tendon Anatomy, Pathologic Classifications, and Injury Risk Factors

1.1 Tendon Microstructure: Normal Anatomy and Changes in Diseased Tendons

Tendons are predominantly composed of water (nearly 55% by weight), with roughly 70% of their dry mass composed mainly of type I collagen (fibrous proteins) [1]. Type I collagen molecules are assembled into filamentous fibrils, which are arranged parallel to the long axis of the tendon in densely packed bundles to create a tissue with a high tensile strength [2]. While collagen is the primary molecule responsible for tendon strength, other non-collagenous components of the extracellular matrix play important roles. Proteoglycans help to resist compressive forces and help modulate collagen fibril formation [3]. Elastins (a protein forming the core of elastic fibers), oriented both longitudinally and transversely to collagen fibers, potentiate elastic deformation and enhance sliding between collagen bundles [4]. The production and degradation of these and other components of tendon extracellular matrix are the responsibility of tenocytes (tendon specific fibroblasts), which react to mechanical stimuli by remodeling the tendon and participating in the events of tendon repair [5]. The cellular processes contributing to tendon homeostasis are crucial to treating tendon pathology. While exercise can result in tendon adaptation, repetitive stimuli in chronic overuse settings may disrupt cellular homeostasis and ultimately lead to altered tissue composition and tissue breakdown [6]. When compared to healthy tendon, diseased tendons have an increased proteoglycan content, an increased ratio of type III to type I collagen, a decrease in total collagen content, molecular modifications to collagen molecules and their interconnections, and an increase in vascular and nerve ingrowth (Fig. 1) [2].

Alterations in tendon microstructure were thought to involve an inflammatory process, making treatment with steroid injections and oral anti-inflammatories seem logical. However, histologic studies have failed to identify a predominate inflammatory pathway in chronic overuse injuries, challenging these treatments [8]. More recent analyses however have described a complex relationship between inflammatory mediators and tendon degeneration [9]. While repetitive stresses can lead to disruption of tendon microfibers, it can also stimulate the release of inflammatory mediators that alter tendon repair pathways. These investigations suggest that ten-

K. A. Schafer (✉) · Z. Zhang · L. C. Schon
Institute for Foot and Ankle Reconstruction, Mercy Hospital, Baltimore, MD, USA
e-mail: kschafe2@mdmercy.com;
zzhang@mdmercy.com; lschon@mdmercy.com

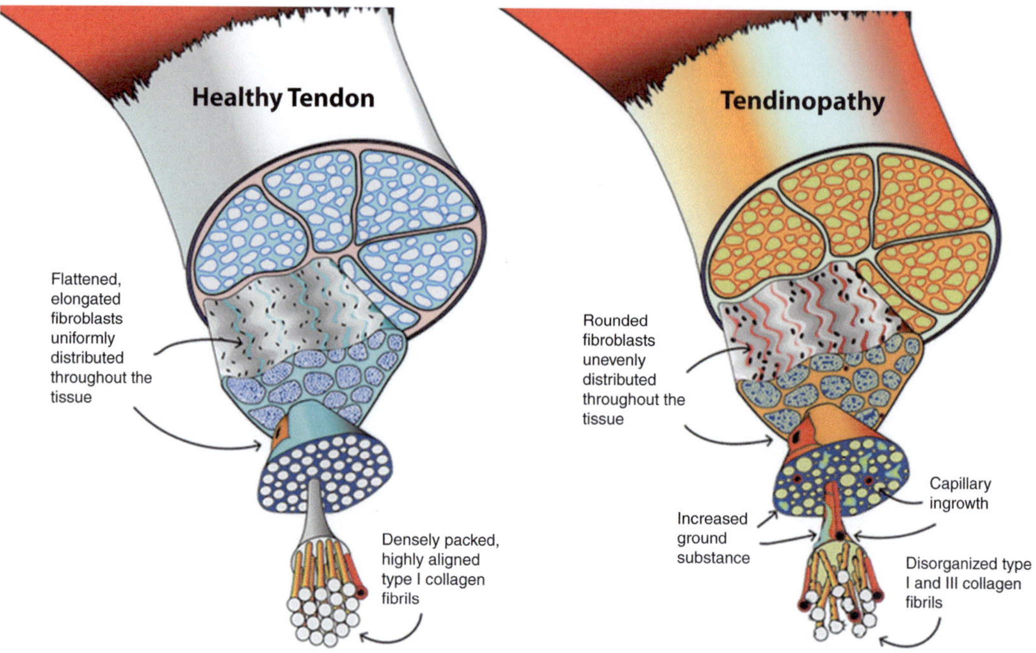

Fig. 1 Tendon microstructure in tendinopathy. Borrowed with permission from Mead et al. [7]

don degeneration and inflammation are intertwined processes at the cellular level and are not mutually exclusive.

1.2 Classifying Tendon Injury: Traumatic Injury, Tendinitis, and Tendinopathy

Tendon injuries occur frequently and can be classified into traumatic ruptures or injuries from mechanical overload. The term "tendinopathy" designates a pathologic tendon and overload injuries can be further described as a tendonitis, tendinosis, or tenosynovitis. Tendonitis indicates clinical and pathological inflammation of the tendon fibers, resulting in tendon microtears [10]. Tendinosis describes degeneration of the collagen bundle without clinical or cellular evidence of inflammation. Tenosynovitis indicates inflammation of the tendon fibers and its sheath and is only possible in tendons with a synovial sheath (peroneals, flexor hallucis longus) but not those with a paratenon (Achilles).

1.3 Extrinsic and Intrinsic Risk Factors for Injury

Contributing factors resulting in an injury can be classified into intrinsic variables that are inherent to the patient, and to extrinsic variables.

Intrinsic variables can be classified into local and systemic conditions and can make a patient more susceptible to developing tendinopathy (Fig. 2). Intrinsic conditions include anatomic, systemic, age related, and genetic conditions. Anatomic alignment and flexibility directly influence the loads experienced by tendons. For example, a cavovarus foot deformity (high arch and medially tilted hindfoot) increases stress on the peroneal tendons and lateral tissues, while a planovalgus foot (flattened arch and laterally tilted hindfoot) overloads the medial tissues and the posterior tibial tendon. Systemic conditions include diabetes, tobacco abuse, obesity, and rheumatologic disorders that result in impaired tendon microstructure and/or impaired tendon recovery after injury. Genetic conditions including Marfan syndrome and Ehlers-Danlos syndrome can result in pathologic laxity of soft tissues. Less joint

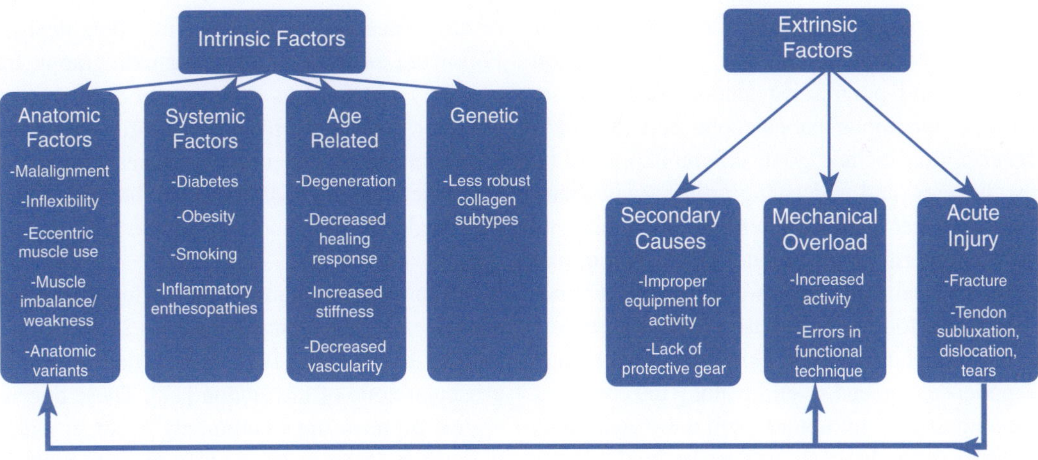

Fig. 2 Intrinsic and extrinsic factors in tendinopathy. Adapted from Federer et al. [11] and borrowed from Schafer et al. [91]. Overview of the various factors that can contribute to tendon injury. As the diagram depicts, acute injury can result in new intrinsic and extrinsic considerations

restraint from more elastic passive stabilizers can secondarily lead to tendon overload.

Extrinsic variables include acute injury, chronic mechanical overload, and environmental factors. An acute overload injury occurs with dynamic, high-impact activity where tendons experience higher loads in a shorter period of time, such as during running and jumping. Such an injury can sometimes permanently alter a patient's anatomy, secondarily resulting in change in a patient's intrinsic conditions (Fig. 2). For example, scar formation after a tendon tear can result in impaired tendon motion and decreased joint flexibility. A chronic mechanical overload condition can occur by increasing basic activities of daily living. The recurrent lower load cyclical stresses overwhelm the remodeling and repair capacity of the tendon. Lastly, environmental factors, including type of footwear, the training surface, and the type training activity, can all contribute to both mechanical overload and acute injury patterns [12, 13], and are important components of the patient history.

1.4 Biomechanics of Tendons

When discussing the different types of training activities, understanding the biomechanics of how tendons function is important as it may help explain how the injury occurred. The muscle-tendon unit is commonly injured during eccentric contraction. This is defined as contracting or tensioning the muscle while it is being lengthened. Concentric contraction indicates that the muscle is being shortened. The peak torque in the muscle-tendon unit is greater during eccentric contraction than during either isometric or concentric contractions where the muscle length stays a constant length or shortens, respectively [14].

After reviewing the general types of tendon injury and the mechanisms for tendon injury, we will now discuss commonly encountered tendon specific conditions. Each of the following sections will discuss the common presentations of each tendon condition and will review the key features of diagnosis and management.

2 Anterior Tibial Tendon

2.1 Pathology and Evaluation

The tibialis anterior tendon is the primary dorsiflexor of the ankle and plays a crucial role in controlling ankle plantarflexion during heel strike via eccentric contraction. These functions are crucial to normal gait and athletic activity.

As previously described, chronic tendinopathy or an acute rupture can occur. In chronic tendinopathy, prior to rupture, combinations of intrinsic and extrinsic factors result in tendon overload and progressive tendon degeneration. Intrinsic conditions that can contribute to tendon degeneration include gout, inflammatory arthritis, diabetes, and underlying arthritis with bony exostoses that abrade the tendon. Many patients develop anterior tibial tendinopathy with minimal or no noticeable symptoms. As a result, it is not uncommon for these patients to present after they have sustained a rupture. However, patients may experience pain and swelling along the course of the tendon prior to rupture, with these symptoms exacerbated by basic repetitive activity.

When examining a patient with chronic tendinopathy, the tendon may appear enlarged. The provider should assess for tenderness along the course of the tendon, pain during resisted dorsiflexion, and power during resisted dorsiflexion. Subtle weakness can be difficult to detect, and it is crucial to compare dorsiflexion strength to the unaffected extremity. It is also important to assess ankle flexibility via the Silfverskiöld test [15] as a tendoachilles or gastrocnemius contracture can create greater resistance to dorsiflexion. Following exam, weightbearing radiographs are routinely obtained to examine for contributing pathology such as midfoot arthritis and bony exostoses. If the diagnosis is unclear, magnetic resonance imaging (MRI) can be obtained to further evaluate the condition of the tendon and detect tenosynovitis.

If the tendon ruptures in the setting of chronic tendinopathy, the typical location is 2–3 cm proximal to its insertion [16], which is defined as the avascular zone of the tendon [17]. These degenerative ruptures most commonly occur in males older than 45 years of age [18], usually without injury or antecedent pain. There is often a delay to diagnosis with patients frequently presenting with a poorly described gait disturbance. Findings on examination include a painless palpable mass at the anterior ankle representing the proximal tendon stump [19], a loss of the normal visual and palpable contour of the tendon during resisted dorsiflexion (Fig. 3), and a foot drop noticeable during gait (steppage gait). Comparing both extremities often demonstrate less supination and

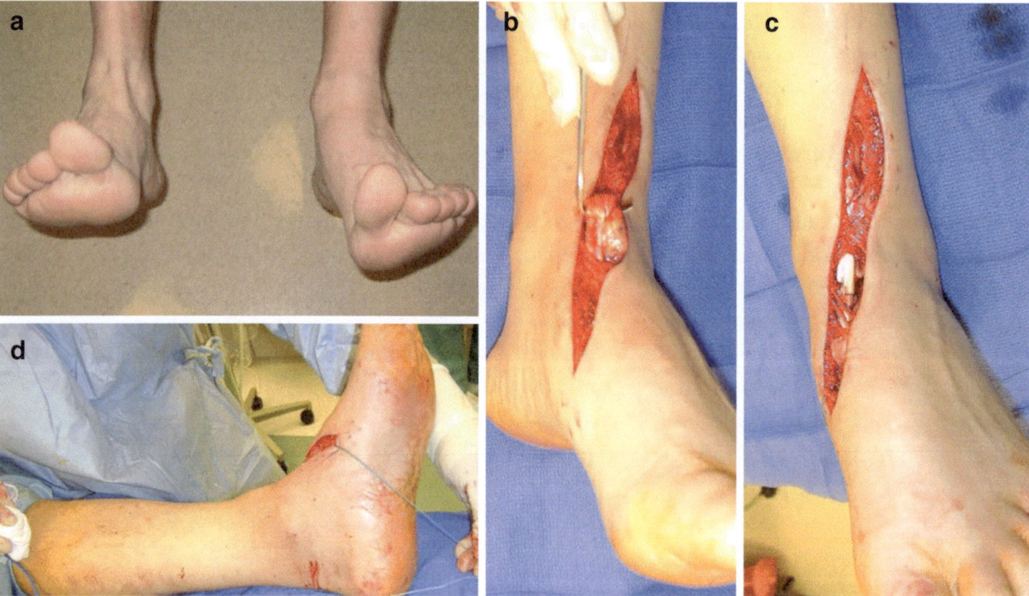

Fig. 3 Tibialis anterior ruptures. (**a**) Clinical photo showing the loss of tendon contour after tendon tear on the patient's left versus the intact right side. (**b**) After surgical incision, the ruptured tendon is localized. (**c**) A tendon repair was performed in this clinical example using a hamstring allograft. (**d**) The repair is tensioned so that the ankle rests in slight dorsiflexion

more eversion of the forefoot with active ankle dorsiflexion due to recruitment of the toe extensors. However, the patient will have less dorsiflexion strength when compared to the noninvolved extremity. In patients with delayed diagnoses, clawing of the toes may be noted, due to the sustained recruitment of the toe extensors for ankle dorsiflexion [20].

Acute ruptures are more apparent at the time of injury. They are less common than tendinopathic ruptures, with the former accounting for 20% of patient presentations [21]. Acute ruptures occur in younger, more active individuals resulting after an eccentric contraction with the ankle in plantarflexion, although penetrating trauma and injury associated with distal tibia fractures have also been described [22, 23]. Swelling, ecchymosis, and tenderness along the tendon are more impressive than in patients with attritional ruptures. In penetrating trauma, extension of the hallux and lesser toes should also be evaluated as these tendons can also be injured. A tendon rupture due to a tibial fracture is rare but can be easily overlooked as lack of dorsiflexion is attributed to antalgic guarding and/or deformity through the fracture [21, 22]. However, a nonpalpable tendon or palpable gap along with an inability to actively dorsiflex should raise suspicion for this injury, warranting additional advanced imaging, such as ultrasound and/or MRI.

In both acute and chronic ruptures, weight-bearing radiographs of the ankle should be obtained routinely to evaluate for additional injury or contributing pathology. Even if the exam is consistent with tendon rupture, an MRI can be helpful to identify the level of the tendon tear and overall condition of the tendon to assist with surgical planning.

2.2 Treatment

In patients with symptomatic tendinopathy prior to rupture, the initial treatment depends upon the severity of symptoms. When the patient is acutely painful, the preferred initial intervention is immobilization in a walking boot during the day and in a night splint when they are resting, along with oral anti-inflammatories and icing for several weeks. The authors recommend against steroid injections given the risk of associated tendon rupture. When pain has improved, patients begin a stretching routine to address calf tightness. When pain is minimal, eccentric strengthening is introduced. If these modalities are ineffective after several months, extracorporeal shockwave therapy (ESWT), platelet rich plasma (PRP) or bone marrow aspirate concentrate (BMAC) injections can be considered in addition to the immobilization to trigger a biologic response, although clinical data is lacking to support routine use of these second line modalities. If these conservative approaches fail, surgical debridement, suture reinforcement, and the use of an Achilles lengthening, to eliminate equinus, can be considered. In low demand patients unable to undergo surgery, a dorsiflexion assist ankle-foot orthosis (AFO) can mitigate tripping risks and can lead to good outcomes when treating tendinopathy or an attritional tendon rupture.

The specific surgical intervention or reconstruction is dependent upon tendon quality, timing from injury, mechanism of rupture, the physical demands of each patient and their medical comorbidities. However, tendon repair or reconstruction is the preferred treatment to restore strength and range of motion in most patients [21]. Outcomes after tendon repair or reconstruction report a high level of satisfaction and marked functional improvement from their preoperative state [16, 23, 24]. In healthy tendons, primary repair is usually possible within 6 weeks of the injury. In injuries where the tendon has avulsed at the insertion, the tendon should be anchored to the medial cuneiform with either a bone tunnel and interference screw, suture button device, or suture anchor [20]. Regardless of the surgical timing, chronic weakness in dorsiflexion and inversion relative to the injured extremity is anticipated [21] and should be discussed preoperatively.

Beyond 6 weeks and in acute attritional ruptures, the feasibility of end-to-end repair should be assessed [20]. Significant tendon gaps after tendon debridement often require reconstructive procedures. Reconstructive procedures have included Z-plasty lengthening [25], free tendon segment transposition/sliding grafts [11], turn down grafts [26], free tendon autograft or allograft (Fig. 3) [27], and tendon transfers [16]. For gaps less than 4 cm [20], local soft tissue reconstructions with tendon lengthening or sliding grafts are possible. For larger gaps, tendon autograft or allograft reconstructions and tendon transfers are favored. In the case of severe atrophy, tendon transfers that add a functional muscular unit are preferred over graft reconstructions.

Post-operatively, all patients are kept in a splint to maintain dorsiflexion for the first 2 weeks. After 2 weeks, they are immobilized in a walking boot during the day and in a night splint when they are sleeping or resting. Weightbearing in a boot brace is typically initiated at 2 weeks. The patients are given strict instructions to avoid active or passive plantarflexion for 3 months. Between 3–6 months, the boot can be gradually eliminated.

3   Achilles Tendon

The Achilles is different from other tendons as it does not have a true synovial sheath but rather a "paratenon." This facilitates tendon gliding and provides vascularization to the epitenon and endotendon [28]. The pathologies of the Achilles can be divided into tendinopathies and traumatic ruptures, which will be discussed in the following sections.

3.1   Tendinopathies: Insertional and Non-insertional

Achilles tendinopathies are the most frequent Achilles tendon disorder [29], and have two primary subtypes: insertional and non-insertional. Insertional tendinopathies involve the calcaneal insertion of the tendon, whereas non-insertional tendinopathies involve the tendon 2–6 cm proximal to its insertion [30].

3.1.1   Insertional Tendinopathy: Pathology and Evaluation

In insertional tendinopathy, patients describe pain at the posterior heel that is exacerbated by inactivity or limits their activity, difficulty with shoe wear, posterior ankle swelling, and often report the development of a "bump," due to the development of insertional osteophytes (enthesophytes). On examination, the tendon is often thickened and painful to palpation. Deep and proximal to the insertion, there may also be a painful retrocalcaneal bursitis, seen in conjunction with a prominent posterosuperior calcaneal prominence (Haglund's deformity). However, retrocalcaneal bursitis and a Haglund's prominence can be present in isolation without insertional tendinopathy. Additionally, one should also evaluate ankle dorsiflexion, with the knee flexed and extended, as decreased dorsiflexion contributes to pathologic tendon loading [31].

After the initial examination, the authors recommend lateral weightbearing radiographs of the ankle. These best profile the development of enthesophytes, intratendinous calcifications, and a Haglund's deformity. It is important to recognize, however, that bone spurs are frequently found in asymptomatic patients [32]. An MRI can be useful to study the size and quality of the tendon, to identify any associated tears, and to detect any adjacent retrocalcaneal bursitis or bony edema. Although MRI studies have been used to determine whether earlier surgical intervention is warranted [33], high-level evidence is lacking to support routine use of MRI scans. Ultrasound assessment for tendon thickening, while more affordable than MRI, has less diagnostic utility in insertional pathology [34] than in noninsertional tendinopathy.

3.1.2   Insertional Tendinopathy: Treatment

Treatment begins with non-operative care. Patients with severe tenderness and marked pain with passive motion and weightbearing respond poorly to immediate strengthening and stretching exercises. Instead, the authors' preference is several weeks of immobilization in an off the shelf solid AFO with wedges or in a hinged brace, placing the foot into an equinus position (approximately 20°). Immobilization is supplemented with oral anti-inflammatories and icing. Once severe pain and tenderness subside (typically 1–2 weeks), physical therapy is initiated. Eccentric strengthening exercises are then the primary intervention [35]. Using limited ankle range of motion eccentric programs (plantarflexion to neutral dorsiflexion) have higher patient satisfaction than a full eccentric motion programs (plantarflexion to below neutral dorsiflexion) [32]. A typical rehabilitation program lasts 12 weeks, although some patients may require longer treatment. The benefit of these exercises is that they are low risk, and affordable as a first line intervention [35]. Active and passive (night splints) stretching to improve range of motion is also a regular component of nonoperative therapy. Use of ESWT has also been studied, with both high energy (single treatment requiring anesthesia) and low energy (multiple in office treatments without anesthetic) proposed when eccentric training fails [35–37]. Additional described treatments include PRP and BMAC injections [35, 38], but high-quality evidence is lacking to support their routine use. The authors strongly recommend against steroid injections given the known risk of complete tendon rupture [39].

When nonoperative treatment fails, the risks and benefits of operative treatment are discussed with the patient. After tendon debridement and retrocalcaneal decompression, patient outcomes are favorable with an estimated satisfaction of 87% [32]. It is important however to discuss the course of recovery with the patient, as full recovery often takes close to 12 months [40]. It is also imperative to discuss potential surgical complications, with complication cited between 6-30% that include scar sensitivity and delayed wound healing [32].

When proceeding with surgical treatment, the most common procedure involves partial detachment of the tendon insertion to allow for tendon debridement (tendon fibers and insertional calcifications), a retrocalcaneal bursectomy, and a Haglund's prominence exostectomy. The tendon is then secured back down to the calcaneus with

bony anchors. When >50% of the tendon is debrided (more commonly in revision cases), a tendon augmentation using the flexor hallucis longus (FHL) or flexor digitorum longus transfer (FDL) is recommended with low morbidity and good functional outcomes reported [41, 42]. The authors' postoperative protocol is identical for insertional tendinopathy, non-insertional tendinopathy, and acute ruptures (please see end of Sect. 3.2.2).

One final point is to address a gastrocnemius contracture. If a preoperative Silfverskiöld test demonstrates a contracture, a gastrocnemius recession can be performed at the start of the procedure to help improve ankle motion and reduce tension on the debrided and repaired tendon. Adjusting the tension on the repair and reconstruction is necessary for a successful functional outcome. Of note, an isolated gastrocnemius recession has been proposed as a stand-alone surgical treatment in patients with Achilles tendinopathy (insertional and noninsertional) with a coexisting gastrocnemius contracture, reporting faster recoveries and lower surgical risks [43]. However, patients should be told that plantarflexion power and endurance are significantly decreased after a recession [43], which may not be tolerated in more active individuals (laborers, athletes).

3.1.3 Noninsertional Tendinopathy: Pathology and Evaluation

Tendinopathy within the body of the Achilles tendon is termed noninsertional tendinopathy. It is the most common Achilles pathology in athletes and occurs with roughly equal frequency to insertional tendinopathy in nonathletes [44]. A tendinosis is the most frequent presentation, although an inflammatory tendinitis can occur with an acute overload event and can be treated like other acute strains. The causes of mechanical overload are similarly multifactorial (Fig. 2). While a hypovascular zone of the tendon has been described in cadaveric studies and suggested as a root cause of tendinopathy [45], this theory has been debated in an in vitro study [46].

Patients complain of pain 2–6 cm proximal to the insertion that increases with activity. It occurs at the beginning and end of exercising, with an intermediate period of reduced pain and dysfunction [30]. There is visible swelling in this area and the tendon may feel thickened and fibrotic and is tender to palpation. A lateral ankle radiograph may aid in identifying intrasubstance calcifications and is obtained routinely by the authors. If the diagnosis is unclear or when surgical treatment is being considered, an MRI can be helpful for evaluating the thickness and length of the diseased tendon. While ultrasound can offer useful information regarding tendon size and tendon quality [47], it requires considerable technical skill and experience. The authors do not routinely use ultrasound and prefer MRI when initial nonoperative treatment fails or the diagnosis is unclear.

3.1.4 Noninsertional Tendinopathy: Treatment

The first line of treatment is nonoperative management with eccentric strengthening [48]. While other modalities have been investigated in combination with eccentric training (prolotherapy, laser therapy, ESWT), no study has shown a definitive benefit compared to eccentric training alone [48]. When eccentric training is ineffective, however, there is evidence to support ESWT [49]. Additional evidence for other treatments like PRP or BMAC injections is needed prior to routine use [50].

When nonoperative management fails, operative treatment, consisting of a tenotomy and debridement, can be considered. Both open and endoscopic debridement have reported good results with an overall patient satisfaction rate of 90% or higher [48]. Additionally, isolated gastrocnemius recession for patients with a gastrocnemius contracture has also been described with favorable outcomes [51]. When debridement results in >50% or complete loss of a segment of tendon, augmentation with a FHL or FDL transfer, attaching tendon to the calcaneus via an anchor, bone tunnel, or suture button is effective [52]. In addition, the authors also perform a tenodesis of any Achilles tendon remnant to the transferred tendon, to add additional power to the transfer.

3.2 Acute and Chronic Achilles Tendon Ruptures

3.2.1 Pathology and Evaluation

Traumatic Achilles tendon ruptures are most seen in males, typically in their 30s or 40s, who participate in recreational or sports intermittently [53]. They often present with complaints of posterior ankle pain, swelling and a "popping" sensation on the back of the leg described as if they were struck from behind.

The physical examination can confirm the diagnosis with a near 100% sensitivity [54]. The Thompson test, performed with the patient in the prone position or on their knees, involves the examiner squeezing the gastrocnemius muscle to elicit a plantarflexion response that occurs if the tendon is in continuity (Fig. 4). This examination maneuver has a sensitivity 0.96 and specificity 0.93 [54]. While the patient is positioned in this fashion, the resting tension of the tendon is also examined by observing the resting dorsiflexion angle of both ankles, as a torn Achilles tendon commonly results in increased resting dorsiflexion (Fig. 4). Other common findings include a palpable defect in the tendon and decreased plantarflexion strength with an inability to perform a single leg heel raise or weakened plantarflex against resistance [54]. If the diagnosis is unclear, plain radiographs, ultrasound, or an MRI study can help to confirm the presence of a partial or complete tear [55]. Radiographs can be helpful in identifying calcifications along the tendon or near the insertion suggesting a pre-existing tendinopathy. An MRI also has increased utility in chronic injuries (>4–6 weeks from injury), as the body quickly fills the palpable gap with scar tissue such that a gap is not clearly palpable.

3.2.2 Treatment

In the acute injury, without pre-existing tendinopathy, several randomized trials have reported similar functional outcomes, strength, and rates of re-rupture for both operative and nonoperative care, when an accelerated (early motion and weightbearing) rehabilitation protocol was followed [56]. However, higher complication rates

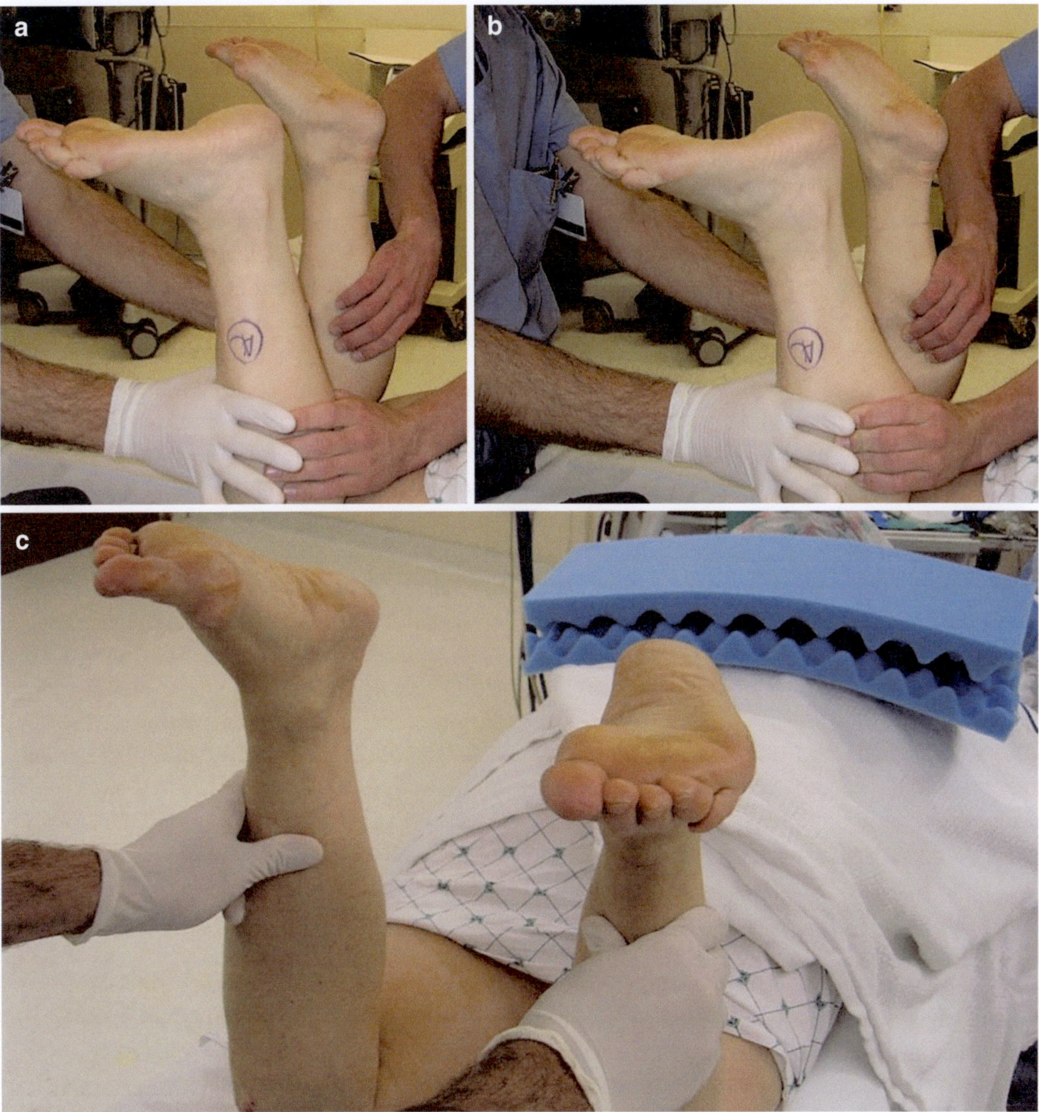

Fig. 4 Acute achilles tendon rupture examination. (**a, c**) On prone exam, there is increased resting dorsiflexion on the right side where the Achilles tendon is torn. (**b**) The gastrocnemius is stimulated with a calf squeeze, and the intact muscle tendon unit on the left creates a plantarflexion response on the left versus no response on the right

(wound complications, infection, and sural nerve damage) have been noted with surgery.

A recent multicenter, randomized controlled trial, however, has shown that surgical treatment reduces the risk of re-rupture (6.2% vs. 0.6% nonsurgical and surgical treatment, respectively), even when early functional rehabilitation is utilized for nonoperative care [57]. Other studies have shown that surgery results in a faster and greater recovery of strength, faster return to work, especially in the military population [58, 59], while avoiding a 2 cm Achilles lengthening seen in nonsurgical patients [60]. Although nonoperative care is a viable option, the authors favor surgical management unless the patient has a pre-existing condition(s) that may increase the risk of postoperative complications (e.g., poorly controlled diabetes or vascular disease).

The optimal rehabilitation protocol, for nonoperative care, has been debated. A meta-analysis utilizing functional rehabilitation (early plantarflexion immobilization followed by controlled motion weightbearing 10 days after injury) was found to be superior to immobilization and delayed motion protocols, resulting in lower rates of re-rupture [56]. However, a meta-analysis comparing these two protocols did not find a difference in re-rupture rates, strength, or ability to return to sport or work [61]. When using nonoperative care, the authors prefer functional rehabilitation, given better patient compliance and satisfaction. The critical time between tendon rupture and beginning nonoperative care is debated, but expert opinion has suggested immobilization in plantarflexion must be initiated within 48 h of injury [62]. The authors favor operative repair when patients present beyond 48 h without plantarflexion immobilization. Our preferred protocol has been previously described by Glazebrook et al. [62].

The critical time for a repair is currently unknown. While no functional differences were detected in repairs performed within 1 week of the injury [63], no study has compared outcomes with later repairs. However, despite a high rate of return to activity with surgery, patients can expect a chronic strength deficit compared to the uninjured extremity [7, 64]. The options for surgical treatment include a traditional open or minimally invasive repair. The latter offers reduced rates of wound complications when compared to open repair, but has equal rates of re-rupture, return to preinjury activity level, time to return to work, and ankle range of motion [65, 66]. However, minimally invasive techniques have reported a greater risk of sural nerve injury and palpable suture knots. In a recent study, approximately one in nine patients undergoing surgery experienced a complication, with overall complication rates similar in open and minimally invasive repairs [67]. These included wound dehiscence, deep and superficial infections, symptomatic venous thromboembolism, sural nerve injury, and re-ruptures.

In chronic ruptures (>4–6 weeks), surgical treatment is indicated unless the patient has low functional demands and significant comorbidities that preclude surgical intervention. Other contraindications include patients with an active infection, severe peripheral vascular disease, and patients who are household or poor community ambulators. These patients are best managed with an AFO. If patients are candidates for a repair, a primary end to end repair is often not possible when the tendon gap exceeds 2 cm [68]. However, there is no consensus regarding the best reconstruction option for each size defect [68]. Techniques for reconstruction include Achilles tendon turndown flaps, a V-Y gastrocnemius fascial advancement, FHL and FDL transfers, bone block Achilles allografts, and free tendon autografts and allografts [68]. Good to excellent results have been described but there is a paucity of comparative studies amongst these techniques. The authors recommend the following algorithm. For chronic cases that have a mild difference in resting tendon tension or less than a 2 cm gap, an end-to-end repair or advancement of the tendon to the calcaneus is performed. For cases with a 2–5 cm gap or moderate difference in resting tendon tension, a V–Y advancement is performed. With a greater than 5 cm gap or severe difference in resting tension, a turndown procedure is performed. If there is inadequate tissue proximally to perform the turndown, an allograft semitendinosus is used to span the void. When any of these scenarios is associated with atrophy of the gastrocnemius-soleus complex, an FDL or FHL tendon transfer is added to augment plantarflexion strength.

The authors' postoperative care, for tendon repairs or reconstructions, is to place patients into a splint in equinus until sutures are removed at 10 days. They are then placed into a hinged boot brace, in 20° of equinus, until 6 weeks postoperatively. While in this plantarflexion boot brace, protected weightbearing with crutches is initiated. After 6 weeks, the ankle can be brought into a neutral position with full weightbearing. During the 3–6 months period, the boot can be gradually eliminated.

4   Peroneal Tendons

The peroneus longus and brevis tendons are the principal foot evertors, but also assist with ankle and forefoot plantarflexion. These tendons have critical functions of opposing inversion to help maintain balance during gait, but also function as dynamic stabilizers of the lateral ankle during rapid inversion events.

4.1 Anatomical Considerations

In most individuals, the peroneus brevis muscle fibers extend more distally than peroneus longus muscle fibers, with brevis muscle extending approximately 16–20 mm above the tip of the fibula [69], or just proximal to the entrance of the tendons into the fibular groove [70]. Extension of the muscle beyond this point is termed a low lying muscle belly and has been hypothesized as a contributing factor in cases of tendon subluxation, tenosynovitis, and tendon tearing [69]. Other variations that may contribute to tendon pathology include accessory muscles within the peroneal sheath. These include the peroneus quartus and quintus and are found within the peroneal tunnel in 10–30% of patients [71]. These accessory muscles and their tendons can cause overcrowding of the peroneal tunnel and produce secondary tendon stenosis or retinacular attrition.

As the tendons course distally, regions of angular change or compression against bony prominences result in localized tendon stress. Prior to an abrupt change in their route at the distal tip of the fibula, the tendons reside posterior to the fibula in a retrofibular groove that is stabilized by a fibrocartilaginous ridge and the superior peroneal retinaculum (SPR). Traumatic injury to the SPR, a shallow fibular groove, and anomalous tendons overcrowding the tendon tunnel have been proposed as causes of SPR incompetence or laxity [70]. When the SPR is torn or lax, the brevis can subluxate laterally over the lateral corner of the fibula. The brevis may then be compressed against this bony prominence with contraction of the overlying peroneus longus [70]. Distal to the fibula, the tendons enter their own separate subsheaths, separated by the peroneal tubercle. At this location, tendon stability is achieved by the inferior peroneal retinaculum. However, the retinaculum and the tubercle may create another

source of compression. This commonly occurs in the setting of a prominent or hypertrophied tubercle and most commonly affects the peroneus longus [72]. A final area of mechanical stress is at the cuboid, where the longus tendon undergoes an angular turn below the cuboid as it courses towards the first metatarsal.

While these mechanical stresses have been described as causes of tendon pathology, regions of tendon hypovascularity have also been suggested as secondary contributing factors. Older cadaveric studies have discussed avascular regions at the retromalleolar groove, affecting the peroneus brevis, and from the distal fibula to peroneal tubercle and at the tendon's entrance into the cuboid tunnel affecting the peroneus longus [73]. However, more recent publications have challenged this hypothesis, showing that both tendons are largely well vascularized by a vincular network [74].

4.2 Tendinopathy

4.2.1 Pathology and Evaluation

Peroneal tendinopathy often presents with pain and swelling at the lateral ankle and hindfoot. Many report no change in activity and cannot describe a precipitating injury. Others may report a history of an ankle inversion injury, which is often associated with patient perceptions of ankle instability. Symptoms are exacerbated by activity and abate with rest. Pain at the posterior aspect of the distal fibula commonly represents peroneus brevis pathology, whereas pain secondary to peroneus longus pathology is more commonly localized to the peroneal tubercle and cuboid tunnel [71]. However, these patterns are not mutually exclusive.

Examination requires careful inspection with patients standing and ambulating as patients with cavovarus alignment and/or metatarsus adductus deformities will chronically overload their peroneal tendons. The course of the tendons should be palpated to assess tenderness, swelling, and tendon thickening. Passive plantarflexion and inversion as well as active plantarflexion and eversion may elicit pain. Resisted eversion or having the patient perform circumduction (circles) of the foot and ankle may result in palpable and/or visible tendon subluxation or dislocation with an incompetent SPR. The stability of the ankle should also be assessed, as lateral ligamentous laxity results in increased work of the peroneal tendons to stabilize the lateral ankle and hindfoot.

Radiographic evaluation should begin with weightbearing radiographs of both the foot and ankle. These are useful to help evaluate alignment, integrity of the neighboring joints, and identify contributing osseous pathology, including a prominent peroneal tubercle or os peroneum. Ultrasound may show a dynamic tendon subluxation, dislocation, tears and instrasheath snapping [75]. An MRI is obtained when the diagnosis is unclear or when symptoms are refractory to nonoperative care. However, a standard ankle MRI with the patient supine may result in increased tendon signal without true pathology secondary to the so-called *magic angle effect*. This occurs when the tendon collagen fibers are oriented 55° relative to the magnetic field, producing an imaging artifact [76]. These effects can be mitigated when the patient is imaged in 20° of plantarflexion [77], or in the prone position [76]. There is less suspicion for imaging artifact if the abnormal tendon signal is appreciated in multiple planes and multiple sequences (T1 and T2 images), and if there is additional pathology including thickening of the tendon or adjacent tenosynovitis.

4.2.2 Treatment

Nonoperative treatment begins with a short period of rest from activity, ice, oral nonsteroidal anti-inflammatories, compression, and immobilization in a boot or stirrup brace limiting inversion and eversion. If a foot deformity exists and is flexible, orthotics or wedges can be used to help correct the deformity and offload the peroneals. Once symptoms have begun to improve with rest and immobilization, the authors begin physical therapy to strengthen the peroneals and other dynamic ankle and hindfoot stabilizers. When rest, immobilization, and therapy fail beyond 3 months, ESWT, PRP, or BMAC injections are

low risk nonsurgical alternatives currently lacking supporting evidence for routine use [78]. Despite reports of intrasheath injection of steroid with modest pain relief and without frequently observed tendon rupture [79], the authors do not offer this treatment to their patients given this potential risk.

After failed nonoperative treatment, surgical treatment can be considered. While tendoscopy can be a useful technique for diagnosis and limited surgical debridement, its use for more involved debridement and tendon repair remains to be defined [71]. Standard treatment consists of an open debridement of the sheath and tendons, with the excision of inflamed tenosynovium and frayed or unhealthy appearing tendon. Pathologic malalignment (cavovarus foot, ankle joint varus, and metatarsus adductus) deformities contributing to tendon overload along with anatomic variants (prominent peroneal tubercle, low lying muscle belly, accessory tendons) may also contribute to pathology and should be addressed.

The traditional teaching has reported that debridement of >50% of either tendon may require a tenodesis to the intact tendon or the use of an allograft/autograft tendon [80]. However, a recent biomechanics study showed that two-thirds of the tendon can be debrided and the intact tendon can still resist physiologic tensile loads [1]. After debridement, the recommendation is to tubularize the remaining tendon, without supplemental augmentation or tenodesis, even if less than 50% remains, as long as the tendon can resist a substantial intraoperative longitudinal stress by the surgeon [80]. When insufficient tendon remains, tenodesis to the noninvolved tendon or an allograft/autograft reconstruction may be needed. Advocates of tenodesis argue that the procedure is simple and does not rely on allograft/autograft healing [81]. Proponents of allograft/autograft reconstruction argue that tenodesis does not restore adequate tension to the tenodesed tendon and that reconstruction is less likely to result in chronic foot imbalance [82].

If there is insufficient tendon for repair or a gap after debridement, the authors' preferred approach is a turndown procedure. In this technique, a long section of the proximal tendon is harvested and flipped distally to fill the void (Fig. 5). Suturing the turned down segment from its distal attachment to the most proximal zone where the turn down was harvested is critical to maintain continuity between the turned down graft and the proximal segment. The authors prefer to preserve the roles of the longus and brevis and perform a tenodesis only in patients with low functional demands. When the longus cannot be salvaged, due to its distal segment, a suture anchor into the fifth metatarsal tuberosity can allow the peroneus longus to function as a second brevis. In the relatively rare scenario when both tendons are irreparable, interposition tendon grafting can be performed if there is adequate

tendon excursion and healthy muscle [83]. If the remaining muscle/tendon unit does not have excursion or the muscle is significantly atrophied, an interposition graft will have minimal function. As such, these conditions require treatment with either an FDL or FHL tendon transfer, resulting in good functional outcomes albeit with residual strength and balance deficits [84]. After any of the above procedures are performed, it is crucial to repair or reconstruct the superior peroneal retinaculum to avoid tendon instability and dysfunction. In addition, it may also be necessary to perform a groove deepening of the fibula. This will unload the tendons, provide adequate space for the reconstruction, and avoid stenosis or potential tendon subluxation.

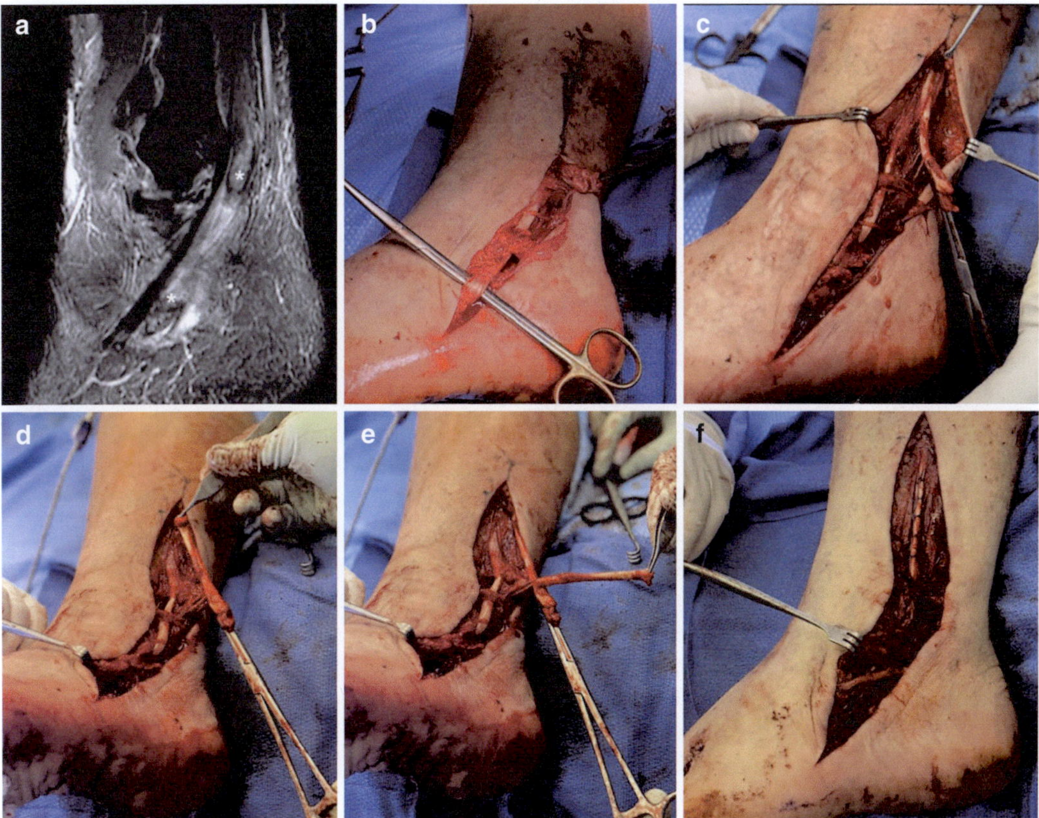

Fig. 5 Peroneal tears and turndown repair. (**a**) A select sagittal MRI showing distal intrasubstance fibrillations of the peroneus brevis and completely torn peroneus longus with a large gap between the proximal and distal tendon stumps. (**b**) Surgical photo showing the intrasubstance tearing with preserved continuity of the frayed peroneus brevis overlying the dissection forceps, and a torn peroneus longus. (**c**) The intact peroneus longus tendon proximally is dissected and isolated. (**d–f**) 50% of the tendon is transected from proximal to distal, allowing the tendon to then be turned down for distal repair

The authors' postoperative protocol is to immobilize the patient in a plantarflexion splint for 10 days after surgery. Patients are then transitioned into a hinged boot brace in equinus for 6 weeks and begin progressive weightbearing and protected motion. In addition, a night splint or brace that protects against passive inversion during sleep is important for the first 3 months. Early protected range of motion is essential to prevent tendon adhesions and involves restricting active and passive dorsiflexion beyond neutral, and avoiding active eversion and passive inversion, to prevent excessive tension on repaired or reconstructed tendons. After 6 weeks, the ankle can be brought into neutral position and progressed to full weightbearing. During months 3–6 the boot can be gradually eliminated. The authors use this protocol after all peroneal tendon reconstruction and repairs (following section). Self-directed physical therapy versus formal therapy is discussed on a patient-by-patient basis.

4.3 Tendon Tears

Peroneal tendon tears can occur acutely during inversion injuries or can develop as part of more chronic tendinopathies. The peroneus brevis is more commonly torn, with longitudinal tears primarily noted at the posterior lateral malleolus [81]. As with previous tendon evaluations, MRI and ultrasound are useful modalities to localize the location and extent of a tear. If a tear is identified but the patient is asymptomatic, no further treatment is required. If symptomatic, however, the treatment algorithm is identical to that discussed above for tendinopathy. When nonoperative care fails and tears treated surgically are deemed repairable, both absorbable and nonabsorbable suture have been used without any clinical difference [85]. If tendon repair isn't possible and reconstruction is required, the same treatment algorithm detailed above is followed. In general, surgery improves outcomes with high patient satisfaction and high rate of return to work, although athletic patients may not return to their prior sporting level [86].

4.4 Instability

4.4.1 Pathology and Evaluation

Peroneal instability, from an incompetent SPR, permits subluxation or dislocation of both tendons. Acute SPR injuries occur during forced dorsiflexion with the hindfoot inverted with simultaneous contraction of the peroneal tendons [71], with forced dorsiflexion during eversion also described as a cause. Patients report a popping sensation at the lateral ankle followed by swelling. This is commonly misdiagnosed and treated as an ankle sprain. In contrast, retinacular attenuation occurs when anatomic variants overcrowd the peroneal tunnel [81], or in the setting of lateral ligament insufficiency with instability [87].

There are five different patterns of instability. The first, and most common, is an elevation of the retinacular attachment from the lateral fibula without complete detachment of either the SPR or fibrocartilaginous rim from the fibula. This creates a potential space for anterior peroneal tendon dislocation [88]. Second, and less common, the SPR elevates from the fibula and the fibrocartilaginous rim and is disconnected from the fibula. Third and even less common, the SPR avulses from the fibula with a cortical fragment producing the so called "fleck sign" [80]. Rarely, in a fourth type of instability, the SPR avulses from the calcaneus [71]. The fifth type of instability, described by Raiken et al., is an intrasheath subluxation injury where either the tendons swap their normal orientation or where the longus tendon displaces through a longitudinal tear of the brevis [75].

In either acute or chronic injury, subluxation or dislocation of the peroneal tendons can be elicited on exam with ankle circumduction or forced dorsiflexion and eversion from a plantarflexed and inverted position. Weightbearing radiographs may reveal the fleck sign, while an MRI and/or ultrasound can help to identify concomitant tendon tears.

4.4.2 Treatment

Treatment of peroneal instability is based upon the patient's level of activity and the chronicity of the injury. In an acute injury, and in a nonathletic patient, where the tendons are reduced into the retromalleolar groove, 6 weeks in a nonweight-bearing cast in slight plantarflexion and inversion can allow the SPR to heal with variable reported success [80, 89]. When acute dislocation occurs in a young and active patient, when the tendons are not reducible, when nonoperative treatment fails, or when peroneal instability is chronic, surgical treatment is recommended.

The surgery consists of reduction of the tendons into the peroneal groove with repair of the SPR to the fibula. In general, repair of the SPR with or without groove deepening has high patient satisfaction [71] and low rates of recurrent instability [90]. Supplemental surgical deep-ening of the retromalleolar groove for added tendon stability is somewhat controversial, with recent literature recommending that acute injuries in athletes and cases of chronic instability be treated with groove deepening, due to higher rate of return to sport [80]. This reflects the authors approach in which the groove is deepened at the posterior fibula via a three-limb osteotomy that allows the cortical surface of the groove to be reflected on a posteromedial cortical hinge. With the cortex reflected, intramedullary bone is removed with a bur, allowing for replacement of the reflected cortical flap into a recessed position that creates a deepened groove (Fig. 6). The

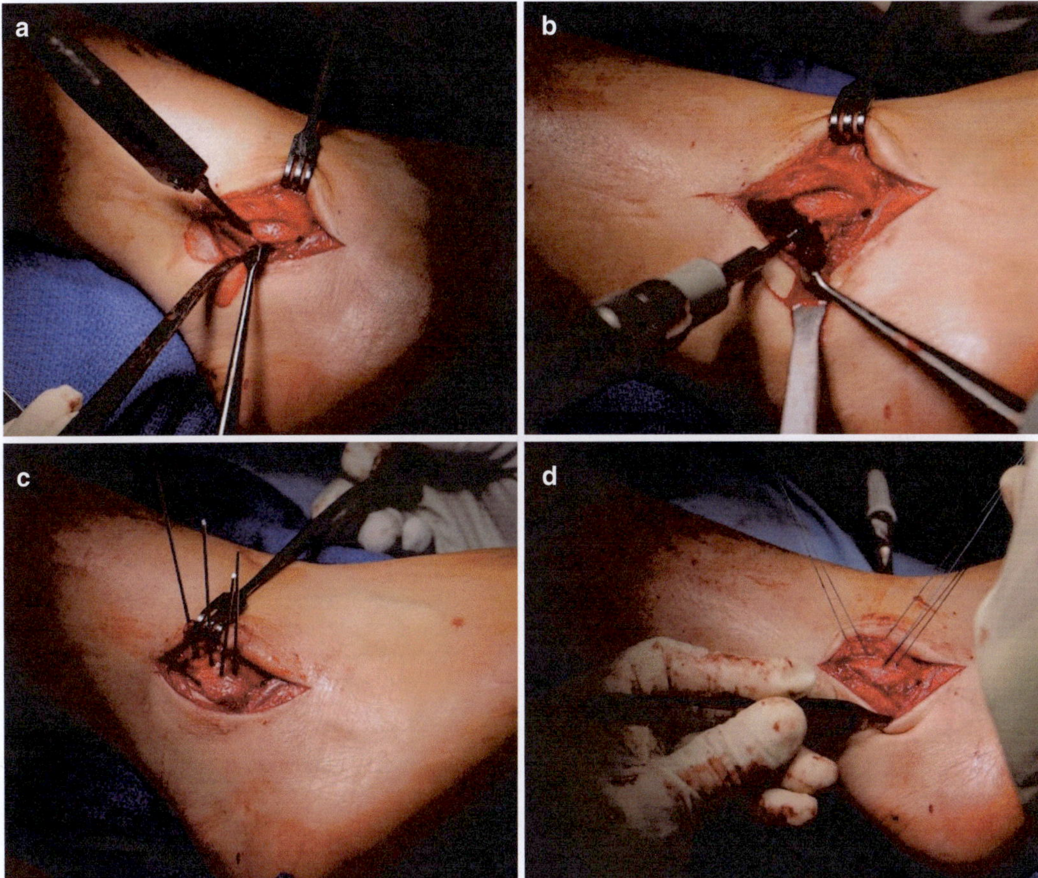

Fig. 6 Technique for fibular groove deepening. (**a**) An osteotome is used to create a cortical window into the medullary cavity of the distal fibula. (**b**) With the cortical window reflected inferiorly, a bur is used to remove intramedullary bone and create a groove. (**c**) With the cortical window replaced and tamped into a depressed position to create a groove, bone tunnels are created with k-wires. (**d**) Sutures are passed through the bone tunnel, into the superior peroneal retinaculum, and then back through the bone tunnel, allowing repair of the SPR to the newly created groove

authors' preferred technique is to then repair the SPR to its anatomic attachment using bone tunnels in the lateral fibula and nonabsorbable suture. In addition, concomitant peroneal tendon tears are addressed as described above. If a peroneal tendon tear is present, the above postoperative protocol is followed. If a groove deepening is performed and a tendon repair or reconstruction is not needed, the patient is splinted in neutral rather than plantarflexion. Similarly, a night splint or brace that protects against passive inversion or plantarflexion during sleep is important for 3 months. After 2 weeks, the patient can be progressed to weightbearing in a boot brace in neutral dorsiflexion. During 3–6 months postoperatively, a cloth brace can be used as the patient transitions from the boot brace.

5 Conclusion

In summary, the spectrum of tendon pathologies affecting ankle function is broad. While each tendon has unique characteristics, there are many common principles in tendon pathophysiology, clinical evaluation, and treatment. Tendinopathy can occur in all tendons, and often involves a change in tendon microstructure secondary to chronic stresses overwhelming the intrinsic repair pathways. While there is no documented evidence of cellular inflammation, inflammatory mediators are likely intimately involved in tendon remodeling and degeneration. In injuries of chronic tendon overload, it is crucial to consider the spectrum of intrinsic and extrinsic factors that are contributing to the patient's presentation. Modifiable factors should be addressed during both nonoperative and operative treatment of the injured tendon. In general, nonoperative care, consisting of a period of immobilization, icing, and anti-inflammatories followed by physical therapy, is appropriate for most tendinopathies. When these treatments fail, debridement and repair, reconstruction, or tendon transfers may be needed to help reduce pain and restore function. In the setting of traumatic injuries resulting in tendon rupture or tendon instability, acute surgical treatment is commonly indicated.

References

1. Thorpe CT, Screen HRC. Tendon structure and composition. Adv Exp Med Biol. 2016;920:3–10. https://doi.org/10.1007/978-3-319-33943-6_1.
2. Xu Y, Murrell GAC. The basic science of tendinopathy. Clin Orthop Relat Res. 2008;466(7):1528–38. https://doi.org/10.1007/s11999-008-0286-4.
3. Parkinson J, Samiric T, Ilic MZ, Cook J, Handley CJ. Involvement of proteoglycans in tendinopathy. J Musculoskelet Neuronal Interact. 2011;11(2):86–93.
4. Grant TM, Thompson MS, Urban J, Yu J. Elastic fibres are broadly distributed in tendon and highly localized around tenocytes. J Anat. 2013;222(6):573–9. https://doi.org/10.1111/joa.12048.
5. Milz S, Ockert B, Putz R. Tenocytes and the extracellular matrix: a reciprocal relationship. Orthopade. 2009;38(11):1071–9. https://doi.org/10.1007/s00132-009-1490-y.
6. Riley G. Tendinopathy–from basic science to treatment. Nat Clin Pract Rheumatol. 2008;4(2):82–9. https://doi.org/10.1038/ncprheum0700.
7. Lantto I, Heikkinen J, Flinkkila T, et al. Early functional treatment versus cast immobilization in tension after achilles rupture repair: results of a prospective randomized trial with 10 or more years of follow-up. Am J Sports Med. 2015;43(9):2302–9. https://doi.org/10.1177/0363546515591267.
8. Khan KM, Cook JL, Kannus P, Maffulli N, Bonar SF. Time to abandon the "tendinitis" myth. BMJ. 2002;324(7338):626–7. https://doi.org/10.1136/bmj.324.7338.626.
9. Millar NL, Murrell GAC, McInnes IB. Inflammatory mechanisms in tendinopathy - towards translation. Nat Rev Rheumatol. 2017;13(2):110–22. https://doi.org/10.1038/nrrheum.2016.213.
10. Bass E. Tendinopathy: why the difference between tendinitis and tendinosis matters. Int J Ther Massage Bodywork. 2012;5(1):14–7. https://doi.org/10.3822/ijtmb.v5i1.153.
11. Reb CW, Stenson JF, Daniel JN. Tibialis anterior tendon reconstruction using augmented half-thickness tendon segment transposition. Foot Ankle Spec. 2017;10(2):144–8. https://doi.org/10.1177/1938640016685825.
12. Calloway SP, Hardin DM, Crawford MD, et al. Injury surveillance in major league soccer: a 4-year comparison of injury on natural grass versus artificial turf field. Am J Sports Med. 2019;47(10):2279–86. https://doi.org/10.1177/0363546519860522.
13. Rowson S, McNally C, Duma SM. Can footwear affect achilles tendon loading? Clin J Sport Med. 2010;20(5):344–9. https://doi.org/10.1097/JSM.0b013e3181ed7e50.
14. Griffin JW. Differences in elbow flexion torque measured concentrically, eccentrically, and isometrically. Phys Ther. 1987;67(8):1205–8. https://doi.org/10.1093/ptj/67.8.1205.

15. Herzenberg JE, Lamm BM, Corwin C, Sekel J. Isolated recession of the gastrocnemius muscle: the Baumann procedure. Foot Ankle Int. 2007;28(11):1154–9. https://doi.org/10.3113/FAI.2007.1154.

16. Ellington JK, McCormick J, Marion C, et al. Surgical outcome following tibialis anterior tendon repair. Foot Ankle Int. 2010;31(5):412–7. https://doi.org/10.3113/FAI.2010.0412.

17. Petersen W, Stein V, Bobka T. Structure of the human tibialis anterior tendon. J Anat. 2000;197(4):617–25. https://doi.org/10.1046/j.1469-7580.2000.19740617.x.

18. Sammarco VJ, Sammarco GJ, Henning C, Chaim S. Surgical repair of acute and chronic tibialis anterior tendon ruptures. J Bone Joint Surg Am. 2009;91(2):325–32. https://doi.org/10.2106/JBJS.G.01386.

19. Lee MH, Chung CB, Cho JH, et al. Tibialis anterior tendon and extensor retinaculum: imaging in cadavers and patients with tendon tear. AJR Am J Roentgenol. 2006;187(2):161–8. https://doi.org/10.2214/AJR.05.0073.

20. Chen J, Kadakia R, Akoh CC, Schweitzer KM. Management of anterior tibialis tendon ruptures. J Am Acad Orthop Surg. 2021;29(16):691–701. https://doi.org/10.5435/JAAOS-D-20-00802.

21. Tickner A, Thorng S, Martin M, Marmolejo V. Management of isolated anterior tibial tendon rupture: a systematic review and meta-analysis. J Foot Ankle Surg. 2019;58(2):213–20. https://doi.org/10.1053/j.jfas.2018.08.001.

22. Ebrahimi FV, Tofighi M, Khatibi H. Closed tibial fracture associated with laceration of tibialis anterior tendon. J Foot Ankle Surg. 2010;49(1):86. https://doi.org/10.1053/j.jfas.2009.08.013.

23. Johansen JK, Jordan M, Thomas M, Walther M, Simatira AM, Waizy H. Surgical treatment of tibialis anterior tendon rupture. Foot Ankle Surg. 2021;27(5):515–20. https://doi.org/10.1016/j.fas.2020.06.011.

24. Fraissler L, Horas K, Bölch S, Raab P, Rudert M, Walcher M. Extensor hallucis longus-transfer for tibialis anterior tendon rupture repair. Oper Orthop Traumatol. 2019;31(2):143–8. https://doi.org/10.1007/s00064-018-0571-7.

25. Goetz J, Beckmann J, Koeck F, Grifka J, Dullien S, Heers G. Gait analysis after tibialis anterior tendon rupture repair using Z-plasty. J Foot Ankle Surg. 2013;52(5):598–601. https://doi.org/10.1053/j.jfas.2013.01.007.

26. Kopriva JM, Cheesborough J, Frick SL. Tendon turndown to bridge a tibialis anterior gap and restore active dorsiflexion after degloving foot injury in a child: a case report. JBJS Case Connect. 2020;10(3):e19.00445. https://doi.org/10.2106/JBJS.CC.19.00445.

27. Karnovsky SC, Desandis B, Papson AK, et al. Tibialis anterior reconstruction with hamstring autograft using a minimally invasive approach.

28. Wu F, Nerlich M, Docheva D. Tendon injuries: basic science and new repair proposals. EFORT Open Rev. 2017;2(7):332–42. https://doi.org/10.1302/2058-5241.2.160075.

29. Järvinen TAH, Kannus P, Maffulli N, Khan KM. Achilles tendon disorders: etiology and epidemiology. Foot Ankle Clin. 2005;10(2):255–66. https://doi.org/10.1016/j.fcl.2005.01.013.

30. Singh A, Calafi A, Diefenbach C, Kreulen C, Giza E. Noninsertional tendinopathy of the achilles. Foot Ankle Clin. 2017;22(4):745–60. https://doi.org/10.1016/j.fcl.2017.07.006.

31. Whitting JW, Steele JR, McGhee DE, Munro BJ. Dorsiflexion capacity affects achilles tendon loading during drop landings. Med Sci Sports Exerc. 2011;43(4):706–13. https://doi.org/10.1249/MSS.0b013e3181f474dd.

32. Chimenti RL, Cychosz CC, Hall MM, Phisitkul P. Current concepts review update: insertional achilles tendinopathy. Foot Ankle Int. 2017;38(10):1160–9. https://doi.org/10.1177/1071100717723127.

33. Nicholson CW, Berlet GC, Lee TH. Prediction of the success of nonoperative treatment of insertional Achilles tendinosis based on MRI. Foot Ankle Int. 2007;28(4):472–7. https://doi.org/10.3113/FAI.2007.0472.

34. Kim DH, Choi JH, Park CH, Park HJ, Yoon KJ, Lee YT. The diagnostic significance of ultrasonographic measurement of the achilles tendon thickness for the insertional achilles tendinopathy in patients with heel pain. J Clin Med. 2021;10(10):2165. https://doi.org/10.3390/jcm10102165.

35. Jarin IJ, Bäcker HC, Vosseller JT. Functional outcomes of insertional achilles tendinopathy treatment: a systematic review. JBJS Rev. 2021;9:6. https://doi.org/10.2106/JBJS.RVW.20.00110.

36. Mansur NSB, Matsunaga FT, Carrazzone OL, et al. Shockwave therapy plus eccentric exercises versus isolated eccentric exercises for achilles insertional tendinopathy: a double-blinded randomized clinical trial. J Bone Joint Surg Am. 2021;103(14):1295–302. https://doi.org/10.2106/JBJS.20.01826.

37. Pinitkwamdee S, Laohajaroensombat S, Orapin J, Woratanarat P. Effectiveness of extracorporeal shockwave therapy in the treatment of chronic insertional achilles tendinopathy. Foot Ankle Int. 2020;41(4):403–10. https://doi.org/10.1177/1071100719898461.

38. Thueakthong W, de Cesar NC, Garnjanagoonchorn A, et al. Outcomes of iliac crest bone marrow aspirate injection for the treatment of recalcitrant Achilles tendinopathy. Int Orthop. 2021;45(9):2423–8. https://doi.org/10.1007/s00264-021-05112-3.

39. Csizy M, Hintermann B. Rupture of the Achilles tendon after local steroid injection. Case reports and consequences for treatment. Swiss Surg. 2001;7(4):184–9. https://doi.org/10.1024/1023-9332.7.4.184.

40. Yontar NS, Aslan L, Can A, Öğüt T. Mid-term results of open debridement and reattachment surgery for insertional Achilles tendinopathy: a retrospective clinical study. Acta Orthop Traumatol Turc. 2020;54(6):567–71. https://doi.org/10.5152/j.aott.2020.18426.

41. de Cesar NC, Chinanuvathana A, da Fonseca LF, Dein EJ, Tan EW, Schon LC. Outcomes of flexor digitorum longus (FDL) tendon transfer in the treatment of Achilles tendon disorders. Foot Ankle Surg. 2019;25(3):303–9. https://doi.org/10.1016/j.fas.2017.12.003.

42. Hunt KJ, Cohen BE, Davis WH, Anderson RB, Jones CP. Surgical treatment of insertional achilles tendinopathy with or without flexor hallucis longus tendon transfer: a prospective, randomized study. Foot Ankle Int. 2015;36(9):998–1005. https://doi.org/10.1177/1071100715586182.

43. Nawoczenski DA, DiLiberto FE, Cantor MS, Tome JM, DiGiovanni BF. Ankle power and endurance outcomes following isolated gastrocnemius recession for achilles tendinopathy. Foot Ankle Int. 2016;37(7):766–75. https://doi.org/10.1177/1071100716638128.

44. Li HY, Hua YH. Achilles tendinopathy: current concepts about the basic science and clinical treatments. Biomed Res Int. 2016;2016:6492597. https://doi.org/10.1155/2016/6492597.

45. Chen TM, Rozen WM, Pan WR, Ashton MW, Richardson MD, Taylor GI. The arterial anatomy of the Achilles tendon: anatomical study and clinical implications. Clin Anat. 2009;22(3):377–85. https://doi.org/10.1002/ca.20758.

46. Knobloch K, Kraemer R, Lichtenberg A, et al. Achilles tendon and paratendon microcirculation in midportion and insertional tendinopathy in athletes. Am J Sports Med. 2006;34(1):92–7. https://doi.org/10.1177/0363546505278705.

47. Tillander B, Gauffin H, Lyth J, Knutsson A, Timpka T. Symptomatic achilles tendons are thicker than asymptomatic tendons on ultrasound examination in recreational long-distance runners. Sports. 2019;7(12):E245. https://doi.org/10.3390/sports7120245.

48. Jarin I, Bäcker HC, Vosseller JT. Meta-analysis of noninsertional achilles tendinopathy. Foot Ankle Int. 2020;41(6):744–54. https://doi.org/10.1177/1071100720914605.

49. Rompe JD, Furia J, Maffulli N. Eccentric loading versus eccentric loading plus shock-wave treatment for midportion achilles tendinopathy: a randomized controlled trial. Am J Sports Med. 2009;37(3):463–70. https://doi.org/10.1177/0363546508326983.

50. Krogh TP, Ellingsen T, Christensen R, Jensen P, Fredberg U. Ultrasound-guided injection therapy of achilles tendinopathy with platelet-rich plasma or saline: a randomized, blinded, placebo-controlled trial. Am J Sports Med. 2016;44(8):1990–7. https://doi.org/10.1177/0363546516647958.

51. Molund M, Lapinskas SR, Nilsen FA, Hvaal KH. Clinical and functional outcomes of gastrocnemius recession for chronic achilles tendinopathy. Foot Ankle Int. 2016;37(10):1091–7. https://doi.org/10.1177/1071100716667445.

52. Drakos MC, Gott M, Karnovsky SC, et al. Biomechanical analysis of suture anchor vs tenodesis screw for FHL transfer. Foot Ankle Int. 2017;38(7):797–801. https://doi.org/10.1177/1071100717702848.

53. Erickson BJ, Mascarenhas R, Saltzman BM, et al. Is Operative treatment of achilles tendon ruptures superior to nonoperative treatment? A systematic review of overlapping meta-analyses. Orthop J Sports Med. 2015;3(4):2325967115579188. https://doi.org/10.1177/2325967115579188.

54. Kou J. AAOS Clinical practice guideline: acute achilles tendon rupture. J Am Acad Orthop Surg. 2010;18(8):511–3. https://doi.org/10.5435/00124635-201008000-00008.

55. Dams OC, Reininga IHF, Gielen JL, van den Akker-Scheek I, Zwerver J. Imaging modalities in the diagnosis and monitoring of Achilles tendon ruptures: a systematic review. Injury. 2017;48(11):2383–99. https://doi.org/10.1016/j.injury.2017.09.013.

56. Soroceanu A, Sidhwa F, Aarabi S, Kaufman A, Glazebrook M. Surgical versus nonsurgical treatment of acute Achilles tendon rupture: a meta-analysis of randomized trials. J Bone Joint Surg Am. 2012;94(23):2136–43. https://doi.org/10.2106/JBJS.K.00917.

57. Myhrvold SB, Brouwer EF, Andresen TKM, et al. Nonoperative or surgical treatment of acute achilles' tendon rupture. N Engl J Med. 2022;386(15):1409–20. https://doi.org/10.1056/NEJMoa2108447.

58. Lantto I, Heikkinen J, Flinkkila T, et al. A prospective randomized trial comparing surgical and nonsurgical treatments of acute achilles tendon ruptures. Am J Sports Med. 2016;44(9):2406–14. https://doi.org/10.1177/0363546516651060.

59. Renninger CH, Kuhn K, Fellars T, Youngblood S, Bellamy J. Operative and nonoperative management of achilles tendon ruptures in active duty military population. Foot Ankle Int. 2016;37(3):269–73. https://doi.org/10.1177/1071100715615322.

60. Heikkinen J, Lantto I, Flinkkila T, et al. Soleus atrophy is common after the nonsurgical treatment of acute achilles tendon ruptures: a randomized clinical trial comparing surgical and nonsurgical functional treatments. Am J Sports Med. 2017;45(6):1395–404. https://doi.org/10.1177/0363546517694610.

61. Zhang YJ, Long X, Du JY, Wang Q, Lin XJ. Is early controlled motion and weightbearing recommended for nonoperatively treated acute achilles tendon rupture? A systematic review and meta-analysis. Orthop J Sports Med. 2021;9(9):23259671211024604. https://doi.org/10.1177/23259671211024605.

62. Glazebrook M, Rubinger D. Functional rehabilitation for nonsurgical treatment of acute achilles tendon rupture. Foot Ankle Clin. 2019;24(3):387–98. https://doi.org/10.1016/j.fcl.2019.05.001.

63. Park YH, Jeong SM, Choi GW, Kim HJ. How early must an acute Achilles tendon rupture be repaired?

Injury. 2017;48(3):776–80. https://doi.org/10.1016/j.injury.2017.01.020.

64. Goren D, Ayalon M, Nyska M. Isokinetic strength and endurance after percutaneous and open surgical repair of Achilles tendon ruptures. Foot Ankle Int. 2005;26(4):286–90. https://doi.org/10.1177/107110070502600404.

65. Grassi A, Amendola A, Samuelsson K, et al. Minimally invasive versus open repair for acute achilles tendon rupture: meta-analysis showing reduced complications, with similar outcomes, after minimally invasive surgery. J Bone Joint Surg Am. 2018;100(22):1969–81. https://doi.org/10.2106/JBJS.17.01364.

66. Rozis M, Benetos IS, Karampinas P, Polyzois V, Vlamis J, Pneumaticos SG. Outcome of percutaneous fixation of acute achilles tendon ruptures. Foot Ankle Int. 2018;39(6):689–93. https://doi.org/10.1177/1071100718757971.

67. Stavenuiter XJR, Lubberts B, Prince RM, Johnson AH, DiGiovanni CW, Guss D. Postoperative complications following repair of acute achilles tendon rupture. Foot Ankle Int. 2019;40(6):679–86. https://doi.org/10.1177/1071100719831371.

68. Schweitzer KM, Dekker TJ, Adams SB. Chronic achilles ruptures: reconstructive options. J Am Acad Orthop Surg. 2018;26(21):753–63. https://doi.org/10.5435/JAAOS-D-17-00158.

69. Mirmiran R, Squire C, Wassell D. Prevalence and role of a low-lying peroneus brevis muscle belly in patients with peroneal tendon pathologic features: a potential source of tendon subluxation. J Foot Ankle Surg. 2015;54(5):872–5. https://doi.org/10.1053/j.jfas.2015.02.012.

70. Sobel M, Geppert MJ, Olson EJ, Bohne WH, Arnoczky SP. The dynamics of peroneus brevis tendon splits: a proposed mechanism, technique of diagnosis, and classification of injury. Foot Ankle. 1992;13(7):413–22. https://doi.org/10.1177/107110079201300710.

71. van Dijk PAD, Kerkhoffs GMMJ, Chiodo C, DiGiovanni CW. Chronic disorders of the peroneal tendons: current concepts review of the literature. J Am Acad Orthop Surg. 2019;27(16):590–8. https://doi.org/10.5435/JAAOS-D-18-00623.

72. Bruce WD, Christofersen MR, Phillips DL. Stenosing tenosynovitis and impingement of the peroneal tendons associated with hypertrophy of the peroneal tubercle. Foot Ankle Int. 1999;20(7):464–7. https://doi.org/10.1177/107110079902000713.

73. Petersen W, Bobka T, Stein V, Tillmann B. Blood supply of the peroneal tendons: injection and immunohistochemical studies of cadaver tendons. Acta Orthop Scand. 2000;71(2):168–74. https://doi.org/10.1080/000164700317413148.

74. van Dijk PAD, Madirolas FX, Carrera A, Kerkhoffs GMMJ, Reina F. Peroneal tendons well vascularized: results from a cadaveric study. Knee Surg Sports Traumatol Arthrosc. 2016;24(4):1140–7. https://doi.org/10.1007/s00167-015-3946-4.

75. Raikin SM, Elias I, Nazarian LN. Intrasheath subluxation of the peroneal tendons. J Bone Joint Surg Am. 2008;90(5):992–9. https://doi.org/10.2106/JBJS.G.00801.

76. Mengiardi B, Pfirrmann CWA, Schöttle PB, et al. Magic angle effect in MR imaging of ankle tendons: influence of foot positioning on prevalence and site in asymptomatic subjects and cadaveric tendons. Eur Radiol. 2006;16(10):2197–206. https://doi.org/10.1007/s00330-006-0164-y.

77. Latt LD, Kuyumcu G, Taljanovic MS. High-resolution ultrasound and MRI imaging of peroneal tendon injuries. In: Sobel M, editor. The peroneal tendons. Cham: Springer; 2020. p. 97–123. https://doi.org/10.1007/978-3-030-46646-6_5.

78. Unlu MC, Kivrak A, Kayaalp ME, Birsel O, Akgun I. Peritendinous injection of platelet-rich plasma to treat tendinopathy: a retrospective review. Acta Orthop Traumatol Turc. 2017;51(6):482–7. https://doi.org/10.1016/j.aott.2017.10.003.

79. Fram BR, Rogero R, Fuchs D, Shakked RJ, Raikin SM, Pedowitz DI. Clinical Outcomes and complications of peroneal tendon sheath ultrasound-guided corticosteroid injection. Foot Ankle Int. 2019;40(8):888–94. https://doi.org/10.1177/1071100719847629.

80. van Dijk PA, Miller D, Calder J, et al. The ESSKA-AFAS international consensus statement on peroneal tendon pathologies. Knee Surg Sports Traumatol Arthrosc. 2018;26(10):3096–107. https://doi.org/10.1007/s00167-018-4971-x.

81. Danna NR, Brodsky JW. Diagnosis and operative treatment of peroneal tendon tears. Foot Ankle Orthopaedics. 2020;5(2):247301142091040. https://doi.org/10.1177/2473011420910407.

82. Pellegrini MJ, Glisson RR, Matsumoto T, et al. Effectiveness of allograft reconstruction vs tenodesis for irreparable peroneus brevis tears: a cadaveric model. Foot Ankle Int. 2016;37(8):803–8. https://doi.org/10.1177/1071100716658469.

83. Redfern D, Myerson M. The management of concomitant tears of the peroneus longus and brevis tendons. Foot Ankle Int. 2004;25(10):695–707. https://doi.org/10.1177/107110070402501002.

84. Seybold JD, Campbell JT, Jeng CL, Short KW, Myerson MS. Outcome of lateral transfer of the FHL or FDL for concomitant peroneal tendon tears. Foot Ankle Int. 2016;37(6):576–81. https://doi.org/10.1177/1071100716634762.

85. Steel MW, DeOrio JK. Peroneal tendon tears: return to sports after operative treatment. Foot Ankle Int. 2007;28(1):49–54. https://doi.org/10.3113/FAI.2007.0009.

86. Demetracopoulos CA, Vineyard JC, Kiesau CD, Nunley JA. Long-term results of debridement and primary repair of peroneal tendon tears. Foot Ankle Int. 2014;35(3):252–7. https://doi.org/10.1177/1071100713514565.

87. Geppert MJ, Sobel M, Bohne WH. Lateral ankle instability as a cause of superior peroneal retinacu-

lar laxity: an anatomic and biomechanical study of cadaveric feet. Foot Ankle. 1993;14(6):330–4. https://doi.org/10.1177/107110079301400604.

88. Oden RR. Tendon injuries about the ankle resulting from skiing. Clin Orthop Relat Res. 1987;216:63–9.

89. Bakker D, Schulte JB, Meuffels DE, Piscaer TM. Non-operative treatment of peroneal tendon dislocations: a systematic review. J Orthop. 2020;18:255–60. https://doi.org/10.1016/j.jor.2019.08.031.

90. van Dijk PAD, Gianakos AL, Kerkhoffs GMMJ, Kennedy JG. Return to sports and clinical outcomes in patients treated for peroneal tendon dislocation: a systematic review. Knee Surg Sports Traumatol Arthrosc. 2016;24(4):1155–64. https://doi.org/10.1007/s00167-015-3833-z.

91. Schafer KA, Adams SB, McCormick JJ. Peroneal tendonitis and tendonopathy. I: Sobel M, ed. The Peroneal Tendons: A Clinical Guide to Evaluation and Management. Springer International Publishing. 2020:183–191. https://doi.org/10.1007/978-3-030-46646-6_9.

Management of Ligament Injuries of the Ankle

Marisa Deliso, Alex Tang, Richard S. Yoon, and Frank A. Liporace

1 Lateral Ankle Injuries (Lateral Ankle Sprain and Chronic Ankle Instability)

1.1 General

1.1.1 Epidemiology

Lateral ankle sprains (LAS) are one of the most common orthopedic injuries encountered with 2 million acute ankle sprains occurring per year in the United States [1]. Ankle injuries can encompass up to 30–50% of all athletic injuries [2]. The sports with the highest reporting of these injuries include basketball, soccer, volleyball, and gymnastics, with injury rates of 1.1 to 1.3/1000 athlete-exposure. The sports with the lowest reporting of these injuries include baseball, softball, and ice hockey at an injury rate of 0.23–0.32/1000 athlete-exposure [3]. The true incidence may be even higher since more than 50% of athletes with ankle sprains do not seek medical treatment [4].

There is conflicting evidence as to whether females are more prone to these injuries than males [3, 5]. Some authors have shown that the risk of ankle sprain is slightly higher for women than men while others show there is no difference [6, 7]. Eighty percent of ankle sprains occur to the lateral ankle [8]. Those ages of 15 and 19 years carry the greatest incidence for ankle sprains at 7.2 per 1000 person-years and over half of all ankle sprains occur in those 10–24 years old [1]. Ankle sprains constitute 7–10% of all admissions to hospital emergency departments and carry a high socioeconomic burden [2, 9]. Annual healthcare costs of acute ankle sprain treatment reach up to $2 billion [1].

1.1.2 Risk Factors

Many studies have investigated risk factors for LAS. These include age, gender, weight, height, body mass index, limb dominance, patient's anatomy (foot type, foot, and ankle alignment, including foot hyper-pronation), laxity (generalized joint laxity, ankle-joint laxity), ankle and first metatarsophalangeal range-of-motion (ROM), muscle strength, muscle-reaction time, balance and proprioception, and previous history of ankle sprain. Other reported risk factors have included sport-related considerations (including type of sport and level of competition, playing on artificial grass, and playing position), type of sport shoe, lack of warm-up stretching, and landing technique after a jump [2, 10]. Previous history of LAS, high body mass index, ankle joint laxity, and impaired balance are the most important risk factors for sustaining ankle injuries [2].

M. Deliso · A. Tang · R. S. Yoon · F. A. Liporace (✉)
Division of Orthopaedic Trauma and Complex Adult Reconstruction, Department of Orthopaedic Surgery, Cooperman Barnabas Medical Center/Jersey City Medical Center – RWJBarnabas Health, Livingston, NJ, USA

© The Author(s), under exclusive license to Springer Nature Switzerland AG 2023
D. Herscovici Jr. et al. (eds.), *Evaluation and Surgical Management of the Ankle*,
https://doi.org/10.1007/978-3-031-33537-2_6

1.1.3 Anatomy

The lateral ankle ligament complex consists of three ligaments: the anterior talofibular ligament (ATFL), the calcaneofibular ligament (CFL), and the posterior talofibular ligament (PTFL) [5] (Fig. 1). The ATFL functions to restrict both internal rotation and adduction while the ankle is plantar flexed. The CFL prevents adduction and inversion of the calcaneus while the ankle is dorsiflexed [11]. The PTFL functions to limit external rotation [11].

In most cases, the ATFL is the first or only ligament affected. Broström found that combined ruptures of the ATFL and the CFL occurred in 20% of cases and that an isolated rupture of the CFL was very rare [2, 12]. The PTFL is usually not injured in an inversion injury of the ankle because its maximal load to failure is three times that of the ATFL and this ligament is lax when the ankle is plantar flexed [5]. Typically, only gross dislocation of the ankle joint will result in PTFL failure, and it is not seen with ankle sprain injuries.

1.1.4 Mechanism of Injury

Lateral ankle sprains occur from excessive inversion and internal rotation of the hindfoot while the leg is held in external rotation [5, 11]. This happens with a plantar-flexed foot that is placed into supination and adduction (inversion) often seen when landing from a jump or turning during activities [5]. A LAS may also occur with or without contact ranging from impact sports or simple tripping event [3].

The order of injury is typically the lateral joint capsule tearing first, followed by rupture of the ATFL. After complete tear of the ATFL, the CFL fibers are disrupted, followed by a variable injury to the PTFL, and, with increasing force, the deltoid ligament [13]. The injury itself can range from a stretch of the ligaments to a partial or complete tear.

1.1.5 Outcomes

Up to 50% of patients with LAS exhibit residual symptoms and recurrence [2]. In a study, following patients for an average of 6.5 years after LAS found that 17–22% of these patients complained of pain, 26–33% of patients demonstrated persistent swelling, and 35–48% of patients reported an unstable feeling. Moreover, among patients with tenderness in the ATFL during the acute phase of the injury, 32% showed tenderness at the same point 7 years post-injury. In athletes with LAS, who were followed for an average of 6.5 years, 4% had to stop their sport activities due to residual symptoms. Similarly, among nonathletes with ankle sprain, 6% were not able to continue their previous occupation and 15% required external support to continue their original occupation [14]. In another study, previously injured young athletes were followed for 3–15 years and, unfor-

Fig. 1 Image depicting the lateral ligaments of the ankle

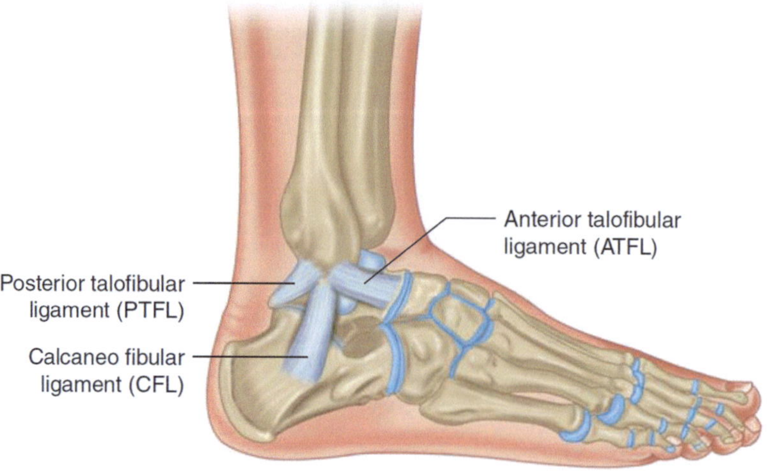

tunately, had more pain and symptoms, poorer self-reported function, ankle-related quality of life, reduced sport participation, balance, and greater fear of pain than those who never sustained an ankle sprain [15].

Recurrent ankle sprains can lead to chronic lateral ankle instability (CLAI) and to significant functional impairment. This can result in a variety of sequelae including an osteochondral injury, chronic pain, and/or a peroneal tendon injury. Accurate assessment and appropriate initial management of the acute ankle sprain may prevent the development of CLAI. However, CLAI may still develop in up to 30% of patients despite adequate nonoperative management [16].

The CLAI may be due to functional and/or mechanical instability and, with repetitive ankle sprains, decreases ankle function and athletic performance. Functional instability is defined by proprioceptive and strength deficits, changes in neuromuscular control, and impaired postural control. It has long been reported that there is an association between muscle weakness and CLAI [16]. In the individual with an ankle sprain, peroneus longus activity decreased in the stance phase during gait, and tibialis anterior activity is increased to compensate.

The normal function of the peroneus longus and soleus, which contribute to landing during jumping activities, are significantly decreased in CLAI patients. Although a recent meta-analysis suggested that concentric eversion strength is decreased in CLAI, there is not yet a consensus regarding the results of inversion and plantar flexion strength [3]. Mechanical ankle instability is defined by laxity of the ankle joint, due to structural damage to any of the three lateral ankle ligaments [11]. In these patients, tibiotalar anterior translation and internal rotation on the injured side were increased compared to the healthy ankle [3].

1.2 Physical Evaluations and Classification

The gold standard for the diagnosis of LAS remains the delayed physical examination (4–5 days post-trauma). Because of the diffuse localization of the pain and swelling within 48 h, the examiner may not be able to differentiate hematoma from edema, and stress maneuvers become less reliable [5]. Physical findings for LAS include tenderness to palpation, hematoma, hemarthrosis, and anterior drawer test (ADT). On physical exam, the patient should be sitting or supine, with both ankles exposed. The uninjured ankle should be examined initially to determine what the patient's baseline exam is. When examining the injured ankle, a thorough exam is necessary.

On inspection, note should be taken on where the patient has swelling and if there is any hematoma or discoloration. On palpation it is important to take note of the particular locations that are tender. ROM may be difficult to assess due to pain. Neurovascular status should be evaluated as with any injury examination. Although tenderness alone may have low specificity, a combination of tenderness, hematoma discoloration, and ADT in the subacute phase (5 days after injury) demonstrate a sensitivity of 96% and a specificity of 84% [17]. Only 14% of individuals without all these findings have a lateral ligament rupture [18].

A special test that can be used for LAS physical examination is the *anterior drawer test*. This is performed by placing one hand to stabilize the anterior distal tibia, and with the foot in approximately 20° of plantar flexion, cupping the patient's calcaneus and placing an anteriorly directed force to the ankle (Fig. 2). Attention should be paid to how much anterior translation occurs to the lateral ankle, and if it is similar to the contralateral side. Again, the uninjured side should be examined first so that a direct comparison can be made. If exam cannot be performed due to patient pain, an ankle block may be considered. One can inject 10 cc of lidocaine just medial to the tibialis anterior and into the ankle joint. This often results in adequate pain relief. Continuing the evaluation, in an ATFL tear, a *dimple sign* may also be visible in the anterior side of the joint in 50% of cases [19] (Fig. 3). During posterior to anterior stress of the talus, negative intra-articular pressure due to the tear causes the subcutaneous tissue to pro-

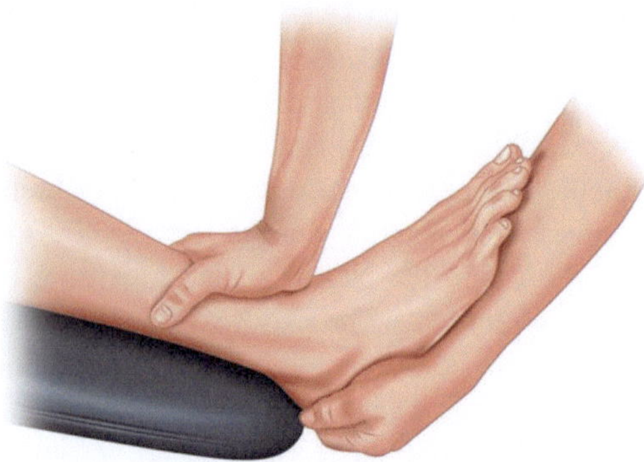

Fig. 2 Image demonstrating the anterior drawer test. This is performed by placing one hand to stabilize the distal tibia (down arrow), and with the foot in approximately 20° of plantar flexion, cupping the patient's calcaneus and placing an anteriorly directed force (up arrow)

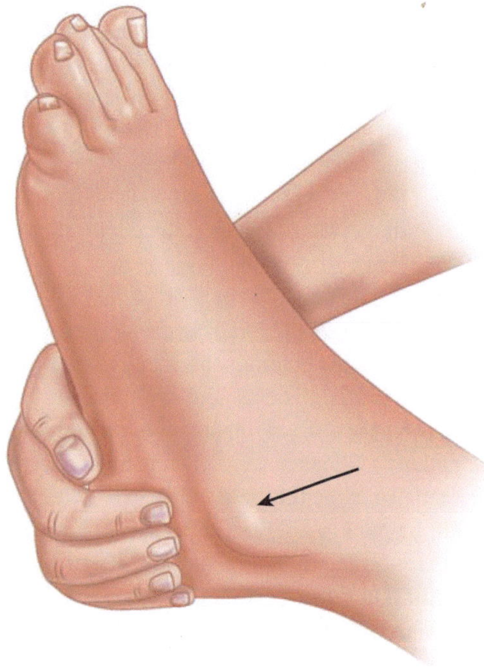

Fig. 3 Image demonstrating a "dimple sign" (depicted by the arrow) which is seen with ATFL tears

duce a divot and create a dimple. Most patients acutely ambulate with an antalgic gait [2]. A previous injury or activity during which the injury occurred, footwear, playing surface, and the use of taping or bracing raise suspicion for LAS [20].

After completion of the physical examination, determining the extent of the injury may help decide the treatment the patient will need. When classifying these injuries, there are several grading and staging systems for lateral ankle ligament injuries, based on anatomical injury, clinical symptoms, trauma mechanism, stability and "severity" of the injury. Hamilton and Kaikkonen introduced a system that incorporates anatomical damage with patient's symptoms (Table 1). However, their classification system is only reliable when made with delayed physical examination [5]. Ottawa rules about the ankle are another useful tool in the evaluation of acute ankle injuries [21]. These rules were established to help physicians decide which patients should have an x-ray following acute ankle injury. These rules suggest that ankle x-rays should be required only if (1) there is any pain or bony tenderness along the distal 6 cm of the posterior edge of tibia or tip of the medial malleolus or (2) pain or bony tenderness along the distal 6 cm of the posterior edge of fibula or tip of the lateral malleolus or (3) the patient is unable to bear weight both immediately following injury and in the emergency department for four steps. While these rules are primarily used to rule out clinically significant ankle fractures, a negative screen can suggest ligamentous injuries that may require further workup depending on the extent of the injury.

1.3 Imaging

1.3.1 X-ray

Radiographic evaluation of the ankle should begin with plain radiographs. This will help to distinguish between a ligamentous and a bony injury. An anteroposterior (AP), oblique, and lateral views of the ankle should be taken. Non-weight-bearing x-rays are acceptable, especially if the patient is in pain. The goal of these radiographs is to exclude a bony injury. In addition to plain radiographs, stress x-rays can be performed that may add more information on the extent of injury. Although often not used, for completeness of a discussion of ankle evaluation, two radiographic stress tests have been reported. These

Table 1 Lateral ankle sprain grading system

Grade	Description	Physical findings	Management
I	Some fibers within the ligament are stretched, but the ligament itself remains intact without laxity	(−) ecchymoses, point tenderness, or loss of function present Decreased ankle motion ≤5° and swelling ≤0.5 cm (−) anterior drawer test, talar tilt test, and stress radiography	Rest, protected weight-bearing, compression, and adhesive taping
II	Involve partial tear of the fibers of the CFL and ATFL with some sign of mild laxity, but overall good stability	(+) Ecchymoses present, point tenderness, and some loss of function present Decreased ankle motion >5° and <10°, swelling >0.5 cm and <2 cm (+) anterior drawer test and (−) talar tilt test and stress radiography	Immobilization followed by aggressive rehabilitation with peroneal strengthening and proprioceptive exercises
III	Complete rupture of the CFL and ATFL ligaments with extensive swelling and ecchymoses. There is instability and the extent of damage is often readily apparent	(++) Extreme ecchymoses, point tenderness, and near total loss of function present Decreased ankle motion ≥10°, swelling ≥2 cm (+) anterior drawer test and talar tilt test Anterior drawer movement >3 mm on stress radiography	Surgical fixation

include the talar tilt test (TTT) and anterior drawer test (ADT) [13].

The TTT measures the angle produced by the tibial plafond and the dome of the talus during forceful inversion of the hindfoot (Fig. 4). A positive test reveals a torn or irreversible stretched lateral ligamentous complex. There is wide disagreement on what constitutes normal tilt of the talus in the ankle. Some studies show that it may range from 5° to 23° of varus tilt in a normal ankle [22, 23]. Comparing both ankles may help to differentiate an abnormal TTT.

The ADT was designed to measure the integrity of the ATFL and may be a more reliable measure than the TTT for diagnosing the extent of ligamentous lateral ankle injuries [13]. It is performed by producing anterior movement of the ankle relative to the distal tibia. This is the same exam maneuver described in the physical exam section, performed with a lateral X-ray. The ADT is measured from the posterior lip of the tibial plafond to the nearest posterior articular surface of the talus. The values for accepted normal subluxation ranges from 2 mm to 9 mm [24, 25]. Again, this should be compared to the contralateral side to determine the difference between ankles.

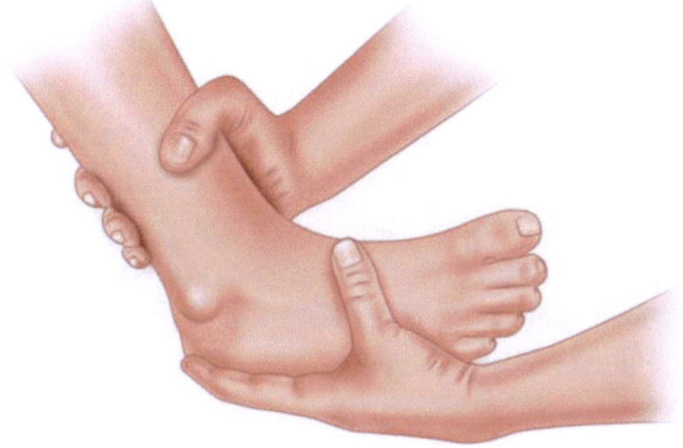

Fig. 4 Image demonstrating the talar tilt test (TTT). The TTT measures the angle produced by the tibial plafond and the dome of the talus during forceful inversion (arrow) of the hindfoot. A positive test reveals a torn or irreversible stretched lateral ligamentous complex

Although high interobserver reliability has been shown on stress X-rays, these examinations often exacerbate pain in the acute phase. In addition, no reports indicate a high sensitivity or specificity for this type of radiographic examination. Some authors feel that ankle stress radiographs are generally unnecessary, unreliable, and outdated for identifying acute ligamentous injuries after ankle sprain. One major reason for this is many studies suggest that ligament laxity, after acute rupture, is not strongly correlated to the development of late symptoms [2, 26].

1.3.2 Ankle Arthrography

Ankle arthrography is not traditionally performed but can be a useful resource in the setting where a magnetic resonance imaging (MRI) is unavailable. Ankle arthrography is performed by injecting approximately 10 cc of contrast material into the ankle joint to identify a ligamentous tear. In a normal exam, the injected contrast will remain within the joint capsule. In up to 10% of cases, the dye may flow into the tendon sheaths of the flexor hallucis longus, flexor digitorum longus, and the subtalar joint, which is not pathological. The dye should not extend beyond the distal end of the lateral malleolus nor should it flow more proximally than 5.5 cm above the distal tip of the fibula [27].

If the ATFL is torn, dye will extravasate anterolaterally. Any extravasation of contrast into the peroneal tendon sheath is abnormal. In most ruptures of the CFL, the medial layer of the peroneal tendon sheath is split longitudinally. If there is flow into the peroneal structures, that is indicative of a tear of both the CFL and ATFL. If the tear in the capsule is very large, there may not be sufficient pressure to force contrast into the sheath even if there is a tear. Therefore, there is a high incidence of false negative rate [13]. In one study, ATFL damage was confirmed by arthrogram in 52% of patients demonstrating tenderness of the ATFL and CFL damage was confirmed in 72% of patients demonstrating tenderness in CFL [3].

This study should not be performed 5 days after the injury. The extravasation of dye may be prevented if performed after 5 days as the tear in the joint capsule or ligament(s) may be closed with blood clots or fibrin tissue.

1.3.3 Ultrasound

Ultrasound can be useful in diagnosing an associated injury during the acute phase, within the first week, and are routinely used in professional athletes [5]. There are reports of up to 95% ATFL and 90% CFL injury diagnostic accuracy [28]. Using ultrasound evaluations for a ligament rupture, has identified a sensitivity is 92% and a specificity of 64%. The positive predictive value is 85% and negative predictive value is 77% [5]. Ultrasound imaging is especially valuable in acute ligamentous injuries, with an accuracy up to 93.8% sensitivity and a 100% specificity, when compared with magnetic resonance imaging (MRI) in diagnosing ATFL tears [29]. The two notable limitations are that acute tears may be difficult to view due to swelling and that its accuracy is highly dependent on the operator and/or equipment [2]. If the images are not interpreted accurately, this often results in a false negative.

1.3.4 MRI

An MRI scan is considered the gold standard for evaluating ligamentous injuries. It can also be useful in diagnosing associated injuries (bone, chondral or tendon) [5]. It is not usually indicated in the routine investigation of acute ankle injuries, within the few weeks, due to high incidence of false-positive findings [2]. In a study, out of 37 complete ATFL tears, 9 were determined to be false positives during surgery (approximately 24%) [30]. As previously stated, it is also useful in detecting osteochondral lesions of the talus and determining whether any injuries occurred to the ankle syndesmotic ligaments [2]. A high percentage of patients identified with ATFL and CFL injuries have also demonstrated injury to the posterior tibialis tendon, peroneus brevis, or peroneus longus [3]. The accuracy of MRI for ATFL partial and complete tears was 74% and 79%, respectively, with a sensitivity and specificity of 64% and 86% for partial tears and 78% and 80% for complete tears, respectively. The accuracy of MRI for CFL partial and complete tears was 66% and 88%, respectively, with a sensitivity and specificity of 41% and 87% for partial tears and 61% and 95% for complete tears, respectively [30].

1.4 Treatment

1.4.1 Nonoperative Management

After performing a physical examination, imaging studies of the ankle, and classifying the ligamentous injury, a discussion with the patient should then be undertaken about the treatment needed to manage the injury. Successful treatment of acute lateral ankle ligament injuries, regardless of grade, can be achieved with individualized aggressive, non-operative measures. Protection, Rest, Ice, Compression, and Elevation (PRICE) therapy is the treatment of choice for the first 4–5 days. This initial approach is designed to reduce pain and swelling. The authors also believe that 2 weeks of immobilization is beneficial, either in an air cast or brace. After 2 weeks, the authors' preferred treatment is the use of a lace-up brace or functional taping, to reduce the risk of recurrent injury. Ankle bracing or taping improves mechanical and functional stability which reduces reinjury rates, improves proprioception, and allows individuals to continue their activities of daily living. Functional taping is typically reserved for athletes, while the majority of patients receive a brace. A study discussing athletes, who have taped or braced after an acute injury, reported 70% fewer ankle injuries compared to individuals without any external support [31]. There is debate between early mobilization versus short-term immobilization upon initial injury. The Collaborative Ankle Support Trial (CAST) study demonstrated faster recovery with a short period of immobilization when compared to treatment solely a compression bandage [32]. Controlling the stress on the ligaments promotes proper orientation of collagen fibers, which allows for full return to activities, between 4 and 8 weeks post-injury [5].

Physical rehabilitation includes proprioceptive training and eversion strengthening of the peroneus brevis, typically beginning 2–3 weeks after the injury, when the swelling decreases. The addition of ultrasound or electrical muscle stimulation have not demonstrated any effectiveness in symptom relief or resolution [2].

In addition to PRICE therapy and acute immobilization, the authors recommend the use of nonsteroidal anti-inflammatory drugs (NSAIDs). This has been shown to provide pain and swelling relief within the first 3 weeks, without any negative long-term effects [5, 11]. Acetaminophen and opioids seem to be equally effective as NSAIDs for pain, swelling, and ROM in the first

2 weeks following acute sprain, although opioids have significantly more adverse effects and should be avoided all together [2].

In addition to the use of PRICE, immobilization, NSAIDs and braces, the treatment of ligamentous injuries has also included biologics (such as platelet-rich plasma (PRP) and hyaluronic acid) injections. These are more recent developments where the efficacy continues to be studied. To date, there is no literature supporting its efficacy in reducing pain and improving functional outcomes to be greater than placebos. As such, further study in this field is warranted.

1.5 Operative Management

Surgery for the repair of acute injuries is not without higher costs, longer recovery times, higher incidences of ankle stiffness, impaired ankle mobility, and increased risk of complications, such as wound-healing problems, nerve damage, and possible infections [26]. Unless the patient is a high performing athlete, surgery is typically not recommended for the management of acute injuries. Although acute repair of the lateral ankle ligaments in grade III injuries in professional athletes may give better results than nonoperative treatment, major reviews have failed to demonstrate a clearly superior treatment approach for LAS between surgical and conservative management [33]. This may be due to a higher proportion of objective stability observed on stress radiography, compared to non-operative treatment, which results in fewer recurrences of LAS [5].

1.5.1 Primary Repair (Broström and Its Modifications)

In patients with chronic lateral ankle instability, the operative standard of care is an anatomic repair of the lateral ligamentous complex. The most common anatomic repair is the use of the Broström procedure and its modifications (Table 2). This approach is used to correct instability that has occurred with chronic injuries to the ATFL and the CFL.

The procedure for isolated ligament repair uses a curved incision over the anterior border of the lateral malleolus or an extensile longitudinal incision along the distal fibula when additional tendon or retinaculum needs to be repaired

Table 2 Surgical techniques about the lateral ankle for anatomic reconstruction

Technique	Utility	Description
Brostrom	Used for isolated ligament repairs	Uses a curved incision over the anterior border of the lateral malleolus or an extensive longitudinal incision along the distal fibula when an additional tendon or retinaculum needs to be repaired The ATFL and CFL are dissected from the surrounding tissue and repaired in a pants-over-vest technique
Gould modification	Increases repair strength by 50%, limits inversion to stabilize the subtalar joint	In addition to the Brostrom procedure, the extensor retinaculum is sutured to the distal fibular and pulled proximally
Karlsson modification	Decreases chronic laxity, promotes ligament-to-bone healing	In addition to the Brostrom procedure, scar tissue is excised, ligaments are sectioned 3-5 mm from their insertions on the fibular and then reattached to the fibula using drill holes or suture anchors

(Fig. 5). The ATFL and CFL are identified at the lateral aspect of the capsule when the tissues are retracted anteriorly. The ATFL and CFL are dissected from the surrounding tissue and repaired in a pants-over-vest technique. To confirm that the repair has not limited the ankle ROM, full dorsi- and plantar flexion should be performed intraoperatively. This procedure is highly effective with 91% of patients reporting good or excellent results, based on the Good Ankle Function Scale [34]. A total of 87% of the patients had full ankle joint ROM restored postoperatively [34].

A second type of ligament repair is the Karlsson technique. This surgical approach is performed by excising scar tissue, sectioning the ligaments 3–5 mm from their insertions on the fibula, and then reattaching them to the fibula using drill holes or suture anchors. The advantage of this technique is that it promotes ligament-to-bone healing versus ligament-to-ligament healing as seen in the Broström procedure. Eighty-eight percent of patients treated with this procedure demonstrated good to excellent functional results, including stability, pain, activity levels, and swelling [35]. Patients with generalized hypermobility, long-standing ligamentous insufficiency, or previous tenodesis surgery are more likely to have unsatisfactory results regardless of technique used [16].

Modifications have also been discussed to improve the strength of these reconstructions. One such technique is the Gould modification [36]. This approach consists of elevating and

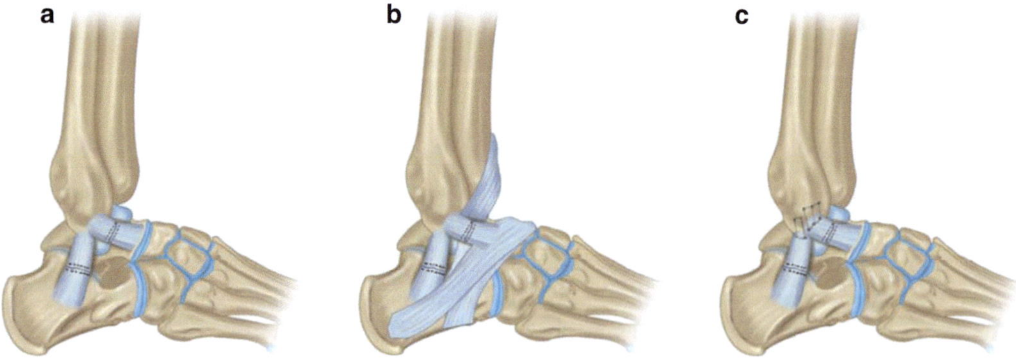

Fig. 5 Image depicting the Broström procedure (**a**) and its modifications, namely the Gould modification (**b**) and the Karlsson modification (**c**)

suturing the extensor retinaculum to the distal fibula by pulling it proximally. The addition of the Gould modification has also been shown to limit inversion of the ankle and to stabilize the subtalar joint with no statistically significant differences of ankle kinematics between repaired ankles and contralateral normal ankles [36].

In patients who present with absent or excessively damaged ligaments, these procedures will likely not be possible or effective. In these situations, an anatomic versus non-anatomic reconstruction must be considered using either allograft, autograft, or tendon transfer [11]. Non-anatomic reconstruction techniques involve rerouting the peroneus brevis tendon through bone tunnels in the distal fibula and include the Watson-Jones, Evans, and Chrisman-Snook procedures (Table 3). These non-anatomic reconstructions have been shown to have poorer long-term outcomes with a greater risk of progression to arthritis, due to alterations in ankle and hindfoot kinematics and the loss of subtalar motion [11, 16].

For anatomic graft reconstructions, the anatomy and mechanics of the ATFL and CFL are recreated via autogenous or allogenic tendon graft placement at the native ligament insertion sites. These are then routed through tunnels in the distal fibula, the talus, and the calcaneus. The tendon grafts can be fixed with interference screws into the tunnels or sutured to themselves [11]. Graft augmentation can also be helpful in patients with CLAI, those that have poor tissue quality, a failed previous repair, generalized ligamentous laxity, and a cavovarus foot deformity. One noted potential risk of both anatomic and non-anatomic reconstructions is an iatrogenic fracture through the fibular tunnels.

1.5.2 Ankle Arthroscopic and Arthroscopic Ligament Repair

Arthroscopy is useful in diagnosing intra-articular conditions associated with CLAI, such as impingement, loose bodies, osteochondral lesions, chondromalacia, and bone spurs [16]. It is commonly performed in combination with open lateral ankle ligament reconstruction, for diagnostic purposes, as well as addressing concomitant intra-articular lesions. In addition, an arthroscopic Broström repair has been shown to restore ankle function equivalent to open repair but with the advantages of smaller scars, less pain, less swelling, less disturbance of cutaneous sensation, and possibly faster recovery [11, 16]. However, this type of repair may be dependent on the surgeon's skill when using this technique.

Table 3 Surgical techniques about the lateral ankle for non-anatomic reconstruction

Technique	Utility	Description
Watson-Jones	Controls internal rotation and anterior displacement of the talus, less effective in controlling talar tilt, restricts subtalar joint motion	Uses a curved incision immediately posterior to the lateral malleolus toward the base of the fifth metatarsal bone. The superior peroneal retinaculum is released to free the peroneus brevis tendon, which is then longitudinally dissected in half until its passage under the apex of the lateral malleolus. Two holes are then drilled into the talus and the lateral malleolus. The peroneus brevis half tendon is passed through the malleolar hole first, and then through the talar hole where its free edge is sutured to the calcaneus
Evans	Allows increased anterior displacement, internal rotation, and talar tilt; restricts subtalar joint motion	The proximal end of the peroneus brevis muscle is sutured to the peroneus longus and transposed anterior to the lateral malleolus where it is passed posteriorly through a drill hole in the distal fibula and then sutured onto itself
Chrisman-Snook	Allows increased internal rotation and anterior displacement of the talus, limits talar tilt, restricts subtalar joint motion	Routes the transferred portion of peroneus brevis tendon along the lateral wall of the os calcis subperiosteally instead of directly drilling a tunnel through the calcaneus

1.6 Post-operative Management

Postoperatively, the authors' approach is to place patients into a non-weight-bearing Arbeitsgemeinschaft für Osteosynthesefragen (AO) splint for the first 2 weeks. After the cast is removed, patients are placed into a removable boot and physical therapy is started focusing on ROM activities, muscle strengthening and proprioceptive training. Partial weight-bearing is begun 4 weeks postoperatively with full weight-bearing allowed at 6 weeks postoperatively. A graduated functional return to a training program is set on an individual basis, aiming for return to training and/or play within 12 weeks of injury [5].

For athletes, return to sport timelines are not well defined and are dependent on the specific injury and the surgery performed. Once 90% of ankle strength has been restored, at approximately 3-months postoperatively, patients may return to play. Ankle bracing or taping for at least 6 months after surgery must be considered for all athletes returning to play as these interventions have been shown to have a 70% decrease in recurrent ankle sprains [11].

2 Medial Ankle Injuries

2.1 General

2.1.1 Epidemiology

Approximately 3–4% of all ankle sprains consist of isolated deltoid ligament injuries [29]. Twelve percent of ankle osteoarthritis cases are the result of medial ligament lesions and 3% are due to combined medial and lateral ligament lesions [29]. The most common cause of recurrent medial ankle instability is an uncorrected hindfoot valgus or pes planovalgus. Inappropriate treatment of both combined or isolated medial ankle sprains can result in chronic rotational ankle instability. In addition, osteochondral lesions (OCL) are often found concurrently with injuries involving the medial ligamentous complex in as high as 20% of cases [29].

2.1.2 Anatomy

The deltoid ligament is the primary stabilizer of the ankle against plantar flexion [29]. It is composed of a superficial and deep layer (Fig. 6). The superficial component deltoid ligament is primarily attached to the anterior colliculus of the medial malleolus and spans both the ankle and the subtalar joints. It consists of the tibionavicular, tibiospring, tibiocalcaneal, and superficial posterior talotibial ligaments. The deep layer is primarily attached to the posterior colliculus of the medial malleolus and the intercollicular groove. It crosses only the ankle joint and consists of the deep anterior and posterior tibiotalar ligaments. The superficial component has been shown to limit external rotation and resist valgus stress of the ankle and hindfoot. The deep component resists ankle eversion and lateral migration of the talus. An additional ligamentous structure, that helps augment the deltoid ligament

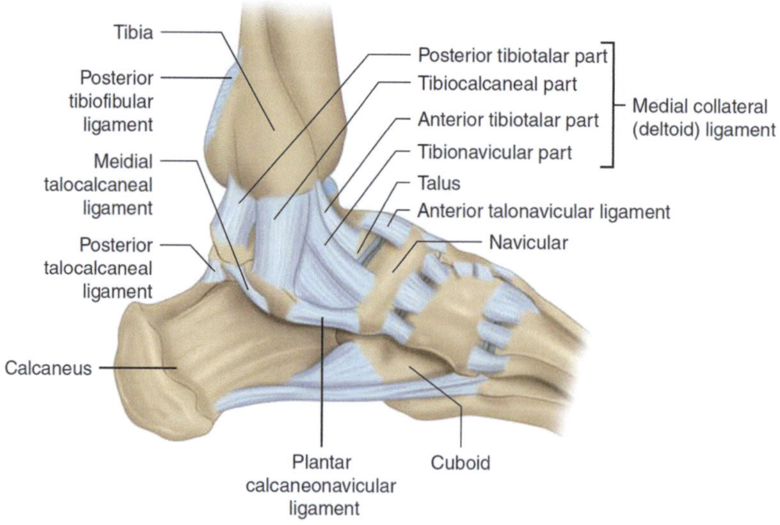

Fig. 6 Image depicting the deltoid ligament of the medial ankle

and aids in stabilization of the medial ankle, is the calcaneonavicular (spring) ligament. It is part of the deltoid ligament complex and consists of two components: the superomedial and inferior ligaments. The spring ligament assists in stabilizing the medial ankle structures of the ankle joint through its connection to the deltoid via the tibiospring ligament [29].

2.1.3 Mechanism

The mechanism of injury is suspected to be a combination of external rotation and eversion of the foot. Alternatively, a fixed foot with an inward twist of the body places stress on the medial ligamentous complex. Deltoid injuries can also occur with pronation and external rotation ankle fractures (Weber C), pronation abduction ankle fractures and less frequently with supination external rotation (Weber B) ankle fractures [29]. It has been reported that the deltoid ligament is involved in up to 40% of ankle fractures [37].

2.1.4 Outcomes

Chronic medial ligamentous instability contributes to chronic medial ankle instability (CMAI). This occurs due to pathologic laxity of the deltoid ligament. The talus falls medially, with talonavicular subluxation, creating a varus deformity in chronic injuries. This contributes to a laxity of the spring ligament and results into the development of pes planus [29]. In addition to chronic ligamentous instability, abnormal bony pathology, seen in patients with a wider talar dome and smaller tibial plafond, can also contribute to chronic mechanical instability [29].

Mechanical ankle instability is defined by laxity of the ankle joint due to the damaged structures, while functional instability is the result of an impaired proprioception and a slowed neuromuscular reflex. However, mechanical instability may result in functional instability. End stage functional instability can be identified when CMAI patients have difficulty maintaining their position during single leg stance [29].

2.2 Physical Examination and Classification

Patients with an acute injury of the deltoid ligament often present with acute swelling, hematoma, and the inability to bear weight. On physical exam, the patient should be sitting or supine, with both ankles exposed. The uninjured ankle should be examined initially to determine what the patient's baseline exam is, similar to the lateral ankle exam. On inspection, note should be taken on where the patient has swelling and if there is any hematoma or discoloration, particularly over the medial ankle complex. On palpation, tenderness will be present over the deltoid complex, just distal to the medial malleolus. ROM may be difficult to assess due to pain. Neurovascular status should be evaluated, as with any injury examination. To evaluate the superficial deltoid ligament, an external rotation test should be utilized, while an eversion stress test is used to assess the deep deltoid ligament [29]. This is performed with the patient in the supine position. One hand is used to stabilize the distal tibia, and with the foot in dorsiflexion, the ankle is either internally or externally rotated.

In CMAI, the patient will complain about the ankle instability. They will demonstrate pain over the anteromedial surface of the ankle, posterior tibial tenderness, and a correctable hindfoot valgus deformity [29]. With the development of intra-articular impingement in CMAI, defined as structures entrapped within the ankle joint during terminal dorsiflexion and/or plantar flexion, mechanical symptoms such as catching, or locking may also be present [29]. Further evaluation of a deltoid injury should be performed with the patient standing. During weight-bearing one should inspect gait and ankle position of the affected ankle, to identify whether there is any planovalgus and abductus of the hindfoot (flat foot with ankle appearing to be pointing inward and heel pointing outward) [29]. After evaluating the ankle for a deltoid injury, the examiner should consider classifying these injuries. Valderrabano et al. classified clinical CMAI into four grades based on increasing severity and ligamentous damage and also created an arthroscopic and intraoperative classification, to determine the severity of the injury [38] (Table 4).

2.3 Imaging

2.3.1 X-ray

Standard ankle radiographs, including supine AP, oblique and lateral views should be used to evaluate the medial ankle clear space, to identify whether there is a bony deltoid avulsion fragment, to assess whether any widening of the syndesmosis has occurred, and whether there are any other associated ankle fractures. Standing views can be utilized to place weight-bearing stress on the ankle complex but is often deferred due to pain.

An increased medial clear space, compared to the contralateral extremity, is indicative of complete tear of the deltoid ligament [39]. Normal medial clear space ranges from 3–4 mm [40]. Other conditions that can be evaluated using plain X-rays include the presence of a foot deformity (such as pes planovalgus and abductus of the hindfoot), OCL of the talus and plafond, bony impingements, and early osteoarthritic changes [29].

2.3.2 Ankle Arthrography

As stated previously, ankle arthrography is not traditionally performed but can be a useful resource in the setting where MRI is unavailable. It is performed by injecting nearly 10 cc of contrast into the ankle joint to identify any ligamentous tears. The injected contrast will remain within the joint capsule if there are no ligamentous injuries present. If the deltoid complex is torn, the dye will extravasate medially. Similar to lateral ligamentous injuries, this should be performed within the first week as fibrinous tissue may block extravasation of dye and effect results.

Table 4 Anatomic, clinical, and arthroscopic classifications of CMAI

Grade	Anatomic classification	Clinical classification	Arthroscopic classification
I	Proximal tear or avulsion (most common)	(+) Giving way (+) Hindfoot valgus/pronation (+) Medial ankle pain (+) Anterolateral ankle pain (−) Posterior tibial dysfunction (+) Flexible deformity	Partial tear of the superficial deltoid ligament, normal deep deltoid ligament (+) Medial malleolus periosteal scar and osteophytes Tibiotalar distance of 2–5 mm (−) Lateral ligament lesion
II	Intermediate tear	(++) Giving way (++) Hindfoot valgus/pronation (++) Medial ankle pain (+) Anterolateral ankle pain (+) Posterior tibial dysfunction (+) Flexible deformity	Ruptured superficial deltoid ligament, partial tear of deep deltoid ligament (++) Medial malleolus Periosteal scar and osteophytes Tibiotalar distance of 2–5 mm (−) Lateral ligament lesion
III	Distal tear or avulsion	(+++) Giving way (+++) Hindfoot valgus/pronation (+++) Medial ankle pain (++) Anterolateral ankle pain (++) Posterior tibial dysfunction (+) Flexible deformity	Ruptured superficial deltoid ligament, partial tear of deep deltoid ligament (+++) Medial malleolus periosteal scar and osteophytes Tibiotalar distance of <5 mm (+) Lateral ligament lesion
IV	N/A	(++++) Giving way (++++) Hindfoot valgus/pronation (++++) Medial ankle pain (+++) Anterolateral ankle pain (+++) Posterior tibial dysfunction (−) Flexible deformity	Ruptured superficial and deep deltoid ligaments (++++) Medial malleolus periosteal scar and osteophytes Tibiotalar distance of <5 mm (+) Lateral ligament lesion

2.3.3 Ultrasound

Ultrasonography is a valuable tool in assessing medial ankle instability. It is not used as often as it is in lateral ligament injuries but may still be useful. The benefits are accessibility, cost, and it can also be performed in real time using joint stress maneuvers to assess for ankle ligament stability and bony impingement [29]. The greatest downfall of this tool is that it is very user dependent which can result in a high false negative if a ruptured deltoid complex is misinterpreted.

2.3.4 MRI

An MRI scan is often used in the diagnosis of acute and chronic medial ankle injuries. It can identify the extent of the injury and associated pathologic conditions, as well as assist in preoperative planning. It has been reported that up to 20% of patients may have false negative MRI findings in the setting of acute deltoid ligament complex injury associated with ankle fractures [41].

2.4 Nonoperative Management

Nonoperative management is often utilized as the initial treatment for isolated deltoid ligament complex injuries. PRICE is encouraged during the first 2 weeks. The use of a soft ankle orthosis, such as air cast or compression wrap, is indicated for simple sprains (grade I) until the patient is pain-free and has reached pre-injury strength levels. This often takes 3–4 weeks. More severe sprains (grades II–III) require eversion avoidance and may require a functional ankle brace that should be worn for at least 6 weeks.

Physical therapy should focus on ROM followed by neuromuscular and strength training, especially of the posterior tibial muscle [29]. Physical therapy should begin after 3–4 weeks of immobilization and should continue until preinjury strength returns, which can be 6–12 weeks after the injury. The use of NSAIDs can also be used as an adjuvant anti-inflammatory and for pain relief, during the first few weeks following injury, and as a method of pain relief during physical therapy sessions.

2.5 Operative Management

Operative treatment may be pursued in patients who have failed to improve with conservative measures, over 6 months in duration [29]. Chronic complaints of instability, recurrent sprains, persistent pain, and a worsening pes planovalgus deformity of the ankle may be an indication for surgical intervention. Treatment options for the deltoid include primary repair, primary repair with augmentation, and occasionally supplementation with bony work if there is fracture or chronic deformity.

Primary repair is dependent on the level of ligament injury and soft tissue structure. The authors' preferred approach is to repair the deltoid ligament from distal to proximal and attach it to the medial malleolus via transosseous sutures or anchors (Fig. 7). Sutures should be tightened with the ankle held at 90° of dorsiflexion. Augmentation reconstruction is an option if the soft tissues are inadequate for a stable direct repair. In settings of posterior tibial tendon insufficiency, a hindfoot reconstruction may be required to augment any posterior tibial tendon reconstruction that is necessary.

In up to 40 % of ankle fractures the deltoid ligament is injured [37]. In patients presenting

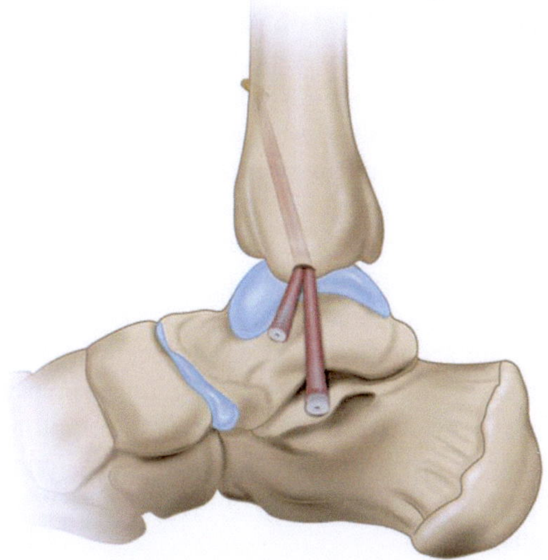

Fig. 7 Image depicting deltoid ligament reconstruction utilizing transosseous sutures and anchors

with both a deltoid ligament injury and a medial malleolus fracture, both ligament repair and fracture fixation are recommended, in certain circumstances [41, 42]. Associated medial malleolus fractures and ligamentous injuries, with a fracture width of less than 17 mm, risk residual deltoid insufficiency despite satisfactory fragment fixation [42]. In lateral malleolar fractures, the medial ligament should heal adequately if the lateral malleolus is well reduced. However, a persistent increase in the medial clear space or a demonstrated intraoperative valgus instability may require surgical exploration and deltoid repair [43].

2.5.1 Arthroscopy

Although not routinely performed, diagnostic arthroscopy can help detect deltoid ligament insufficiency and evaluate anatomic structural abnormalities within the deltoid, spring ligament, and posterior tibial tendon. Many studies support visualizing the deltoid ligament complex and associated injuries intraoperatively prior to surgical intervention [29, 37].

2.6 Post-operative Management

For the first 6 weeks, the authors' preference is to put the patient into a high stabilizing walking boot and placed on partial weight-bearing protocols. The boot will maintain the ankle at 90° (neutral position) and physical therapy, focusing on ROM, should begin after the 2 week post-operative visit. After 6 weeks, the authors recommend discontinuation of the boot and utilization of a sneaker with a soft ankle orthosis (compression wrap air cast), until 12 weeks post-operative. After ROM, physical therapy should focus on proprioception, coordination, and muscle strengthening exercises [29]. A graduated functional return to training program is set on an individual basis aiming for return to activities within 12-weeks post-injury [5].

3 Syndesmotic Injuries

3.1 General

3.1.1 Epidemiology

The syndesmosis refers to the ligaments of the ankle that connect the tibia and fibula. In the United States, it is estimated that there are nearly 6500 syndesmotic injuries per year [44]. The majority of these injuries occur in those 18–34 years of age but affects individuals of all ages. In the athlete, a study that looked at European professional soccer teams, revealed that 7% of all ankle injuries (both fractures and sprains) sustained by players were isolated syndesmotic injuries [45]. Syndesmotic injuries can be in isolation, known as high ankle sprains, or with associated ankle fractures. High ankle sprains encompass up to 12% of all ankle sprains in the common population and 25% of ankle sprains sustained in collision sports [46]. In individuals with lateral ankle sprains, the rate of additional syndesmotic injury was nearly 18% [47]. This underscores the need for a careful examination of ankle injuries, regardless of the reported mechanism of injury, particularly given the possibility of concomitant ligamentous injury.

Approximately 10% of all ankle fractures are associated with syndesmotic damage. If the patient's ankle fracture requires operative fixation, nearly 20% have been found to have an associated syndesmotic injury [48]. When breaking down incidence, using the Danis-Weber classification of lateral malleolus fractures, a Weber A injury (inferior to level of syndesmosis) is rarely associated with syndesmotic injury (less than 3%). A Weber B (at level of syndesmosis) and Weber C (superior to syndesmosis) have been shown to have a 30–40% incidence and up to 80% incidence, respectively [49].

3.1.2 Risk Factors

A variety of risk factors have been explored. A frequently investigated factor, gender, is not determined to be a risk factor for injury [50].

Sports that may expose the individual to high-speed collisions, high torque cutting, and jumping may increase risk of syndesmotic injury. Other risk factors include artificial surfaces and uneven terrains [46]. Mechanisms of injury other than those observed in sporting activities include falls or tripping accidents with twisting weight-bearing injuries and motor vehicle accidents.

3.1.3 Anatomy

The ligaments that compose the syndesmosis (Fig. 8) are the anterior-inferior tibiofibular ligament (AITFL), interosseous ligament, interosseous membrane, posterior-inferior tibiofibular ligament (PITFL), transverse tibiofibular ligament, and inferior transverse ligament. The tibia has a concave triangular groove, just above the lateral articular surface, described as the incisura that the fibula lies in. The syndesmosis maintains this important relationship between the tibia and fibula and preserves ankle stability.

The AITFL runs from the distal anterolateral tibial (Chaput's) tubercle to the distal anterior (Wagstaffe's) tubercle on the fibula. The PITFL runs from the posterolateral tibial tubercle to the posterolateral malleolus, above the digital fossa. The inferior transverse ligament runs from the posterolateral tibia to the posteromedial distal fibula. The interosseous membrane runs from the tibia periosteum to the fibula down to the tibiotalar joint. At that level, it is known as the interosseous ligament [46, 51].

3.1.4 Mechanism of Injury

Typically, injuries to the syndesmosis occur when an external rotation force is applied to a dorsiflexed ankle. The talus then places a lateral force on the fibula, separating the fibula from the tibia. This results in the fibula externally rotating and displacing posteriorly. If the foot is pronated during the external rotation, it often results in injury to the AITFL. If the foot is in neutral, it often affects the deltoid [52]. Up to 55% of high ankle sprains may be caused by a collision injury while the foot is externally rotated and planted on the ground [53].

3.2 Physical Evaluations and Classification

On physical exam, the patient should be sitting or supine, with both ankles exposed. Historically, the patient will often complain of feeling a dif-

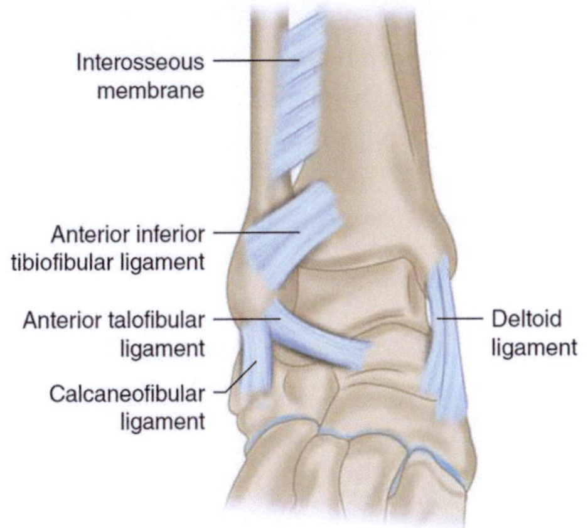

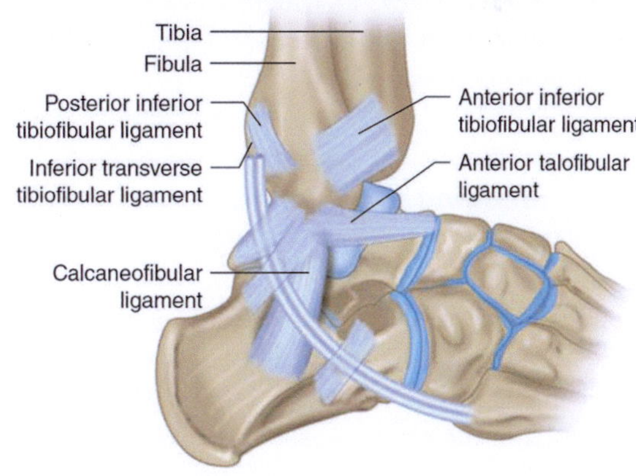

Fig. 8 Image depicting the syndesmotic ligaments of the ankle, which is composed of several structures including the anterior-inferior tibiofibular ligament (AITFL), interosseous membrane (IOM), posterior-inferior tibiofibular ligament (PITFL), and transverse tibiofibular ligament (TTFL)

fuse, generalized ankle pain. On inspection, determine if the patient has swelling and whether there is any hematoma or discoloration about the ankle. This is diffuse and often seen at the level of the ankle joint but it can extend to the junction of the distal third of the leg. On palpation, patients often have tenderness at the tibiofibular joint that extends proximally. ROM may be difficult to assess due to pain. Neurovascular status should be evaluated as with any injury examination.

Special maneuvers that can be used for a syndesmotic injury include *the squeeze test, the tibiofibular shuck or Cotton test, abduction and external rotation test* and the *fibular translation test*. A complete explanation of how to perform these tests and references is listed in chapter "Evaluation of Ankle Pain".

Regarding classification, there is no definitive agreed upon system. In all, the sprain is classified from Grade 1 to 3, with 3 being the most severe. Grade 1 is described as mild injury with a stable joint and normal X-rays. Grade 2 is a moderate injury and indicates that there has been a partial ligament disruption, with positive provocative exams, but normal X-rays. There is no established agreement on if there is ankle stability in this grade of sprains. The authors believe this is an unstable injury and treat it as so. Grade 3 is a severe, complete injury to the syndesmotic ligaments. X-rays show a widened clear space between the tibia and fibula and provocative exams that are positive.

3.3 Imaging

3.3.1 Plain Radiography

Standard ankle radiographs, including supine AP, oblique and lateral views should be used to evaluate the medial ankle clear space, if any widening (diastasis) of the syndesmosis has occurred, and to determine whether there are any associated ankle fractures. Some may find weight-bearing X-rays helpful to place stress on the syndesmotic ligaments and evaluate for tibiofibular diastasis. The three factors used to evaluate this diastasis is tibiofibular clear space, tibiofibular overlap and medial clear space. On the mortise view the nor-

mal values for each are <6 mm, >1 mm, and <4 mm, respectively [54].

The tibiofibular clear space is measure from the lateral border of the posterior tibial malleolus to the medial border of the distal fibula, 1 cm above the plafond. This can be measured on the AP or mortise view with normal <6 mm. This is the authors' preferred method of measurement as it is not affected by ankle rotation. The tibiofibular overlap is measured from the anterior tibial tubercle's lateral edge and the medial distal fibula. Normal value on the AP is >6 mm and the mortise is >1 mm. Because this measurement is affected by foot rotation it is not as reliable. Medial clear space is measured from the lateral edge of the medial malleolus to the medial border of the talus. This is measured on the mortise view and normal is <4 mm. As it can only be accurately measured on the mortise view, it is affected by ankle rotation. If there are any questions about abnormal findings, a comparison view of the non-injured contralateral extremity should also be taken.

3.3.2 Ankle Arthrography and Ultrasound

Unlike with medial and lateral ligamentous complex injuries, ultrasound and ankle arthrography are not diagnostic modalities commonly utilized for syndesmosis evaluation. Ankle arthrography has limited value in syndesmotic injury and, has previously been stated, is often used for lateral ankle injury suspicions and sometimes medial. Ultrasound may have a role in the future to determine tibiofibular diastasis but is not often useful at this point in time.

3.3.3 MRI

As with near all soft tissue ligamentous injury, MRI is the most accurate tool for diagnosis. It is fundamental to confirming suspicion when there is doubt on simply clinical exam and plain radiographs [54]. An MRI has a sensitivity, specificity, and accuracy of 100%, 93%, and 96%, respectively for diagnosing AITFL ruptures and 100%, 100%, and 100%, respectively, for diagnosing PITFL tears [46]. MRI also can diagnose associated injuries of the bone, cartilage, other ligaments and tendons.

3.4 Nonoperative Management

Grade I stable, purely ligamentous injuries are treated nonoperatively. PRICE therapy is a mainstay of this treatment. They are placed in a supportive CAM boot and remain non-weight-bearing for the first 4 days, to allow the acute inflammation and pain to reside. The patient is then instructed to continue the CAM boot but begin weight-bearing as tolerated and may remove the boot and begin active ROM [46]. After the first week, and after the inflammation has subsided, the patient may discontinue the boot and replace it with a soft brace or ace wrap. Patients will continue to weight bear as tolerated, continue their ROM exercises, and begin a strengthening program. Some patients may benefit from NSAIDs, as a pain reliever for the first week. Patients often do not need formal physical therapy but if they have not fully recovered within 4–6 weeks, physical therapy may be started.

3.5 Operative Management

Unstable syndesmotic injuries should be treated with operative management. The authors believe this includes Grade 2 and Grade 3 high ankle sprains and nearly all fractures with concomitant syndesmotic injuries. The treatment involves stabilization of the syndesmosis, and reduction and fixation of the fractures.

The fracture should be anatomically reduced and fixed first, then syndesmotic stability should be assessed. This is performed under fluoroscopy. The authors' preference is to use an external rotation stress test, or the cotton hook test can be used intraoperatively. The Cotton hook test is performed by translating the fixed fibula laterally via a clamp [55]. Both tests assess for widening of the syndesmosis. If normal parameters are not restored, the surgeon should proceed with syndesmotic stabilization.

There are two common methods for syndesmotic fixation: screw fixation and suture button fixation [56].

3.5.1 Screw Fixation

Screw fixation, under fluoroscopic guidance, is used most commonly, but there is no consensus on screw size, number of screws, number of cortices, and need for implant removal [56]. Either 3.5 mm or 4.5 mm screws are used and are placed 2–5 cm proximal to the ankle joint and parallel to the articular surface. Due their size and strength, 4.5 screws break less often although such a rigid construct may not be a benefit. They are easier to remove but often leave a larger defect, which may create a stress on the fibula, resulting in a fracture. Regardless of the screw size used, there is no difference between a three to four cortex fixation, in regard to loss of reduction, screw breakage, or the need for implant removal [57].

3.5.2 Suture Button

A newer surgical implant with a promising future is the use of an endobutton (suture) device. A strong (fiber wire) suture loop is secured between two metal buttons that are placed on the outer cortices of the tibia and fibula, or through a fibular plate. It is placed in the same location and trajectory as the syndesmotic screws. It is then tensioned after placed appropriately. This construct is less rigid than screws and may allow the tibiofibular joint more physiologic motion.

3.5.3 Arthroscopy

Arthroscopy may be used as a diagnostic tool to assess syndesmosis. A length-labeled prob or small shaver can be used to measure the diastasis and determine instability [46]. If there is instability diagnosed, the surgeon may proceed with the stabilization methods described above. Arthroscopy is also beneficial in that it can diagnose other concurrent lesions the patient may have sustained such as osteochondral lesions or medial and lateral ligament injuries. In addition, it can also be used to confirm syndesmotic reduction under direct visualization.

3.6 Post-operative Management

The authors preference is to have the patient splinted in a short leg AO splint, which is a posterior splint with stirrup, for 2–3 weeks, non-weight-bearing. At the first postoperative visit (at 2–3 weeks), the splint is removed, and the patient is placed in a removable CAM boot. The patient is to remain non-weight-bearing for approximately 6 weeks postoperatively to allow proper healing but may begin gentle ROM at 3–4 weeks. After 6 weeks postoperatively, patient may begin weight-bearing. Patient with poorly controlled diabetes or other factors such as smoking, alcohol use, vascular disease, or neuropathy, may require longer timelines of immobilization and non-weight-bearing. Although some surgeons remove these screws routinely, the authors reserve the additional procedure, the earliest at 3–4 months postoperatively, and only for those who are experiencing irritation or reduced ROM.

4 Conclusion

Ligamentous ankle injuries are one of the most commonly diagnosed musculoskeletal injuries. These include lateral ankle sprains (LAS), medial ankle sprains (MAS), and syndesmotic injuries, any of which may occur as an isolated or associated with an ankle fracture. The LAS typically occurs from excessive inversion and internal rotation of the foot while the opposite is true for MAS. Syndesmotic injuries occur during supination or pronation with external or internal rotation about the ankle. All these injuries may present with significant pain, swelling, decreased range-of-motion, and inability to bear weight. They are diagnosed with special physical examination maneuvers along with plain radiography, used to rule out associated fractures, or magnetic resonance imaging to identify the extent of ligamentous injury. While most ankle sprains resolve using non-operative care, recurrent sprains and subsequent chronic ankle instability, with significant functional impairment may develop in some individuals. In cases of significant or chronic instability, operative management is warranted.

References

1. Waterman BR, Owens BD, Davey S, et al. The epidemiology of ankle sprains in the United States. J Bone Jt Surg Ser A. 2010;92(13):2279–84.
2. Halabchi F, Hassabi M. Acute ankle sprain in athletes: clinical aspects and algorithmic approach. World J Orthop. 2020;11(12):534–58.
3. Kobayashi T, Gamada K. Lateral ankle sprain and chronic ankle instability: a critical review. Foot Ankle Spec. 2014;7(4):298–326. Available from https://pubmed.ncbi.nlm.nih.gov/24962695/.
4. McKay GD, Goldie PA, Payne WR, et al. Ankle injuries in basketball: injury rate and risk factors. Br J Sports Med. 2001;35(2):103–8.
5. van den Bekerom MPJ, Kerkhoffs GMMJ, McCollum GA, et al. Management of acute lateral ankle ligament injury in the athlete. Knee Surg Sport Traumatol Arthrosc. 2013;21(6):1390–5.
6. Beynnon BD, Vacek PM, Murphy D, et al. First-time inversion ankle ligament trauma: the effects of sex, level of competition, and sport on the incidence of injury. Am J Sports Med. 2005;33(10):1485–91.
7. Doherty C, Delahunt E, Caulfield B, et al. The incidence and prevalence of ankle sprain injury: a systematic review and meta-analysis of prospective epidemiological studies. Sports Med. 2014;44(1):123–40.
8. Gerber JP, Williams GN, Scoville CR, et al. Persistent disability associated with ankle sprains: a prospective examination of an athletic population. Foot Ankle Int. 1998;19(10):653–60.
9. Viljakka T, Rokkanen P. The treatment of ankle sprain by bandaging and antiphlogistic drugs. Ann Chir Gynaecol. 1983;72(2):66–70.
10. Tyler TF, McHugh MP, Mirabella MR, et al. Risk factors for noncontact ankle sprains in high school football players: the role of previous ankle sprains and body mass index. Am J Sports Med. 2006;34(3):471–5.
11. Camacho LD, Roward ZT, Deng Y, et al. Surgical management of lateral ankle instability in athletes. J Athl Train. 2019;54(6):639–49.
12. Broström L. Sprained ankles. V. Treatment and prognosis in recent ligament ruptures. Acta Chir Scand. 1966;132(5):537–50.
13. Boruta PM, Bishop JO, Braly WG, et al. Acute lateral ankle ligament injuries: a literature review. Foot Ankle Int. 1990;11(2):107–13.
14. Verhagen RAW, de Keizer G, van Dijk CN. Long-term follow-up of inversion trauma of the ankle. Arch Orthop Trauma Surg. 1995;114(2):92–6.
15. Owoeye OBA, Whittaker JL, Toomey CM, et al. Health-related outcomes 3-15 years following ankle sprain injury in youth sport: what does the future hold? Foot Ankle Int. 2022;43(1):21–31.
16. Ferkel E, Nguyen S, Kwong C. Chronic lateral ankle instability: surgical management. Clin Sports Med. 2020;39(4):829–43.
17. Van Dijk CN, Lim LSL, Bossuyt PMM, et al. Physical examination is sufficient for the diagnosis of sprained ankles. J Bone Jt Surg Ser B. 1996;78(6):958–62.

18. Ivins D. Acute ankle sprain: an update. Am Fam Physician. 2006;74(10):1714–20.
19. Aradi AJ, Wong J, Walsh M. The dimple sign of a ruptured lateral ligament of the ankle: brief report. J Bone Joint Surg Br. 1988;70(2):327–8.
20. Chen ET, McInnis KC, Borg-Stein J. Ankle sprains: evaluation, rehabilitation, and prevention. Curr Sports Med Rep. 2019;18(6):217–23.
21. Stiell IG. Decision rules for the use of radiography in acute ankle injuries. Refinement and prospective validation. JAMA. 1993;269(9):1127–32.
22. Cox CJS, Hewes TF. "Normal" talar tilt angle. Clin Orthop Relat Res. 1979;140:37–41.
23. Chrisman OD, Snook GA. Reconstruction of lateral ligament tears of the ankle. An experimental study and clinical evaluation of seven patients treated by a new modification of the Elmslie procedure. J Bone Joint Surg Am. 1969;51(5):904–12.
24. Laurin CA, Ouellet R, St-Jacques R. Talar and subtalar tilt: an experimental investigation. Can J Surg. 1968;11(3):270–9.
25. Al-Mohrej OA, Al-Kenani NS. Chronic ankle instability: current perspectives. Avicenna J Med. 2016;06(04):103–8.
26. Karlsson J, Sancone M. Management of acute ligament injuries of the ankle. Foot Ankle Clin. 2006;11(3):521–30.
27. Emerson R. Surgical treatment of third-degree lateral ankle ligament ruptures to ensure stability. J Am Osteopath Assoc. 1978;78(4):273–80.
28. Peetrons P, Creteur V, Bacq C. Sonography of ankle ligaments. J Clin Ultrasound. 2004;32(9):491–9.
29. Alshalawi S, Galhoum AE, Alrashidi Y, et al. Medial ankle instability: the deltoid dilemma. Foot Ankle Clin. 2018;23(4):639–57.
30. Tan DW, Teh DJW, Chee YH. Accuracy of magnetic resonance imaging in diagnosing lateral ankle ligament injuries: a comparative study with surgical findings and timings of scans. Asia-Pac J Sport Med Arthrosc Rehabil Technol. 2017;7:15–20.
31. Dizon JMR, Reyes JJB. A systematic review on the effectiveness of external ankle supports in the prevention of inversion ankle sprains among elite and recreational players. J Sci Med Sport. 2010;13(3):309–17.
32. Lamb SE, Marsh JL, Hutton JL, et al. Mechanical supports for acute, severe ankle sprain: a pragmatic, multicentre, randomized controlled trial. Lancet. 2009;373(9663):575–81.
33. Kerkhoffs GMMJ, Handoll HHG, De Bie R, et al. Surgical versus conservative treatment for acute injuries of the lateral ligament complex of the ankle in adults. Cochrane Database Syst Rev. 2007;2:CD000380.
34. Roos EM, Brandsson S, Karlsson J. Validation of the foot and ankle outcome score for ankle ligament reconstruction. Foot Ankle Int. 2001;22(10):788–94.
35. Karlsson J, Bergsten T, Lansinger O, et al. Surgical treatment of chronic lateral instability of the ankle joint. A new procedure. Am J Sports Med. 1989;17(2):268–73.
36. Wainright WB, Spritzer CE, Lee JY, et al. The effect of modified Broström-Gould repair for lateral ankle instability on in vivo tibiotalar kinematics. Am J Sports Med. 2012;40(9):2099–104.
37. Hintermann B, Boss A, Schäfer D. Arthroscopic findings in patients with chronic ankle instability. Am J Sports Med. 2002;30(3):402–9.
38. Valderrabano V, Hintermann B. Diagnostik und Therapie der medialen Sprunggelenkinstabilität. Arthroskopie. 2005;18(2):112–8.
39. Close JR. Some applications of the functional anatomy of the ankle joint. J Bone Joint Surg Am. 1956;38(4):761–81.
40. Gibson PD, Ippolito JA, Hwang JS, et al. Physiologic widening of the medial clear space: what's normal? J Clin Orthop Trauma. 2019;10(1):S62–4.
41. Yu GR, Zhang MZ, Aiyer A, et al. Repair of the acute deltoid ligament complex rupture associated with ankle fractures: a multicenter clinical study. J Foot Ankle Surg. 2015;54(2):198–202.
42. Tornetta P. Competence of the deltoid ligament in bimalleolar ankle fractures after medial malleolar fixation. J Bone Jt Surg Ser A. 2000;82(6):843–8.
43. Harper MC. The deltoid ligament. An evaluation of need for surgical repair. Clin Orthop Relat Res. 1988;226:156–68.
44. Vosseller JT, Karl JW, Greisberg JK. Incidence of syndesmotic injury. Orthopedics. 2014;37(3):e226.
45. Lubberts B, D'Hooghe P, Bengtsson H, et al. Epidemiology and return to play following isolated syndesmotic injuries of the ankle: a prospective cohort study of 3677 male professional footballers in the UEFA Elite Club Injury Study. Br J Sports Med. 2019;53(15):959–64.
46. Hunt KJ, Phisitkul P, Pirolo J, et al. High ankle sprains and syndesmotic injuries in athletes. J Am Acad Orthop Surg. 2015;23(11):661–73.
47. De César PC, Ávila EM, De Abreu MR. Comparison of magnetic resonance imaging to physical examination for syndesmotic injury after lateral ankle sprain. Foot Ankle Int. 2011;32(12):1110–4.
48. Pogliacomi F, De Filippo M, Casalini D, et al. Acute syndesmotic injuries in ankle fractures: from diagnosis to treatment and current concepts. World J Orthop. 2021;12(5):269–92.
49. Kennedy JG, Soffe KE, Vedova PD, et al. Evaluation of the syndesmotic screw in low Weber C ankle fractures. J Orthop Trauma. 2000;14(5):359–66.
50. Prakash AA. Epidemiology of high ankle sprains: a systematic review. Foot Ankle Spec. 2020;13(5):420–30.
51. Hermans JJ, Beumer A, De Jong TAW, et al. Anatomy of the distal tibiofibular syndesmosis in adults: a pictorial essay with a multimodality approach. J Anat. 2010;217(6):633–45.
52. Wei F, Villwock MR, Meyer EG, et al. A biomechanical investigation of ankle injury under excessive external foot rotation in the human cadaver. J Biomech Eng. 2010;132(9):091001.
53. Nussbaum ED, Hosea TM, Sieler SD, et al. Prospective evaluation of syndesmotic ankle sprains without diastasis. Am J Sports Med. 2001;29(1):31–5.

54. Tourné Y, Molinier F, Andrieu M, et al. Diagnosis and treatment of tibiofibular syndesmosis lesions. Orthop Traumatol Surg Res. 2019;105(8):S275–86.
55. Cotton F. Dislocations and joint-fractures. JAMA J Am Med Assoc. 1910;55(22):1916.
56. Schepers T. Acute distal tibiofibular syndesmosis injury: a systematic review of suture-button versus syndesmotic screw repair. Int Orthop. 2012;36(6):1199–206.
57. Moore JA, Shank JR, Morgan SJ, et al. Syndesmosis fixation: a comparison of three and four cortices of screw fixation without hardware removal. Foot Ankle Int. 2006;27(8):567–72.

Management of Entrapment Neuropathies of the Foot and Ankle

Toni M. McLaurin

Entrapment neuropathies of the foot and ankle are uncommon but can result in considerable disability and distress to patients as they are frequently mis- and underdiagnosed. Any of the five nerves innervating the foot and ankle—tibial, superficial and deep peroneal, sural, and saphenous—may be involved along with their branches. Although symptoms are most often sensory in nature, motor changes may also occur.

Entrapment neuropathies occur when a nerve is compressed either by an anatomic structure or by a space-occupying lesion. Although the entrapment can arise within the foot and ankle, it can also happen along the entire course of the involved nerve. It is important to differentiate these more "local" entrapment neuropathies from lumbar nerve root impingement producing radiculopathy, peripheral neuropathy due to systemic diseases like diabetes mellitus, or pain resulting from peripheral vascular disease. Although uncommon with entrapment neuropathis, these other causes should be considered when symptoms are bilateral as this is uncommon with entrapment neuropathies. Symptoms can range from mild paresthesias or intermittent pain to much more debilitating pain and significant motor findings such as weakness and muscle wasting. Since the diagnosis is made based on clinical findings, the physician treating these problems must have a thorough understanding of the anatomy and how patients with these entrapment neuropathies present to ensure that a correct diagnosis can be made and an appropriate treatment plan developed.

1 Tibial Nerve Entrapment

The tibial nerve is a terminal branch of the sciatic nerve that courses deep to the soleus along with the posterior tibial vessels and passes posterior to the medial malleolus. In 93% of the population, it divides into two main branches, the medial and lateral plantar nerves, and a third smaller medial calcaneal branch that provides sensation to the heel and medial hindfoot [1]. Compression may occur anywhere along the entire course of the nerve or at any of its branches.

1.1 Tarsal Tunnel Syndrome

Tarsal tunnel syndrome (TTS) is one of the more familiar entrapment neuropathies identified in the foot and ankle. Although previously described in the literature, it was first identified and named as a discrete entity by Keck in 1962 [2]. It is sometimes referred to as tibial nerve dysfunction or

T. M. McLaurin (✉)
Orthopedic Service Bellevue Hospital Center,
New York, NY, USA

Department of Orthopaedic Surgery, NYU Langone Health, New York, NY, USA
e-mail: toni.mclaurin@nyulangone.org

© The Author(s), under exclusive license to Springer Nature Switzerland AG 2023
D. Herscovici Jr. et al. (eds.), *Evaluation and Surgical Management of the Ankle*,
https://doi.org/10.1007/978-3-031-33537-2_7

posterior tibial nerve neuralgia and is due to compression of the tibial nerve within the tarsal tunnel. The tarsal tunnel is a narrow fibro-osseous space that contains the posterior tibial neurovascular bundle, plus the tendons of tibialis posterior, flexor digitorum longus, and flexor hallucis longus. It extends from approximately 10 cm proximal to the tip of the medial malleolus to the sustentaculum tali distally. It is bordered anterosuperiorly by the medial malleolus and laterally by the distal tibia, talus, and calcaneus. The roof of the tunnel is the flexor retinaculum or lancinate ligament. The tunnel extends from the proximal to distal extent of the retinaculum (Fig. 1), where the tibial nerve exits and bifurcates into the medial and lateral plantar nerves which then pierce the abductor hallucis fascia (Fig. 2). As this tunnel is fully enclosed, anything that decreases the volume of the tunnel or increases the pressure within the tunnel will compress the nerve. The compression may involve the tibial nerve itself (proximal TTS) or one or more of the terminal branches (distal TTS) [3]. Typically, the tibial nerve branches within the tarsal tunnel but distal entrapments may occur distal to the tunnel proper and are considered a separate entity.

1.1.1 Proximal Tarsal Tunnel Syndrome

Etiology

Tibial nerve entrapment can be due to space-occupying lesions like a ganglion, lipoma, or exostosis, as well as tenosynovitis, accessory musculature within the tunnel (abductor hallucis or flexor digitorum longus), and neurilemmomas. Venous varicosities within the tarsal tunnel may also act as space-occupying lesions and are one

Fig. 1 Course of the posterior tibial nerve through the tarsal tunnel. The Γ indicates the flexor retinaculum. The π indicates a potential site of entrapment of the medial plantar nerve at the knot of Henry

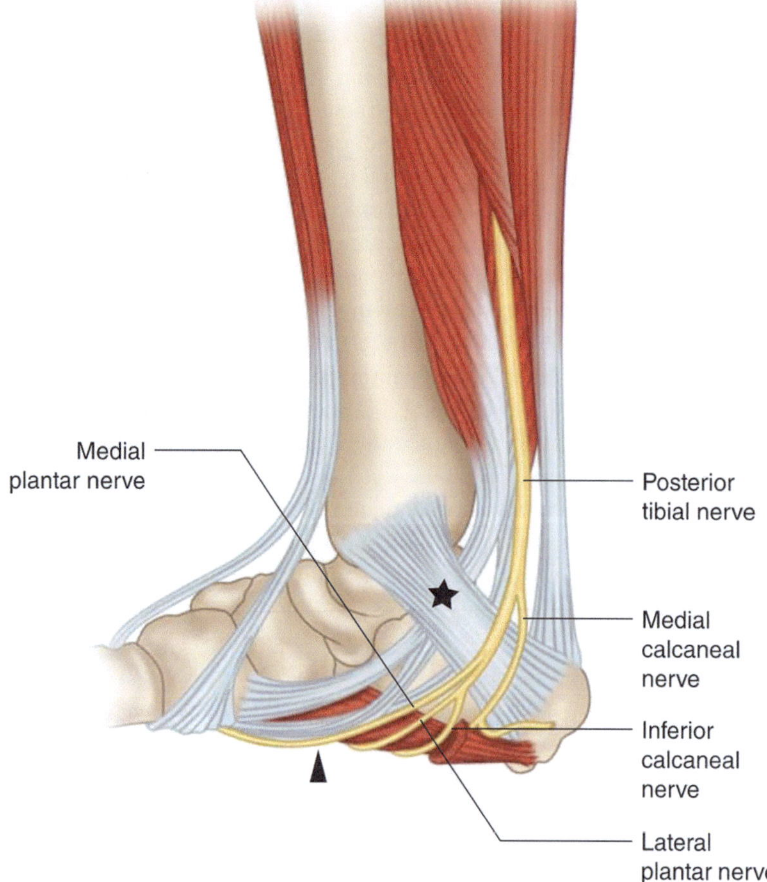

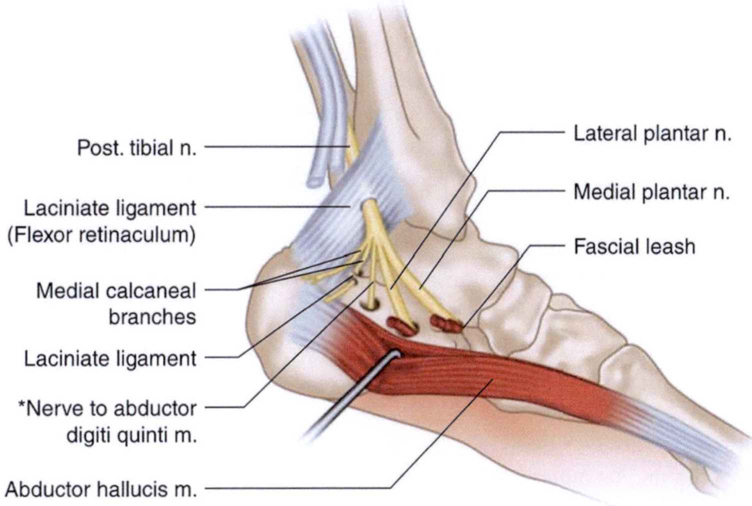

Fig. 2 The medial, lateral and inferior calcaneal (nerve to abductor digiti quinti) nerves as the they pierce the abductor hallucis fascia

of the more common causes [4]. In addition, trauma resulting in bony or cartilaginous prominences or thickening of the floor of the retinaculum can also contribute to decreasing the volume of the tunnel, resulting in compression. It is also hypothesized that significant hindfoot valgus or pes planus predisposes to some patients developing TTS, as this change in foot position would increase the pressure within the tunnel. Although increases in pressure have been demonstrated, the relationship of this to *symptomatic* tarsal tunnel remains unproven, and a truly causative relationship to TTS has not yet been clearly shown [5, 6]. Systemic issues, such as inflammatory arthropathies, obesity, and lower leg edema, may also cause TTS.

Diagnosis

Patients with proximal TTS present with diffuse pain along the medial ankle and plantar surface of the foot. This pain may be exacerbated by activity and relieved by rest and is usually present (and often worse) at night. Unfortunately, the patient's description of the pain may be vague and difficult to characterize when they present with an insidious onset of heel and plantar foot pain [1, 7]. Patients may describe the pain as burning, shooting, tingling, numbing, or an electric sensation. They may also complain of pain radiating proximally into the calf (known as the

Valleix phenomenon of retrograde radiation of pain from an entrapment neuropathy) or distally into the plantar aspect of the foot [3]. In addition, they may also note intermittent plantar paresthesias.

On physical examination, the patient must first be evaluated standing to assess heel and foot alignment with particular attention to valgus malalignment. The patient is then seated for the remainder of the examination. On palpation, there may be a point where a sensation of "pins and needles" is elicited distally when tapping along the course of the nerve. The recreation of this pins and needles sensation when tapping at a particular point is referred to as a positive Tinel's sign and can indicate a site of nerve compression. Despite a low sensitivity (23–67%), the Tinel's sign has a high specificity (95–99%) and remains a useful initial diagnostic tool [8]. Patients may also report pain with deep palpation in the area of the tarsal tunnel. In later stages, there may be intrinsic muscle wasting, especially noticeable in the abductor hallucis. The examination should also proceed more proximally, especially in patients with a history of a failed tarsal tunnel release, as soleal sling syndrome can mimic TTS symptoms including calf pain, plantar numbness, and paresthesias [3]. However, patient with soleal sling syndrome may also present with flexor hallucis longus weakness. Soleal sling syndrome is the result of the tibial nerve being entrapped proximally in a fibrous sling at the origin of the soleus muscle. It can be differentiated from TTS on physical examination by eliciting pain with palpation of the posterior calf at the level of the soleal sling, approximately 9 cm below the popliteal flexion crease (Fig. 3).

To identify a proximal TTS, the examiner may use the dorsiflexion-eversion test. This is a provocative maneuver where the ankle is maximally dorsiflexed and everted while the toes are maximally dorsiflexed at the metatarsophalangeal joints (Fig. 4). This position is held for 5–10 s, and patients are questioned about any change in their pain and/or numbness [9]. In addition, the nerve is palpated for tenderness along its course and the presence of a positive Tinel's sign is assessed. A majority of patients with TTS will describe immediate onset or worsening of the pain with new onset or worsening of numbness within a few seconds, along with increased tenderness on palpation of the nerve and a more pronounced Tinel's sign while the foot is held in this position. As many of the signs and symptoms of TTS can be nonspecific, this provocative maneuver may help increase the sensitivity of the physical examination.

Further evaluation of the patient should always include plain radiographs to assess for any bony abnormalities and a computed tomographic (CT) to better evaluate the tarsal tunnel (Fig. 5). Magnetic resonance imaging (MRI) and ultrasound can also be used to assess for any soft tissue etiologies causing increased pressure within the tarsal tunnel. As with most foot and ankle entrapment neuropathies, the main value in electrodiagnostic testing in the diagnosis of TTS is in ruling out more proximal pathology as a cause. With respect to findings in TTS, electromyographic (EMG) studies have been shown to have a high false positive rate when testing the intrinsic muscles of the foot, and nerve conduction velocity (NCV) studies have been shown to have a high false-negative rate. In an evidence-based review of electrodiagnostic techniques in the evaluation of tarsal tunnel syndrome, it was also shown that nerve conduction studies (NCS) were abnormal in some but not all patients, with sen-

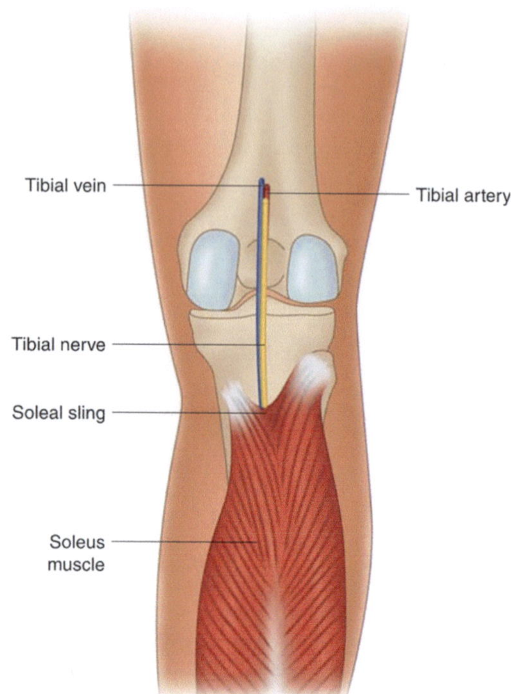

Fig. 3 The tibial nerve as it passes under the soleal sling which can act as a proximal site of entrapment

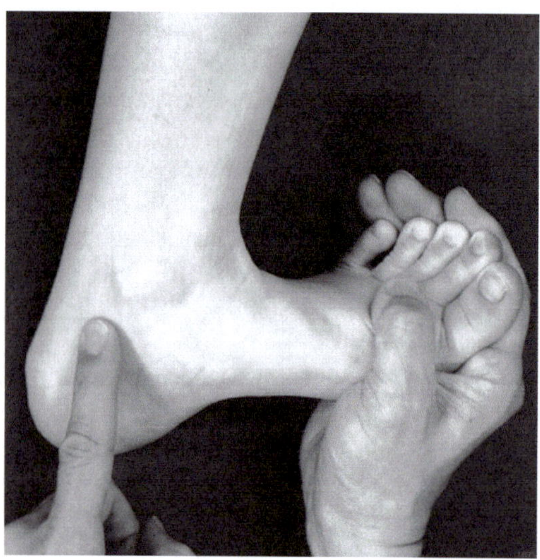

Fig. 4 The dorsiflexion-eversion test: the ankle is maximally dorsiflexed and everted while the toes are maximally dorsiflexed at the metatarsophalangeal joints. The finger is palpating over the course of the tibial nerve which may elicit tenderness or a positive Tinel's sign. (Kinoshita M, Okuda R, Morikawa J, Jotoku T, Abe M. *JBJS*. 2001;83(12):1835-1839)

Fig. 5 The bony prominence of a tarsal coalition as a potential cause of TTS. (Takakura Y, Kitada C, Sugimoto K, Tanaka Y, Tamai S. *J Bone Joint Surg Br.* 1991;73(1):125-128)

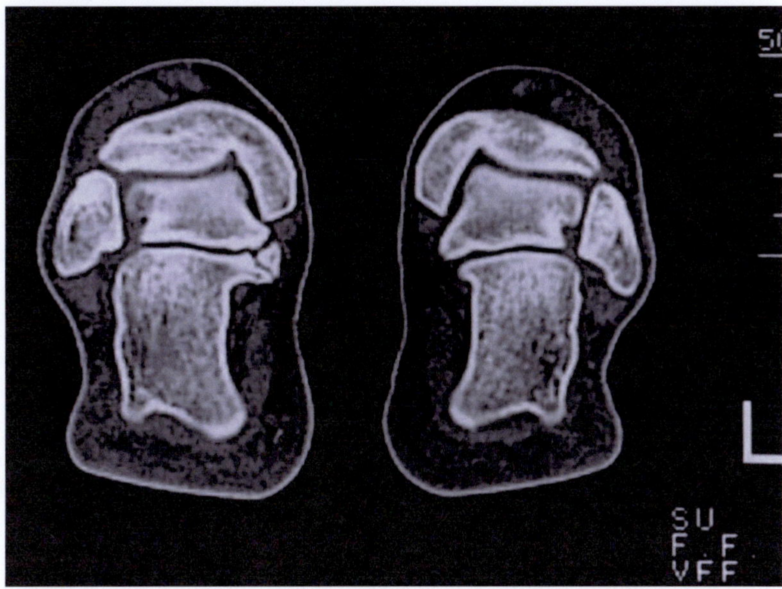

sory NCS potentially more likely to be abnormal than motor NCS. However, the authors were unable to determine the true sensitivity or specificity of these tests [7, 10].

Management

Nonsurgical management is always the first line of treatment in almost all compressive neuropathies of the foot and ankle. Management may include nonsteroidal anti-inflammatory drugs (NSAIDs), activity modifications, night splinting/orthotics, physical therapy, and modification or discontinuation of any compressive clothing or footwear. Corticosteroid injections may provide symptomatic relief, but this tends to be short-lived.

Surgical management is indicated for those patients who do not improve with non-operative measures as well as for those with identifiable space-occupying lesions. Decompression requires release of the entire flexor retinaculum and the fascia over the abductor hallucis and can be performed open, endoscopically, or with ultrasound guidance through multiple small incisions [11, 12]. Success rates are reported in the literature as anywhere from 44 to 96% mainly due to the heterogeneity in factors such as patient selection, timing of surgical interven-

tion, and technique of decompression [13, 14]. Results are best for those patients with space-occupying lesions that are excised, and some authors have noted that patients with a strongly positive Tinel's sign pre-operatively have better outcomes. Conversely, those patients with sensory deficits and absence of a Tinel's sign showed a limited chance of regaining nerve function [15]. Correlation of improved results with earlier decompression has also been suggested [3, 16]. Although surgical management should not be the first line of treatment in TTS, decompression should also not be delayed unnecessarily once conversative measures have not been effective.

1.1.2 Distal Tarsal Tunnel Syndrome

Medial Plantar Nerve Entrapment (Jogger's Foot)

Etiology

Medial plantar nerve (MPN) entrapment may occur at multiple sites. The nerve may be compressed between the abductor hallucis fascia and its origin at the navicular and calcaneus, between the abductor hallucis muscle belly and the knot of Henry (Fig. 1), or as it passes through the medial intermuscular septum. It has been termed "Jogger's Foot" as it is associated with the repetitive trauma of running, especially in patients with increased heel valgus and foot pronation, with inflammation occurring at the entrapment site [17, 18].

Diagnosis

Patients with MPN entrapment present with complaints of a burning heel and medial arch pain. Pain may radiate distally to the plantar surfaces of the first, second, and third toes and proximally into the medial heel and ankle. A standing examination is necessary to evaluate hindfoot valgus. A positive Tinel's sign may be elicited at the plantar border of the navicular tuberosity, and dysesthesias may be present along the heel, medial arch, and plantar aspects of the first through third toes. A diagnostic injection with local anesthetic at the entrapment point may be helpful in differentiating this from other cases of heel pain such as calcaneal bursitis and plantar fasciitis [17]. The patient should also be questioned about whether or not they use any rigid arch supports as these may place additional pressure on the entrapment site.

Plain radiographs are important to rule out any bony abnormalities or foot deformities as sources of entrapment. An MRI may show soft tissue space-occupying lesions and also denervation edema of the abductor hallucis and flexor digitorum brevis which are both innervated by the MPN. There is no clear role for electrodiagnostic studies in the diagnosis of MPN entrapment.

Management

Treatment is mainly non-operative consisting of NSAIDs, rest, and physical therapy. Patients should avoid the use of arch supports and for runners; attention should be focused on shoewear that avoids any medial compression and improving the running posture with emphasis on striking more on the lateral border of the foot. If non-operative management fails to relieve the pain, then surgical decompression is indicated. The deep fascia of the abductor hallucis is released from its origin on the calcaneus to the knot of Henry. It is recommended that the release extends proximally to include the flexor retinaculum and tibial nerve as compression of this branch may begin within the actual tarsal tunnel not just distal to it [3].

Lateral Plantar Nerve Entrapment (Baxter Neuropathy)

Etiology

The first branch of the lateral plantar nerve (LPN), also called the inferior calcaneal branch, nerve to the abductor digiti quinti (ADQ), or Baxter's nerve, may be compressed at primarily two distinct sites. The nerve enters underneath the fascia of the abductor hallucis muscle, passes through its fascial leash, and exits distally beneath its inferior fascial edge. It then makes a sharp 90° turn laterally to pass under the calcaneus. It is the only nerve branch that lies deep to the abductor hallucis and flexor digitorum brevis (FDB) muscles and travels superficial to the quadratus plantae (QP) along the medial aspect of the calcaneus. It provides motor function to the ADQ and occasionally to the FDB and to the lateral half of the QP muscles. It is also provides sensation to the lateral plantar skin, calcaneal periosteum, and long plantar ligament. This nerve may be entrapped either as it passes between the deep fascia of the abductor hallucis muscle and the medial plantar margin of the quadratus plantae muscle or where the nerve passes anterior to the medial calcaneal tuberosity (Fig. 6) [7, 19]. This is an entity noted to be commonly seen in athletes and has been associated with hypertrophy of the abductor hallucis and FDB and may be exacerbated in the setting of a hyperpronated foot. There may also be an association with heel spurs [19].

Diagnosis

Patients present with complaints of chronic medial heel pain and may also describe a sharp, burning pain just distal to the medial calcaneal tuberosity, making this presentation easily confused with plantar fasciitis, heel pain syndrome, and fat pad disorders [20]. However, the pain tends to be more proximal and medial and may radiate proximally along the medial ankle or distally and laterally across the plantar aspect the foot. Paresthesias typically are not present [1, 3]. Palpation over the nerve deep to the abductor hallucis should reproduce the symptoms and may also cause radiation of the pain proximally or distally [20]. Palpation should also continue proximally and distally to rule out other potential entrapment sites. Plain radiography may help identify any bony etiologies of the entrapment. An MRI can identify space-occupying lesions, show abductor hallucis hypertrophy, demonstrate plantar fasciitis with a medial spur, and reveal surrounding soft tissue edema. All of these findings indicate the possibility of inferior calcaneal nerve entrapment. Although abductor

digiti quinti atrophy is a frequent incidental MRI finding, in patients with chronic heel pain, this finding may represent a missed diagnosis of inferior calcaneal nerve entrapment [18]. Electrodiagnostic studies may help confirm the presence of a compressive neuropathy but do not otherwise add much to the diagnosis. It is often not possible to differentiate between inferior calcaneal entrapment and entrapment of the lateral plantar nerve more proximally as it exits the tarsal tunnel.

Management

Initial management is non-operative and includes NSAIDs, rest, and physical therapy. However, if symptoms persist for more than 3 months, surgical decompression should be performed. Typically, release of the superficial and deep fascia of the abductor hallucis overlying the nerve are adequate but it is recommended that the nerve continue to be followed distally and released from any entrapment caused by the medial plantar fascia, FDB, or QP (Fig. 7) [3, 7]. Earlier literature also recommended excision of any heel spurs that may be present, but more recent reports state this generally is not necessary [3, 7, 19, 20]. Although these series are small due to the uncommon nature of this problem, high rates of good to excellent results of surgical decompression have been reported [3, 7, 20].

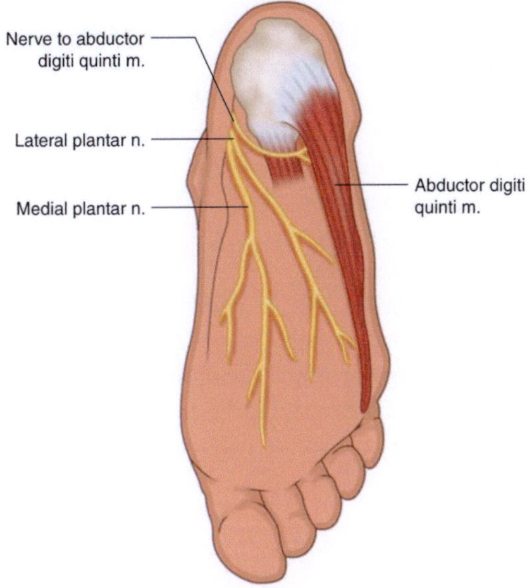

Fig. 6 Plantar view of the nerve to the abductor digiti quinti (inferior calcaneal nerve) as it turns sharply and passes in front of the calcaneus

Fig. 7 Release of the inferior calcaneal nerve as it passes deep to the abductor hallucis and superficial to the quadratus plantae

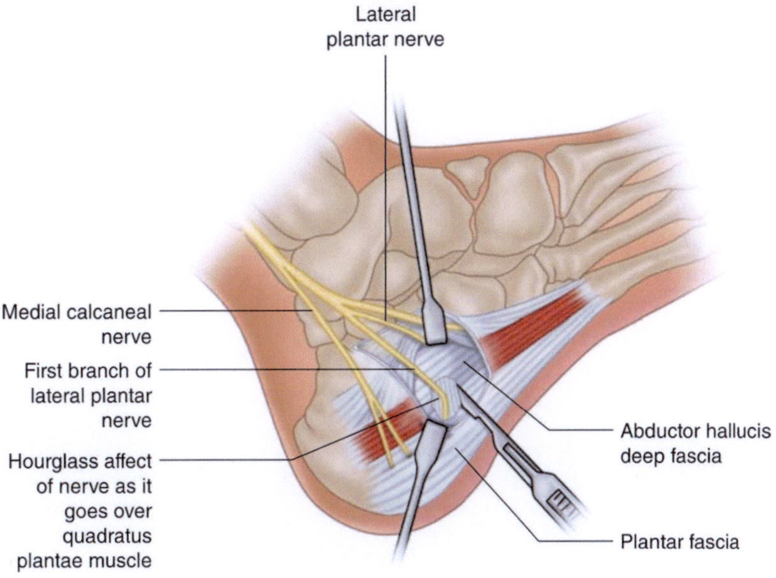

1.2 Common Digital Nerve Entrapment (Morton's Neuroma)

1.2.1 Etiology

The entity commonly known as Morton's neuroma is actually an entrapment neuropathy of the plantar digital nerve and not a true neuroma. It is caused by entrapment and crushing of the nerve between the metatarsal heads just plantar and distal to the transverse metatarsal ligament. It is most common in the third web space but does also occur in the second and fourth webspaces. Although it is referred to as an interdigital neuroma, histologically, there is actually degeneration of the myelinated fibers, thickening, and fibrosis of the epineurium and perineurium with thickening of the walls of the epineural and endoneural vessels. This is in contrast to the proliferative changes that are seen in a true neuroma [21]. It is unclear why most lesions occur in the third webspace, but there are three principle theories:

First, the third web space is between the stable first through third metatarsals and the more mobile fourth and fifth rays potentially increasing the risk of entrapment. Second, both the second and third web spaces are smaller, increasing the likelihood of entrapment. Lastly, an accessory interconnecting branch from the LPN to the MPN occurs here in some individuals causing an increase in overall neural diameter and potentially increasing the risk of tethering and entrapment (Fig. 8) [1]. Women are affected more than men, and compression of the forefoot, as occurs with narrow toe box shoes, is often cited as a cause of Morton's neuroma and the reason for its prevalence in women.

1.2.2 Diagnosis

Patients usually present with the classic complaint of plantar pain between the metatarsal heads which is worsened with high heels or narrow toe box shoes and may be relieved by removing the shoe or walking barefoot. Patients often

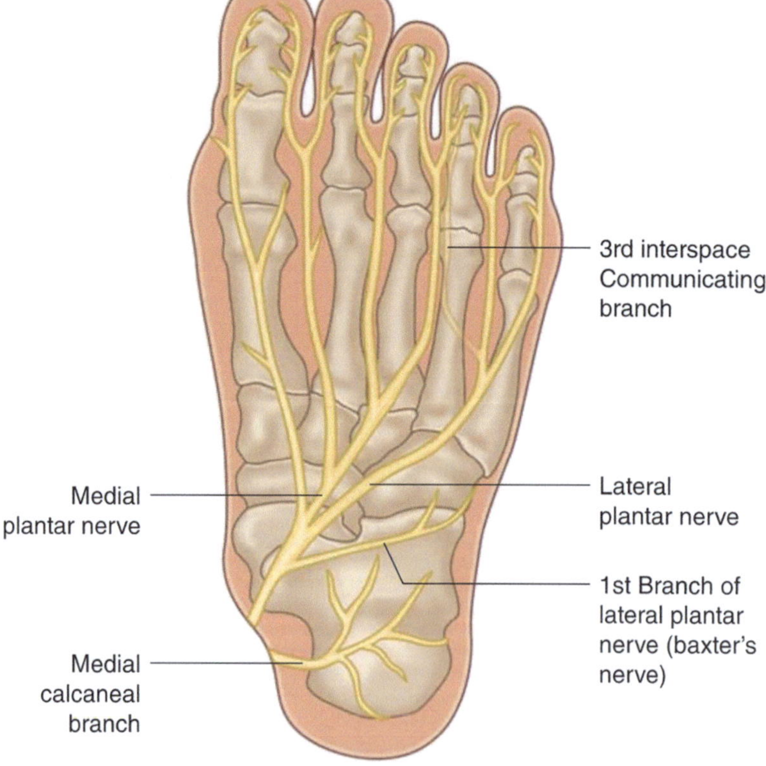

Fig. 8 The dotted line indicates the possible accessory interconnecting branch from the lateral plantar nerve to the medial plantar nerve which occurs in the third web space potentially increasing the overall nerve diameter

describe a burning or electrical pain that may radiate to the toes affected by the involved digital nerve. They may also describe the sensation of walking or standing on a pebble [1, 3]. On physical examination, there is usually pain with direct pressure placed between the metatarsal heads on the plantar foot or with squeezing the metatarsal heads together. A Mulder's click may be elicited when these maneuvers are performed sequentially. Forcing the neuroma from between the metatarsal heads into the sole of the foot can often produce a palpable click or clunk and may recreate the pain [1, 22]. A local anesthetic injection can be helpful in confirming the diagnosis. Standing AP and lateral plain radiographs should be obtained to rule out bony abnormalities or degenerative changes. Both ultrasound and MRI have been shown to have very high sensitivity and specificity, but the diagnosis is mainly clinical [1]. There is no role for electrodiagnostic studies.

1.2.3 Management

Non-operative management consists of NSAIDs, shoewear modifications, orthotics, and the use of a metatarsal pad placed proximal to the neuroma to offload it. Corticosteroid injections have good outcomes for short-term relief, but this does not persist. Previous interest in serial injections with an alcohol sclerosing agent has faded as the results have been disappointing, and there is concern for damaging surrounding tissues [1, 3].

Operative management is indicated when pain persists despite non-operative intervention. Traditionally, surgery has consisted, not of surgical decompression, as with most other entrapment neuropathies, but with excision of the neuroma through either a dorsal or plantar approach. Results are quite variable with poor results reported as ranging from 3 to 40% [3]. The most common complication is recurrence of the pain either due to inadequate nerve resection or inadvertent resection of the wrong tissue, usually a lumbrical tendon or digital artery [3, 21]. Even with successful pain relief, the area around the resected neuroma remains partially anesthetic which may be troubling to some patients. The release of the anterior edge of the deep intermeta-

carpal ligament without resection of the neuroma was initially described in 1979 and treatment by local decompression is being revisited as some authors again question the role of, and need for, nerve excision for a pathology that is not actually a neuroma [23–25]. Isolated division of the inter-metacarpal ligament has also been advocated. This avoids the potential complications of neuroma resection including loss of sensation, loss of sweat production, or neuroma development at the nerve stump [1, 24]. In addition, the incidence of postoperative neurogenic symptoms has been shown to be lower with neurolysis than with neurectomy. Postoperative outcomes have also been shown to improve when dorsal transposition of the nerve is performed along with the neurolysis [25].

2 Peroneal Nerve

2.1 Anterior Tarsal Tunnel Syndrome (Deep Peroneal Nerve Entrapment)

2.1.1 Etiology

The term anterior tarsal tunnel syndrome was first used by Marinacci in 1968 to describe the rare entrapment of the deep peroneal nerve (DPN) as it crosses in front of the ankle to the foot [26]. The anterior tarsal tunnel is a fibro-osseus flattened space lying between the inferior extensor retinaculum and the fascia overlying the talus and navicular. The DPN is a branch of the common peroneal nerve (CPN) that runs between the tibialis anterior and the extensor hallucis longus (EHL). As it passes under the superior extensor retinaculum, approximately 1 cm proximal to the ankle joint, it divides into a medial and a lateral branch. Both branches travel under the inferior extensor retinaculum, a Y-shaped band anterior to the ankle, with the lateral branch providing motor function to the extensor digitorum brevis (EDB) and sensation to the ankle joint and the lateral tarsal joints (Fig. 9). The medial branch travels dorsally with the dorsalis pedis and gives sensation to the first web space. Contents of the anterior tarsal tunnel include the dorsalis pedis

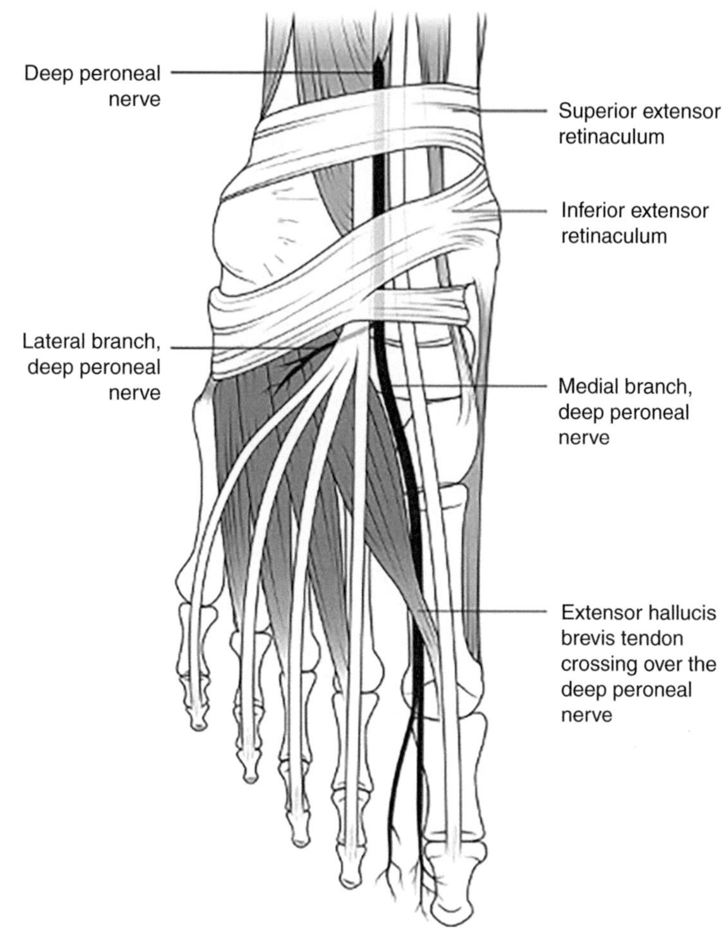

Fig. 9 The course of the deep peroneal nerve as it passes under the superior and inferior extensor retinaculi and gives off its sensory medial branch and lateral branch that provides motor function to the extensor digitorum brevis and sensation to the ankle and lateral tarsal joints. (Pomeroy G, Wilton J, Anthony S. *JAAOS.* 2015;23(1):58-66)

artery and vein and the tendons of the EHL, tibialis anterior, extensor digitorum longus, and peroneus tertius [26–28]. As the tarsal tunnel is a flattened, very superficial, and unprotected space, the most common cause of ATTS is compression of either branch of the DPN by compression on the dorsum of the foot or anything that further narrows the space. Some of the more commonly reported etiologies include trauma, resulting in fibrosis or bony deformities, osteophytes around the talonavicular or second tarsometatarsal joints, space-occupying lesions, such as a ganglion or even tight shoewear (Fig. 10) [1, 3, 28].

2.1.2 Diagnosis

Symptoms of ATTS most commonly involve the medial branch. Patients present with complaints of a burning pain over the dorsum of the foot radiating to the first and second toes occasionally accompanied by paresthesias radiating to the first web space. Symptoms may be exacerbated by excessive plantarflexion and may radiate proximally [28]. On physical examination, there may be local tenderness over the nerve and a positive Tinel's sign. Patients with compression of the lateral branch typically report dorsal foot pain radiating to the region of the lateral tarsometatarsal joints [3]. Wasting of the EDB implies more proximal compression of the DPN above its bifurcation, and evaluation of DPN neuropathy should always involve the more proximal leg with consideration of a common peroneal nerve etiology [28]. A diagnostic injection of local anesthetic can help better identify the site of compression.

Radiographic evaluation should include weight-bearing foot X-rays to evaluate for bony

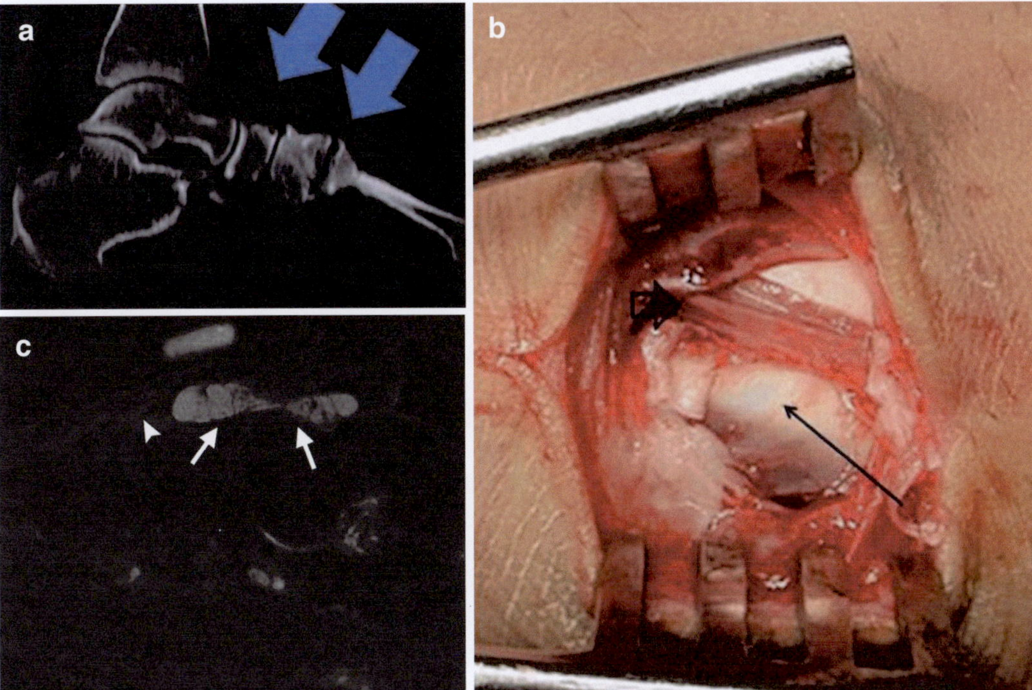

Fig. 10 A CT scan (**a**) and clinical image (**b**) of midfoot osteophytes (black arrow) causing compression of the deep peroneal nerve. (**c**) A ganglion (white arrows) may also cause compression. (**a**, **b**) Yassin M, Garti A, Weissbrot M, Heller E, Robinson D. *The Foot.* 2015;25(3):148-151; (**c**) Donovan A, Rosenberg ZS, Cavalcanti CF. *Radiographics.* 2010;30(4):1001-1019

deformity and MRI if a space-occupying lesion is suspected. Ultrasound can also be used to detect anatomic causes, such as scarring, lesions, bony deformities narrowing the canal, and can be used dynamically to identify tethering of the nerves during movement [29]. Electrodiagnostic studies may show an increased latency and reduced distal velocity, but with preserved proximal function. However, these findings are neither sensitive nor specific for symptomatic ATTS [28, 29].

2.1.3 Management

Conservative management, beginning with shoewear modification, should always be one of the first and most obvious lines of treatment. Also, the usual mainstays of NSAIDs, physical therapy, and possibly bracing to address any ankle instability should be utilized. Surgical management is reserved for those rare cases that do not respond to conservative management and can be performed open or arthroscopically [30]. The nerve

is released from the inferior extensor retinaculum to its entry into the deep fascia, and any associated osteophytes or lesions are also excised. Attempts should be made to avoid full release of the retinaculum to prevent bowstringing of the enclosed tendons, but if it is necessary for complete decompression of the nerve, then a Z-plasty of the retinaculum should be performed to avoid this complication [1].

2.2 Superficial Peroneal Nerve Entrapment

2.2.1 Etiology

The superficial peroneal nerve (SPN) is the second branch of the common peroneal nerve. It travels in the lateral compartment of the leg and innervates the peroneus longus and brevis and gives sensation to the dorsum of the foot aside from the first web space. However, in 14–17% of patients it may travel in the anterior compartment which becomes an important fact when considering treatment [31]. The nerve exits the fascia 10–15 cm proximal to the tip of the lateral malleolus, and this is where the entrapment occurs as the nerve becomes subcutaneous (Fig. 11) [18]. The cause of the entrapment can be a thickened fascial tunnel due to prior injury and scarring, a fascial defect with muscle herniation, or a space-occupying lesion, most often a lipoma. There is also an association with severe ankle sprains as the SPN is put on stretch with an inversion injury. Due to its tethered anteromedial position, when the foot is inverted and plantar flexed as occurs during an ankle sprain, a traction injury to the SPN can result [3, 29, 32]. This same position occurs repeatedly in patients with lateral ligament deficiency or functional ankle instability,

and they may also present with symptoms of entrapment due to repetitive traction strain on the SPN. Perineural fibrosis of the SPN at the level of the ankle has also been reported even in children and adolescents following a first acute severe inversion ankle sprain [33]. This is a rare entrapment neuropathy, reported in only about 3.5% of patients with chronic leg pain and can easily go undiagnosed [31].

2.2.2 Diagnosis

Patients present with pain, tingling, numbness, and paresthesias over the dorsolateral aspect of the foot. Confoundingly, they may also present with anterolateral leg pain radiating from the calf into the top of the foot which can be confused with exertional compartment syndrome or a more proximal L5 radiculopathy, so it is important to localize the pain appropriately [1, 29, 34]. This is especially true as the symptoms are often worsened with activity, similar to exertional compartment syndrome. On physical examination, pressure at the entrapment point can elicit retrograde pain up the calf [29]. There may be a positive Tinel's sign just anterior to the lateral malleolus. If there is muscle herniation or a fascial defect, there may be a mass or swelling at the site that worsens with use and is painful to palpation. Tenderness may also be elicited by inverting and plantarflexing the ankle and then tapping on the nerve as it exits the deep fascia. A maneuver to recreate the symptoms is referred to as Styf's provocative test. This involves palpating the fascial defect while the patient is actively dorsiflexing and everting the foot against resistance, a move that elicits pain [1, 35]. It is also important to assess ankle stability as this can also be a dynamic cause of SPN entrapment as noted above. Local anesthetic injections may also help with diagnosis.

Plain radiographs are important to rule out any bony abnormalities, and MRI can detect space-occupying lesions. Electromyographic studies may show a decrease in nerve conduction velocities but are neither specific nor sensitive. However, they can help differentiate SPN entrapment from more proximal neuropathies.

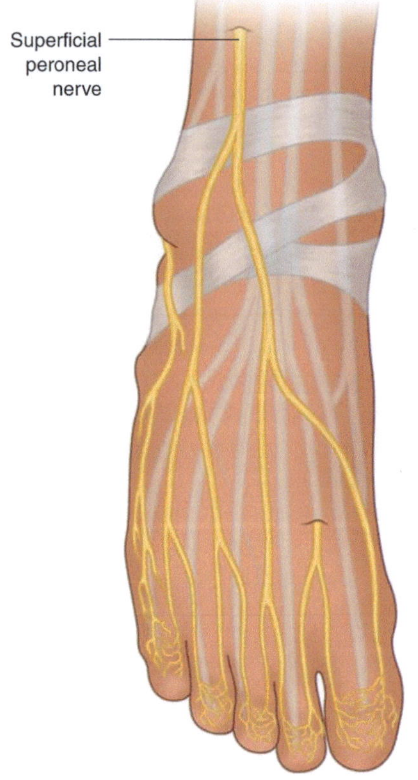

Fig. 11 The superficial peroneal nerve exiting the fascia—a potential entrapment site

2.2.3 Management

Conservative management consists of NSAIDs, shoewear modification, and physical therapy for ankle instability rehabilitation if indicated. A lateral wedge shoe insert orthotic may be helpful as it decreases supination of the foot and stretch on the nerve. In addition to diagnostic local anesthetic injections, steroid injections have often been reported to result in short-term symptom relief. In addition, peripheral nerve stimulation has been reported to give relief, especially with ultrasound-guided placement for lead implantation [29, 36]. The very superficial nature of the SPN makes it a good candidate for this technique.

Surgical decompression is indicated when conservative measures fail. It is often recommended that surgical release be performed within 2–3 months of onset of symptoms, but good results of decompression have been seen after longer time intervals [33]. The decompression involves fasciectomy over the site of compression with neurolysis and a concomitant fasciotomy to release the entire lateral compartment proximally to the fibular head and distally to the retinaculum [1, 3, 35]. In addition, it is important to have determined the exact site of compression pre-operatively. Some patients may require distal release of the fascia of the *anterior* compartment along with the lateral fasciotomy and release of the septum between the two compartments if the SPN travels in the anterior rather than lateral compartment [3, 29, 31]. As it can be difficult to determine clinically if both compartments are involved in the entrapment, some authors recommend routinely releasing both compartments [31]. If ankle instability is a contributing factor and not improved with physical therapy, this may also need to be addressed with surgical reconstruction.

3 Sural Nerve Entrapment

3.1 Etiology

Sural nerve entrapment was first described by Pringle in 1974, and isolated sural neuropathy remains an uncommon diagnosis [37]. The sural nerve is a pure sensory nerve with a variable anatomic makeup. Most commonly, it is formed by the joining of the medial sural nerve branch of the tibial nerve and either the peroneal communicating nerve or the lateral sural cutaneous nerve, both of which are branches of the CPN. It may also originate directly from the tibial nerve or the CPN [18]. It passes between the two heads of the gastrocnemius and exits the deep fascia in the middle third of the calf. It then continues subcutaneously lateral to the Achilles tendon, onto the lateral border of the foot. It provides sensation to the lateral surface of the heel, the lateral border of the fifth metatarsal, and sometimes the fifth toe and 4th web space [1]. Entrapment of the nerve can occur anywhere along its course with the most common sites of compression occurring along the lateral border of the ankle, talus, calcaneus, and base of the fifth metatarsal. Entrapment is usually secondary to trauma such as direct contusion and the subsequent soft tissue scarring or bony due to a bony overgrowth from fractures along its course [3, 18]. Severe ankle sprains, ankle instability, and space-occupying lesions may also result in entrapment. Atraumatic entrapment at the level of the superficial sural aponeurosis where the nerve exits the fascia may also occur. This can be due to the presence of a fibrous arch that thickens the superficial sural aponeurosis (Fig. 12) and is more commonly seen in athletes, possibly due to greater sural muscle mass and/or repetitive microtrauma [38].

3.2 Diagnosis

Patients present complaining of pain, burning, numbness, or aching in the posterolateral leg, lateral ankle, or lateral foot. Paresthesias along the lateral foot are common and palpation along the nerve distally can elicit pain. There may be a Tinel's sign present, but its absence does not rule out sural nerve entrapment. Plantarflexion and inversion of the ankle may also recreate the pain [3, 18]. Patients with compression at the superficial sural aponeurosis may present with chronic calf pain that often radiates into the lateral foot. As the nerve exits the fascia near the musculotendinous junction of the Achilles tendon, reproduc-

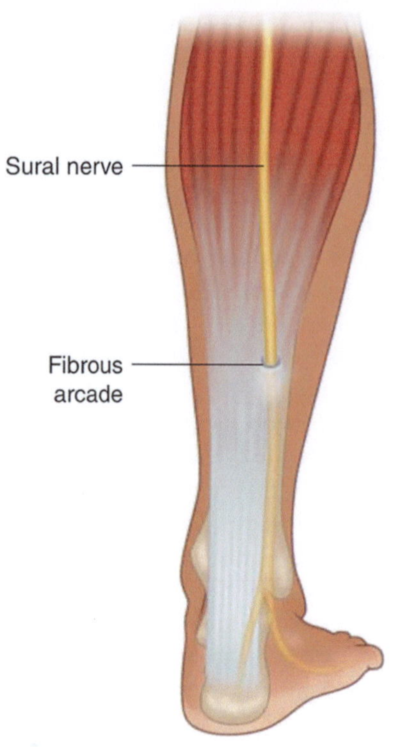

Fig. 12 A fibrous arcade at the superficial sural aponeurosis that may act as an atraumatic entrapment site of the sural nerve

tion of the pain with direct pressure over this area can also help pinpoint the aponeurosis as the site of entrapment [38].

Plain radiographs will help diagnose any bony abnormalities. MRI can identify space-occupying lesions, such as a ganglion that may be causing compression and may also be able to identify the site of compression. Electrodiagnostic studies show decreased nerve conduction velocity but are more important for ruling out more proximal pathology, such as an S1 radiculopathy.

3.3 Management

Conservative management with NSAIDs, physical therapy including desensitization and neural gliding techniques, and shoewear modification should always be tried first. Importantly, any predisposing ankle instability needs to be addressed as well with bracing and physical therapy. Due to the superficial location of the sural nerve, peripheral nerve stimulation with ultrasound-guided placement of the leads may provide good pain relief [36]. Patients with entrapment at the superficial sural aponeurosis may not respond well to conservative management and may require a more proximal decompression of the fibrous thickening. Any ankle instability that is present but not improved by physical therapy should be addressed surgically with appropriate reconstruction.

4 Saphenous Nerve Entrapment

4.1 Etiology

Entrapment neuropathies of the saphenous nerve are very rare. The saphenous nerve is an entirely sensory branch of the femoral nerve. It exits through the adductor canal in the thigh and divides into an infrapatellar and a descending branch. The infrapatellar branch supplies the skin over the lower knee while the descending branch continues to the foot where its two terminal branches supply the medial ankle and medial midfoot. The nerve is usually entrapped more proximally in Hunter's canal or due to trauma at some point along its length. Distal entrapment of the nerve is rare [1, 3].

4.2 Diagnosis

Although entrapment of the nerve tends to occur more proximally in the leg, resulting in thigh, medial knee, and calf pain, patients may also present with pain and paresthesias over the dorsum of the medial foot, especially the first ray. The presence of medial knee and calf pain and isolation of the medial forefoot pain to the 1st ray only can help different this entrapment from the similar foot symptoms seen with ATTS [1]. There should be no associated motor weakness as this is a purely sensory nerve. Any finding of weakness should steer the diagnosis toward a more proximal etiology, such as L3/L4 radiculopathy [1, 3]. A Tinel's sign at any point along the course of the nerve may aid in the diagnosis along with a diagnostic injection of local anesthetic. Radiographic evaluation with plain X-rays and CT or MRI is performed to rule out bony pathology or soft tissue lesions. Electrodiagnostic studies are of little value in making the diagnosis other than identifying more proximal etiologies.

4.3 Management

Conservative management is the mainstay of treatment for saphenous nerve entrapment. Along with NSAIDs, corticosteroid injections around Hunter's canal may be beneficial [1]. More distal entrapment is most often due to trauma or scarring from surgery and may be improved with surgical decompression and neurolysis if non-operative management has failed [1, 3].

Summary Although rare, entrapment neuropathies of the foot and ankle can be a source of significant morbidity and often go undiagnosed or misdiagnosed for prolonged periods of time. An understanding of the anatomy of the nerves to the foot and ankle as well as careful attention to symptoms and physical examination findings can help identify the nerve involved and the source or site of entrapment. Plain radiographs are helpful in showing any bony deformities or abnormalities that may be causing compression, and MRI studies can identify space-occupying lesions. Electrodiagnostic studies are most useful in helping to rule out other, more proximal pathologies such as lumbosacral disc disease or more proximal nerve involvement. Most entrapment neuropathies of the foot and ankle respond well to conservative management including NSAIDs, bracing/orthotics, physical therapy, shoewear modification and addressing any underlying pathologies, such as ankle instability. Corticosteroids have been recommended only for short-term relief, and more superficial nerves such as the SPN and sural nerve may respond well to peripheral nerve stimulation.

Surgical decompression is indicated when all conservative measures have failed and may have better results in some nerves if performed within 3 months of onset of symptoms or as soon as failure of conservative management has been confirmed. Complete release of any tight soft tissue structures and excision of bony prominences or soft tissue lesions is required for adequate decompression. For many of the entrapment sites, decompression can be performed open, arthroscopically or under ultrasound guidance. Neurolysis should also be performed. Only in the case of a Morton's neuroma has neurectomy routinely been recommended, but this may be changing as good results from decompression and neurolysis are proving to be much better than those from neurectomy with fewer negative side effects. Consideration of an entrapment neuropathy should be part of the assessment for any patient presenting with a history of often vague but persistent pain, burning, and aching in the foot or ankle, especially if management addressing more proximal pathologies has not been helpful.

References

1. Williams THD, Robinson AHN. Entrapment neuropathies of the foot and ankle. Orthopaed Trauma. 2009;23(6):404–11.
2. Keck C. The tarsal-tunnel syndrome. JBJS. 1962;44(1):180–2.
3. Pomeroy G, Wilton J, Anthony S. Entrapment neuropathy about the foot and ankle: an update. JAAOS. 2015;23(1):58–66.
4. Sammarco GJ, Chang L. Outcome of surgical treatment of tarsal tunnel syndrome. Foot Ankle Int. 2003;24(2):125–31.
5. Daniels TR, Lau JT, Hearn TC. The effects of foot position and load on tibial nerve tension. Foot Ankle Int. 1998;19(2):73–8.
6. Bracilovic A, Nihal A, Houston VL, Beattie AC, Rosenberg ZS, Trepman E. Effect of foot and ankle position on tarsal tunnel compartment volume. Foot Ankle Int. 2006;27(6):431–7.
7. Lareau CR, Sawyer GA, Wang JH, DiGiovanni CW. Plantar and medial heel pain: Diagnosis and management. JAAOS. 2014;22(6):372–80.
8. Ho T, Braza ME. Hoffmann tinel sign. StatPearls. 2022. Available https://www.ncbi.nlm.nih.gov/books/NBK555934/.
9. Kinoshita M, Okuda R, Morikawa J, Jotoku T, Abe M. The dorsiflexion-eversion test for diagnosis of tarsal tunnel syndrome. JBJS. 2001;83(12):1835–9.
10. Patel AT, Gaines K, Malamut R, Park TA, Toro DR, Holland N. Usefulness of electrodiagnostic techniques in the evaluation of suspected tarsal tunnel syndrome: an evidence-based review. Muscle Nerve. 2005;32(2):236–40.
11. Iborra A, Villanueva M, Sanz-Ruiz P. Results of ultrasound-guided release of tarsal tunnel syndrome: a review of 81 cases with a minimum follow-up of 18 months. J Orthop Surg Res. 2020;15(1):30.
12. Iborra Á, Villanueva-Martínez M, Barrett SL, Rodríguez-Collazo ER, Sanz-Ruiz P. Ultrasound-guided release of the tibial nerve and its distal branches: a cadaveric study. J Ultrasound Med. 2019;38(8):2067–79.
13. Doneddu PE, Coraci D, Loreti C, Piccinini G, Padua L. Tarsal tunnel syndrome: Still more opin-

ions than evidence. Status of the art. Neurol Sci. 2017;38(10):1735–9.

14. McSweeney SC, Cichero M. Tarsal tunnel syndrome—a narrative literature review. Foot. 2015;25(4):244–50.

15. Ahmad M, Tsang K, Mackenney PJ, Adedapo AO. Tarsal tunnel syndrome: a literature review. Foot Ankle Surg. 2012;18(3):149–52.

16. Takakura Y, Kitada C, Sugimoto K, Tanaka Y, Tamai S. Tarsal tunnel syndrome. Causes and results of operative treatment. J Bone Joint Surg Br. 1991;73(1):125–8.

17. Rask MR. Medial plantar neurapraxia (jogger's foot): report of 3 cases. Clin Orthop Relat Res. 1978;134:193–5.

18. Donovan A, Rosenberg ZS, Cavalcanti CF. MR imaging of entrapment neuropathies of the lower extremity. Part 2. The knee, leg, ankle, and foot. Radiographics. 2010;30(4):1001–19.

19. Baxter DE, Thigpen CM. Heel pain—operative results. Foot Ankle. 1984;5(1):16–25.

20. Baxter DE, Pfeffer GB. Treatment of chronic heel pain by surgical release of the first branch of the lateral plantar nerve. Clin Orthop Relat Res. 1992;279:229–36.

21. Johnson JE, Johnson KA, Unni KK. Persistent pain after excision of an interdigital neuroma. Results of reoperation. JBJS. 1988;70(5):651–7.

22. Mulder JD. The causative mechanism in Morton's metatarsalgia. J Bone Joint Surg. 1951;33(1):94–5.

23. Gauthier G. Thomas Morton's disease: a nerve entrapment syndrome. A new surgical technique. Clin Orthop Relat Res. 1979;142:90–2.

24. Villas C, Florez B, Alfonso M. Neurectomy versus neurolysis for Morton's neuroma. Foot Ankle Int. 2008;29(6):578–80.

25. Choi JY, Hong WH, Kim MJ, Chae SW, Suh JS. Operative treatment options for Morton's neuroma other than neurectomy – a systematic review. Foot Ankle Surg. 2021;28(4):450–9.

26. Marinacci AA. Neurological syndromes of the tarsal tunnels. Bull Los Angel Neurol Soc. 1968;33(2):90–100.

27. Liu Z, Zhou J, Zhao L. Anterior tarsal tunnel syndrome. J Bone Joint Surg. 1991;73(3):470–3.

28. Logullo F, Ganino C, Lupidi F, Perozzi C, Di Bella P, Provinciali L. Anterior tarsal tunnel syndrome: a misunderstood and a misleading entrapment neuropathy. Neurol Sci. 2014;35(5):773–5.

29. Fortier LM, Markel M, Thomas BG, Sherman WF, Thomas BH, Kaye AD. An update on peroneal nerve entrapment and neuropathy. Orthop Rev. 2021;13(2):24937.

30. Yassin M, Garti A, Weissbrot M, Heller E, Robinson D. Treatment of anterior tarsal tunnel syndrome through an endoscopic or open technique. Foot. 2015;25(3):148–51.

31. Rosson GD, Dellon AL. Superficial peroneal nerve anatomic variability changes surgical technique. Clin Orthop Relat Res. 2005;438:248–52.

32. O'Neill PJ, Parks BG, Walsh R, Simmons LM, Miller SD. Excursion and strain of the superficial peroneal nerve during inversion ankle sprain. JBJS. 2007;89(5):979–86.

33. Falciglia F, Basiglini L, Aulisa AG, Toniolo RM. Superficial peroneal nerve entrapment in ankle sprain in childhood and adolescence. Sci Rep. 2021;11(1):15123.

34. Bowley MP, Doughty CT. Entrapment neuropathies of the lower extremity. Med Clin N Am. 2019;103(2):371–82.

35. Styf J. Entrapment of the superficial peroneal nerve. Diagnosis and results of decompression. J Bone Joint Surg Br. 1989;71(1):131–5.

36. Hanyu-Deutmeyer A, Pritzlaff SG. Peripheral nerve stimulation for the 21st century: sural, superficial peroneal, and tibial nerves. Pain Med. 2020;21(Suppl 1):S64–7.

37. Pringle RM, Protheroe K, Mukherjee SK. Entrapment neuropathy of the sural nerve. J Bone Joint Surg Br. 1974;56(3):465–8.

38. Fabre T, Montero C, Gaujard E, Gervais-Dellion F, Durandeau A. Chronic calf pain in athletes due to sural nerve entrapment. A report of 18 cases. Am J Sports Med. 2000;28(5):679–82.

Part III

Fractures

Classification of Ankle Fractures

Ross Taylor

1 Introduction

Systems of fracture classification create of order out of chaos and facilitate rational inferences and treatment decisions based on related injury patterns, each of which share common anatomic or biomechanical characteristics. These characteristics form the basis for the two most used ankle fracture classification systems, the Danis–Weber and the Lauge–Hansen systems, respectively. The Danis–Weber System was subsequently incorporated into the AO/OTA (AO Foundation/Orthopaedic Trauma Association) classification, creating an exhaustive and detailed catalogue of ankle fractures. The recently recognized significance of the posterior malleolus in fracture stability has led to creation of several excellent classification systems describing fractures of the posterior malleolus, and the Mason and Malloy Classification of posterior malleolar fractures provides valuable diagnostic and treatment insights. Each of these classification systems are discussed in this chapter.

Fracture classification is useful only if the process guides clinical decision-making. Michelson et al. have demonstrated the importance of stability in determining treatment indications, with surgery largely reserved for unstable fractures. Stability of the ankle is determined by integrity of the syndesmotic and deltoid ligaments, as well as the medial, lateral, and posterior malleolus [1]. While neither the Lauge–Hansen nor Danis–Weber AO/OTA classifications are prescriptive of treatment, each stage, type, subtype, and group have implications regarding fracture stability. Each classification system may provide the greatest insights when used in combination with the other or in combination with fracture classifications of the posterior malleolus [2–7].

2 Danis–Weber Classification

The Danis–Weber Classification System of Ankle Fractures evolved from the introduction of the 3-level anatomic system introduced by Danis in 1949, which distinguished fracture types based on the level of the fibula fracture relative to the tibia-talar joint line [8]. This classification system was based on the early concept that the fibula is the key to ankle stability [9]. In 1972, Weber modified Danis' original classification to reference each of the three-alphabetically designated fracture types by the location of the anterior fibular fracture line relative to the syndesmosis (Fig. 1) [10]. Each of the three types is outlined below.

R. Taylor (✉)
Department of Orthopaedic Surgery, HCA Florida Osceola Hospital, University of Central Florida, Kissimmee, FL, USA
e-mail: Ross.Taylor@HCAHealthcare.com

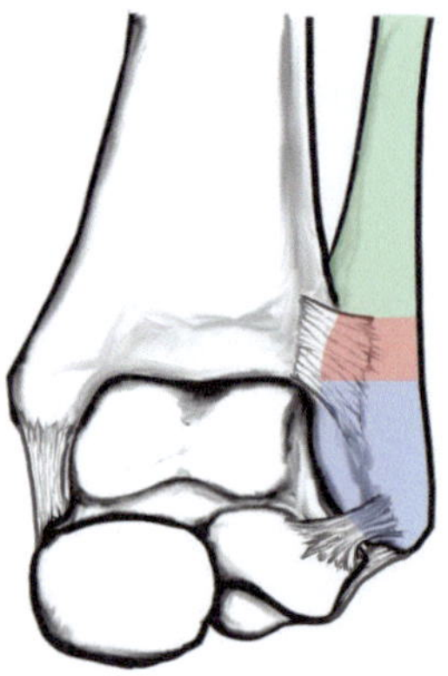

Fig. 1 Danis-Weber Classification System. Danis-Weber type-A fractures occur below the level of the tibiotalar joint (blue area). Danis-Weber type-B fractures occur at the level of the syndesmosis (red area). Danis-Weber type-C fractures occur above the level of the syndesmosis (green area)

2.1　Danis–Weber Type-A

Ankle fractures in which the fibula fracture occurs at or below the syndesmosis. These are the second most common type of ankle fracture, accounting for up to 38% of such injuries [11, 12]. These occur in isolation or in combination with fracture of the medial or posterior malleolus. When medial malleolar fractures are present, these are typically vertical and may be associated with impaction of the medial tibial plafond adjacent the fracture, as seen in Lauge–Hansen supination-adduction stage II injuries [10]. Danis–Weber A fractures usually result from forced adduction of the ankle, and as such are unlikely to involve injury to the syndesmotic or deltoid ligaments [10].

2.2　Danis–Weber Type-B

Ankle fractures in which the fibula fracture occurs through the syndesmosis. Accounting for up to 52% of ankle fractures, these injuries are usually the result of rotational forces and are therefore most closely associated with Lauge–Hansen supination-external rotation or pronation-external rotation type injuries [11, 12]. As such, this type of injury is more likely than Danis–Weber type-A fractures to be associated with fracture of the medial malleolus or deltoid ligament rupture, and the presence of a Danis–Weber type B fibula fracture should alert the clinician to the possibility of syndesmotic instability, as may be seen in up to 50% of cases [10, 13, 14].

2.3　Danis–Weber Type-C

Ankle fractures in which the fibula fracture occurs above the syndesmosis. These are the least common of the Danis–Weber fracture types yet are the most likely of the three types to represent an unstable injury, due to concomitant injuries to the syndesmosis and medial side of the ankle [11, 12]. Hinds et al. demonstrated that almost 57% of these injuries are Lauge–Hansen pronation-external rotation type injuries, and greater than 35% are supination-external rotation type [15]. Recognition of this fracture type is important, as Danis–Weber type C fractures are almost always part of an unstable fracture pattern [16].

2.4　Utility of the Danis Weber Classification

The Danis–Weber Classification System simple has good reliability as measured by low intra and inter-observer variation and is easy to apply, but alone provides limited information related to fracture outcomes [17–20]. Lacking recognition of injuries to the medial side of the ankle, this system was devised under the obsolete assumption that the distal fibula was the key to the stability of the ankle mortise. Since that time, numerous authors have demonstrated the importance of concomitant injuries to the medial side of the ankle [17, 18, 21]. Pathoanatomic factors, such as syndesmotic injury, deltoid ligament injury, or coexisting fractures of the medial or posterior malleolus, which may occur commonly in the presence of Danis–Weber type-B or C fibula fractures, are not accounted for in the Danis–Weber Classification System [7, 22]. The Danis–Weber Classification System is simple and reproducible, but provides limited useful information regarding the prognosis and treatment of ankle fractures.

3 AO/OTA Classification System

The Danis–Weber Classification was incorporated into the Association Osteosynthesis (AO Foundation)/Orthopaedic Trauma Association (OTA) Fracture Classification (AO/OTA Classification) with the inception of this system in 1996 [23]. This system standardizes fracture terminology by converting all fractures in the human body into a reproducible alpha-numeric code such that fractures of the malleolar region of the distal tibia and fibula are assigned the numeric designation of 44.

When combined with the Danis–Weber Classification System to denote the level of the fibular fracture relative to the syndesmosis, malleolar fractures are divided into three types:

Type 44A—infrasyndesmotic fibula fracture (Fig. 2)
Type 44B—transsyndesmotic fibula fracture (Fig. 3)
Type 44C—suprasyndesmotic fibula fracture (Fig. 4).

Each of these three fracture types is then divided again into three-numerically designated groups, depending on the presence or absence of coexisting fractures, ligamentous disruptions, or fracture comminution. Finally, each group is further classified into three subgroups, which is delineated by a decimal point, based on the presence of fractures or ligamentous injuries in addition to those specified at the group level [24].

The AO/OTA Fracture Classification adds qualification codes that injury morphology specific to certain fracture subgroups. These qualifications may delineate the precise location of disruption of the syndesmosis, such as whether disruption of the anterior syndesmosis has

occurred at the fibular insertion (Wagstaffe's Tubercle) or at the tibial origin (Chaput's Tubercle) with certain groups of 44B-type fractures. Similar designations are present to convey the presence or absence of syndesmotic instability or the location of proximal fibular injury with certain groups of 44C-type fractures. These qualification codes trail the subgroup number in parenthesis, ultimately creating a highly specific fracture classification with 27-different injury subtypes, with multiple qualifiers possible within certain subtypes (Table 1).

Universal modifiers are available as well, which provide a single numeric code to denote variables applicable to fractures, such as displacement, dislocation, or systemic factors, such as osteoporosis. Additional lower-case letters within the modifier may be added to denote the direction of displacement or dislocation. Multiple modifiers may be used for any fracture, and modifiers are separated by commas and denoted within square brackets. While complex, the AO/OTA allows for the precise alphanumeric designation of all fractures and dislocations in the human body and even specifies metabolic conditions that may affect the fracture using universal modifiers. The reader is encouraged to reference the full range of available modifiers at: https://journals. lww.com/jorthotrauma/Fulltext/2018/01001/ Introduction__Fracture_and_Dislocation.1.aspx

3.1 Utility of the AO/OTA Classification

The AO/OTA Classification greatly increases the power of Danis–Weber System, by adding additional fracture groups, subgroups, and subtypes to each of the three Danis Weber fracture types. While this level of detail is ideal for research and fracture registries, this level of specificity creates complexity, and this system cannot always be applied using radiographic criteria alone. The authors of the AO/OTA System confirm that classification depends not only on radiographic findings but may also require CT or MRI for accurate classification. Furthermore, complete classification may not be possible "until the operative pro-

a

Group classification 44A1: Infrasyndesmotic isolated lateral injury

b

Group classification 44A2: Infrasyndesmotic lesion with medial malleolar fracture

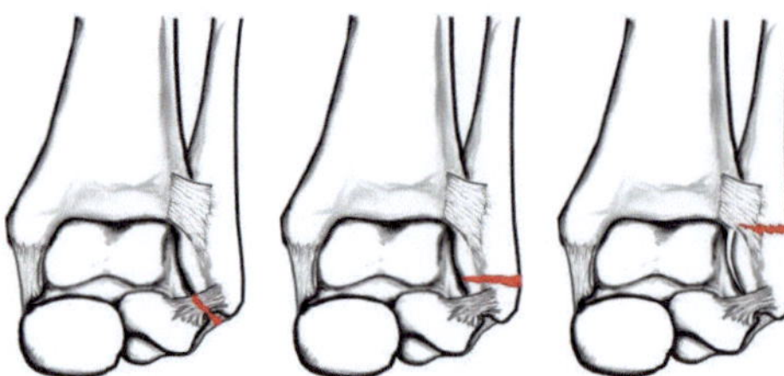

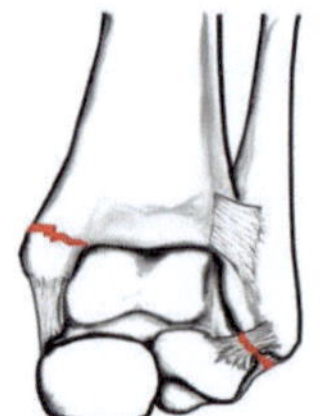

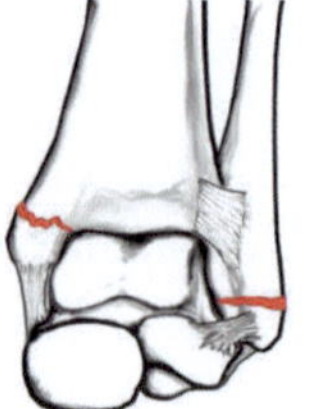

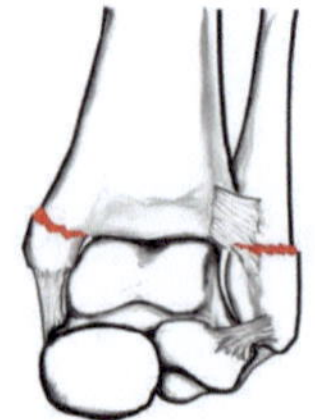

Subgroup 44A1.1: Rupture lateral collateral ligament

Subgroup 44A1.2: Avulsion fracture tip of lateral malleolus

Subgroup 44A1.3: Transverse fracture of lateral malleolus

Subgroup 44A2.1: Rupture lateral collateral ligament with medial malleolar fracture

Subgroup 44A2.2: Avulsion fracture tip of lateral malleolus with medial malleolar fracture

Subgroup 44A2.3: Transverse fracture of lateral malleolus with medial malleolar fracture

c

Group classification 44A3: Infrasyndesmotic lesion with posterior malleolar fracture

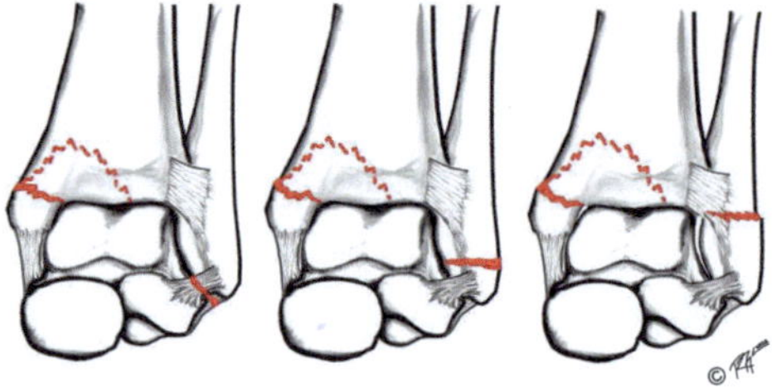

Subgroup 44A3.1: Rupture lateral collateral ligament with medial malleolar and posteromedial fracture

Subgroup 44A3.2: Avulsion fracture tip of lateral malleolus with medial malleolar and posteromedial fracture

Subgroup 44A3.3: Transverse fracture of lateral malleolus with medial malleolar and posteromedial fracture

Fig. 2 OA/OTA Type 44A: Tibia/fibula, malleolar segment, infrasyndesmotic fibula injury. (**a**) Group classification 44A1: Tibia/fibula, malleolar segment, infrasyndesmotic isolated lateral injury (shaded in blue). (**b1**) Subgroup classification 44A1.1: Rupture lateral collateral ligament. (**b2**) Subgroup classification 44A1.2: Avulsion fracture of the tip of the lateral malleolus. (**b3**) Subgroup classification 44A1.3: Transverse fracture of the lateral malleolus. (**c**) Group classification 44A2: infrasyndesmotic lesion with medial malleolar fracture. (**c1**) Subgroup classification 44A2.1: Rupture lateral collateral ligament with medial malleolar fracture. (**c2**) Subgroup classification 44A2.2: Avulsion fracture of the tip of the lateral malleolus with medial malleolar fracture. (**c3**) Subgroup classification 44A2.3: Transverse fracture of the lateral malleolus with medial malleolar fracture. Group classification 44A3: infrasyndesmotic fibula injury with a posterior malleolar fracture (dashed line). Subgroup classification 44A3.1: Rupture lateral collateral ligament with a posteromedial fracture (dashed line). Subgroup classification 44A3.2: Avulsion fracture of the tip of the lateral malleolus with a posteromedial fracture (dashed line). Subgroup classification 44A2.3: Transverse fracture of the lateral malleolus with a posteromedial fracture (dashed line)

a Group classification 44B1: Transsyndesmotic isolated fibula fracture

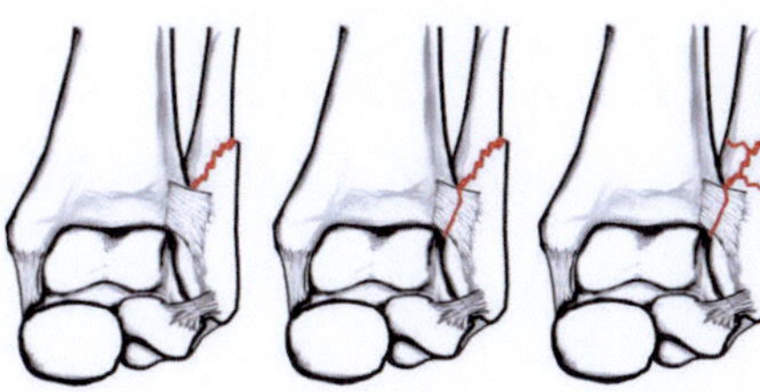

b Group classification 44B2: Transsyndesmotic fibula fracture with medial lesion

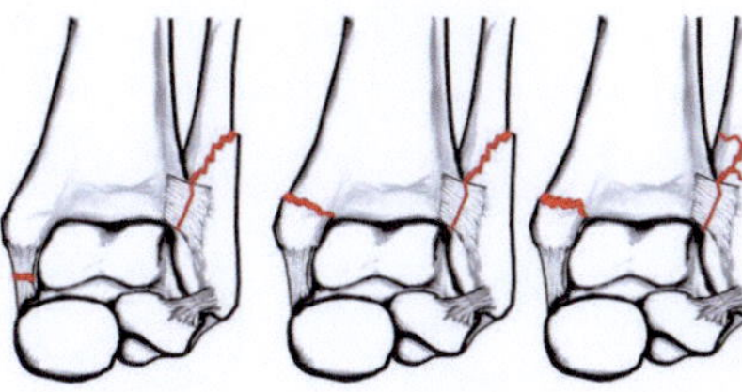

Subgroup 44B1.1: Simple fibula fracture

Subgroup 44B1.2: Simple fibula fracture with injury to the syndesmosis

Subgroup 44B1.3: Wedge or multifragmentary fibula fracture with injury to the syndesmosis

Subgroup 44B2.1: Simple fibula fracture with rupture of deltoid and injury to the syndesmosis

Subgroup 44B2.2: Simple fibula and medial malleolus fracture with injury to the syndesmosis

Subgroup 44B2.3: Wedge or multifragmentary fibula and medial malleolus fracture with injury to the syndesmosis

Available qualifications: n,o,u

Available qualifications: n,o,u

Available qualifications: n,o,u

Available qualifications: n,o,u

Available qualifications: n,o,u

c Group classification 44B3: Transsyndesmotic fibula fracture with medial lesion and fracture of posterolateral rim of tibia (Volkmann's Fragment)

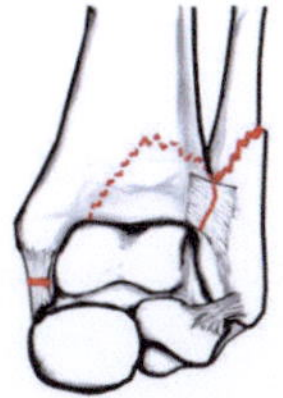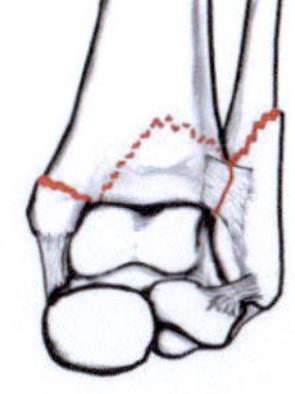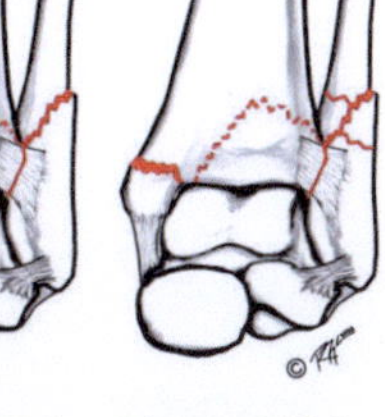

Subgroup 44B3.1: Simple fibula and posterolateral fracture (Volkmann's Fragment) with rupture of deltoid and injury to the syndesmosis

Available qualifications: n,o,u

Subgroup 44B3.2: Simple fibula and posterolateral fracture (Volkmann's Fragment) with medial malleolus fracture and injury to the syndesmosis

Available qualifications: n,o,u

Subgroup 44B3.3: Wedge or multifragmentary fibula and posterolateral fracture (Volkmann's Fragment) and injury to the syndesmosis

Available qualifications: n,o,u

Fig. 3 OA/OTA Type 44B: Tibia/fibula, malleolar segment, transsyndesmotic fibula fracture. (**a**) Group classification 44B1: Isolated fibula fracture (shaded in pink). (**b1**) Subgroup classification 44B1.1: Simple fibula fracture. Qualifications: n,o,u. (**b2**) Subgroup classification 44B1.2: With injury to the anterior syndesmosis. Available qualifications: n,o,u. (**b3**) Subgroup classification 44B1.3: Wedge or multifragmentary fibula fracture. Available qualifications: n,o,u. (**c**) Group classification 44B2: Transsyndesmotic fibula fracture with a medial malleolus fracture. (**c1**) Subgroup classification 44B2.1: With a rupture of the deltoid ligament and anterior syndesmosis. Available qualifications: n,o,u. (**c2**) Subgroup classification 44B2.2: With a medial malleolus fracture and a rupture of the anterior syndesmosis.

Available qualifications: n,o,u. Illustrated example: fracture shown as #2 would be classified as 44B2.2(n), due to fracture of Chaput's Tubercle. (**c3**) Subgroup classification 44B2.3: Wedge or multifragmentary fibula fracture with medial injury. Available qualifications: r,s,u. Group classification 44B3: Transsyndesmotic fibula fracture with a medial injury and fracture of the posterolateral rim (Volkmann's fragment) (dashed line). Subgroup classification 44B3.1: Simple, with a deltoid ligament rupture. Available qualifications: n,o,u. Subgroup classification 44B3.2: Simple medial malleolus fracture. Available qualifications: n,o,u. Subgroup classification 44B3.3: Wedge or multifragmentary fibula fracture with fracture of the medial malleolus. Available qualifications: n,o,u

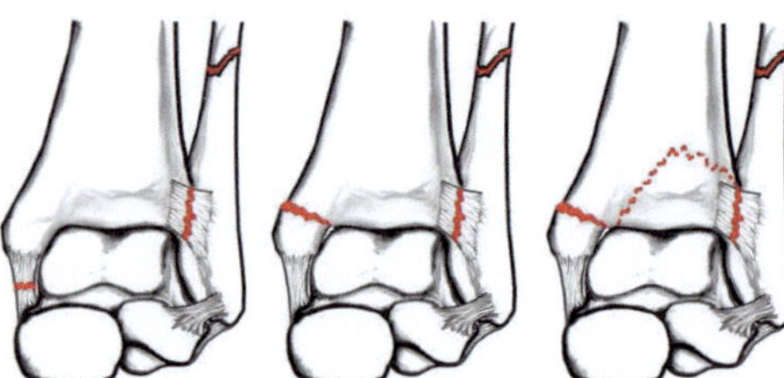
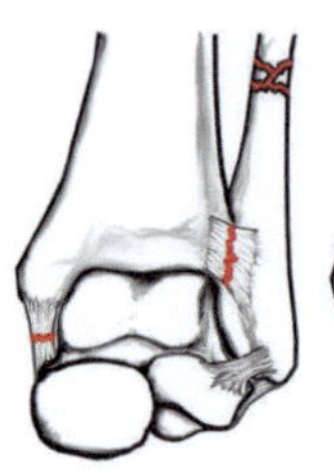
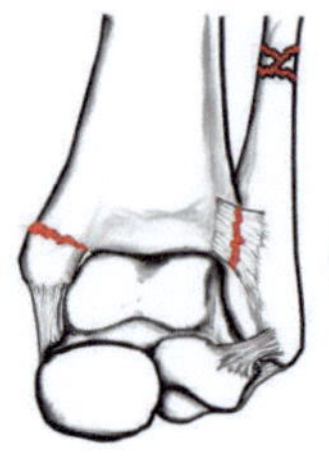
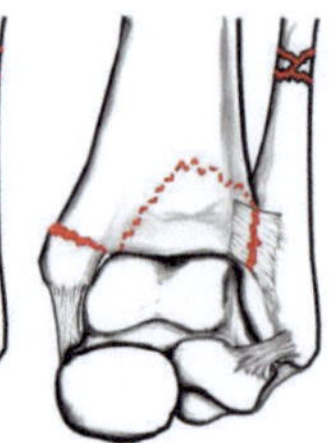

a Group classification 44C1: Simple suprasyndesmotic fibula fracture

b Group classification 44C2: Wedge or mulitfragmentary fibula fracture

Subgroup 44C1.1:
Simple diaphyseal fibula fracture with rupture of deltoid ligament and injury to the syndesmosis

Subgroup 44C1.2:
Simple diaphyseal fibula fracture and medial malleolus fracture with injury to the syndesmosis

Subgroup 44C1.3:
Simple diaphyseal fibula and medial malleolus fracture and posterolateral rim fracture (Volkmann's Fragment) with injury to the syndesmosis

Subgroup 44C2.1:
Wedge or multifragmentary fibula fracture with rupture of deltoid and injury to the syndesmosis

Subgroup 44C2.2:
Wedge or multifragmentary fibula and medial malleolus fracture with injury to the syndesmosis

Subgroup 44BC.3:
Wedge or multifragmentary fibula and medial malleolus fracture and posterolateral rim fracture (Volkmann's Fragment) with injury to the syndesmosis

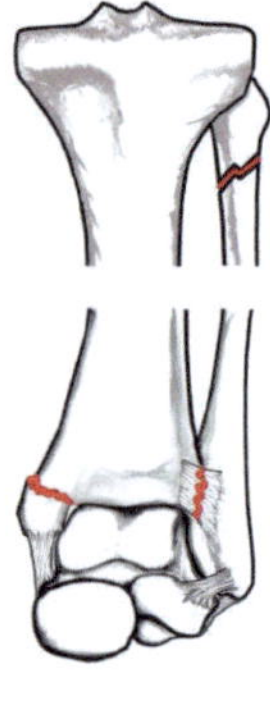
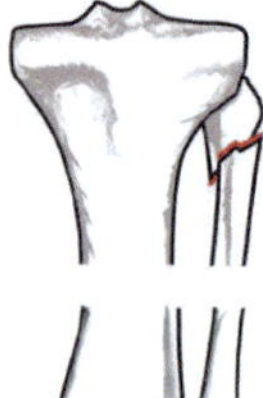
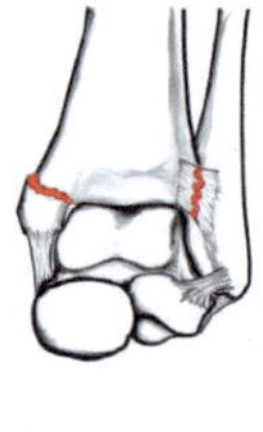
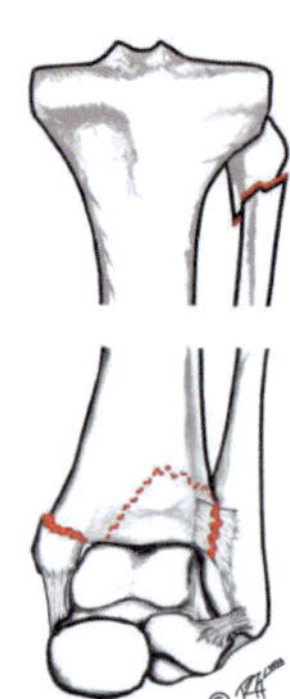

c Group classification 44C3: Proximal fibula injury

Subgroup 44C3.1:
Proximal fibula injury and medial lesion with injury to the syndesmosis

Subgroup 44C3.2:
Proximal fibula injury with shortening and medial lesion with injury to the syndesmosis

Subgroup 44C3.3:
Proximal fibula injury with shortening and posterolateral rim fracture (Volkmann's Fragment) with medial lesion and injury to the syndesmosis

Fig. 4 OA/OTA Type 44C: Tibia/fibula, malleolar segment, suprasyndesmotic fibula fracture. (**a**) Group classification 44C1: Simple diaphyseal fibula fracture (shaded in green). (**b**1) Subgroup classification 44C1.1: With a rupture of the deltoid ligament. (**b**2) Subgroup classification 44C1.2: With a fracture of the medial malleolus. (**b**3) Subgroup classification 44C1.3: With a medial and a posterior malleolus fracture (dashed line). (**c**) Group classification 44C2: Wedge or multifragmentary diaphyseal fibula fracture. (**c**1) Subgroup classification 44C2.1: With a rupture of the deltoid ligament. (**c**2) Subgroup classification 44C2.2: With a fracture of the medial malleolus. (**c**3) Subgroup classification 44C2.3: With a fracture of the medial and posterior malleolus (dashed line). Group classification 44C3: Proximal fibula injury. Subgroup classification 44C3.1: With a medial side injury. Subgroup classification 44C3.2: With shortening and a medial side injury. Subgroup classification 44C3.3: With a medial side injury and a posterior malleolus fracture (dashed line)

Table 1 OTA Fracture qualifications

Qualification	Injury morphology
n	Tillaux–Chaput tubercle fracture
o	Wagstaffe–Le Fort avulsion fracture
p	Fibula neck fracture
q	Proximal tibio-fibular dislocation
r	Rupture of the deltoid ligament
s	Fracture of the medial malleolus
t	Syndesmosis stable
u	Syndesmosis unstable

cedure is completed and the fracture fully visualized" [23]. The high degree of specificity inherent to the AO/OTA system renders it less reproducible than other systems [12, 20, 22].

The addition of the AO/OTA subclasses to the Danis–Weber Classification System provides additional information pertaining to prognosis. The AO/OTA Fracture Classification is designed in an hierarchical manner, such that fracture severity increases within each of the Danis–Weber Groups from A to C. Similarly, within each group, injury severity increases from 1 to 3. As such, the ability of the AO/OTA Classification System to predict injury outcome has been studied. Kennedy demonstrated a significantly worse outcome with Danis–Weber type C fractures than either type A or B [25]. Sung et al. demonstrated a correlation between negative outcomes as measures using FAOS scores and injury severity as determined by AO/OTA subgroup [26].

The addition of the AO/OTA System to the Danis–Weber Classification improves the specificity of this classification and has thus contributed greatly to the understanding of how anatomic variables influence the treatment and outcomes of ankle fractures. Ultimately, the Danis–Weber/OA/OTA Classification may be more useful in combination with the Lauge–Hansen System.

4 Lauge–Hansen Classification

The Lauge–Hansen System classifies ankle fractures according to mechanism of injury using a two-part nomenclature to describe ankle fractures according to the position of the foot at the time of injury (supination or pronation) and the direction of the deforming force that creates the defined injury (external rotation, adduction or abduction) [27]. Using these principles, the Lauge–Hansen Classification System outlines four fracture types and up to four successive stages of injury for each type.

Supination injuries are characterized by initial injury to the tensioned lateral or anterolateral structures, while pronation injuries result in initial injury to the tensioned medial side. After initial injury, the direction of the deforming force determines the sequence of injury to the stabilizing bony and ligamentous structures of the ankle. This system allows the clinician to associate observed fracture patterns with potentially unseen underlying bony and ligamentous injuries on which are based the need for stress testing, advanced imaging, or surgical treatment. Not all fractures neatly fit into the Lauge–Hansen Classification System, but up to 90% or more do [15]. Each of the Lauge–Hansen type is examined below.

4.1 Supination-External Rotation (SER) (Fig. 5)

When external rotation is applied to the supinated foot, the initial structure to fail is the laterally tensioned anterior inferior tibiofibular ligament (SER stage I) (Fig. 5a). This is followed by fracture of the lateral malleolus (SER stage II) (Fig. 5b), then by rupture of the posterior tibiofibular ligament (PITFL) or fracture of the posterior malleolus (SER stage III) (Fig. 5c), followed finally by fracture of the medial malleolus or deltoid ligament injury (SER stage IV) (Fig. 5d). SER type injuries are the most common Lauge–Hansen fracture type, with series citing an incidence of between 50% and 65% of ankle fractures [11, 28].

SER injuries may be recognized by the character of the fibula fracture, which are typically spiral to variably oblique and are oriented from anteroinferior to posterosuperior. Originating within 4 cm of the tibiotalar joint, the height and length of the fibular fracture in SER III injuries may be predictive of syndesmotic instability, with longer

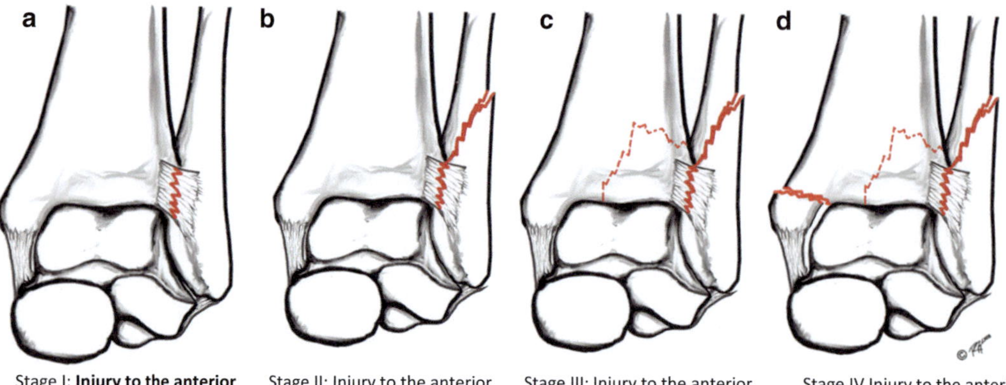

Fig. 5 Lauge-Hansen supination-external rotation type fractures. (**a**) Stage I: Anterior syndesmotic injury with rupture of the anterior tibiofibular ligament (ATFL). (**b**) Stage II: Addition of a fracture of the lateral malleolus. (**c**) Stage III: Addition of rupture of the posterior tibiofibular ligament (PTFL) or fracture of the posterior malleolus (dashed line). (**d**) Stage IV: Addition of fracture of the medial malleolus or deltoid ligament

fractures encompassing more of the insertion of the anterior syndesmotic ligaments [15, 28, 29]. The reported incident of syndesmotic instability in SER III injuries is highly variable, between 30% and 75%, and these injuries may require stress testing to determine the need for surgical treatment [28, 30, 31]. SER IV injuries are unstable, with fracture of the fibula, complete disruption of the syndesmosis, and injury to the deltoid ligament or fracture of the medial malleolus [28].

4.2 Supination-Adduction (SAD) (Fig. 6)

When adduction is applied to the supinated foot, injury begins with the tensioned lateral side and progresses medially. The first stage of SAD injuries is transverse fracture of the tensioned lateral malleolus or rupture of the lateral ankle ligaments (SAD stage I) (Fig. 6a). Continued adduction of the unrestrained talus results in a vertical fracture of the medial malleolus, and articular impaction of the medial tibial plafond may occur (SAD stage II) (Fig. 6b). SAD I injuries, as evidenced by Danis–Weber A transverse or short oblique fracture of the fibula below the level of the syndesmosis, are typically stable unless

accompanied by fracture of the medial malleolus, as seen in SAD II injuries [28]. Supination adduction injuries occur in 20% or less of ankle fractures [10]. Supination adduction injuries have a worse outcome than other rotational ankle injuries and represent a transitional pattern between rotational ankle fractures and pilon fractures. This is discussed in more detail in chapter "Management of Fractures of the Tibial Plafond".

4.3 Pronation-External Rotation (PER) (Fig. 7)

External rotation of the pronated foot results in initial injury to the tensioned medial side, with either rupture of the deltoid ligament or fracture of the medial malleolus, which typically fractures in an oblique pattern (PER stage I) (Fig. 7a). Injury then progresses in an externally rotating direction to next include rupture of the anterior inferior talofibular ligament (AITFL) (PER stage II) (Fig. 7b), followed by a fracture of the fibula at or above the level of the syndesmosis (PER stage III) (Fig. 7c). In the final and most severe stage of pronation-external rotation injuries, rupture of the PITFL or fracture of the posterior malleolus at the origin of the PITFL (PER stage IV) (Fig. 7d).

Fig. 6 Lauge-Hansen supination-adduction type fractures. (**a**) Stage I: Oblique fracture of the lateral malleolus or rupture of the lateral ankle ligaments. (**b**) Stage II: Addition of vertical fracture of the medial malleolus with or without articular impaction of the medial tibial plafond

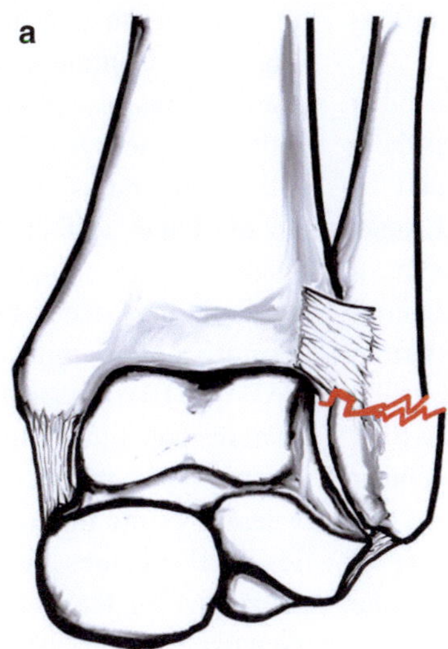

Stage I: **Fracture of the lateral malleolus or fracture of the distal fibula**

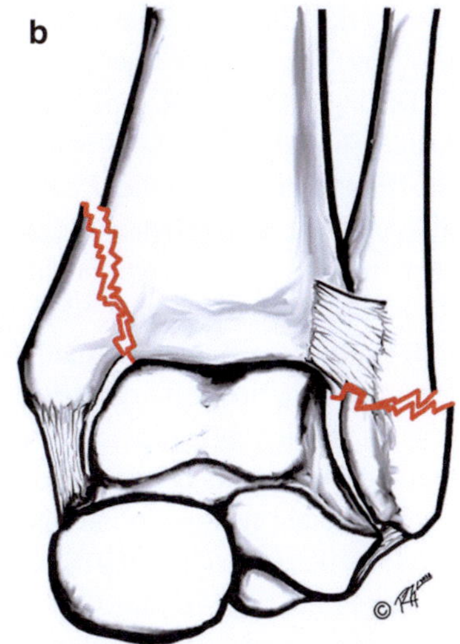

Stage II: Fracture of the lateral malleolus or rupture of the lateral ankle ligaments and **fracture of the medial malleolus with or without articular impaction of the medial distal tibia**

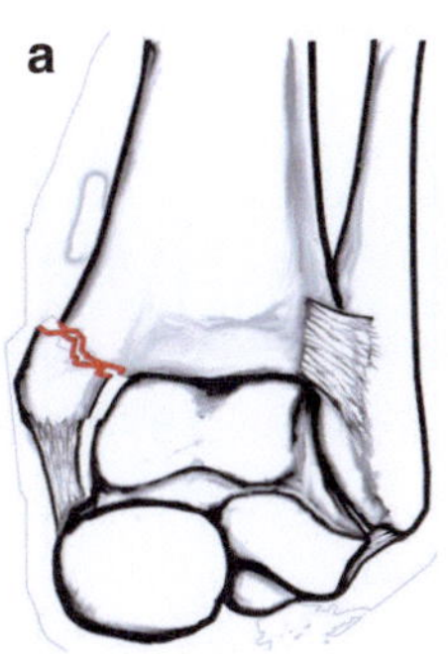

Stage I: Rupture of the deltoid ligament or **fracture of the medial malleolus**

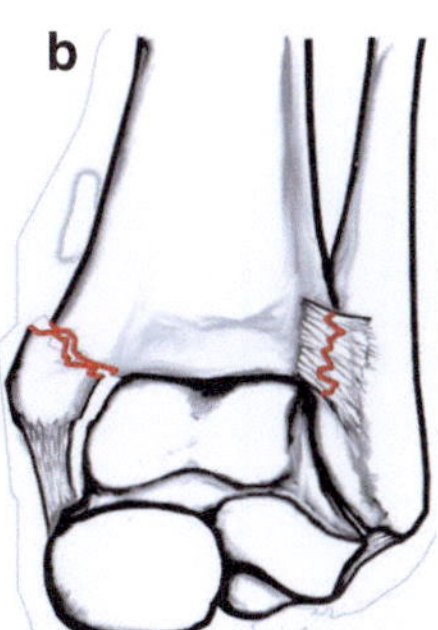

Stage II: Rupture of the deltoid ligament or fracture of the medial malleolus with **anterior syndesmotic injury**

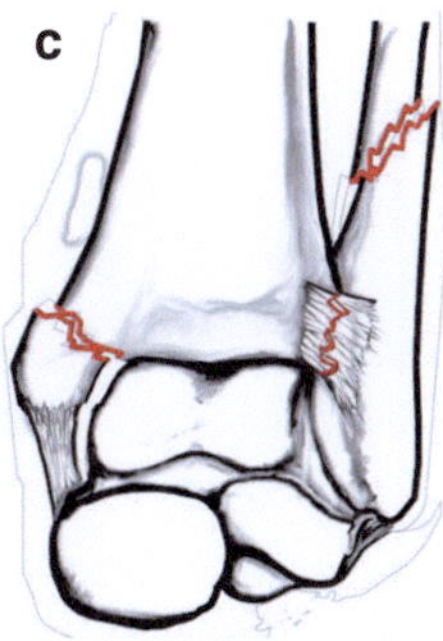

Stage III: Rupture of the deltoid ligament or fracture of the medial malleolus with anterior syndesmotic injury (propagating to the level of the fibula fracture) and **oblique fracture of the distal fibula**

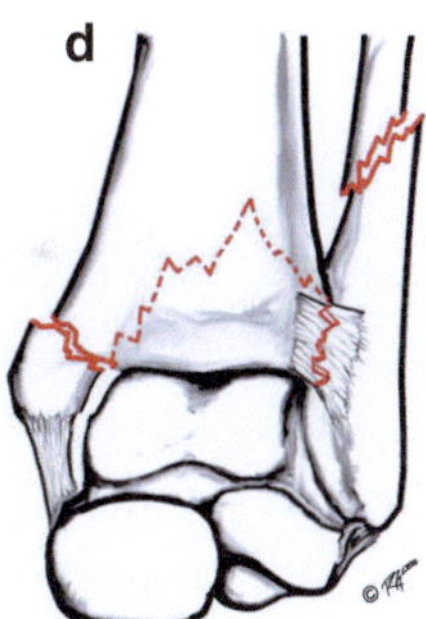

Stage IV Rupture of the deltoid ligament or fracture of the medial malleolus with anterior syndesmotic injury (propagating to the level of the fibula fracture) and oblique fracture of the distal fibula with **rupture of the PITFL or fracture of the posterior malleolus**

Fig. 7 Lauge-Hansen pronation-external rotation type fractures. (**a**) Stage I: Rupture of the deltoid ligament or fracture of the medial malleolus. (**b**) Stage II: Addition of anterior syndesmotic injury with rupture of the ATFL. (**c**) Stage III: Addition of oblique fracture of the fibula, with syndesmotic injury propagating to the level of the fracture. (**d**) Stage IV: Addition of rupture of the PTFL or fracture of the posterior malleolus

Most series cite an incidence of PER fractures as less than 20% of ankle fractures [10, 11].

Distinguishing PER type injuries from other Lauge–Hansen type injuries is important, as these injuries are often unstable. PER injuries may be differentiated radiographically from other Lauge–Hansen types by the directionality and height of the fibula fracture. Unlike SER type fractures, PER type fibula fractures usually progress from anterosuperior to posteroinferior, and typically originate from a more proximal location than SER types. Hinds et al. demonstrated that a fibular fracture height relative to the tibiotalar joint line of >35 mm demonstrated a 91% sensitivity in predicting a PER stage III injury, which may indicate the need for surgical management [15, 31].

4.4 Pronation-Abduction (PAB) (Fig. 8)

Abduction of the pronated foot results in initial injury of the tensioned medial side, with resultant rupture of the deltoid ligament or transverse fracture of the medial malleolus (PAB stage I) (Fig. 8a). Continued abduction of the unrestrained talus results in a laterally directed force with subsequent injury to the AITFL or avulsion of the ligamentous origin of the AITFL with fracture of Chaput's Tubercle (PAB stage II) (Fig. 8b). Finally, a short oblique or transverse fracture of the fibula may occur above the level of the syndesmosis, often with significant comminution (PAB type III) (Fig. 8c) [27]. Pronation-abduction fractures constitute a minority of Lauge–Hansen fracture types, with a reported incidence of 10% or less. Despite the low incidence of these injuries, PAB fractures are commonly open, with the sharp edge of the tibial proximal fracture fragment exposed through the relatively thin and tensioned soft tissue envelope [10, 32].

It is important to distinguish Lauge–Hanson pronation-type fractures from supination injuries. Unlike supination fractures, which are characteristically Danis–Weber type-B fractures oriented obliquely from anterior-inferior to posterior-superior, pronation fractures are more likely to originate above the syndesmosis and are oriented

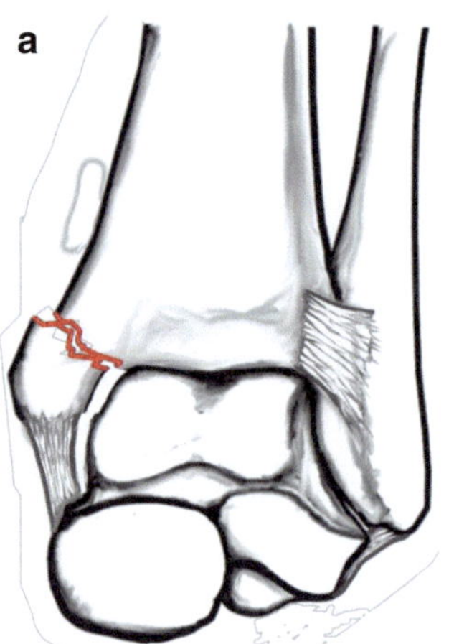

Stage I: Rupture of the deltoid ligament or **fracture of the medial malleolus**

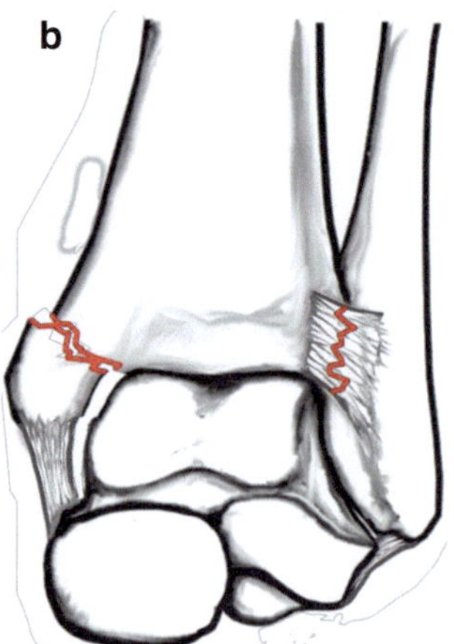

Stage II: Rupture of the deltoid ligament or fracture of the medial malleolus with **anterior syndesmotic injury or fracture of Chaput's Tubercle**

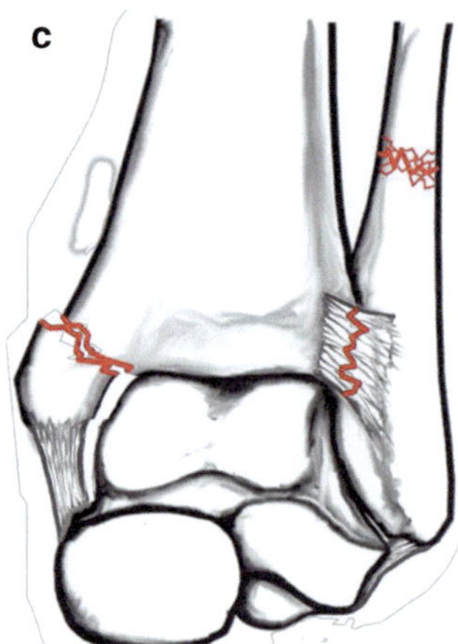

Stage III: Rupture of the deltoid ligament or fracture of the medial malleolus with anterior syndesmotic injury or fracture of Chaput's Tubercle and **transverse or comminuted fracture of the fibula**

Fig. 8 Lauge-Hansen pronation-abduction type fractures. (**a**) Stage I: Rupture of the deltoid ligament or fracture of the medial malleolus. (**b**) Stage II: Anterior syndesmotic injury with rupture of the ATFL or fracture of Chaput's Tubercle. (**c**) Stage III: Transverse or comminuted fracture of the fibula, with syndesmotic injury propagating to the level of the fracture

obliquely from anterior-superior to posterior-inferior. Pronation fractures are generally higher in energy and are more likely than supination-type injuries to be unstable due to fracture of the medial malleolus or injury to the deltoid ligament [28, 33].

4.5 Utility of the Lauge–Hansen Classification

Critics of the Lauge–Hansen Classification System challenge its validity, due to an inability of authors to reproduce the originally described injury patterns using modern force reproduction techniques [6, 34, 35]. Such criticism is not surprising, given that the original work of Lauge–Hansen involved the manual application of a deforming force to cadaveric ankles that were secured to a board using commercial nails [35]. Modern techniques have allowed authors to review injury videos available on social media and correlate the observed mechanism of action to the corresponding radiographs. These studies have shown a poor correlation between radiographic fracture pattern and observed mechanism of injury [36, 37]. Michelson et al. recreated SER injuries using a system of force plates and transducers, yet these authors were unable to reliably generate injuries to the AITFL or PITFL or recreate the corresponding fractures of each ligamentous origin, that could render an advanced stage SER fracture unstable, as is implied in the original Lauge–Hansen description [6, 38].

Despite questions regarding the validity of the Lauge–Hansen Classifications as it relates to mechanism of injury, this classification system outlines reproducible patterns of ligament injury associated with individual Lauge–Hansen types that may impact treatment. Warner et al. found a greater than 85% correlation between Lauge–Hansen stage and injuries to the deltoid ligament or syndesmosis using MRI and operative findings [39]. This insight allows the surgeon to understand which fracture patterns are likely to be associated with ligamentous injuries that may render a given fracture unstable.

Greater complexity renders the Lauge–Hansen Classification System less reproducible than more simple systems such as the Danis–Weber Classification. Nielson et al. examined intra and inter-observer variability in classifying 118 ankle fractures using the Lauge–Hansen System and demonstrated agreement in only 82% of paired observations when considering Lauge–Hansen Type, and this agreement declined to less than 65% when agreement among Lauge–Hansen Stage was sought [40]. This may be because findings that determine staging, such as disruption of the deltoid ligament or AITFL, are not seen on plain radiographs.

In final analysis, the Lauge–Hansen system is a comprehensive mechanical classification system of fractures that has contributed greatly to the understanding and study of ankle fractures, particularly through the recognition of reliably recurring injury patterns that may result in instability of the ankle. Furthermore, definite inferences can be made regarding fracture stability and the need for surgical treatment based on Lauge–Hansen type and stage.

5 Mason and Malloy Classification of Fractures of the Posterior Malleolus

Up to 46% of Weber B and C ankle fractures include injuries to the posterior malleolus [41]. Traditionally, indications for surgical treatment of posterior malleolus fractures were based on the percent involvement of the articular surface, with 25% being commonly cited as the threshold for repair [16, 42–45]. More recently, Gardner et al. have demonstrated the importance of direct repair of the posterior malleolus in restoring syndesmotic stability through restoration of the origin of the PITFL, without discounting the role of the extent of articular involvement [46, 47]. As such, Haraguchi, Bartonocek, and most recently Mason and Malloy have developed posterior malleolus fracture classification systems, each of which recognize similar recurring fracture patterns [34, 46, 48–50]. Unlike fractures of the medial and lateral malleolus, fractures of the posterior malleolus are uniquely difficult to visualize on plain radiographs, and CT scan is required to understand the morphology of these fractures [49, 51, 52]. Using information gained from CT scan, the Mason and Malloy Classification System of posterior malleolus fractures may be used to provide important insights into the management of these complex fractures [38].

5.1 Mason and Malloy Type-1 Fracture

These fractures represent avulsion fractures of the posterior inferior tibiofibular ligament (PITFL) from the posterolateral distal tibia caused by external rotation of the talus within the mortise and typically involve less than 11% of the articular surface (Fig. 9a) [34]. These fractures commonly result in syndesmotic instability, the diagnosis of which may require an internal rotation stress test to detect widening of the tibiofibular clear space [38]. This fracture type is typically accompanied by an oblique distal fibula fracture and medial injury, as seen in Lauge–Hansen SER IV injury [53].

5.2 Mason and Malloy Type 2 Fractures

Type-2 fractures are characterized by a large posterolateral fragment that involves the incisura fibularis. Mason and Malloy recognized two grades of severity, based on the degree of external rotation of the talus within the ankle mortise.

Type-2A injuries are initiated by external rotation of the talus within the ankle mortis, causing bony abutment of the talus on the posterolateral tibial plafond, resulting in a large posterolateral fracture fragment. Mason and Malloy type-2A fractures are associated with a low fibular fracture, medial injury, and variably result in syndesmotic disruption. The single large posterolateral fragment produced by type-2A fractures has been found to be associated with Lauge–Hansen Type SER injuries (Fig. 9b) [19].

Type 2B injuries result from continued external rotation of the talus within the ankle mortise and propagation of the posterolateral fracture characteristic of type-2A fractures along a second fracture line 45° to the first, extending into the medial malleolus (Fig. 9c) [38]. These injuries commonly result in syndesmotic instability, due to complete disruption of the PITFL origin

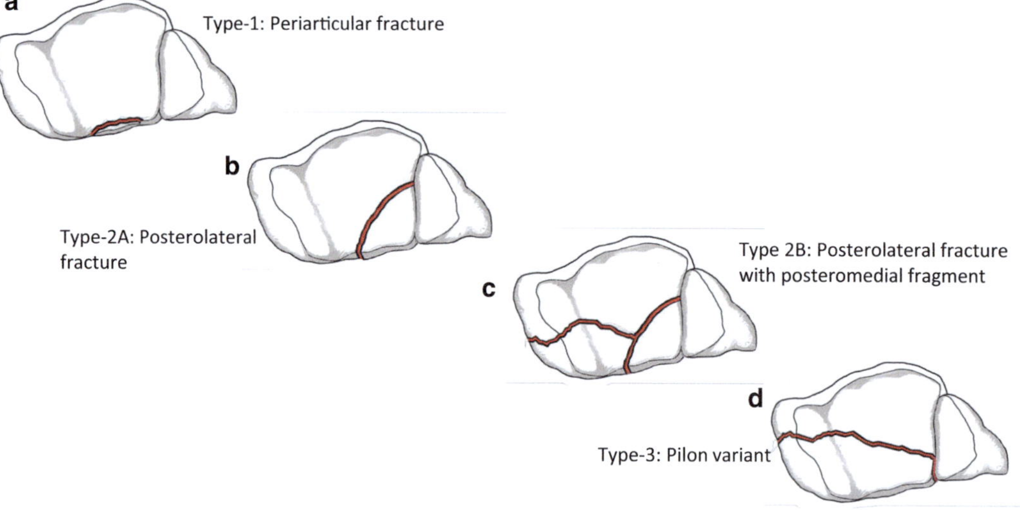

Fig. 9 Mason and Malloy Classification of posterior malleolus fractures. (**a**) Type-1: Periarticular fracture. (**b**) Type-2A: Posterolateral fracture. (**c**) Type-2B: Posterolateral fracture with posteromedial fragment. (**d**) Type-3: Pilon variant

from the posterior malleolus in combination with medial injury. Mason and Malloy Type-2B fractures are associated with advanced Lauge–Hansen Type PER injuries and are universally unstable [53, 54].

5.3 Mason and Malloy Type-3 Fracture

Characterized as a high-oblique fracture of the posterior tibial plafond, these injuries occur frequently in conjunction with a long coplanar fibula fracture (Fig. 9d). This fracture type is a pilon variant and is theorized by Mason to be caused by axial loading of the plantar-flexed talus. The syndesmosis remains stable due to the intact syndesmotic association between the large posterior tibial fragment and the long posterior fibular attachment, even though these fractures typically involve a large portion of the articular surface of the distal tibia.

5.4 Utility of the Mason and Malloy Classification

The Mason and Malloy Classification is useful in directing the surgical approach to repairing the posterior malleolus when needed to restore syndesmotic stability or articular congruity. Type-1 fractures require indirect syndesmotic repair using traditional syndesmotic fixation through a lateral approach, while restoration of the ligamentous origin of the PITFL through open reduction and internal fixation of the posterior malleolus may be preferable for type 2 or 3 fractures. Type-2A fractures are best approached posterolaterally, with the patient positioned prone. A posteromedial approach is advised for Type-2B fractures, and fracture-specific repair, usually with visualization through the coplanar distal fibula fracture is preferable for type-3 fractures [55]. Open reduction and fixation of the posterior malleolar origin of the PITFL has been shown to provide significantly improved syndesmotic stability compared to traditional syndesmotic screws [46].

Classification systems of posterior malleolar fractures provide an adjunctive tool in evaluating ankle fractures and may provide useful guidance regarding treatment. Once posterior malleolar involvement is identified on plain radiographs, as may be seen with advanced Lauge–Hansen SER or PER injuries, CT scanning may be used to identify the posterior malleolar fracture pattern, as outlined in this chapter, to guide surgical decision making.

6 Conclusion

The two most commonly used classification systems for ankle fractures are the Danis–Weber AO/OTA Classification System and the mechanistic Lauge–Hansen Classification System. The Danis–Weber Classification has the advantage of simplicity and may be combined with the Lauge–Hansen Classification System. The incorporation of the Danis–Weber classification into the AO/OTA system provides additional specificity through the addition of distinct fracture groups, subgroups, qualifications, and general modifiers, which render this classification ideal for use in research and fracture registries. The Lauge–Hansen Classification has the advantage of describing reliably reoccurring injury patterns and assigned stages of severity, which may be used to identify underlying unstable osseoligamentous injury patterns that may impact treatment. The Mason and Malloy Classification of Posterior Malleolus Fractures provides a framework for understanding fractures of the posterior malleolus and may provide insights into fracture stability and is useful in guiding surgical approach. Most importantly, each of the classification systems described in this chapter may be used to singly or in combination to guide diagnostic and treatment decisions.

References

1. Boden SD, Labropoulos PA, McCowin P, Lestini WF, Hurwitz SR. Mechanical considerations for the syndesmosis screw. A cadaver study. J Bone Joint Surg Am. 1989;71(10):1548–55.
2. Michelson JD, Magid D, McHale K. Clinical utility of a stability-based ankle fracture classification system. J Orthop Trauma. 2007;21(5):307–15.

3. Pakarinen H. Stability-based classification for ankle fracture management and the syndesmosis injury in ankle fractures due to a supination external rotation mechanism of injury. Acta Orthop Suppl. 2012;83(347):1–26.

4. Pakarinen HJ, Flinkkil TE, Ohtonen PP, Ristiniemi JY. Stability criteria for nonoperative ankle fracture management. Foot Ankle Int. 2011;32(2):141–7.

5. Fox A, Wykes P, Eccles K, Barrie J. Five years of ankle fractures grouped by stability. Injury. 2005;36(7):836–41.

6. Michelson J, Solocoff D, Waldman B, Kendell K, Ahn U, Ankle fractures. The Lauge-Hansen classification revisited. Clin Orthop Relat Res. 1997;345:198–205.

7. Delaney JP, Charlson MD, Michelson JD. Ankle fracture stability-based classification: a study of reproducibility and clinical prognostic ability. J Orthop Trauma. 2019;33(9):465–71.

8. Müller ME, Perren SM, Allgöwer M, Müller ME, Schneider R, Willenegger H. Manual of internal fixation: techniques recommended by the AO-ASIF group. Berlin: Springer Science & Business Media; 1991.

9. Muller MAM, Schneider R, Willenegger H. Manual of internal fixation. Techniques recommended by the AO Group. New York: Springer; 1979.

10. Lindsjo U. Classification of ankle fractures: the Lauge-Hansen or AO system? Clin Orthop Relat Res. 1985;199:12–6.

11. Court-Brown CM, McBirnie J, Wilson G. Adult ankle fractures—an increasing problem? Acta Orthop Scand. 1998;69(1):43–7.

12. Rydberg EM, Zorko T, Sundfeldt M, Moller M, Wennergren D. Classification and treatment of lateral malleolar fractures—a single-center analysis of 439 ankle fractures using the Swedish fracture register. BMC Musculoskelet Disord. 2020;21(1):521.

13. Hopkinson WJ, St Pierre P, Ryan JB, Wheeler JH. Syndesmosis sprains of the ankle. Foot Ankle. 1990;10(6):325–30.

14. El-Rosasy M, Ali T. Realignment-lengthening osteotomy for malunited distal fibular fracture. Int Orthop. 2013;37(7):1285–90.

15. Hinds RM, Schottel PC, Berkes MB, Little MT, Helfet DL, Lorich DG. Evaluation of Lauge-Hansen designation of Weber C fractures. J Foot Ankle Surg. 2014;53(4):434–9.

16. Broos PL, Bisschop AP. Operative treatment of ankle fractures in adults: correlation between types of fracture and final results. Injury. 1991;22(5):403–6.

17. Pettrone FA, Gail M, Pee D, Fitzpatrick T, Van Herpe LB. Quantitative criteria for prediction of the results after displaced fracture of the ankle. J Bone Joint Surg Am. 1983;65(5):667–77.

18. Michelson JD, Magid D, Ney DR, Fishman EK. Examination of the pathologic anatomy of ankle fractures. J Trauma. 1992;32(1):65–70.

19. Bhimani R, Ashkani-Esfahani S, Lubberts B, Kaiser P, Kerkhoffs G, Waryasz G, et al. Utility of WBCT to diagnose syndesmotic instability in patients with Weber B lateral malleolar fractures. J Am Acad Orthop Surg. 2021;30:e423.

20. Ramos LS, Goncalves HM, Freitas A, Oliveira MP, Lima DMS, Carmargo WS. Evaluation of the reproducibility of Lauge-Hansen, Danis-Weber, and AO classifications for ankle fractures. Rev Bras Ortop (Sao Paulo). 2021;56(3):372–8.

21. Harper MC. Ankle fracture classification systems: a case for integration of the Lauge-Hansen and AO-Danis-Weber schemes. Foot Ankle. 1992;13(7):404–7.

22. Alexandropoulos C, Tsourvakas S, Papachristos J, Tselios A, Soukouli P. Ankle fracture classification: an evaluation of three classification systems: Lauge-Hansen, A.O. and Broos-Bisschop. Acta Orthop Belg. 2010;76(4):521–5.

23. Meinberg EG, Agel J, Roberts CS, Karam MD, Kellam JF. Fracture and dislocation classification compendium-2018. J Orthop Trauma. 2018;32(Suppl 1):S1–S170.

24. Malleolar segment. J Orthop Trauma. 2018;32:S65–S70.

25. Kennedy JG, Johnson SM, Collins AL, DalloVedova P, McManus WF, Hynes DM, et al. An evaluation of the weber classification of ankle fractures. Injury. 1998;29(8):577–80.

26. Sung KH, Kwon SS, Yun YH, Park MS, Lee KM, Nam M, et al. Short-term outcomes and influencing factors after ankle fracture surgery. J Foot Ankle Surg. 2018;57(6):1096–100.

27. Lauge-Hansen N. Fractures of the ankle. II. Combined experimental-surgical and experimental-roentgenologic investigations. Arch Surg. 1950;60(5):957–85.

28. Chun DI, Kim J, Kim YS, Cho JH, Won SH, Park SY, et al. Relationship between fracture morphology of lateral malleolus and syndesmotic stability after supination-external rotation type ankle fractures. Injury. 2019;50(7):1382–7.

29. Pankovich AM. Maisonneuve fracture of the fibula. J Bone Joint Surg Am. 1976;58(3):337–42.

30. Kortekangas TH, Pakarinen HJ, Savola O, Niinimaki J, Lepojarvi S, Ohtonen P, et al. Syndesmotic fixation in supination-external rotation ankle fractures: a prospective randomized study. Foot Ankle Int. 2014;35(10):988–95.

31. Jeong BO, Kim TY, Baek JH, Song SH, Park JS. Assessment of ankle mortise instability after isolated supination-external rotation lateral malleolar fractures. J Bone Joint Surg Am. 2018;100(18):1557–62.

32. Kahan J, Brand J, Schneble C, Li D, Saad M, Kuether J, et al. Open pronation abduction ankle fractures associated with increased complications and patient BMI. Injury. 2020;51(4):1109–13.

33. Hinds RM, Tran WH, Lorich DG. Maisonneuve-hyperplantarflexion variant ankle fracture. Orthopedics. 2014;37(11):e1040–4.

34. Haraguchi N, Armiger RS. A new interpretation of the mechanism of ankle fracture. J Bone Joint Surg Am. 2009;91(4):821–9.
35. Shariff SS, Nathwani DK. Lauge-Hansen classification—a literature review. Injury. 2006;37(9):888–90.
36. Rodriguez EK, Kwon JY, Herder LM, Appleton PT. Correlation of AO and Lauge-Hansen classification systems for ankle fractures to the mechanism of injury. Foot Ankle Int. 2013;34(11):1516–20.
37. Kwon JY, Chacko AT, Kadzielski JJ, Appleton PT, Rodriguez EK. A novel methodology for the study of injury mechanism: ankle fracture analysis using injury videos posted on YouTube.com. J Orthop Trauma. 2010;24(8):477–82.
38. Mason LW, Marlow WJ, Widnall J, Molloy AP. Pathoanatomy and associated injuries of posterior malleolus fracture of the ankle. Foot Ankle Int. 2017;38(11):1229–35.
39. Warner SJ, Garner MR, Hinds RM, Helfet DL, Lorich DG. Correlation between the Lauge-Hansen classification and ligament injuries in ankle fractures. J Orthop Trauma. 2015;29(12):574–8.
40. Nielsen JO, Dons-Jensen H, Sorensen HT. Lauge-Hansen classification of malleolar fractures. An assessment of the reproducibility in 118 cases. Acta Orthop Scand. 1990;61(5):385–7.
41. Jehlicka D, Bartonícek J, Svatos F, Dobiás J. Fracture-dislocations of the ankle joint in adults. Part I: epidemiologic evaluation of patients during a 1-year period. Acta Chir Orthop Traumatol Cech. 2002;69(4):243–7.
42. de Souza LJ, Gustilo RB, Meyer TJ. Results of operative treatment of displaced external rotation-abduction fractures of the ankle. J Bone Joint Surg Am. 1985;67(7):1066–74.
43. Hartford JM, Gorczyca JT, McNamara JL, Mayor MB. Tibiotalar contact area. Contribution of posterior malleolus and deltoid ligament. Clin Orthop Relat Res. 1995;320:182–7.
44. Macko VW, Matthews LS, Zwirkoski P, Goldstein SA. The joint-contact area of the ankle. The contribution of the posterior malleolus. J Bone Joint Surg Am. 1991;73(3):347–51.
45. McDaniel WJ, Wilson FC. Trimalleolar fractures of the ankle. An end result study. Clin Orthop Relat Res. 1977;122:37–45.
46. Gardner MJ, Brodsky A, Briggs SM, Nielson JH, Lorich DG. Fixation of posterior malleolar fractures provides greater syndesmotic stability. Clin Orthop Relat Res. 2006;447:165–71.
47. Miller MA, McDonald TC, Graves ML, Spitler CA, Russell GV, Jones LC, et al. Stability of the syndesmosis after posterior malleolar fracture fixation. Foot Ankle Int. 2018;39(1):99–104.
48. Drijfhout van Hooff CC, Verhage SM, Hoogendoorn JM. Influence of fragment size and postoperative joint congruency on long-term outcome of posterior malleolar fractures. Foot Ankle Int. 2015;36(6):673–8.
49. Bartonicek J, Rammelt S, Kostlivy K, Vanecek V, Klika D, Tresl I. Anatomy and classification of the posterior tibial fragment in ankle fractures. Arch Orthop Trauma Surg. 2015;135(4):505–16.
50. Langenhuijsen JF, Heetveld MJ, Ultee JM, Steller EP, Butzelaar RM. Results of ankle fractures with involvement of the posterior tibial margin. J Trauma. 2002;53(1):55–60.
51. Gonzalez O, Fleming JJ, Meyr AJ. Radiographic assessment of posterior malleolar ankle fractures. J Foot Ankle Surg. 2015;54(3):365–9.
52. Vosoughi AR, Jayatilaka MLT, Fischer B, Molloy AP, Mason LW. CT analysis of the posteromedial fragment of the posterior malleolar fracture. Foot Ankle Int. 2019;40(6):648–55.
53. Yi Y, Chun DI, Won SH, Park S, Lee S, Cho J. Morphological characteristics of the posterior malleolar fragment according to ankle fracture patterns: a computed tomography-based study. BMC Musculoskelet Disord. 2018;19(1):51.
54. Bartoníček J, Rammelt S, Tuček M. Posterior malleolar fractures: changing concepts and recent developments. Foot Ankle Clin. 2017;22(1):125–45.
55. Mason LW, Kaye A, Widnall J, Redfern J, Molloy A. Posterior malleolar Ankle fractures: an effort at improving outcomes. JB JS Open Access. 2019;4(2):e0058.

Preoperative Management and Evaluation of Ankle Fractures

Rahul Vaidya and James Mueller

1 Introduction

There are approximately 135,000 ankle fractures per year in the United States [1]. The most common age is between the age of 10 and 19 years which account for 23.5% of ankle fractures. In these patients it's most commonly a cause of sporting injuries. In older individuals the most common mechanism is due to low energy falls. Women are affected about 56% of cases. Mechanisms of injury include falls in just over 50%, sports injuries in about 20%, other exercise misadventures in 17%, jumping, trauma, and other make up the remaining causes [1]. The purpose of this chapter is to provide guidelines for the evaluation and treatment of ankle fractures particularly in the perioperative period to optimize their care.

2 Relevant Anatomy

The ankle joint is a hinge synovial joint that is formed by the articulation of the talus, tibia, and fibula. Together the distal end of the tibia and fibula form the ankle mortise, in which the talus is held by ligaments. There are two articulations: one between the fibula and tibia and a second between the fibula, tibia, and talus [2]. The ankle works in concert with the subtalar joint to act as a modified hinged joint which can plantar flex, dorsiflex, glide, and roll. The malleoli are the medial and lateral bony constraints of the ankle joint. Both these medial and lateral constraints serve as the attachments for the medial and lateral ligamentous complex (Fig. 1a, b). The talar body is wider in the front than the back and thus has increased stability in the ankle joint when the ankle is dorsiflexed. In contrast, when the ankle is plantar flexed there is less congruency with the talus and there is more mobility in varus and valgus [3].

Stability of the joint is maintained by three lateral ligaments; the anterior talofibular, calcaneofibular, and the posterior talofibular ligament. These lateral ligaments help to prevent varus displacement of the talus in the ankle mortise and act as a stop to internal rotation of the ankle. They stabilize the subtalar joint as well as prevent varus and limit lateral opening of the subtalar joint. There is a strong medial deltoid ligament complex which has a superficial and deep component. This ligament prevents valgus and extreme external rotation of the talus in the ankle mortise. There are also the ligaments that maintain the intimate relationship of the fibula and tibia: the anterior tibiofibular and posterior tibiofibular ligaments as well as the interosseous

R. Vaidya
Department of Orthopaedic Surgery, Wayne State University, Detroit, MI, USA

J. Mueller (✉)
Department of Medical Education, Garden City Hospital, Garden City, MI, USA

© The Author(s), under exclusive license to Springer Nature Switzerland AG 2023
D. Herscovici Jr. et al. (eds.), *Evaluation and Surgical Management of the Ankle*,
https://doi.org/10.1007/978-3-031-33537-2_9

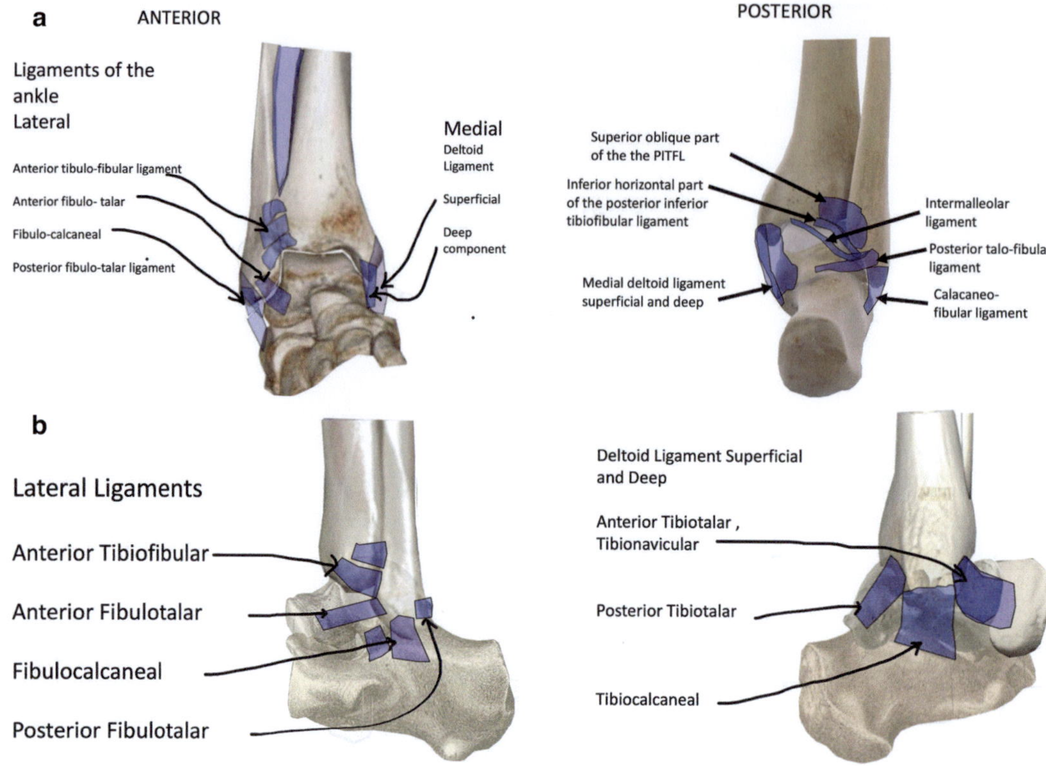

Fig. 1 Ligamentous constraints of the ankle (**a**) Anterior (**b**) Posterior

membrane [2]. The distal tibiofibular joint is a diarthrodial joint between the tibia and the fibula for approximately the first 1.5 cm above the ankle joint. Although this is a synovial joint, very little movement occurs because of the constraints mentioned above [2].

The muscles and tendons that move the ankle joint can be divided by their location into plantar flexors and dorsiflexors. Inversion and eversion are complex movements of the hind foot which encompass the ankle, subtalar, talo-navicular, and calcano-cuboid joints. Inversion is performed by all muscles medial (primarily tibialis anterior and tibialis posterior) and eversion primarily by the peroneal muscles [2].

3   Presentation

Ankle fractures typically present with immediate onset of ankle pain with localized or general swelling. They may be accompanied by bruising,

joint deformity, and an inability to bear weight [4]. Ankle sprains and fractures may present similarly, however, treatment is often different. Differentiating the two is paramount in obtaining a successful outcome.

4   History

The history and physical exam are the cornerstones of the orthopedic encounter. The history often describes the mechanism of injury which may be inversion, eversion, plantar flexion, dorsiflexion, or a complex movement which combines those motions (supination or pronation). The force and velocity involved and weight bearing or position of the foot during the traumatic force can result in a variety of different injury patterns. The history taker should also ask if there are wounds that could signify an open fracture, if the ankle was dislocated and relocated at the scene, if there are any neurovascular changes such as numbness or inability to move the ankle or toes, or if there is severe pain out of proportion which may be indicative of compartment syndrome of the foot or lower leg.

The past medical history is used to elucidate previous ankle injuries, comorbidities that might influence treatment such as pre-existing mobility impairment (e.g.—use of a walking aid), diabetes +/− peripheral neuropathy, peripheral vascular disease, renal disease, osteoporosis, and risk factors such as smoking and alcohol overuse [5].

5 Examination

Examination starts with inspection for deformity, open wounds, and current skin condition. This may include bruising, swelling, or blisters. Palpation is performed sequentially over the medial and lateral malleolus, the proximal fibula, and the interosseous membrane [5, 6]. Pain with palpation or squeeze of the interosseous membrane can indicate a syndesmotic injury such as the Maisonneuve injury—a proximal fibula fracture with tearing of the interosseous membrane and distal tibiofibular syndesmosis. Tenderness over the malleoli is suggestive of a fracture rather than a sprain [7]. A neurovascular exam is essential. Pulses should be felt at the dorsalis pedis and posterior tibial artery and documented. A sensory exam of the foot and a motor exam including flexion, extension, pronation, and supination should be performed in order to establish if there is any neurologic deficit or tendon injury. Comparison should be made to the opposite non injured limb when possible. Severe swelling in the foot may be a sign of a compartment syndrome of the foot. It's important to identify any concomitant hind foot or mid foot injury which can be missed by focusing on a significant ankle injury. Documentation of positive findings as well as pertinent negatives should be thorough.

It may be difficult to distinguish between fracture and sprain in ankles which present with pain but are not clinically deformed. The Ottawa ankle rules [7] help decide which patients need to be imaged. These rules state that an X-ray is required only if there is malleolar tenderness or pain with an inability to weight bear immediately in the emergency department for four steps, bony tenderness of the posterior tibial fibular joint, or bony tenderness at the tips of the medial and lateral malleoli. Together, these have a sensitivity of almost 100% with the specificity of 39.8% and have been shown to reduce the use of radiographs, which are unnecessary in 30 to 40% of patients [8].

5.1 The Dislocated or Subluxed Ankle Joint

Clinically deformed ankles require urgent reduction and splinting [5]. Radiographs should not be performed before reduction if they will cause an unacceptable delay [5], although often the radiographs are completed before the orthopedic team is consulted. A neurovascular exam should be performed prior to and after the reduction. Reduction can be done with intra-articular injection of local anesthetic or with IV conscious sedation per hospital protocol. Reduction can be done with the patient in the supine position by stabilizing the leg with one hand and placing traction on the heel. The foot is then rotated into the reduced position by eversion or inversion according to the position of the dislocation. Reduction may be accompanied by a palpable clunk. The splinting material should be gathered and prepared prior to performing the reduction maneuver so that the splint can be applied immediately after the joint is reduced. Alternatively, Quigley's method of ankle reduction can often be accomplished without anesthetic, although it is usually used with ankle injection [9]. The patient's knee is bent over a bolster and a stockinette is applied from above the knee over the foot and then suspended from an IV pole, positioned on the opposite side of the bed. Webril around the proximal portion of the stockinette prevents it from sliding. Once the leg is allowed to hang and relax for a minute, the ankle will often self-reduce or require just a gentle push to relocate. With the leg held in its flexed knee and dorsiflexed ankle position one can then apply padding and a posterior slab with side stirrups, molding the foot into the reduced position (Fig. 2). A picture of one version of the Quigley technique is shown in chapter "Emergency Management of Ankle Fractures".

Prompt reduction minimizes the risk of skin necrosis and also reduces pain and swelling [9]. After reduction, neurovascular exam is repeated, and radiographs should be performed to verify that the talus is seated under the plafond of the tibia. If adequate alignment is not achieved, one may consider repeating the attempt in the emergency department or proceeding to the operating room, but multiple attempts at closed reduction should be avoided. Difficulty with closed reduction is often related to inadequate technique or inadequate anesthesia (local +/− sedation), however, sometimes there are anatomic blocks to reduction. Tendons and ligaments can become dislocated or subluxed into the joint space blocking the reduction (Fig. 3).

5.2 Open Ankle Fractures

Patients with open ankle fractures make up 1.5% of all ankle fractures [10]. In the emergency department, thorough irrigation is unnecessary, but any gross contamination should be removed by flushing with sterile saline. The size, location, and quality of the open wound should be documented, occasionally with sketches or photographs. The fracture site should be covered with saline soaked gauze wrapped loosely with an occlusive dressing while waiting to proceed with surgery. The ankle should then be reduced and splinted in a similar manner as described above. Intravenous antibiotics should be given within 1 h of injury and tetanus status ascertained and updated as necessary [10]. Surgical debridement of open fracture wounds should be accomplished within 24 h per institutional protocol, and for severely contaminated wounds 6 to 12 h is preferable. Fixation and definitive soft tissue coverage should be performed at the first operation if there is no soft tissue loss [11].

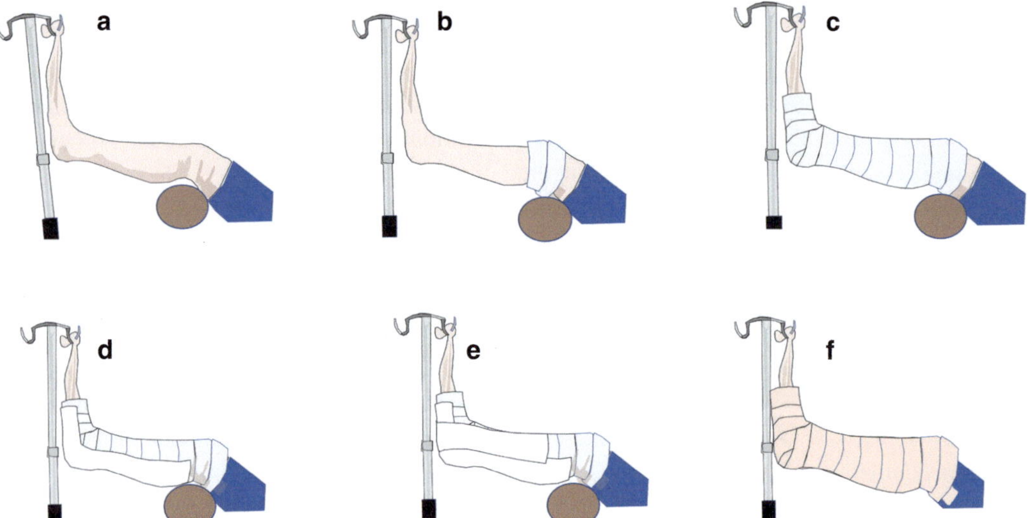

Fig. 2 Quigleys method of ankle reduction (**a**) The leg is covered in a stockinette and hung from an IV pole at the end of the bed or stretcher with a bolster under the knee which allows a small amount of knee bend (**b**) Webril is applied at the top of the lower leg to prevent the stockinette from sliding off . Hanging the leg allows gravity to gradually reduce the ankle on its own or with a gentle push once the muscles relax (**c**) The leg is then covered with adequate padding (**d**) 10 to 12 layers of plaster bandage is wet and placed posteriorly (**e**) Followed by lateral stirrups (**f**) Ace bandages are placed to cover the plaster

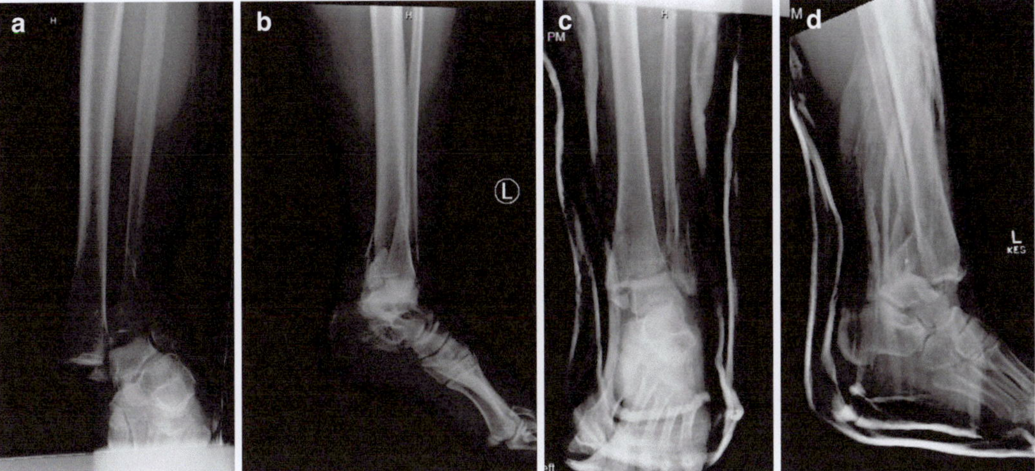

Fig. 3 This trimalleolar fracture-dislocation underwent a failed attempt at closed reduction and splinting in the emergency department. Images A and B are AP and lateral pre-reduction images of the ankle fracture-dislocation. Images C and D show are post reduction views revealing the joint still dislocated in the splint. Both AP and lateral views are needed after any manipulation attempt to verify adequate reduction

6 Radiographic Evaluation

6.1 X-Rays

Standard X-rays should be performed and include a lateral and mortise view [12]. A mortise view is an anteroposterior image of the leg in 15–20° of internal rotation. Poor X-rays should be repeated. Standard measurements have been described to identify subluxation of the talus, the fibular length, and rotation (Fig. 4). In isolated lateral malleolar fractures, stress views may be used to identify associated medial sided ligamentous injuries. A gravity or manual stress view has been described to distinguish stable ankle fractures from unstable ankle fractures [13] (Fig. 5). With "isolated" medial injuries, or those with proximal tenderness, a full-length tibia and fibula X-ray may help identify a proximal fibular fracture when a Maisonneuve injury has occurred. Radiographic parameters have been developed to describe the mortise and relations to the talar articular surfaces: superior clear space (SC), medial clear space (MC), and lateral clear space [14]. These should be symmetrical. The length of the fibula can be determined by the dime sign, the talocrural angle, and/or images of the contralateral ankle as a template [14, 15] (Fig. 4).

6.2 CT Scan

Computerized topography (CT scan) is useful for the assessment of complex ankle fractures, especially those involving the posterior malleolus and/or comminuted malleolar fractures [6, 16]. A CT scan can help identify more complicated injury patterns including pilon injuries, osteo chondral lesions, small intra-articular fragments, impaction of the articular surface, and associated hind foot injuries (Fig. 6). It can also assist in preoperative planning to determine the fixation sequence, strategy, and implants. However, CT scanning is not necessary for all ankle fractures, if the fracture morphology is clear on plain films.

6.3 Ultrasound

The use of Ultrasound in ankle injuries by properly trained practitioners can help identify ligamentous injuries (partial and complete), vascular injuries and tendinous injuries around

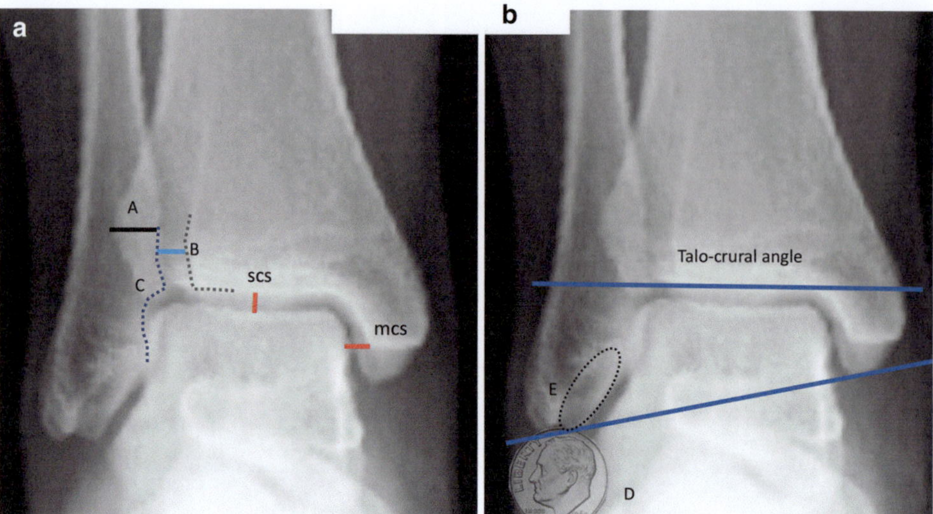

Fig. 4 Radiographic measurements on the AP X-ray. (**a**) Label A image a: Tibiofibular overlap is the overlapping area between the anterior distal tibial prominence and the medial edge of the distal fibula Normal >10 mm. (**b**) Label B image a: Tibiofibular clear space is measured 1 cm above the ankle joint and reflects syndesmotic injury and is measure between the deepest point of the fibular groove of the tibia and the medial fibula the average is 4.6 mm on the AP, >6 mm is abnormal an indicative of syndesmotic disruption. (**c**) Label C image a: The Shenton's line of the ankle correlates to appropriate fibular length when reducing a fibula to its normal length. (**d**) Label D image b: The dime sign is a useful radiographic sign of fibular length on the AP view. It correlates to an unbroken curve connecting the recess in the distal tip of the fibula and the lateral process of the talus when the fibula is out to length. (**e**) Label E image b: The fibular oval is a sign of fibular rotation and can be compared to the normal side when restoring fibular alignment. (**f**) The Talo-crural angle (image b) is formed by a line drawn parallel to the articular surface of the distal tibia to a line connecting the tips of both malleoli. Normal it measures fibula 8–15°. This angle should be within 2–5° of the opposite side. (**g**) Label SCS image b: Superior Clear Space (SCS) is measured between the tibia and talus at the lowest point of the tibial plafond. Normal is symmetrical to the medial and lateral clear space on the mortise view. (**h**) Label mcs image b: Medial clear space (MCS) is measured from the talus to the medial malleolus at the medial colliculus . An absolute value of >5 mm, or 2 mm > the SCS, is abnormal and indicates a deltoid ligament disruption

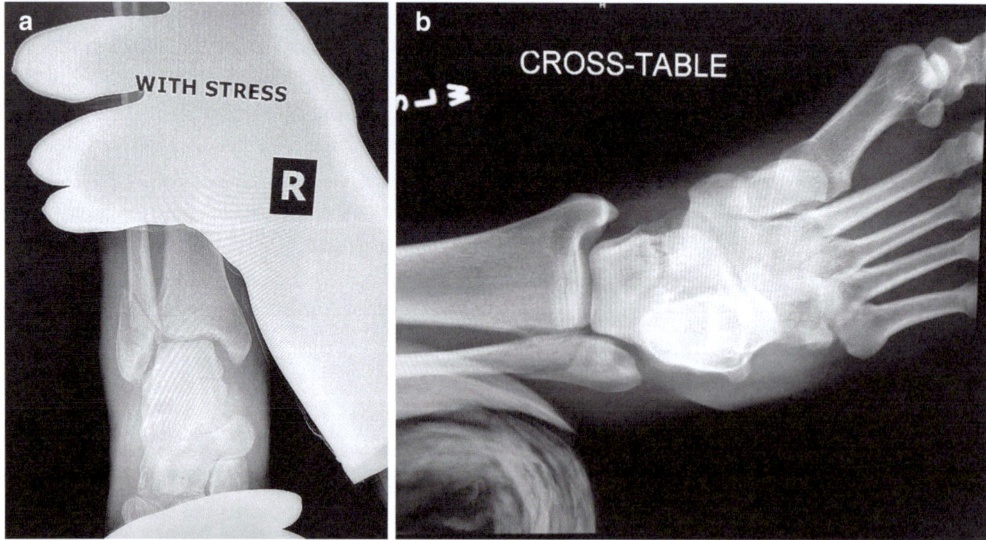

Fig. 5 (**a**) A positive manual stress view with widening of the medial clear space (**b**) gravity stress view has been demonstrated to distinguish stable ankle fractures from unstable ankle fractures without manipulating again with widening of the medial clear space as compared to the superior clear space

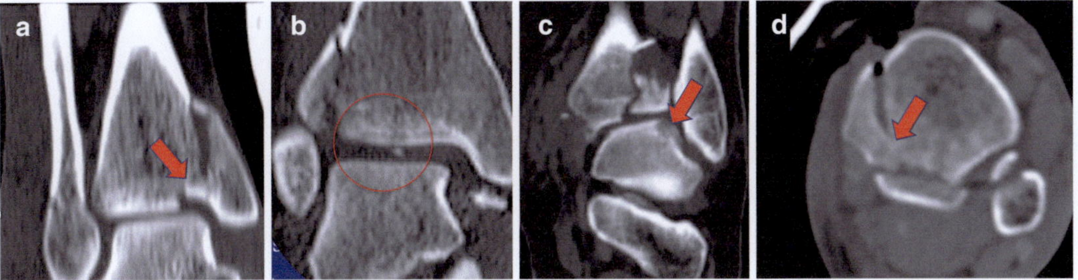

Fig. 6 CT scan demonstrating (**a**) marginal impaction (**b**) loose body (**c**) osteochondral lesion of the talus (**d**) a complex posterior malleolar fracture

the ankle joint. It may obviate the need for stress radiographs and confirm exam findings [17, 18].

6.4 MRI

The utility of magnetic resonance imaging (MRI) in ankle injuries is fairly similar to that ultrasound; namely: ligamentous and osteochondral injuries. However, it is much less dependent on the skill of the technologist administering the exam. It can help identify ligamentous, tendon injuries and is particularly useful in identifying early osteochondral injuries [19]. It is not routinely necessary in most acute ankle fractures.

7 Management

For the most part, ankle fractures are not emergent cases. The exceptions are severely contaminated open fractures, irreducible dislocations, deformity with ischemic skin, neurovascular compromise, and compartment syndrome. Once the ankle joint is adequately reduced and splinted, and the decision is made for surgical treatment, the timing of surgery may be semi-elective, and determined by patient desire, OR availability, and surgeon schedule. If the soft tissues are too swollen for safe incisions, the surgical procedure may be delayed. It is imperative that the leg be elevated above the heart continuously during the waiting period. In some cases that can be accomplished at the patient's place of residence if the patient has adequate assistance and seems likely to comply. In other cases, the surgeon may want to admit the patient to the hospital to ensure that the patient and limb condition is optimized. During the waiting period, tobacco use should be avoided, nutritional status should be optimized, and adequate pain control provided. In patients with risk factors, consideration should be given to prophylaxis against venous thromboembolism.

Definitive surgical fixation of ankle fractures will be detailed in subsequent chapters. The decision regarding open or closed treatment revolves around characteristics of the fracture pattern (stable vs. unstable), as well as characteristics of the patient (risk/benefit profile) [20]. The overall question of fracture stability is relatively simple: will the talus move in a normal range of motion under physiologic load even though the ankle is fractured? Stable fractures include isolated lateral malleolus fractures; most bimalleolar fractures, bimalleolar equivalent injuries and trimalleolar fractures are unstable [21]. Stable fracture patterns are typically treated nonoperatively in a weightbearing cast or controlled ankle motion (CAM) boot. Unstable fracture patterns are better managed operatively. It is relatively easy to diagnose bimalleolar and trimalleolar fractures based on plain X-rays alone, however, the bimalleolar equivalent fractures require a more nuanced approach.

The deltoid ligament is the most important ligament for stability in the ankle [20, 21]. When this ligament is disrupted, the talus can subluxate out of the ankle mortise under physiologic load. It is this medial sided injury that often dictates instability, and furthermore the indication for operative intervention. Isolated medial malleolus injuries, bimalleolar, and trimalleolar fractures, and bimalleolar equivalent fractures all have medial sided injuries that compromise the stability of the ankle joint.

In patients with an isolated lateral malleolus fracture, it is imperative to determine stability, typically using some form of stress X-ray to evaluate the talus in the mortise. This can be either a manual external rotation stress view, in which the proximal calf is stabilized with one hand and the foot is gently but firmly externally rotated while a radiograph of the mortise is taken or a gravity stress view, in which the leg is positioned in external rotation with the foot unsupported, as in over a bolster [13]. With these stress X-rays the medial clear space is compared to the superior and lateral clear spaces and evaluated for widening. If there is widening, this is indicative of a medial sided injury and diagnosed overall as a bimalleolar equivalent fracture (Fig. 5).

8 Soft Tissue Swelling and Blisters

When the patient has a compromised soft tissue envelope it will be necessary to delay the definitive care of the ankle fracture. This is often evident by blisters which form on the skin (Fig. 7). If stable on post reduction X-rays in the splint, surgery can wait until the soft tissues have calmed down. However, if the ankle is not reduced, this will cause the soft tissues to remain swollen for an inordinate amount of time. Repeat closed reduction can be attempted in the office, or the patient should be brought back to the OR for a closed or open reduction and external fixation [22]. One or 2 failed reductions should be followed by an intraoperative attempt. In the case of a difficult reduction or an unstable one, an external fixator is a good choice for maintaining reduction while waiting for the swelling to calm down [22]. The foot should be elevated and cryotherapy and/or a pneumatic pedal pump applied to help reduce swelling [23].

When reduced, the soft tissue swelling takes anywhere between 5 days to 3 weeks to calm down [24]. When the skin is no longer shiny, the

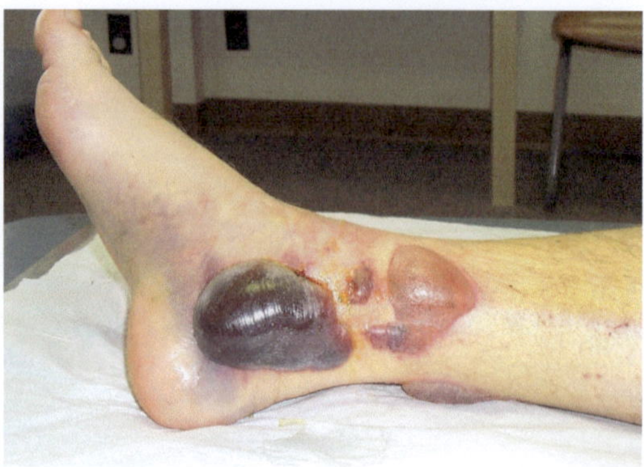

Fig. 7 An ankle fracture with severely compromised soft tissue envelope. Extensive hemorrhagic fracture blisters preclude surgical incision. The skin is tight and has deep ecchymosis

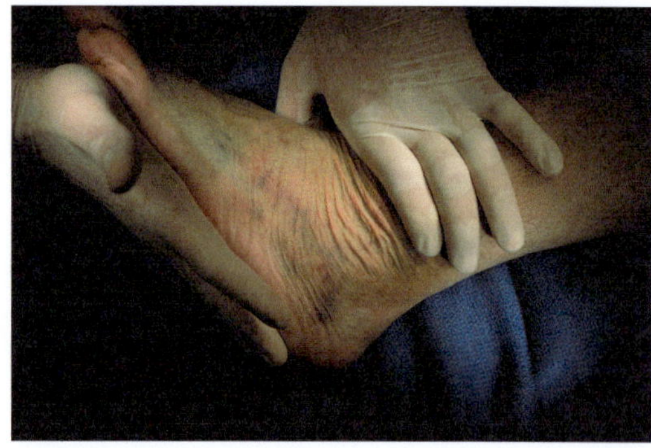

Fig. 8 The wrinkle test. Despite some bruising, the skin of the ankle is soft, mobile, and forms wrinkles easily when gently manipulated. This skin will tolerate surgical incision

blisters have resolved or epithelialized, and the skin is soft and mobile enough to wrinkle with gentle manual manipulation, it is safer to proceed with surgery (Fig. 8). External fixation of the ankle can be accomplished with a delta frame (two pins placed from anterior to posterior in the tibia connected to a transverse pin through the calcaneus with bars in a triangular configuration) or "traveling traction" (a transverse pin through the proximal tibia connected to a transverse pin in the calcaneus with two parallel bars). Our preferred technique for reduction with an external fixator is traveling traction as the pull of the fixator maintains the position of the foot and talus below the distal tibia [25, 26] (Fig. 9).

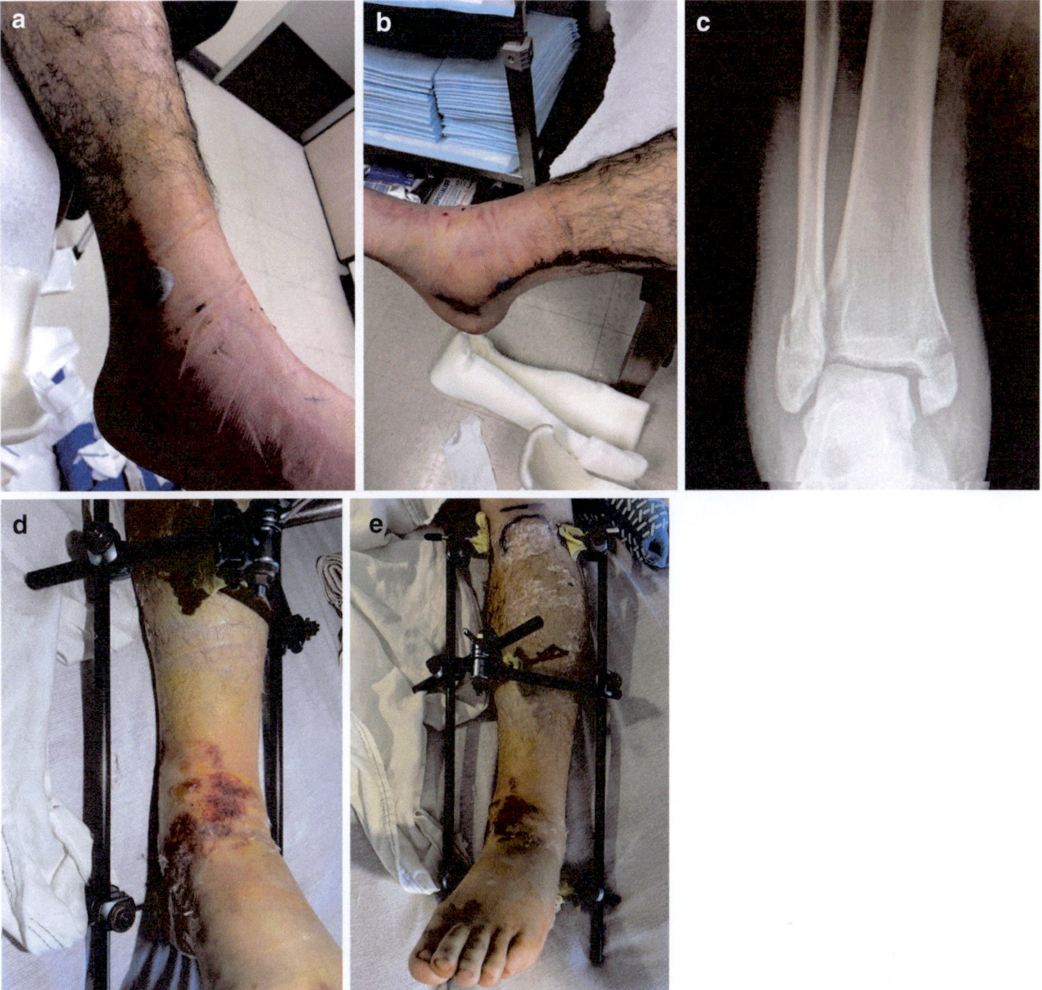

Fig. 9 (**a**, **b**) An ankle fracture that presented with swelling and blisters. The options for treatment were splinting if a good reduction was achieved and wait for the swelling to resolve for surgery in 5 days to 3 weeks. (**c**) In this case a good reduction was achieved. If a good reduction cannot be achieved or maintained, or if the soft tissues will require care and close monitoring, the patient is taken to the OR for re-reduction and external fixation. (**d**, **e**) This frame configuration is a hybrid between the 2 types, travelling traction with a supplemental anterior pin for more stability

9 Special Considerations

Co-morbidities that might influence treatment choice and outcome should be documented [5]. These include pre-existing immobility, diabetes, peripheral neuropathy, peripheral vascular disease, osteoporosis, renal disease, smoking, and alcohol.

9.1 Vascular Disease

Vascular insufficiency or peripheral vascular disease can delay healing of bone and soft tissue. It is important to be mindful of this comorbidity and caution must be exercised before applying a tourniquet during surgery in these patients. Most operating room guidelines recommend the documentation of pulses prior to applying a tourniquet and certainly that documentation should be done in the ED initially and after every manipulation. In patients without palpable pulses, surgery without a tourniquet is recommended [27]. Patients with peripheral vascular disease have a 1.65 times the odds ratio of having complications after an operatively treated ankle fracture [28]. If an adequate reduction can be achieved and maintained for 4 to 6 weeks, surgery can be avoided even in bimalleolar injuries. In patients who have vascular disease identified on presentation, consultation with a vascular surgeon may be useful for pre-operative work-up. In a non-emergent setting, endovascular correction of obstructions may be considered to enhance the chances or bone and wound healing [29].

9.2   Diabetes

Patients with complicated diabetes have a 2.3 times odds ratio for complications after the fixation of ankle fractures [28]. These patients can be tested for HbA1c levels and if their level is $\geq 6.5\%$ it appears to be predictive of an increased risk and complication rates [28].

These patients are at risk for presenting late and with deformity if they lack sensation in their feet. This can be confirmed via the standard 5.07 Semmes-Weinstein monofilament test. This may lead to much more difficult surgery or a Charcot joint [30]. In this case primary fusion may need to be considered [31]. These issues are discussed in detail in chapter "Management of Acute Diabetic ankle Fractures".

9.3   Smoking

Cigarette smoking entails a higher risk for cardiopulmonary dysfunction and impaired healing of soft tissue and bone [32]. Current active smokers should be encouraged to stop smoking, and enrolled in tobacco cessation programs if available and the patient is willing. It may be helpful to carefully explain the specific adverse effects of smoking on healing after this injury, as many smokers are used to people telling them they should stop, and they tend to tune that advice out. It may be useful to tell them that they can consider it a temporary restriction, until the wound and bone are healed. After surgery these patients should be watched carefully for wound healing issues as well as delayed or non-union.

9.4   Osteoporosis

Osteoporosis presents a specific problem with reduction and fixation. Sharp clamps and forceful reductions may turn simple fractures into a comminuted mess. Thus, alternative strategies with buttress or antiglide plating to reduce the fibular or medial malleolar fracture may be helpful. Locking screws and other fixed angle devices may also help increase fixation strength, intramedullary wires may provide interdigitation in the fibula, and screws that traverse the syndesmosis using 4 cortices may enhance the fixation strength [33]. These techniques are discussed in subsequent chapters.

9.5   Hematological Issues and Drugs of Anticoagulation

Many elderly patients present with anticoagulation for prior arrythmia or thromboembolic disease. They use a mix of drugs from warfarin, low molecular heparin, the direct oral anticoagulants (DOACs—dabigatran, rivaroxaban, apixaban, edoxaban) or Aspirin (ASA). There needs to be a balance between reducing the risk of thromboembolism and preventing excessive surgical bleeding. Preoperative consultation with the appropriate service (e.g. cardiology or internal medicine) can optimize medications for surgery or bridge the patients with shorter acting anticoagulants. The optimal plan is dependent on the procedure and perceived risk. Tables 1 and 2 show the commonly used anticoagulants and their reversal agents with dosages.

Table 1 Anticoagulants with their reversal agents and dosages

Drug	Reversal agent	Dosing
Vitamin K antagonist (warfarin)	Vitamin K Prothrombin complex concentrate (PCC) Fresh frozen plasma	10 mg IV [34] See next table for weight and international normalized ratio (INR) based dosing See next table for weight and INR based dosing
Heparin	Protamine sulfate	<1/2 h: 1–1.5 mg/100 units of heparin 30–120 min: 0.5–0.75 mg/100 units of heparin >2 h: 0.25–0.375 mg/100 units of heparin
Low molecular weight heparin	Protamine sulfate	1 mg per mg enoxaparin (if enoxaparin given within 8 h) If >8 h or bleeding continues after 4 h after first dose, give 0.5 mg protamine per mg enoxaparin [35]
Dabigatran	Idarucizumab	Idarucizumab 5 g i.v. in two bolus doses of 2.5 g i.v. no more than 15 min apart [34]
Factor Xa inhibitors: Apixaban, rivaroxaban, edoxaban	Andexanet alpha	Bolus over 15–30 min, followed by 2 h infusion Rivaroxaban (last intake >7 h before) or apixaban: 400 mg bolus, 480 mg infusion @ 4 mg/min Rivaroxaban (last intake <7 h before or unknown) or enoxaparin or edoxaban: 800 mg bolus, 960 mg infusion at 8 mg/min [34]

Table 2 Dosing of 4F-PCC and FFP for reversal of warfarin based on INR level

Baseline INR	4 factor PCC dose: IU/kg body weight	FFP mL/kg body weight
2 to ≤4	25	10
4 to ≤6	35	12
>6	50	15

Max dose ≤5000 IU of PCC or ≤1500 mL of FFP

surgery. Immediately following dialysis is usually the best time for an intervention when electrolytes and fluid balance is optimized [36]. In open fractures or dislocations surgery may need to be performed on an emergent basis and consultation with the anesthesiologist as to the duration of surgery will help achieve the best outcome. Often staged surgery can be performed once the patient has dialysis.

9.7 Polytrauma with an Ankle Fracture

The guideline for the treatment of polytrauma is Advanced Trauma Life Support (ATLS®) protocol. This focuses on stabilizing life and limb threatening injuries [37]. The initial orthopedic component of the exam focuses on the pelvis, spine, long bones, open fractures, and compartment syndrome. As a part of the examination limb perfusion status is noted and gross fractures and dislocations are reduced. Ankle fractures and dislocations are not commonly found in the polytrauma population, but still exist [38]. These should be reduced and splinted. Serial examinations are required as the patient continues to be resuscitated and limb swelling exacerbates. The swelling can cut off tenuous blood supply and a compartment syndrome can develop.

9.6 Renal Failure

Patients who are in impending renal failure or in renal failure with regularly scheduled dialysis should have an internal medicine or nephrology consult and may need to be optimized prior to

References

1. Scheer RC, Newman JM, Zhou JJ, Oommen AJ, Naziri Q, Shah NV, Pascal SC, Penny GS, McKean JM, Tsai J, Uribe JA. Ankle fracture epidemiology in the United States: patient-related trends and mechanisms of injury. J Foot Ankle Surg. 2020;59(3):479–83. https://doi.org/10.1053/j.jfas.2019.09.016.

2. Moore KL, Dalley AF, Agur AMR. Clinically oriented anatomy. 7th ed. Philadelphia, PA: Lippincott Williams & Wilkins; 2014.

3. McKeon JMM, Hoch MC. The ankle-joint complex: a kinesiologic approach to lateral ankle sprains. J Athl Train. 2019;54(6):589–602.

4. Slimmon D, Brukner P. Sports ankle injuries—assessment and management. Aust Fam Physician. 2010;39(1–2):18–22.

5. British Orthopaedic Association Standards for Trauma. The management of ankle fractures. 2016. https://www.boa.ac.uk/resources/boast-12-pdf.html. Accessed Mar 2022.

6. Lampridis V, Gougoulias N, Sakellariou A. Stability in ankle fractures: diagnosis and treatment. EFORT Open Rev. 2018;3(5):294–303.

7. Stiell IG, Greenberg GH, McKnight RD, Nair RC, McDowell I, Worthington JR. A study to develop clinical decision rules for the use of radiography in acute ankle injuries. Ann Emerg Med. 1992;21(4):384–90.

8. Bachmann LM, Kolb E, Koller MT, Steurer J, Ter Riet G. Accuracy of Ottawa ankle rules to exclude fractures of the ankle and mid-foot: systematic review. Br Med J. 2003;326(7386):417–9.

9. Mordecai S, Al-Hadithy N. Management of ankle fractures. BMJ. 2011;343:d5204. https://doi.org/10.1136/bmj.d5204.

10. Juto H, Nilsson H, Morberg P. Epidemiology of adult ankle fractures: 1756 cases identified in Norrbotten County during 2009–2013 and classified according to AO/OTA. BMC Musculoskelet Disord. 2018;19(1):441. https://doi.org/10.1186/s12891-018-2326-x.

11. Peterson DL, Schuurman M, Geamanu A, Padela MT, Kennedy CJ, Wilkinson J, Vaidya R. Early definitive care is as effective as staged treatment protocols for open ankle fractures caused by rotational mechanisms: a retrospective case-control study. J Orthop Trauma. 2020;34(7):376–81. https://doi.org/10.1097/BOT.0000000000001734.

12. Vangsness CT, Carter V, Hunt T, Kerr R, Newton E. Radiographic diagnosis of ankle fractures: are three views necessary? Foot Ankle Int. 1994;15(4):172–4. https://doi.org/10.1177/107110079401500403.

13. Ashraf A, Murphree J, Wait E, Winston T, Wooldridge A, Meriwether M, Wilson J, Grimes JS. Gravity stress radiographs and the effect of ankle position on deltoid ligament integrity and medial clear space measurements. J Orthop Trauma. 2017;5:270–4. https://doi.org/10.1097/BOT.0000000000000817.

14. Egol KA, Koval KJ, Zuckerman JD, Technologies O, Inc. Handbook of fractures. Philadelphia: Wolters Kluwer Health; 2015.

15. Abarca M, Besa P, Mora E, Palma J, Lira MJ, Filippi J. The use of intraoperative comparative fluoroscopy allows for assessing sagittal reduction and predicting syndesmosis reduction in ankle fractures. Foot Ankle Surg. 2022;28:750. https://doi.org/10.1016/j.fas.2021.10.003.

16. Leung KH, Fang CX, Lau TW, Leung FK. Preoperative radiography versus computed tomography for surgical planning for ankle fractures. J Orthop Surg (Hong Kong). 2016;24(2):158–62. https://doi.org/10.1177/1602400207.

17. Allen GM, Wilson DJ, Bullock SA, Watson M. Extremity CT and ultrasound in the assessment of ankle injuries: occult fractures and ligament injuries. Br J Radiol. 2020. Epub 2019 Dec 4. PMID: 31742428; PMCID: PMC6948070.;93(1105):20180989. https://doi.org/10.1259/bjr.20180989.

18. Esmailian M, Ataie M, Ahmadi O, Rastegar S, Adibi A. Sensitivity and specificity of ultrasound in the diagnosis of traumatic ankle injury. J Res Med Sci. 2021. PMID: 34084193; PMCID: PMC8106407.;26:14. https://doi.org/10.4103/jrms.JRMS_264_20.

19. Özcan S, Koçkara N, Camurcu Y, Yurten H. Magnetic resonance imaging and outcomes of osteochondral lesions of the talus associated with ankle fractures. Foot Ankle Int. 2020. Epub 2020 Jul 2.;41(10):1219–25. https://doi.org/10.1177/1071100720937243.

20. Michelson JD. Ankle fractures resulting from rotational injuries. J Am Acad Orthop Surg. 2003;11(6):403–12.

21. Michelson JD, Magid D, McHale K. Clinical utility of a stability-based ankle fracture classification system. J Orthop Trauma. 2007;21(5):307–15. https://doi.org/10.1097/BOT.0b013e318059aea3.

22. Rammelt S, Endres T, Grass R, Zwipp H. The role of external fixation in acute ankle trauma. Foot Ankle Clin. 2004;9(3):455–74. https://doi.org/10.1016/j.fcl.2004.05.001.

23. Thordarson DB, Ghalambor N, Perlman M. Intermittent pneumatic pedal compression and edema resolution after acute ankle fracture: a prospective, randomized study. Foot Ankle Int. 1997;18(6):347–50. https://doi.org/10.1177/107110079701800607.

24. Sirkin M, Sanders R, DiPasquale T, Herscovici D Jr. A staged protocol for soft tissue management in the treatment of complex pilon fractures. J Orthop Trauma. 2004;18(8 Suppl):S32–8. https://doi.org/10.1097/00005131-200409001-00005.

25. Shah K, Johnson J, O'Donnell S, Gil J, Born C, Hayda R. External fixation in the Emergency Department for pilon and unstable ankle fractures. J Am Acad Orthop Surg. 2019;27(12):e577–84. https://doi.org/10.5435/JAAOS-D-18-00080.

26. Watson JT, Moed BR, Karges DE, Cramer KE. Pilon fractures. Treatment protocol based on severity of soft tissue injury. Clin Orthop Relat Res. 2000;375:78–90.

27. Sharma JP, Salhotra R. Tourniquets in orthopedic surgery. Indian J Orthop. 2012;46(4):377–83. https://doi.org/10.4103/0019-5413.98824.

28. SooHoo NF, Krenek L, Eagan MJ, Gurbani B, Ko CY, Zingmond DS. Complication rates following open reduction and internal fixation of ankle fractures. J Bone Joint Surg Am. 2009. PMID: 19411451.;91(5):1042–9. https://doi.org/10.2106/JBJS.H.00653.

29. Aigner R, Lechler P, Kolia Boese C, Bockman B, Ruchholtz S, Frink M. Standardized pre-operative diagnostics and treatment of peripheral arterial disease reduce wound complications in geriatric ankle fractures. Int Orthop. 2018. Epub 2017 Dec 14.;42(2):395–400. https://doi.org/10.1007/s00264-017-3705-x.

30. Lavery LA, Lavery DC, Green T, Hunt N, La Fontaine J, Kim PJ, Wukich D. Increased risk of nonunion and Charcot Arthropathy after ankle fracture in people with diabetes. J Foot Ankle Surg. 2020. PMID: 32600558.;59(4):653–6. https://doi.org/10.1053/j.jfas.2019.05.006.

31. Ebaugh MP, Umbel B, Goss D, Taylor BC. Outcomes of primary Tibiotalocalcaneal nailing for complicated diabetic ankle fractures. Foot Ankle Int. 2019. Epub 2019 Aug 18. PMID: 31423816.;40(12):1382–7. https://doi.org/10.1177/1071100719869639.

32. Chang CJ, Jou IM, Wu TT, Su FC, Tai TW. Cigarette smoke inhalation impairs angiogenesis in early bone healing processes and delays fracture union. Bone Joint Res. 2020. Published 2020 May 16.;9(3):99–107. https://doi.org/10.1302/2046-3758.93.BJR-2019-0089.R1.

33. Giannoudis PV, Schneider E. Principles of fixation of osteoporotic fractures. J Bone Joint Surg Br. 2006. PMID: 17012413.;88(10):1272–8. https://doi.org/10.1302/0301-620X.88B10.17683.

34. Moia M, Squizzato A. Reversal agents for oral anticoagulant-associated major or life-threatening bleeding [published correction appears in intern Emerg med. 2019 Nov 27]. Intern Emerg Med. 2019;14(8):1233–9. https://doi.org/10.1007/s11739-019-02177-2.

35. Medscape. protamine (Rx). https://reference.medscape.com/drug/protamine-343746. Accessed May 2022.

36. Nickolas TL, Leonard MB, Shane E. Chronic kidney disease and bone fracture: a growing concern. Kidney Int. 2008;74(6):721–31. https://doi.org/10.1038/ki.2008.264.

37. Advanced Trauma Life Support. Student course manual. 10th ed. Chicago, IL: American College of Surgeons; 2018.

38. Briet JP, Houwert RM, Smeeing DPJ, Dijkgraaf MGW, Verleisdonk EJ, Leenen LPH, Hietbrink F. Differences in classification between mono- and Polytrauma and low- and high-energy trauma patients with an ankle fracture: a retrospective cohort study. J Foot Ankle Surg. 2017. PMID: 28633779.;56(4):793–6. https://doi.org/10.1053/j.jfas.2017.04.012.

Emergency Management of Ankle Fractures

Abhishek Ganta and Kenneth A. Egol

1 Introduction

Ankle fractures are some of the most common lower extremity injuries treated by orthopedic surgeons [1]. They typically occur in a bi-modal distribution with more severe fracture dislocations and open injuries occurring from high energy injuries in younger populations and lower energy injuries occurring in the geriatric population [2]. However, recent studies have demonstrated that the incidence of ankle fractures in the elderly population has had a significant rise since 2000 [3, 4]. Open fractures in this cohort are associated with increased complications and have a significant impact on health care costs [5].

While most patients with ankle fractures can be treated as an outpatient, there are circumstances which require urgent treatment, including admission and inpatient management [6]. These include displacement compromising skin viability, dislocation of the tibiotalar joint, neurovascular compromise, and severe soft tissue injury, including open fractures.

A. Ganta (✉) · K. A. Egol
Division of Orthopedic Trauma Surgery, Department of Orthopedic Surgery, NYU Langone Health, NYU Langone Orthopedic Hospital, New York, NY, USA

Department of Orthopedic Surgery, Jamaica Hospital Medical Center, Queens, NY, USA
e-mail: Abhishek.Ganta@nyulangone.org; Kenneth.egol@nyulangone.org

2 Emergency Room Work Up and Management

Initial assessment of an ankle injury requires history, physical examination and, often, radiographic imaging. Radiographs should be obtained if there is gross deformity, bony tenderness along the malleolar region or along the foot, and if the patient is unable to bear weight [7]. The mechanism of injury is important and includes both low energy twisting mechanisms and higher energy mechanisms such as falls from height, motor vehicle accidents, and pedestrian struck [2]. These higher energy mechanisms can indicate the likelihood of severe soft tissue compromise, compartment syndrome, pilon variations of ankle fractures, and associated injuries to the foot, as well as other musculoskeletal injuries (Fig. 1a, b) [8].

Obtaining a medical history can help direct post-operative management of the patient. Poorly controlled diabetics and patients with severe vascular disease are at risk of significant complications post-operatively even in simple ankle fracture patterns [9, 10]. Furthermore, a history of tobacco use, drug or alcohol abuse, and psychiatric illnesses can alert the physician to increased risk of post-operative complications [11].

Examination should begin with the knee at the fibular head and work distally. Careful inspection of the limb for scars, deformity, skin integrity,

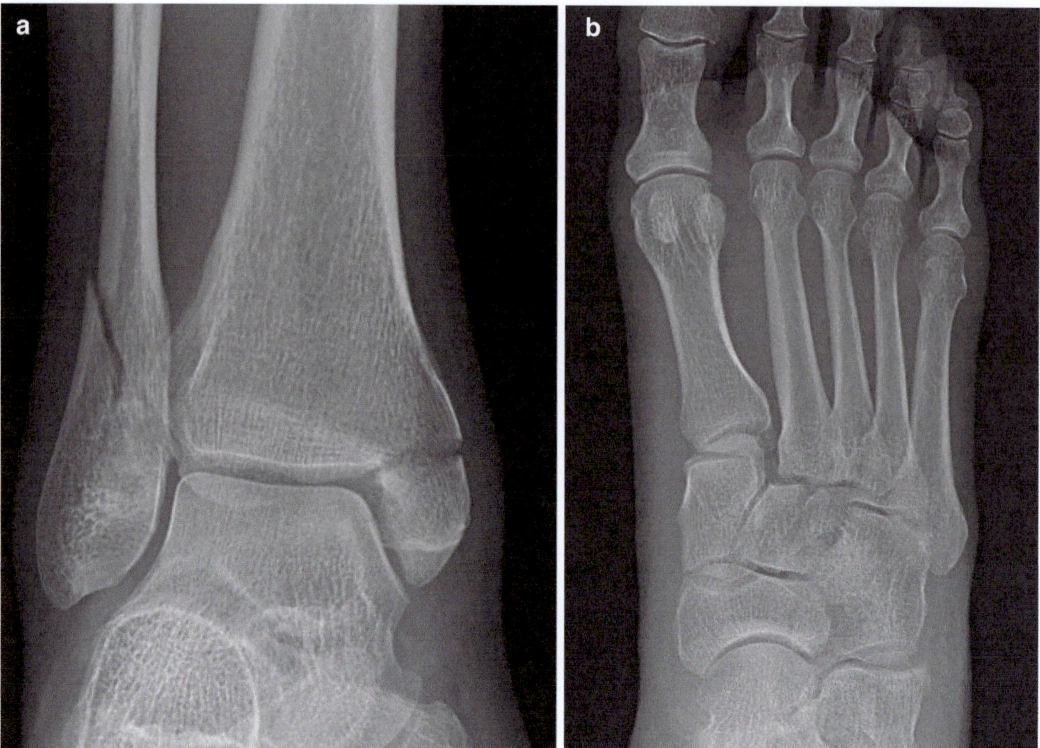

Fig. 1 (**a**, **b**) Patient is a 70-year-old male who had a forklift injury to the right ankle. He sustained a combined ankle and midfoot injury. (**a**) AP radiograph of the right ankle demonstrates a bi-malleolar ankle fracture. (**b**) AP of the right foot demonstrates incongruity of the first tarsometatarsal joint and widening of the Lisfranc Joint

open wounds, and any blisters should be noted and documented. Given the subcutaneous nature of the medial malleolus, skin blistering and compromise typically can be found in this area. Blanched, taut skin without capillary refill due to displacement of the ankle is an emergent condition requiring reduction to maintain viability of skin in this crucial area. Do not overlook the skin and soft tissues around the posterior aspect of the ankle. Palpation of the foot can help identify concomitant hindfoot, midfoot, and forefoot injuries such as calcaneus fractures and Lisfranc fractures. Palpation of the posterior tibial and dorsalis pedis pulses should be performed both before and after reduction and splinting. If the ankle is dislocated, the dorsalis pedis pulse may be diminished due to vessel kinking from the anterior displacement of the tibia relative to the talus. Expedient reduction will restore flow back to this vessel.

The ankle trauma series consist of three standard radiographs: the AP, lateral, and mortise (Fig. 2a–c). A full length tibia film should sometimes be obtained, if physical examination is suggestive or unclear, as proximal fibula fractures may not be fully visualized on the ankle radiographs [12].

Contra-lateral films can be obtained for a frame of reference as well in the emergency room or intra-operatively as there can be substantial variability in anatomy (Fig. 3) [13].

In isolated fibula fractures with medial signs and/or symptoms, a gravity stress or a stress external rotation examination should be performed to assess competency of the medial malleolar ligamentous complex (Fig. 4a–d) [14]. It is important to avoid a plantarflexed position as it can result in apparent but not true widening of the medial ligamentous complex due to narrowing of the talus posteriorly [15].

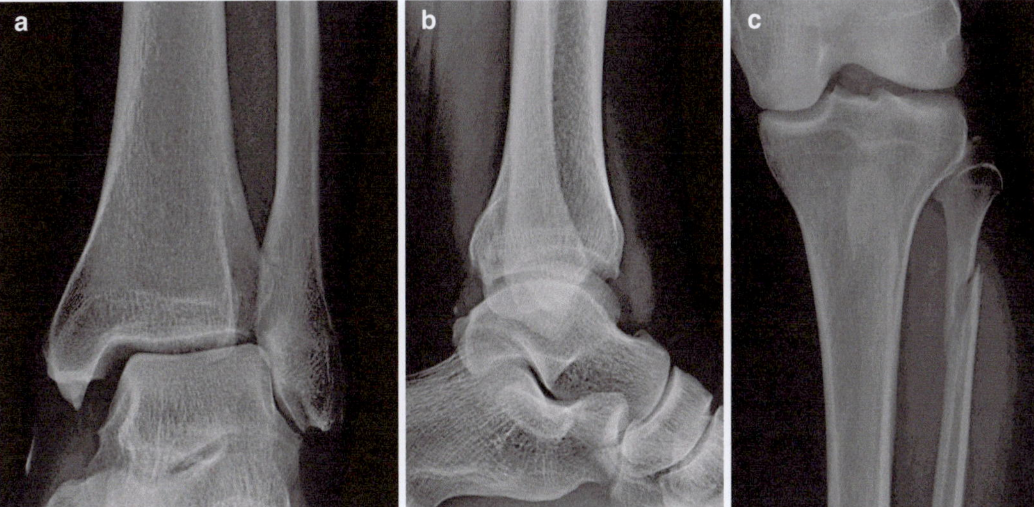

Fig. 2 (**a–c**) Patient is a 44-year-old male s/p fall on ice who sustained a left ankle injury with widening of the medial and tibia-fibula clear space on his injury films. (**a** and **b**) AP and Lateral imaging of the left ankle demonstrating widening of the medial clear space and lateral shifting of the talus. Of note there is a posterior malleolus fracture as well. (**c**) AP of the tibia demonstrates a proximal fibula fracture indicated a Maisonneuve ankle injury

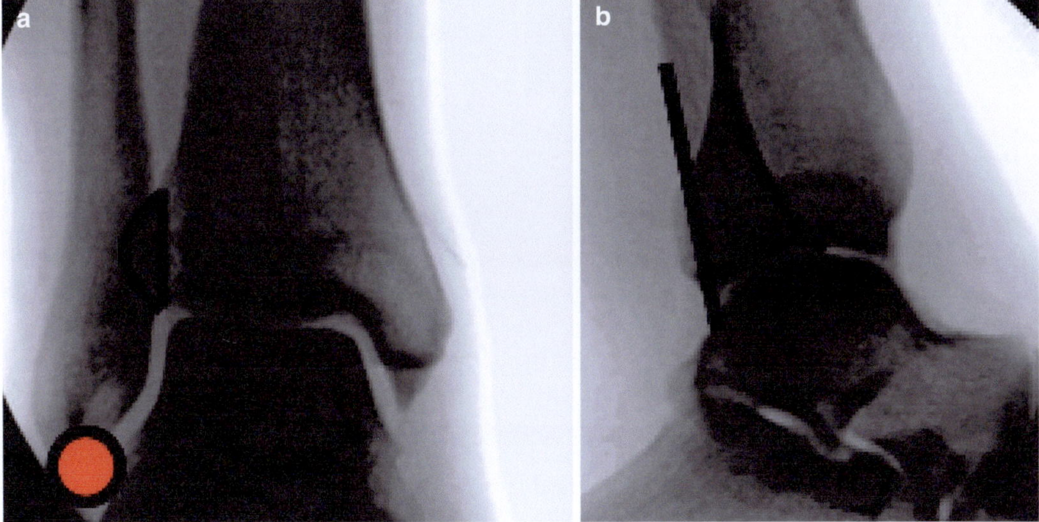

Fig. 3 (**a, b**) Intra-operative fluoroscopy of the contralateral ankle is used to assess fibular length and anatomic relationship of the fibula to the tibia. (**a**) Demonstrates the relationship of the distal tibia to the talus and the amount of overlap of the tibia and fibula on a mortise view. (**b**) Lateral fluoroscopy demonstrates how the fibula sits within the posterior aspect of the tibia

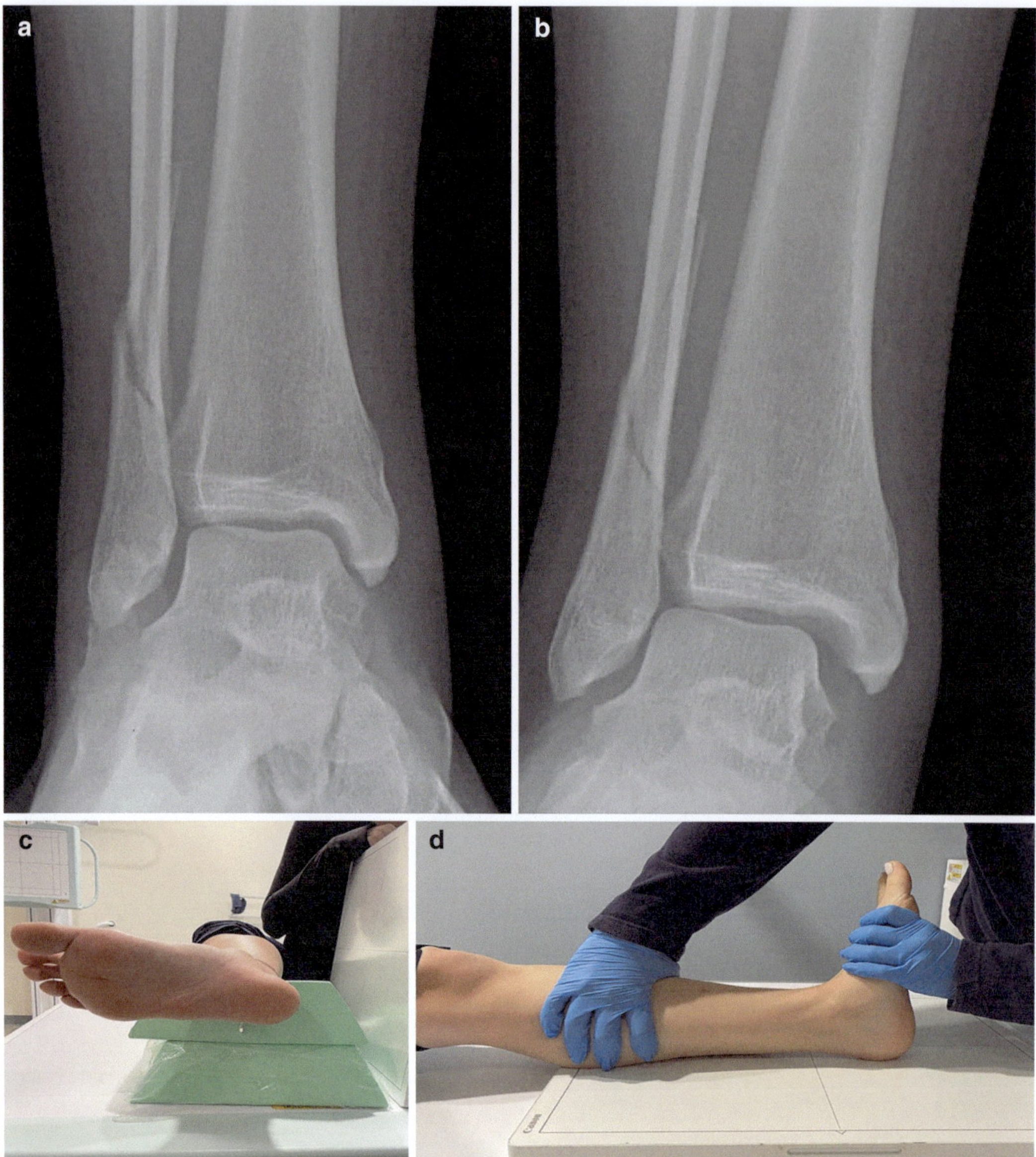

Fig. 4 (**a**, **b**) Patient is a 35-year-old man that slipped and fell on ice and sustained a right unstable lateral malleolus above the level of the syndesmosis. (**a**) Mortise view of the ankle demonstrate no lateral translation of the talus and no medial clear space widening. (**b**) External rotation stress view of the ankle demonstrates interval clear space widening and lateral translation of the talus. (**c**) This clini-cal picture demonstrates a gravity stress external rotation view where the foot is externally rotated due to its weight. The XR cassette is placed behind ankle. (**d**) This clinically demonstrates the technique of a manual stress external rotation stress where the foot is dorsiflexed and externally rotated

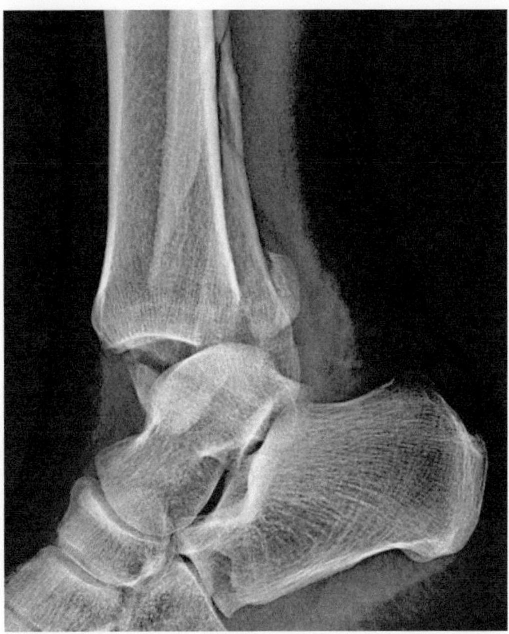

Fig. 5 Patient is a 31-year-old male that was bicyclist struck by a car and sustained a tri-malleolar ankle fracture dislocation. Note that the talus dislocates posteriorly following the posterior malleolus fracture displacement

Dislocated or subluxated tibiotalar joints should be reduced urgently to alleviate soft tissue tenting and pressure and splinted to maintain reduction. Typically, the talus will dislocate posteriorly while the tibia translates anteriorly especially in the presence of large posterior malleolus fractures (Fig. 5).

Reduction requires manual traction with anterior translation of the talus and supination of the foot. Closed reduction and splinting can be done with a single person; however, it requires coordination with the emergency room team. Closed reduction may require the following: (1) Sedation, (2) Analgesia, (3) Muscle relaxation, and (4) appropriate material to maintain reduction [12]. The ED team should be available to provide sedation and relaxation. A tibiotalar ankle block given within the tibiotalar joint can also provide additional analgesia [16]. A 10 cc syringe is used and 10 cc of 1% lidocaine is injected into the medial axilla of the ankle with a 22gauge needle. Given the capsular disruption, the lidocaine can spread along the fracture hematoma well. Multiple reductions should be avoided as they are painful and damaging to the joint, so splinting materials should be gathered and adequate assistance be present to allow immediate application of stabilizing immobilization to prevent re-dislocation. Prior to reduction, an "AO" short leg splint should be pre-measured and rolled out and ample webril padding should be available. The authors prefer 3–4 layers of webril padding on the splinted injury and 10 layers of plaster for both the posterior slab and sugar tong U mold. Plaster is preferable to fiberglass as a splinting material due to superior molding ability.

Once the set up for splinting is completed and the patient has adequate relaxation and analgesia, the knee should be bent to help relax the gastrocnemius/soleus complex. A Quigley maneuver can be used to not only assist with the reduction but also to suspend the extremity to allow independent splint placement [17]. The use of Quigley requires an IV pole and a cast stockinette. The IV pole is placed behind the contra-lateral shoulder while the patient is in a supine position. A long stockinette is placed around the ankle above the knee and tied to the IV pole. Alternatively a kerlix that can be attached to the great toe and second toe. This not only relaxes the gastrocnemius/soleus complex but also provides an anterior directed force on the talus. Placement of the IV pole posterior to the contra-lateral shoulder allows for supination of the foot as well (Fig. 6).

Once the ankle is reduced and the plaster splint is applied, a firm mold is applied to maintain reduction. While molding, care should be taken to avoid pressure points. Molding of a splint should be done with the flat surfaces of the palm and not fingers. The molds on the splint should be placed laterally along the base of the heel and medially above the medial malleolus to hold the mortise reduced (Fig. 7a–d).

After reduction is performed and the splint has dried appropriately, radiographs of the ankle should be obtained to ensure that the mortise is reduced. Axial imaging with a CT scan be obtained after reduction to look for marginal impaction in supination adduction type fractures and also to evaluate the morphology and size of posterior malleolus fractures as well (Fig. 8a–d) [18, 19]. MRI has been used in research studies to evaluate the competency of the deltoid ligament as well as osteochondral lesions; however, its use in clinical practice is unnecessary.

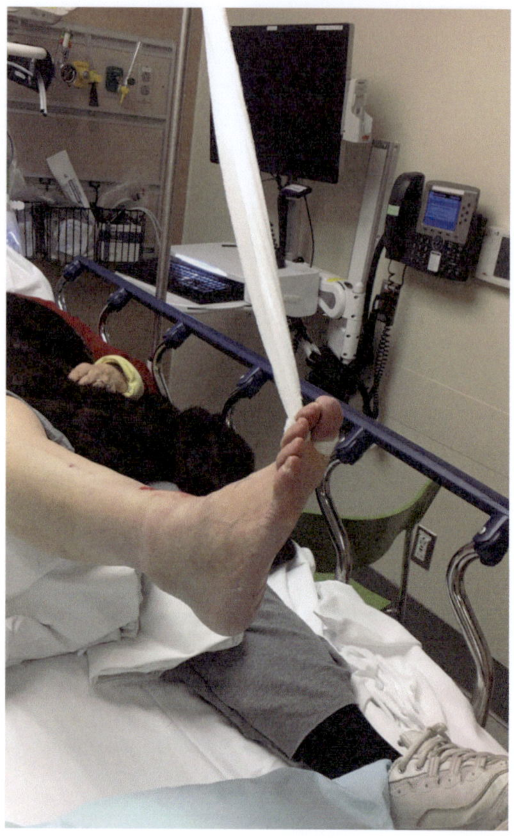

Fig. 6 This image demonstrates the use of a modified Quigley maneuver to help reduce and maintain reduction of an ankle fracture dislocation. Note that the IV pole along the contra-lateral should allow the foot to supinate. The knee remains flexed under sheets or pillows to relax the gastrocnemius/soleus complex. The reduction can be finetuned and a splint can be applied without the need for multiple assistants. A stockinette can also be used

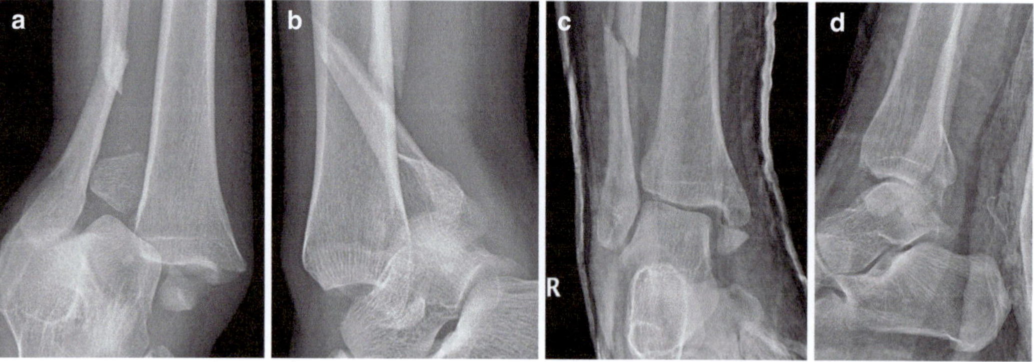

Fig. 7 (**a–d**) Patient is a 32 year old male who sustained a tri-malleolar ankle fracture dislocation after falling off an electric scooter. (**a, b**) AP and lateral of the ankle demonstrate a posterolateral dislocation of the talus with a large posterior malleolus fracture. (**c, d**) Demonstrates interval reduction and placement of an AO splint. Note the plaster mold along the medial aspect of the tibia and laterally along the calcaneus

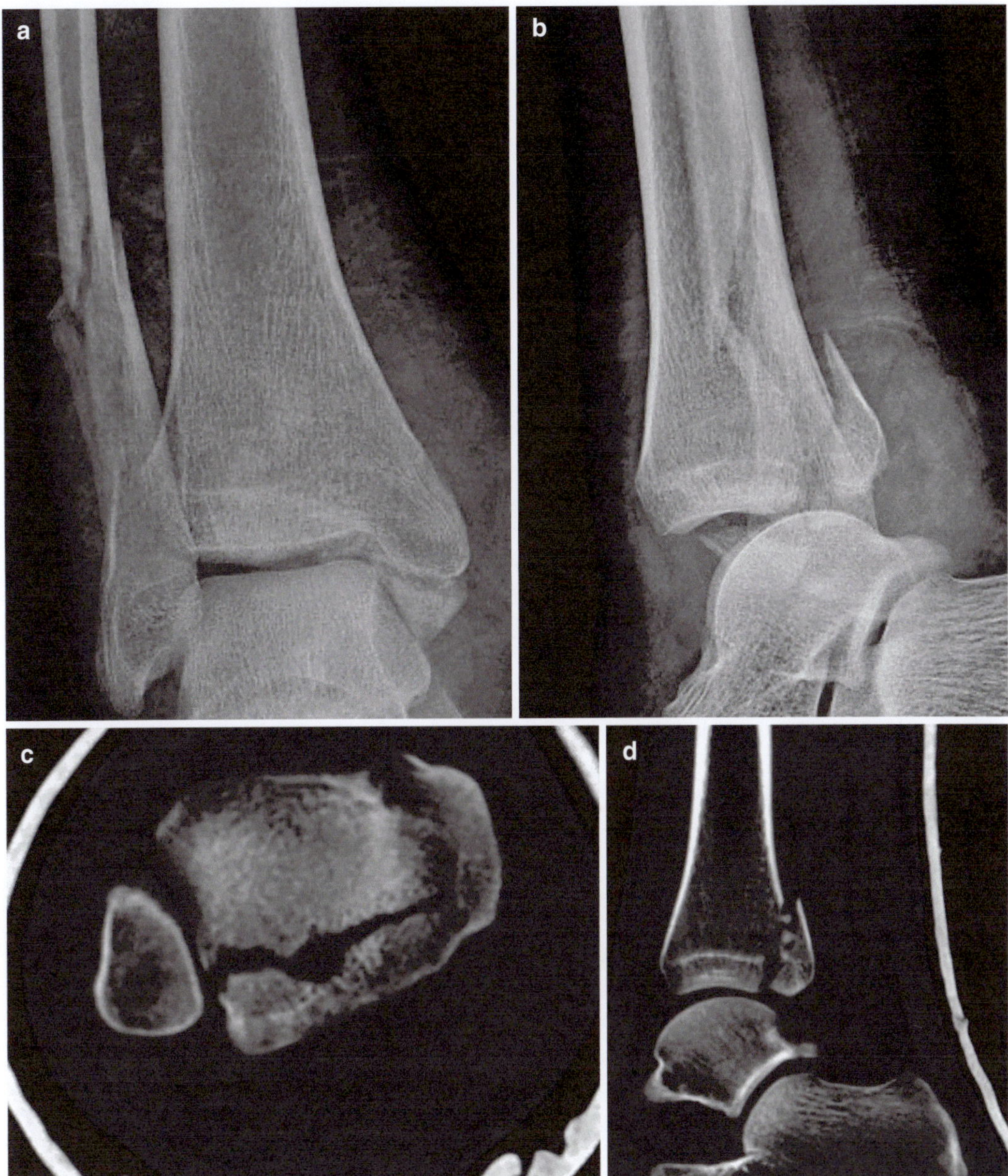

Fig. 8 (**a–d**) Patient is an 18-year-old male s/p twisting injury to the right ankle while playing soccer sustaining a right tri-malleolar fracture dislocation. (**a, b**) AP and lateral of the right ankle demonstrate a tri-malleolar fracture dislocation with a large posterior malleolus fracture. (**c, d**) Post-reduction axial and sagittal CT scan of the ankle demonstrate medial extension of the posterior malleolus fracture as well as marginal impaction that is not fully appreciated on radiographs

3 Irreducible Ankle Fractures

While the majority of ankle fractures can be closed reduced and splinted, there are reports of ankle fractures that are irreducible. The patients that have these injuries usually present after a high energy mechanism such as a fall from height or a motor vehicle accident; however, there are cases of these that occur from a ground level fall or twisting mechanism. The fracture pattern typically involves a fibula fracture consistent with a pronation injury [20]. The continued appearance of a disproportionately wide medial clear space before and after an adequate reduction attempt should suggest the possibility of soft tissue interposition (Fig. 9a, b).

Most interposition occurs when the medial structures such as the posterior tibial tendon dislocates from its groove posteriorly and gets entrapped laterally at the level of the syndesmosis [20]. This results in an anterior and laterally subluxated talus. Other structures that can be entrapped in this region include the anterior tibialis tendon as well as the entire posteromedial tendons and neurovascular bundle [21, 22].

Concern and presence of entrapment can be confirmed with a CT scan; however, advanced imaging is often not needed. Repeated attempts at closed reduction may be damaging and should be limited; if concern about entrapped structures persist, the patient should be taken to the OR expeditiously for open reduction. While ankle procedures typically start with lateral sided fixation, if there is concern for entrapment, a medial approach can be utilized first [23]. This allows for interposed tissue to removed so that the ankle joint can be reduced.

4 Soft Tissue Injuries: Open Fractures

Open fractures comprise about 1.5–3% of all ankle fractures and typically occur in younger patients with high energy mechanisms [24]. However, there has been a substantial increase of these open

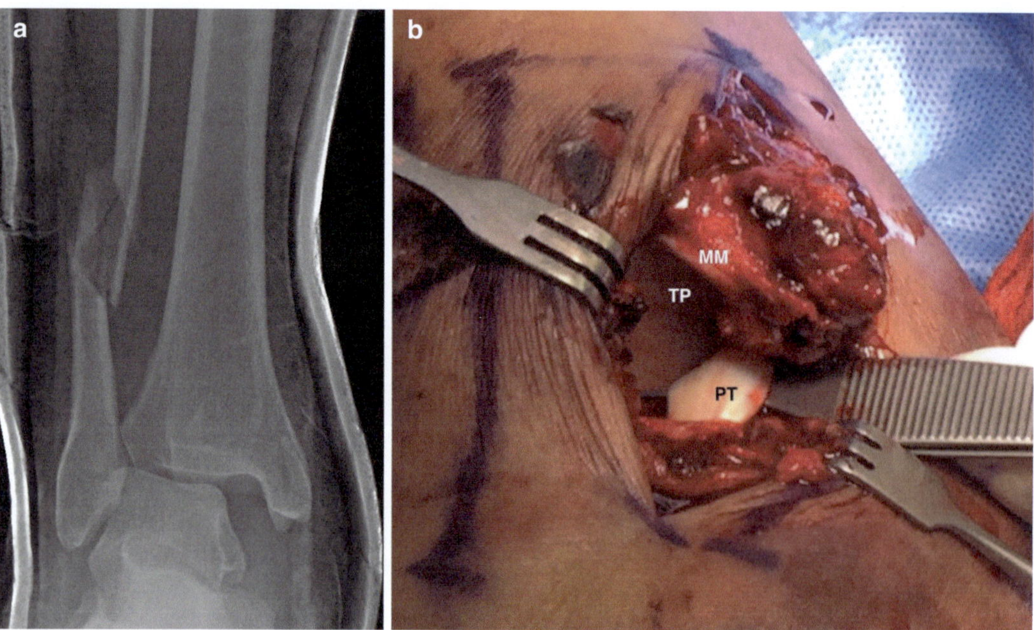

Fig. 9 (**a**, **b**) Patient is a 57-year-old male who had an irreducible ankle fracture following a fall and twist from a two-step height. (Courtesy of Dr. Sanjit R. Konda). (**a**) Mortise view of the ankle after multiple reduction attempts demonstrate persistent widening of the medial clear space and lateral subluxation of the talus. (**b**) Intra-operative image of the wound demonstrates displacement of the posterior tibial tendon within the axilla of the medial malleolus preventing reduction. *TP* tibial plafond, *PT* posterior tibial tendon, *MM* medial malleolus

injuries in geriatric patients from ground level falls or low energy mechanism. This can be attributed to the fact that this population has diminished skin tensile strength leading to open fractures even with low energy falls (Fig. 10a, b) [25].

Most open wounds result from a tensile failure along the medial aspect of the tibia. The wound is typically transverse or stellate in nature regardless of the presence of medial malleolus fracture . Rarely, does the open wound involve the lateral malleolus or the posterior aspect of the ankle. Emergency room management of these injuries includes removal of any gross contamination before reduction and protecting the medial skin from damage or entrapment during reduction. The wound should be covered with a sterile saline soaked gauze [26]. Intravenous antibiotics should be administered within 60 min of arrival with a first-generation cephalosporin for Gustilo Anderson type 1 and type 2 fractures. Gram negative coverage may be considered for type III fractures as well as for gross contamination [27, 28].

The authors prefer acute internal fixation after irrigation and debridement of these injuries [29, 30]. Lacerations may need to be extended longitudinally to allow adequate access, but careful placement of incisions is necessary with consideration of future needs. The ankle should be gently re-dislocated during irrigation and debridement to allow irrigation of the articular surface and into the incisura with several liters of low flow saline. Primary closure of the open wound is recommended if possible, as it has been associated with improved outcomes and lower rate of infection [31]. At times, immediate closure can have increased tension on the traumatic wound. The use of Allgöwer-Donati closure demonstrates superior incisional prefusion compared to vertical mattress; however, this may not correlate to any clinical difference [32]. While incisional wound vacs can be applied to areas at risk, its routine usage may not confer any clinical benefit even in open fractures [33, 34]. External fixation is reserved for fractures that require a second look due to contamination or as damage control for poly traumatized patient (Fig. 11). In the setting of severe bone loss/comminution or if the ankle remains unstable, an external fixator can be used to supplement internal fixation [25].

If the wound cannot be closed, a negative pressure dressing (wound VAC) can be placed and a delayed closure can be performed with either a local rotational flap or a free flap. The patient should remain on antibiotics until coverage, which ideally should be within 7 days [35].

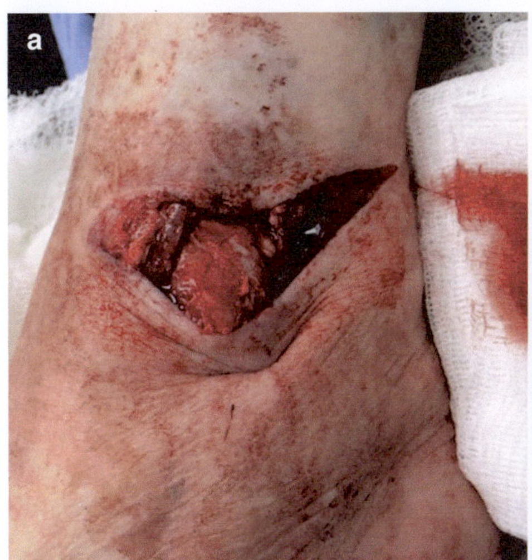
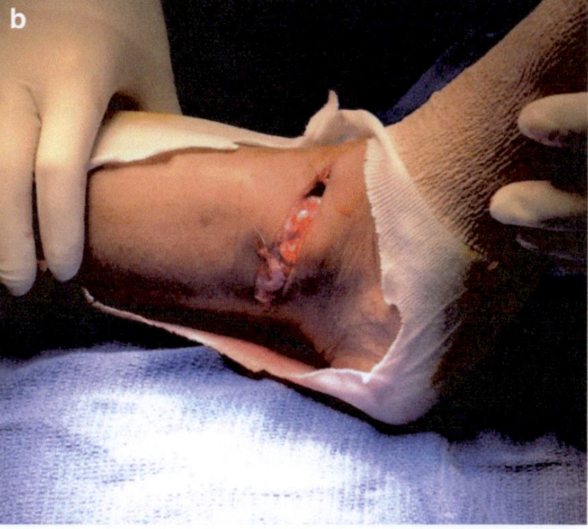

Fig. 10 (a) Patient is an 87-year-old woman who has a history of lung cancer that required chemotherapy, insulin dependent diabetes, and coronary artery disease who had a ground level fall sustaining a large transverse wound over the medial ankle. (b) Patient is a 40-year-old female with no past medical history who sustained a similar transverse wound over her medial malleolus from a motor vehicle accident.

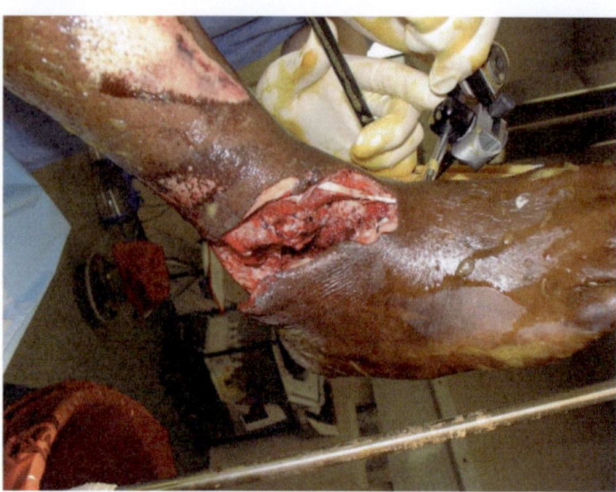

Fig. 11 Clinical images demonstrate a severely contaminated open ankle fracture with soft tissue compromise. Due to this, the patient was treated with initial external fixation and serial debridement until they were amenable to internal fixation

Delaying wound closure or coverage longer than 7 days may increase risk of infection.

5 Soft Tissue Injury: Closed Fractures

Closed fractures can also have severe skin damage that precludes acute fixation for days or even weeks [35]. The presence of fracture blisters at the site of surgical incisions may require a staged approach with careful monitoring of soft tissues as immediate fixation is associated with increased wound complications. The injured limb should be strictly elevated in the hospital. Treatment of fractures with blisters with a defined protocol is generally recommended [36].

There are two main types of fracture blisters: serous (clear filled) and hemorrhagic (blood filled). These types differ in the depth of soft tissue injury. Blood-filled blisters have a greater degree of dermal-epidermal separation and injury (Fig. 12a, b).

Fracture blisters may develop 24–72 h post-injury and be first noticed upon removal of the

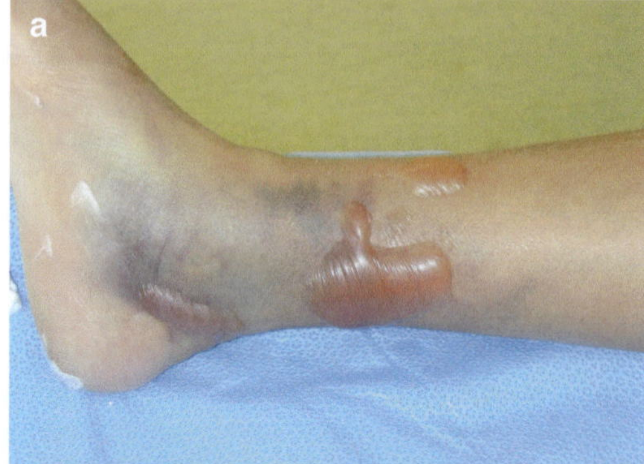

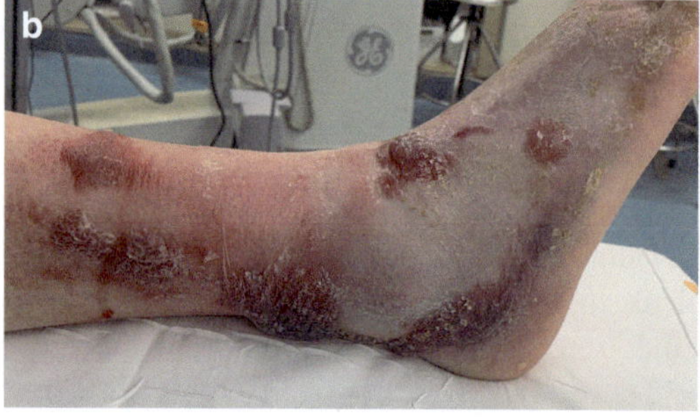

Fig. 12 (**a**) Clinical image of a 43-year-old female who sustained a rotational ankle injury with several serous filled fracture blisters. (**b**) Clinical image of a 70-year-old female with history of severe lower extremity neuropathy who sustained a ground level fall and has developed hemorrhagic fracture blisters. Note the difference in appearance of the fracture blisters

splint [37]. They can be circumferential around the ankle. To adequately visualize and monitor the soft tissues, the authors prefer to place a delta frame external fixator for unstable patterns in the presence of fracture blisters around planned surgical incisions [38]. This allows for maintained reduction of the ankle mortise and allows inspection of the entire ankle. If the ankle is unstable or the mortise continues to subluxate with the external fixation in place, smooth Steinmann pins can be from the calcaneus into the tibia either trans-articular or posteriorly out of the dome of the talus for additional stability (Fig. 13a–c) [39].

The blisters should be unroofed with sterile scissors and trimmed back to the point of healthy

Fig. 13 (**a**) Clinical image of a 30-year-old male with an open ankle fracture dislocation that was placed in a delta frame external fixator. This construct consists of two half pins in the tibia and two centrally threaded pins in the calcaneus. (**b**, **c**) Fluoroscopic images of an 86-year-old female with a tri-malleolar ankle fracture dislocation that was treated with stabilization with percutaneous Steinmann pins to allow for reduction and soft tissue stabilization prior to definitive treatment.

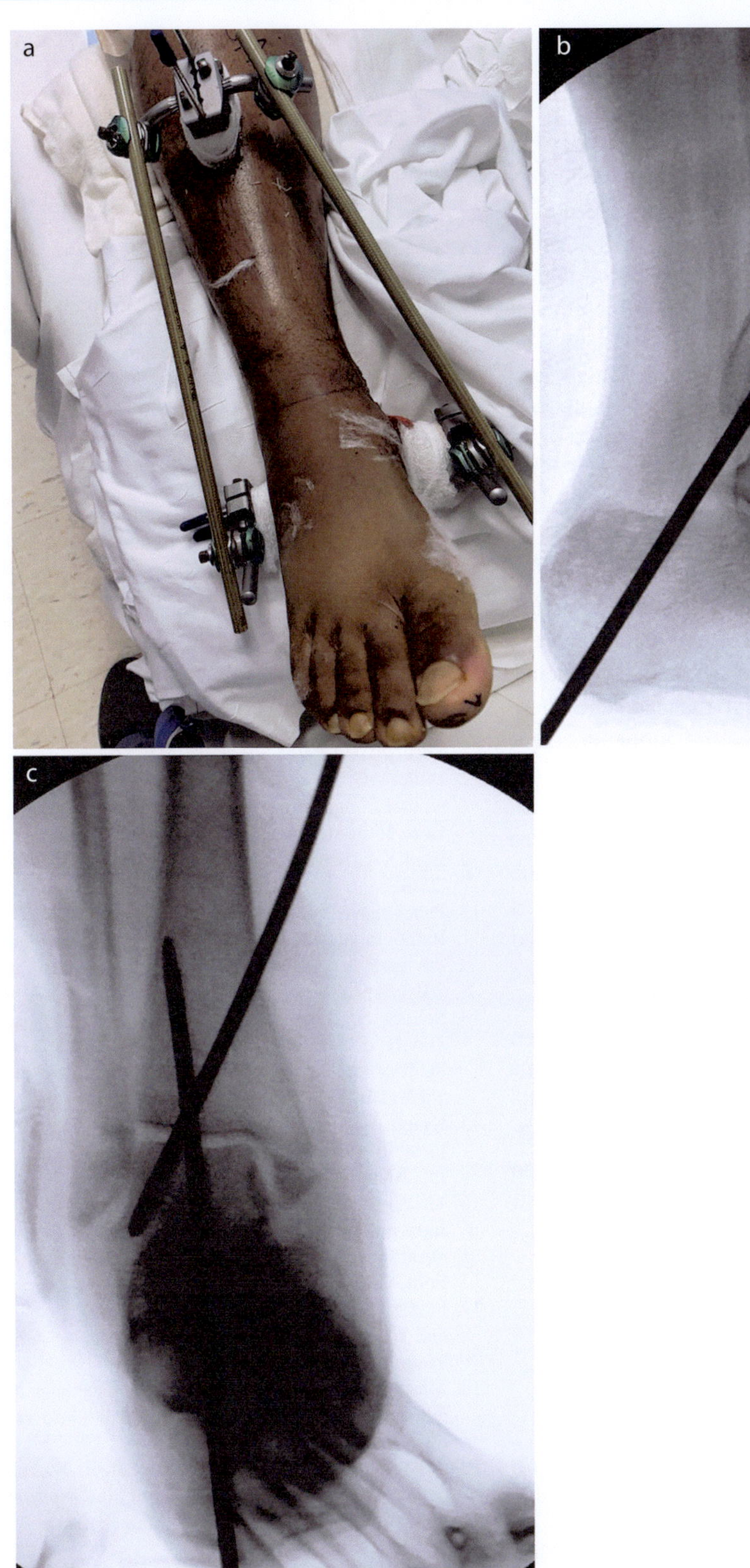

tissue. After this, Xeroform dressings can be applied to blistering area. The authors prefer to leave these on for a week. The dressings should then be changed regularly, ideally twice a day but at the minimum daily [36] . Patients with hemorrhagic blisters tend to take longer for the skin to re-epithelialize. Clinically, re-epithelialization occurs when the granulation type tissue that is present becomes replaced by a full epithelial layer and the blister is no longer evident. The patients should be counseled that definitive fixation should likely be delayed until full epithelization occurs.

6 Conclusion

While the majority of ankle fractures and fracture dislocations can be reduced and splinted in the emergency department and sent home with semi-elective outpatient surgical management, there are circumstances that require more emergent inpatient management. Clinicians should be aware of radiographic findings consistent with irreducible ankle fractures as these may require more urgent open reduction to mitigate soft tissue compromise. Furthermore, high energy injuries or severe fracture dislocations even in ground level falls may pre-dispose patients to soft tissue compromise. Open fractures should be urgently debrided in the operating room and temporized or definitively fixed in a timely fashion to mitigate complications. The lacerations should be closed, or the wounds covered as soon as possible. Fractures associated with blistering or deep abrasion of the skin need early care of the soft tissue envelope and may require delayed fixation.

References

1. Scheer RC, Newman JM, Zhou JJ, et al. Ankle fracture epidemiology in the United States: patient-related trends and mechanisms of injury. J Foot Ankle Surg. 2020;59:479–83.
2. Briet JP, Houwert RM, Smeeing DPJ, et al. Differences in classification between mono- and polytrauma and low- and high-energy trauma patients with an ankle fracture: a retrospective cohort study. J Foot Ankle Surg. 2017;56:793–6.
3. Kannus P, Palvanen M, Niemi S, et al. Increasing number and incidence of low-trauma ankle fractures in elderly people: Finnish statistics during 1970-2000 and projections for the future. Bone. 2002;31:430–3.
4. Strauss EJ, Egol KA. The management of ankle fractures in the elderly. Injury. 2007;38(Suppl 3):S2–9.
5. Toole WP, Elliott M, Hankins D, et al. Are low-energy open ankle fractures in the elderly the new geriatric hip fracture? J Foot Ankle Surg. 2015;54:203–6.
6. Qin C, Dekker RG, Helfrich MM, et al. Outpatient management of ankle fractures. Orthop Clin North Am. 2018;49:103–8.
7. Bachmann LM, Kolb E, Koller MT, et al. Accuracy of Ottawa ankle rules to exclude fractures of the ankle and mid-foot: systematic review. BMJ. 2003;326:417.
8. Tarkin IS, Sop A, Pape H-C. High-energy foot and ankle trauma: principles for formulating an individualized care plan. Foot Ankle Clin. 2008;13:705–23.
9. Manway JM, Blazek CD, Burns PR. Special considerations in the management of diabetic ankle fractures. Curr Rev Musculoskelet Med. 2018;11:445–55.
10. Saleh H, Konda S, Driesman A, et al. Wound-healing issues following rotational ankle fracture surgery: predictors and local management options. Foot Ankle Spec. 2019;12:409–17.
11. Miller AG, Margules A, Raikin SM. Risk factors for wound complications after ankle fracture surgery. J Bone Joint Surg Am. 2012;94:2047–52.
12. Egol KA, Koval KJ. Handbook of fractures. 6th ed; 2020.
13. Panchbhavi VK, Gurbani BN, Mason CB, et al. Radiographic assessment of fibular length variance: the case for "Fibula Minus". J Foot Ankle Surg. 2018;57:91–4.
14. Schock HJ, Pinzur M, Manion L, et al. The use of gravity or manual-stress radiographs in the assessment of supination-external rotation fractures of the ankle. J Bone Joint Surg Br. 2007;89:1055–9.
15. Kragh JF, Ward JA. Radiographic indicators of ankle instability: changes with plantarflexion. Foot Ankle Int. 2006;27:23–8.
16. MacCormick LM, Baynard T, Williams BR, et al. Intra-articular hematoma block compared to procedural sedation for closed reduction of ankle fractures. Foot Ankle Int. 2018;39:1162–8.
17. Skelley NW, Ricci WM. A single-person reduction and splinting technique for ankle injuries. J Orthop Trauma. 2015;29:e172–7.
18. Mason LW, Marlow WJ, Widnall J, et al. Pathoanatomy and associated injuries of posterior malleolus fracture of the ankle. Foot Ankle Int. 2017;38:1229–35.
19. Alluri RK, Hill JR, Donohoe S, et al. Radiographic detection of marginal impaction in supination-adduction ankle fractures. Foot Ankle Int. 2017;38:1005–10.
20. Stevens NM, Wasterlain AS, Konda SR. Case report: irreducible ankle fracture with posterior tibialis ten-

don and retinaculum, deltoid ligament, and antero-medial joint capsule entrapment. J Foot Ankle Surg. 2017;56:889–93.

21. Pankovich AM. Fracture-dislocation of the ankle. Trapping of the postero-medical ankle tendons and neurovascular bundle in the tibiofibular interosseous space: a case report. J Trauma. 1976;16:927–9.

22. Natoli RM, Summers HD. Irreducible ankle fracture-dislocation due to tibialis anterior subluxation: a case report. J Foot Ankle Surg. 2015;54:268–72.

23. Karim A, So E, Taylor BC, et al. Ankle fracture fixation: medial or lateral first? J Foot Ankle Surg. 2019;58:75–9.

24. Bugler KE, Clement ND, Duckworth AD, et al. Open ankle fractures: who gets them and why? Arch Orthop Trauma Surg. 2015;135:297–303.

25. Rammelt S. Management of ankle fractures in the elderly. EFORT Open Rev. 2016;1:239–46.

26. Hulsker CCC, Kleinveld S, Zonnenberg CBL, et al. Evidence-based treatment of open ankle fractures. Arch Orthop Trauma Surg. 2011;131:1545–53.

27. Halawi MJ, Morwood MP. Acute management of open fractures: an evidence-based review. Orthopedics. 2015;38:e1025–33.

28. Garner MR, Sethuraman SA, Schade MA, et al. Antibiotic prophylaxis in open fractures: evidence, evolving issues, and recommendations. J Am Acad Orthop Surg. 2020;28:309–15.

29. Hong-Chuan W, Shi-Lian K, Heng-Sheng S, et al. Immediate internal fixation of open ankle fractures. Foot Ankle Int. 2010;31:959–64.

30. Peterson DL, Schuurman M, Geamanu A, et al. Early definitive care is as effective as staged treatment protocols for open ankle fractures caused by rotational mechanisms: a retrospective case-control study. J Orthop Trauma. 2020;34:376–81.

31. Jenkinson RJ, Kiss A, Johnson S, et al. Delayed wound closure increases deep-infection rate associated with lower-grade open fractures: a propensity-matched cohort study. J Bone Joint Surg Am. 2014;96:380–6.

32. Shannon SF, Houdek MT, Wyles CC, et al. Allgöwer-Donati versus vertical mattress suture technique impact on perfusion in ankle fracture surgery: a randomized clinical trial using intraoperative angiography. J Orthop Trauma. 2017;31:97–102.

33. Petrou S, Parker B, Masters J, et al. Cost-effectiveness of negative-pressure wound therapy in adults with severe open fractures of the lower limb: evidence from the WOLLF randomized controlled trial. Bone Jt J. 2019;101-B:1392–401.

34. Cook R, Thomas V, Martin R, et al. Negative pressure dressings are no better than standard dressings for open fractures. BMJ. 2019;364:k4411.

35. Pincus D, Byrne JP, Nathens AB, et al. Delay in flap coverage past 7 days increases complications for open tibia fractures: a cohort study of 140 north American trauma centers. J Orthop Trauma. 2019;33:161–8.

36. Strauss EJ, Petrucelli G, Bong M, et al. Blisters associated with lower-extremity fracture: results of a prospective treatment protocol. J Orthop Trauma. 2006;20:618–22.

37. Tosounidis TH, Daskalakis II, Giannoudis PV. Fracture blisters: pathophysiology and management. Injury. 2020;51:2786–92.

38. Wawrose RA, Grossman LS, Tagliaferro M, et al. Temporizing external fixation vs splinting following ankle fracture dislocation. Foot Ankle Int. 2020;41:177–82.

39. Meijer RPJ, Halm JA, Schepers T. Unstable fragility fractures of the ankle in the elderly: Transarticular Steinmann pin or external fixation. Foot (Edinb). 2017;32:35–8.

Management of Unimalleolar Ankle Fractures

Patrick M. Pallitto, Andrew T. Chen, and Robert F. Ostrum

1   Introduction

Fractures about the ankle are among the most common injuries encountered by the orthopedist, representing 10% of all fractures [1–3]. The mechanics of the ankle, discussed elsewhere, benefit from review when discussing fractures. The joint functions as a mobile mortise and tenon hinge joint with essentially one degree of freedom. The tenon of the joint is the talus, which articulates with the tibial plafond (including the posterolateral projection known as the posterior malleolus), medial malleolus, and distal fibula (lateral malleolus). An important consideration when specifically discussing unimalleolar ankle fractures is the axis of the joint line, as the medial malleolus is both shorter and more anterior, and the joint is in an average of between 18.8 and 21.5 degrees of external rotation, with reference to the axis of the knee [4]. The weightbearing load is shared throughout the tibial plafond, with about one sixth of the load then being distributed through the fibula [5, 6].

P. M. Pallitto · A. T. Chen · R. F. Ostrum (✉)
Department of Orthopaedics, University of North Carolina, Chapel Hill, NC, USA
e-mail: Patrick.Pallitto@unchealth.unc.edu; andrew_chen@med.unc.edu; robert_ostrum@med.unc.edu

2   Assessment of Unimalleolar Ankle Fractures

As with all injuries, the clinical evaluation should be thorough and complete. History surrounding the injury should include mechanism and timing of the injury as well as any concomitant injuries. Pre-existing comorbidities play an important role in clinical decision making and particular attention should be paid to those that may impact bone quality (Table 1) as well as the presence of diabetes, peripheral vascular disease, and/or neuropathy which may alter sensory function. As with all injuries, the remaining extremities should be evaluated, paying particular attention to any tenderness to palpation about the knee and proximal tibia/fibula to rule out ipsilateral proximal injuries. The physical examination should include a thorough evaluation and documentation in the chart of skin integrity, swelling and deformity, and a complete neurovascular examination.

As with all injuries, physical exam is important. It has been demonstrated that the clinical sign of tenderness medially has a positive predictive value (PPV) of 50% and the absence of tenderness has a negative predictive value (NPV) of 66% [7]. Furthermore, the absence of combined tenderness and bruising has a NPV of 39%. Not all ankle injuries warrant radiographs. The inability to bear weight for four steps and bony tenderness at the ankle, defined as within 6 cm proximal to the tip of either the medial or lateral malleoli,

© The Author(s), under exclusive license to Springer Nature Switzerland AG 2023
D. Herscovici Jr. et al. (eds.), *Evaluation and Surgical Management of the Ankle*,
https://doi.org/10.1007/978-3-031-33537-2_11

warrant imaging but it is first paramount to insure there is not a midfoot injury or similar alternative diagnosis [8]. The standard radiographic images of the ankle include the AP, the lateral and the mortise view. It is important to examine fibular length, utilizing markers such as Shenton's line

Table 1 Risk factors for osteoporosis and fractures

- Smoking
- Excessive alcohol intake (>3 units/day)
- Low body weight (BMI <19)
- Early menopause
- Genetic factors
  - Race
  - Family history hip fracture
- Diseases
  - Thyrotoxicosis
  - Rheumatoid arthritis
  - Primary hyperparathyroidism
  - Cushing syndrome
  - Hypogonadism
  - Anorexia nervosa
  - Cancer
  - Chronic liver disease
  - Celiac disease
  - Cystic fibrosis
  - Epilepsy
- Drugs
  - Corticosteroids
  - Thyroxine
  - Gonadotrophin releasing hormone agonists
  - Sedatives
  - Anticonvulsants

Courtesy Rockwood and Green's fractures in adults

and the dime sign (Fig. 1), as well as the medial clear space, tibiofibular overlap, tibiofibular clear space, and talar tilt. Since fibula fractures are often in the sagittal plane, the lateral view may be the only indication that there is distal fibular translation or angulation. The stress view is of particular importance in the evaluation of isolated lateral malleolus fractures. These may be performed via gravity or manual stress; the latter requiring increased provider time and more radiation exposure and the former requiring adequate x-ray technician education. The technique for stress views is simple. A patient is placed supine on the x-ray table with the leg held in 20 degrees of internal rotation to produce a mortise view. The rotation of the proximal calf is secured with one hand, while a firm, but gently progressive external rotation force is applied to the forefoot and a radiograph is taken. The same effect can be achieved with the patient in lateral decubitus on the x-ray table with the injured limb down and the foot hanging free from the end of the table [9] (Figs. 2 and 3).

Interpretation of stress views is somewhat controversial with several criteria proposed for instability. The ankle mortise can be deemed unstable if stress increases the medial clear space to or above 5 mm [10]. An increase of 3 mm from the contralateral ankle may be interpreted as demonstrating instability, though this requires bilateral films and the accompanying increase in cost and radiation. The clear space on the mortise

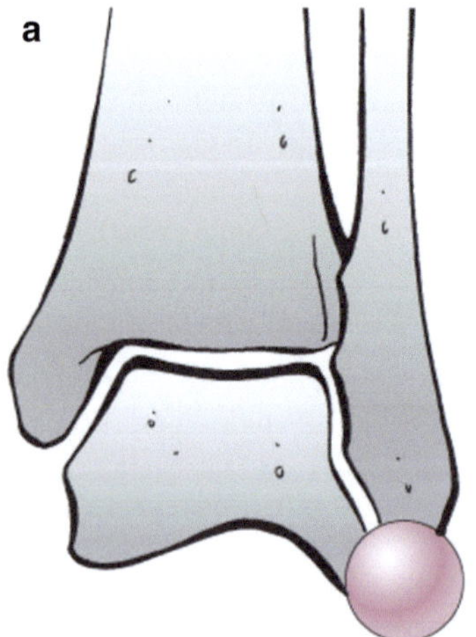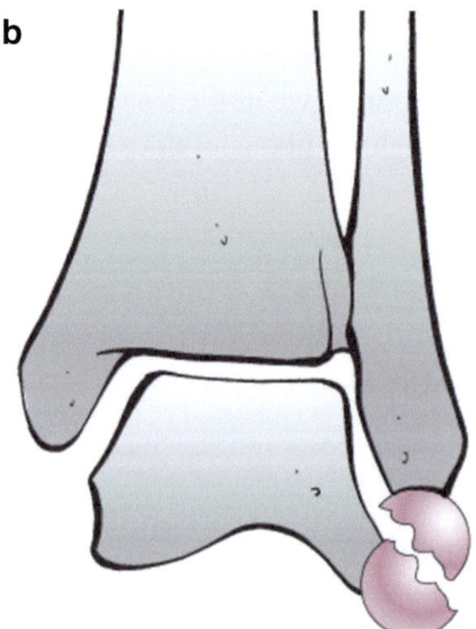

Fig. 1 The dime sign indicated by the distal tip of the fibula and lateral process of the talus. An intact dime sign (**a**) indicates appropriate fibular length while a disruption (**b**) indicates fibular shortening. (Courtesy Rockwood and Green's fractures in adults)

Fig. 2 Patient positioning and technique for gravity stress views. (Courtesy Rockwood and Green's fractures in adults)

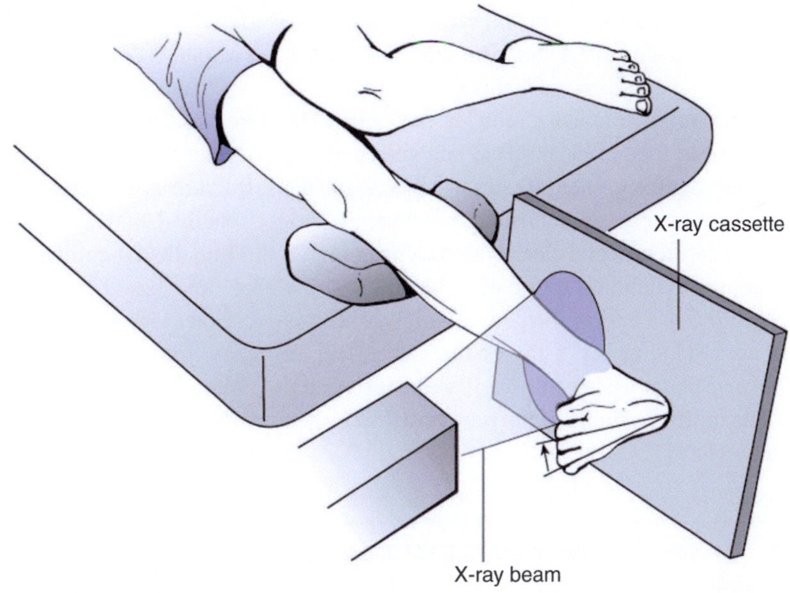

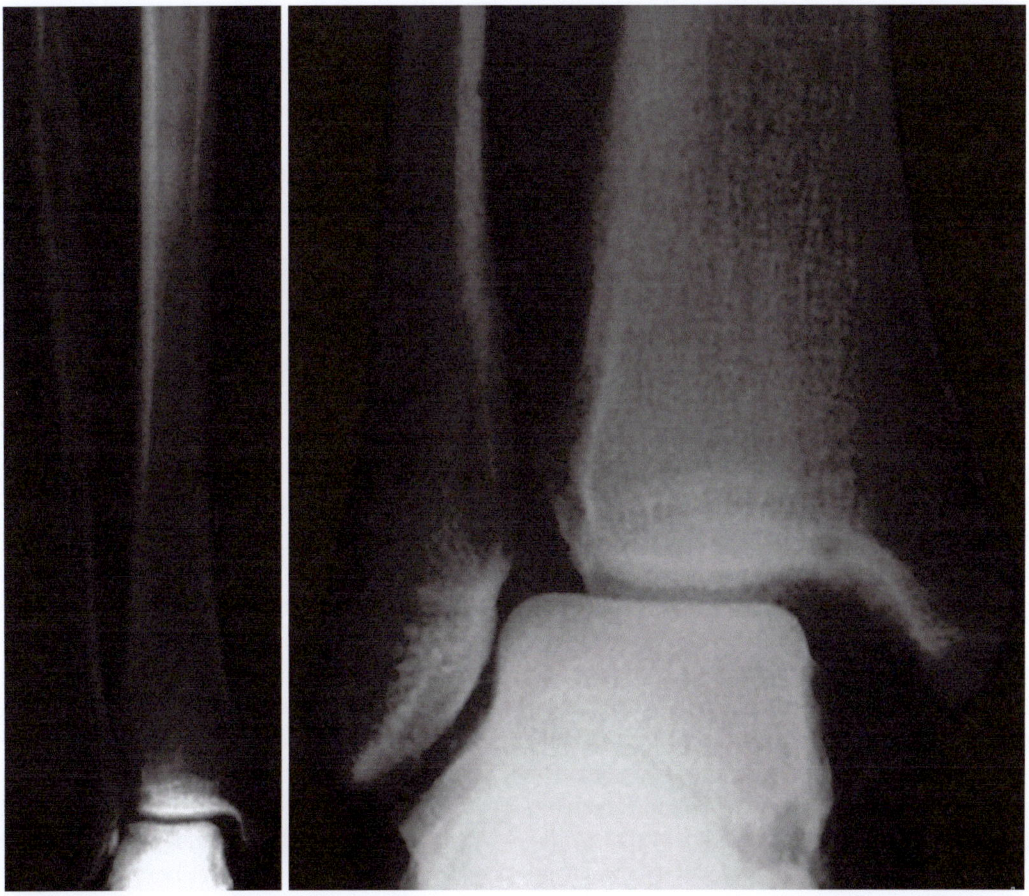

Fig. 3 Stress radiographs demonstrating syndesmotic injury with medial clear space widening. (Courtesy Rockwood and Green's fractures in adults)

view should be congruent and symmetrical all the way around the talar dome from medial to lateral. Any increase or decrease in this space is indicative of subluxation or dislocation of the talus. The increase in medial clear space is a surrogate for deltoid ligament integrity and stability of the ankle. Despite these published numbers, no specific cutoff for medial clear space has been shown to equate to deltoid rupture on ankle arthroscopy [11]. Another option for determining stability is to do a standing AP x-ray of the ankle with an isolated fibula fracture to see if widening occurs of the mortise, similar to the previously described stress tests [12].

3   Lateral Malleolar Fractures

A true isolated lateral malleolar fracture that is associated with a stable mortise will heal without significant functional consequence and can be treated conservatively. These fractures do not result in tibiotalar incongruence or abnormal ankle kinematics, even if there is some degree of minor deltoid ligament injury [13] Bauer et al. reported 98% of patients with supination external rotation (SER) stage 2 ankle fractures showed no evidence of OA at 30 years and studies by Kristensen and Hanson corroborate this with 95% of patients reporting good functional outcomes at 21 years [14]. Management of true isolated lateral malleolar fractures focuses on allowing rapid return to mobilization and normal function. Elastic bandaging, air stirrup devices, and walking boots have all been shown to be well tolerated. No significant differences have been found between these options beyond 3 months post injury [15, 16]. Some minor radiographic displacement of lateral malleolar fractures does not impair clinical outcomes [17]. In the setting of a truly isolated lateral malleolus fracture, we prefer air stirrups as patient tolerance is high, ankle motion is encouraged, and they allow for removal for evaluation of skin in more vulnerable patients. Immediate weightbearing of stable injuries is permissible and our protocol is to wean the immobilization device by around 4 weeks post-injury. We do not routinely recommend physical

therapy unless a range of motion or gait deficit is present.

While a true isolated lateral malleolus may be treated conservatively, disruption of the deltoid ligament in association with a lateral malleolus fracture is associated with instability and functionally behaves as a bimalleolar ankle fracture ("bimalleolar equivalent"). This situation may be obvious based on significant deformity or dislocation on the initial presentation. Other times, it may not be immediately obvious, if there is no significant displacement on the initial injury films. Assessment of the integrity of the deltoid is both clinical and radiographic. Clinical signs include medial swelling, bruising, and tenderness. In addition to clinical signs, a "walking test", in which there is no talar shift following a week of ambulation, proves stability [18]. It is the author's preferred method for an apparent isolated lateral malleolus fracture to radiographically stress the ankle (manual or gravity) and make an operative decision based on the results. MRI studies are not routinely obtained. In a small study of 21 patients, Koval followed patients suspected of having a medial sided injury in addition to a lateral malleolar fracture [18]. They underwent manual stress views and were shown to have 5 to 8 mm of medial clear space. All patients underwent MRI and were shown to have superficial deltoid rupture, though only 2 had a concomitant deep deltoid rupture, the remaining 19 had partial deep deltoid injuries. The 19 without complete deep deltoid injuries underwent conservative management with full weightbearing in a boot and each went on to make a complete recovery. This information suggests that functional instability cannot be gauged simply from clinical or radiographic measurements and the integrity of the deep deltoid may be paramount in determining stability. The treatment algorithm for treating these fractures hinges on determining whether the medial structures remain truly stable. Lateral malleolus fractures that are associated with an unstable mortise allow for talar shift, which has functional implications. While a stable lateral malleolus fracture can be treated nonoperatively, the addition of a complete deltoid injury demands operative consideration and may initially be difficult to diagnose without obvious displacement on initial plain radiographs.

In contrast to the above, the progression to a lateral malleolar fracture with syndesmotic disruption, a complete deltoid injury, or a combination of the two portends a worse prognosis with conservative care if unrecognized as it allows for talar tilt, talar shift and altered ankle mechanics. Distal fibular injuries with involvement of the syndesmosis result in lower functional, SMFA and AOFAS, and higher pain scores than those without. The only significant predictor of outcomes found in a syndesmotic injury is the adequacy of the reduction of the syndesmosis. Malreduction of the syndesmosis leads to lower SMFA scores [19]. The generally accepted fixation of the syndesmosis involves screw placement approximately 2 cm above the tibiotalar joint line, without violating the cartilage of the syndesmosis, as this balances proximity and syndesmotic cartilage violation and there is evidence that screw placement closer to the syndesmosis leads to less widening. There are a wide variety of syndesmotic fixation methods which can be employed during fixation of a lateral malleolus fracture. Further discussion of syndesmotic injury, reduction methods and fixation techniques can be found in chapter "Management of Bimalleolar Ankle Fractures".

4 Lateral Malleolus Fixation

The approach and fixation for isolated distal fibula fractures may be carried out either with a posterior anti-glide or lateral plate fixation utilizing lag screws and neutralization plating techniques [20]. Depending on the fibula fracture morphology and location, plating has expanded to include buttress, bridge, and compression techniques with a myriad of plate designs based on fracture pattern. Considerations with any of these techniques is limited by the soft tissue envelope of the ankle, with rates of infection and wound dehiscence between 5 and 26% [21, 22]. Risks of the lateral approach to the distal fibula include the superficial peroneal nerve and fixation distally is often limited to only unicortical screws. To avoid the issues associated with lateral plating, Weber described posterior buttress plating for fractures with the typical postero-superior to anteroinferior obliquity. Posterior to anterior screws in this plate placement affords the added benefit of bicortical screws and lack of risk of intraarticular penetration or peroneal tendon irritation. With posterior plate placement and a posterior to anterior screw just proximal to the apex of the fracture, this buttress plate performs as an antiglide mechanism to protect against fracture displacement with any further external rotation [23]. Sometimes this mechanical construct can be used even without screws distal to the fracture, but it is advisable to obtain at least one if possible. Typically, a 1/3 tubular plate is used for this purpose and a lag screw can be placed through the plate from posterior to anterior if desired. There is a larger soft tissue envelope over the plate in this location and the posterior antiglide plate has been shown to be biomechanically stronger, however a tradeoff is the risk of peroneal tendon irritation distally (Fig. 4, [24–26]). Peroneal tendon irritation was associated with low plate placement and protruding screws in the distal hole and some have recommended that the most distal screw hole be left empty, when able, and that hardware be removed early but careful plate and screw placement can avoid these issues [26]. In patients with vulnerable soft tissues, minimally invasive techniques such as MIPO plating, may be of benefit, though these techniques prove to be quite challenging with potentially high rates of nonunion (Fig. 5) [27].

In poor quality bone, increasing the number of total screws and utilization of multiple locking screws may be necessary. Like other fractures and anatomic locations, locking plates and screws afford the benefit of increased pullout strength with the possible tradeoff of increased wound complications documented at the fibula [22]. In addition, the use of multiple trans-syndesmotic screws may be beneficial in osteoporotic and diabetic ankle fractures [28]. Intramedullary nail and screw fixation may also have a role in certain lateral malleoli fracture morphologies without a need for syndesmotic fixation. In these cases, a variety of fibular intramedullary fixation devices can be employed, ranging from specifically designed fibular intramedullary nails to screw fixation (Figs. 6 and 7). Fibular nails have been shown to have equal outcomes to lateral plating

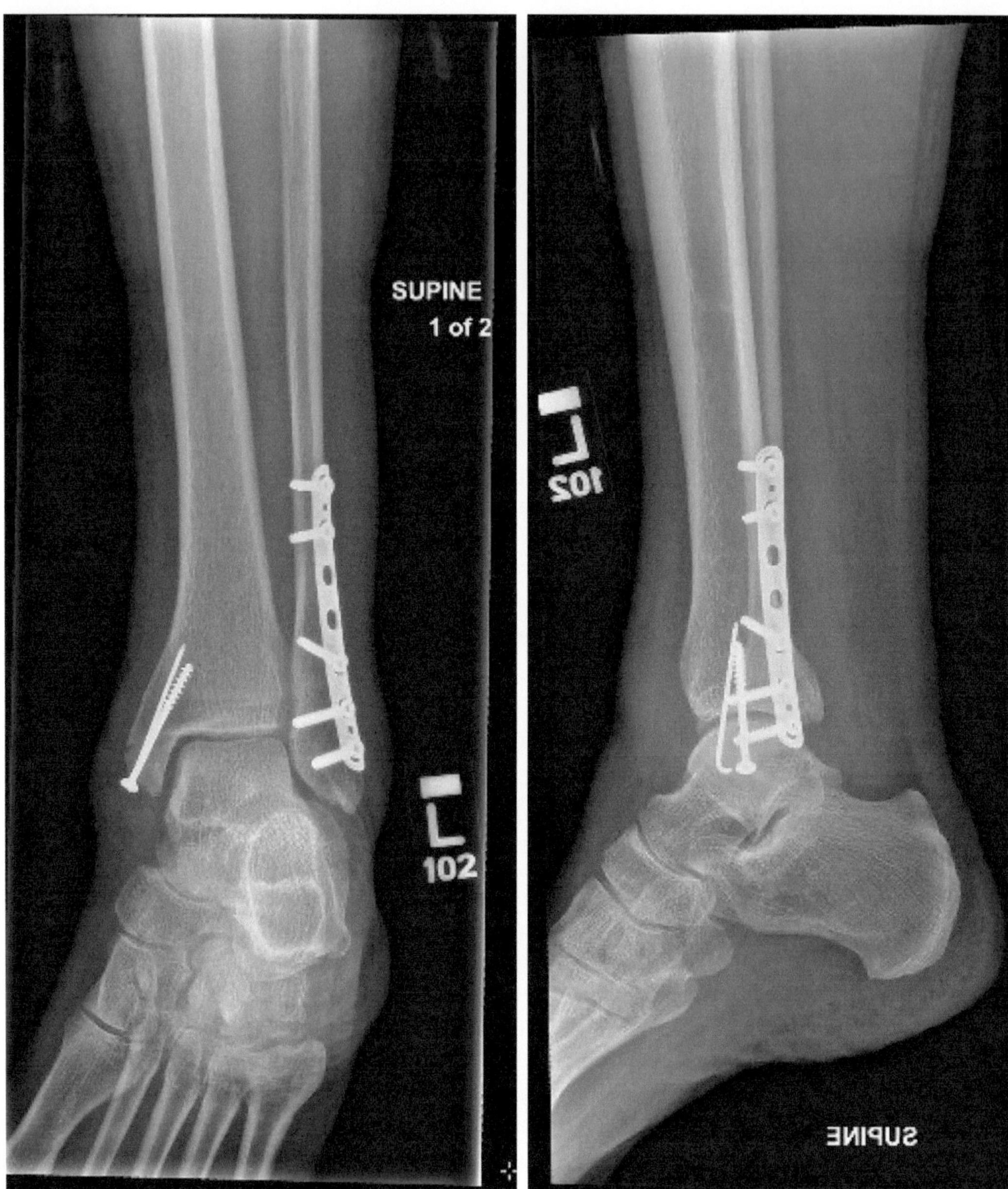

Fig. 4 Antiglide plating of the distal fibula. (Courtesy Dr. Robert F. Ostrum)

patients in one prospective randomized trial, though this only included a total of 125 patients with a variety of "unstable ankle fractures" [29].

In addressing the syndesmosis, anatomic reduction is important and malreduction remains high, with some studies reporting up to 50% malreduction rate [30]. Malreduction secondary to off-axis clamping has been cited as a potential cause. In a study of ideal clamp position for accurate syndesmotic fixation it has been shown that the medial tine should be placed in the anterior third of the tibia on the lateral view to reduce syndesmotic malreduction. Care should be taken not to over-compress if electing to clamp the syndesmosis as this may lead to malreduction [30]. Firmly reducing the fibula into the tibial incisura

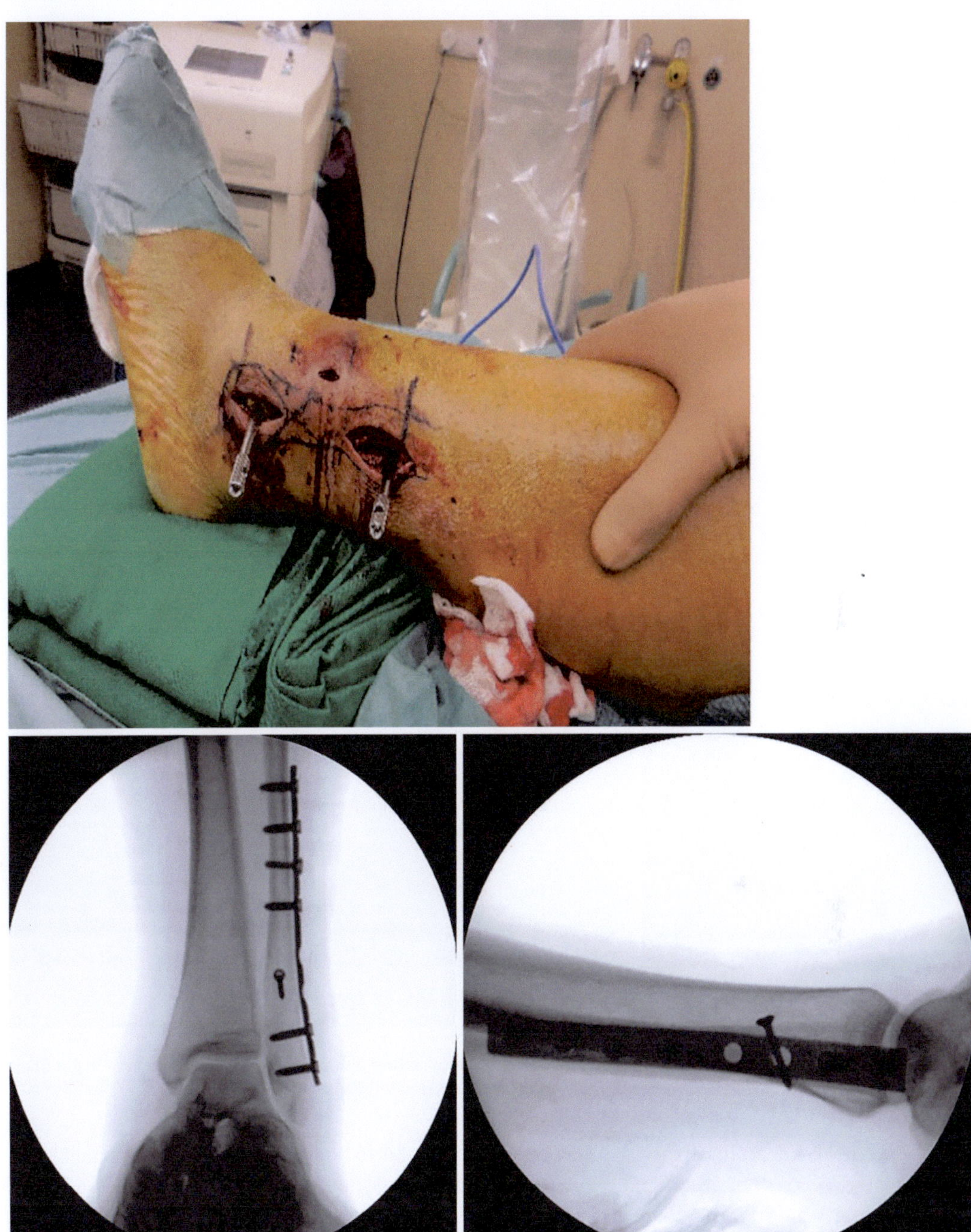

Fig. 5 Distal fibula fracture intraoperative photos and radiographs demonstrating two incision minimally invasive plate osteosynthesis. (Hess F, Sommer C. Minimally invasive plate osteosynthesis of the distal fibula with the locking compression plate: First experience of 20 cases. J Orthop Trauma. 2011;25 (2):110–115)

with the grip of the surgeon's hand is safer. When examining for accurate reduction, Tornetta et al. demonstrated that visualizing the articular surface at the lateral shoulder of the mortise through a small incision is a more reliable method for assessing reduction when compared to looking at

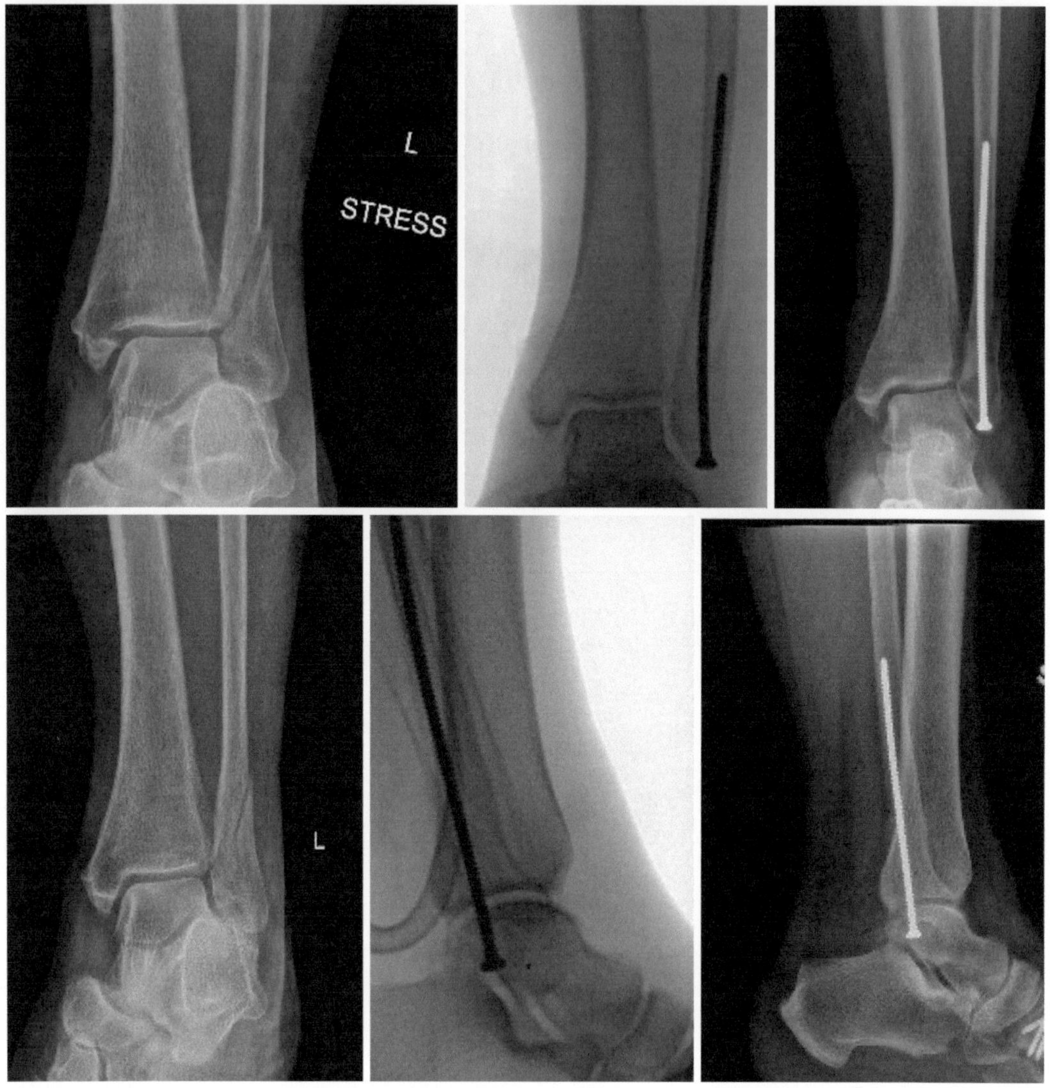

Fig. 6 Injury, intraoperative, and postoperative radiographs demonsrating intramedullary screw fixation of distal fibula fixation with long 3.5 mm screw. (Courtesy of Dr. Andrew T. Chen)

the incisura [31]. Regarding fixation, it has been shown that two 3.5 mm tricortical screws are equivalent at 1 year with quadricortical 4.5 mm screws in terms of function, pain, and dorsiflexion [32]. The tricortical screws may not need to be removed if they loosen or break allowing for more normal ankle motion. There has been increasing literature on bioabsorbable screws which have shown good to excellent results thus far, but data remains limited. Suture button fixation has been shown to have similar or better functional scores and faster return to work when compared to screw fixation in some small studies, though many outcome score differences did not reach statistical significance and complication rates have been shown to be as high as 25% [33, 34]. Syndesmotic fixation with the TightRope device (Arthrex Inc., Naples, FL) was shown to have a malreduction rate half of that of two 3.5 mm screws in a small randomized controlled trial (Fig. 7) [33]. While early results are encouraging, larger and higher quality studies are still lacking regarding suture fixation for syndesmotic injury.

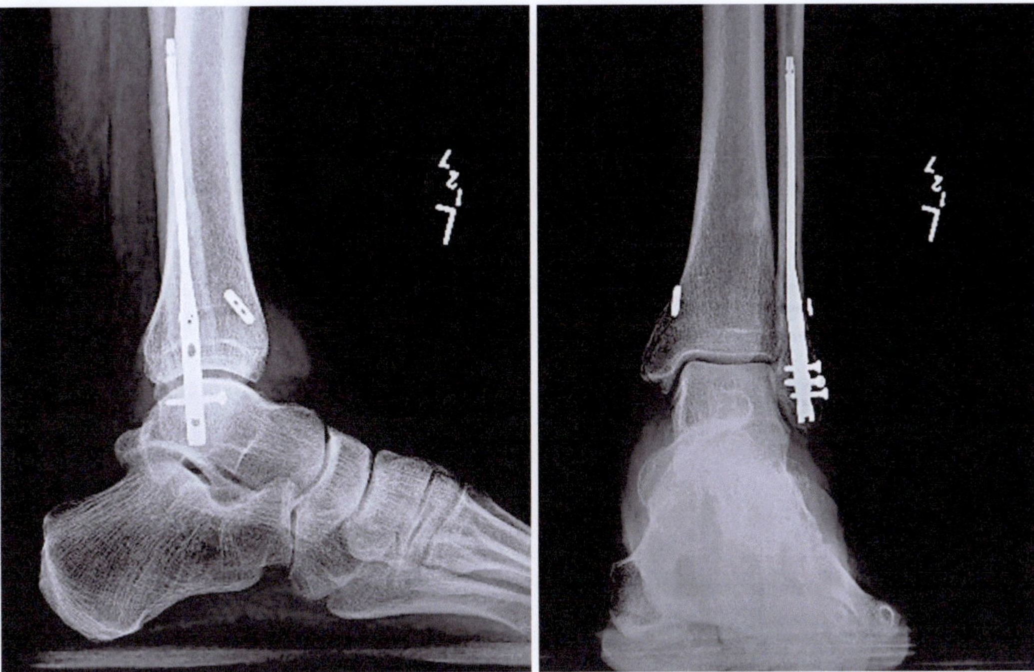

Fig. 7 Postoperative radiograph of distal fibula fracture with syndesmotic injury repaired with intramedullary nail device as well as suture button sydesmotic fixation. (Courtesy Dr. Trapper A Lalli)

5 Medial Malleolar Fractures

Truly isolated medial malleolar fractures may be adequately treated nonoperatively if they do not involve the weight bearing surface. It is important to recognize the complex anatomy of the deltoid ligament and its significance in medial malleolar fractures. The deltoid has two components: the superficial deltoid arising from the anterior colliculus and deep deltoid from posterior colliculus. The deep deltoid is critical in preventing lateral displacement of talus in the setting of medial malleolar fractures and, if intact, may allow for adequate nonoperative treatment. Herscovici et al. reviewed functional and radiographic outcomes of 57 patients with an isolated medial malleolus who were immobilized with a below knee non-weightbearing cast for 6 weeks followed by progressive weightbearing and PT [35]. Despite many fractures showing displacement, even up to 6 mm, only two went on to progress to nonunion and no patient demonstrated development of osteoarthritis (OA) or displace-

ment of the mortise. An important consideration in the evaluation and treatment of the medial malleolus is the location of the fracture. Tornetta et al. reported that anterior colliculi fractures found on plain X-ray fared better with conservative than operative management, suggesting that anterior colliculus fracture is a radiographic surrogate for fractures with only superficial and not deep deltoid involvement [36]. Fractures which exit through the plafond into the tibiotalar joint may benefit from operative fixation, particularly if there is displacement and articular step-off.

6 Medial Malleolus Fixation

Fixation of the medial malleolus depends primarily on the size of the fragment. Screw fixation, tension band wiring, and plate fixation have all been described . The most commonly used technique is cancellous lag screw fixation, which can be augmented with washers in comminuted or soft bone. Two parallel screws, one screw plus one K wire in very small fragments, are typically used to allow for rotational control, though single screws have also been shown to be effective [37]. In a study comparing two partially threaded 4.0 cannulated screws to two fully threaded bicortical 3.5 mm screws for medial malleolar fixation, the 3.5 mm bicortical screws demonstrated statistically significantly greater pullout strength [38]. In a study of one versus two screws by Buckley et al., single screw fixation demonstrated no difference in operating room time, SF36, or Ankle Hindfoot Scale at all follow-up time points [39]. Implant cost also becomes a factor, with cannulated screws affording some perceived ease of use at a cost of approximately 12x that of solid screws. Screws inserted posterior to the anterior colliculus place the posterior tibial tendon at significant risk for injury or abutment [40]. For small fragments, tension band wiring (TBW) (Fig. 8) can achieve good compression and biomechanical studies have shown them to be stronger under tension than unicortical screws [41, 42]. Ostrum et al. reported on a cohort of 32 patients with TBW at 1 year follow-up in which

there were no cases of nonunion and only a single case of malunion [43]. Symptomatic hardware remains the greatest concern with this technique with rates of near 10% [44]. A specific pattern to recognize and treat is the vertical medial malleolar fracture of supination-adduction (SAD) injuries. This fixation must control the shear component of the forces acting on the medial malleolus and requires buttress plating of the medial malleolus. An under-contoured plate on the medial side can maintain reduction of the articular segment and prevent further shear, a key component of this construct is the anti-glide screw at the apex on the fragment, similar in function to the anti-glide plate on the posterior lateral malleolus (Fig. 9). These medial malleolar fractures need to be closely inspected for plafond impaction at the time of fixation and lag screws close to he joint should be used to compress the articular cartilage. Avoidance of intraarticular screw penetration depends on fluoroscopy collinear with the medial joint space on the AP image. The SAD pattern is discussed further in chapter "Management of Fractures of the Tibial Plafond".

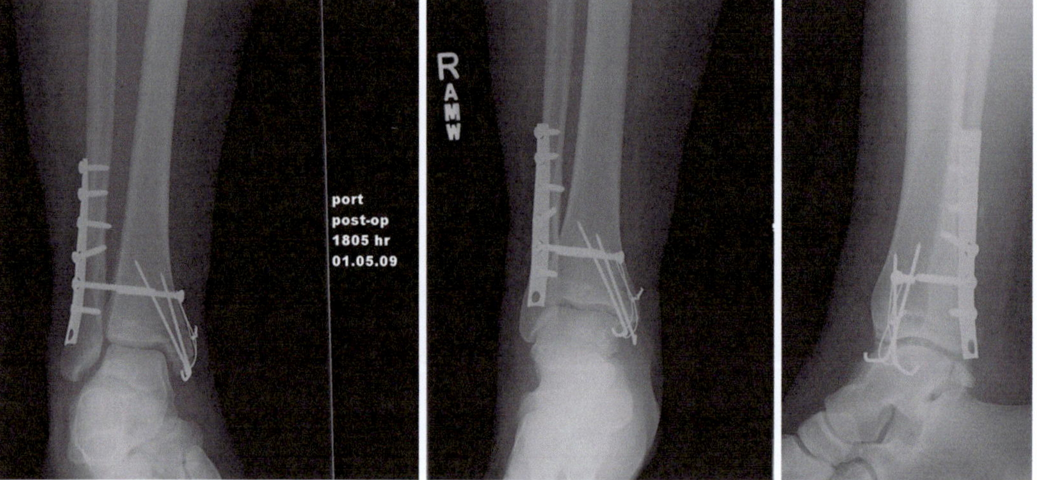

Fig. 8 Postoperative radiographs of bimalleolar ankle fracture dislocation with medial malleolus tension band wire fixation. (Courtesy Dr. Robert Ostrum)

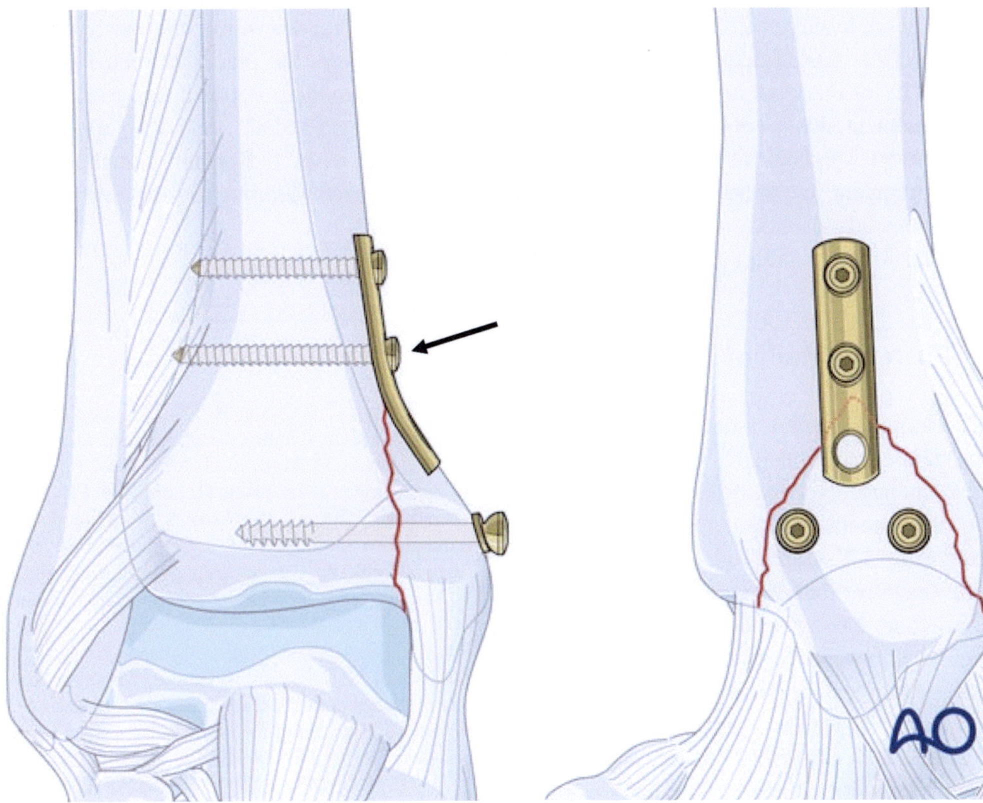

Fig. 9 Antiglide plating of vertical medial malleolus fracture with independent lag screw fixation. The most distal plate screw, or axilla screw (arrow), remains the most crucial to the function to the antiglide concept. (Courtesy AO Surgery reference)

7 Management of Isolated Posterior Malleolar Fracture

Management of posterior malleoli fractures has several controversial aspects. Posterior malleolus (PM) fracture as part of a trimalleolar fracture pattern is discussed in detail in the chapter "Trimalleolar Ankle Fractures". They can also be seen in conjunction with spiral fractures of the distal tibial shaft. An isolated posterior malleolus fracture is exceedingly rare. Two small studies, one involving 54 patients and the other involving approximately 300, have found poor outcomes in the short term; others have not found any predictive value in terms of functional outcome or late OA [45, 46]. One concern is the loss of the posterior malleolus as a stabilizing structure, leaving the ankle exposed to posterior tibiotalar sublux-

ation and a reduction in total contact area reduction. Cadaveric structures indicate that loss of up to 50% of the posterior malleolus does not correlate with significant posterior instability in the presence of maintained medial and lateral structures [47–49]. Some studies demonstrated better clinical and radiographic outcomes when patients with fractures involving >25% of the joint surface on plain films were addressed operatively, while others demonstrated no difference in reduction, union, complications, and late OA, though these were not isolated posterior malleolus fractures [50, 51]. An additional complicating factor is the ability to determine the size of the posterior malleolus fracture in the first place. It has been shown that estimating the true size of a posterior malleolar fragment is difficult on plain radiographs, and posterior malleolar fractures benefit from CT scan to assist in the decision-making process for possible surgery [52]. While it is frequently stated that those fractures which involve more than 25% of the joint surface benefit from operative treatment, this is not based on solid evidence and many surgeons use other factors in addition to fragment size to decide upon surgery. This is discussed in more detail in chapter "Trimalleolar Ankle Fractures".

8 Posterior Malleolus Fixation

While posterior malleolus fixation and surgical criterion remain controversial, in our practice, surgery is indicated for fractures which involve >25% of the articular surface apparent on lateral radiographs or CT scan. Additional considerations for operative fixation include syndesmotic injury, articular incongruence or impaction, or posterior talar instability. Surgical stabilization may consist of open (posterior) or percutaneous screw placement (anterior) after reduction, in many cases with posterior buttress plating. Reduction of posterior malleolus fractures should be anatomic as nonanatomic fractures have a high rate of OA [53]. A specific consideration is the posterior malleolus fracture in the setting of syndesmotic widening. Gardner et al. compared posterior malleolar fixation to syndesmotic screw fixation and found that PM fixation restored 70% of the pre-injury stiffness while syndesmotic screw fixation only restored 40% of that value [54]. The approach to, and fixation of, the posterior malleolus is dictated by fracture morphology. Screws and posterior buttress plate fixation have both been shown to have good outcomes, though little biomechanics evidence is available [55, 56]. Fractures which are amenable to percutaneous fixation are generally best stabilized by an anteromedial to posterolateral screw trajectory to ensure adequate capture of the fracture fragment in our hands, though posterior to anterior percutaneous screw fixation has also been described [57]. In further displaced or impacted fractures which require open reduction, both a posteromedial and posterolateral approach can be utilized. The posteromedial approach makes use of the plane between the flexor hallicus longus (FHL) and the

neurovascular bundle while the posterolateral approach employs the plane between FHL and the peroneal tendons. While it has been shown that the posteromedial approach allows for greater exposure of the posterior malleolus, it does so with increased risk to the neurovascular structures [55].

References

1. Court-Brown CM, Caesar B. Epidemiology of adult fractures: a review. Injury. 2006;37(8):691–7.
2. Court-Brown CM, McBirnie J. Adult ankle fractures-an increasing problem? Acta Orthop. 1998;69:43–7.
3. Kannus P, Palvanen M, Niemi S, et al. Increasing number and incidence of low-trauma ankle fractures in elderly people: Finnish statistics during 1970–2000 and projections for the future. Bone. 2002;31(3):430–3.
4. Putnam SM, Linn MS, Spraggs-Hughes A, McAndrew CM, Ricci WM, Gardner MJ. Simulating clamp placement across the trans-syndesmotic angle of the ankle to minimize malreduction: a radiological study. Injury. 2017;48(3):770–5. Epub 2017 Jan 13. PMID: 28131483; PMCID: PMC5478166. https://doi.org/10.1016/j.injury.2017.01.029.
5. Lambert KL. The weight-bearing function of the fibula. A strain gauge study. J Bone Joint Surg Am. 1971;53(3):507–13.
6. Takebe K, Nakagawa A, Minami H, et al. Role of the fibula in weight-bearing. Clin Orthop Relat Res. 1984;184:289–92.
7. DeAngelis NA, Eskander MS, French BG. Does medial tenderness predict deep deltoid ligament incompetence in supination-external rotation type ankle fractures? J Orthop Trauma. 2007;21(4):244–7.
8. Stiell IG, Greenberg GH, McKnight RD, Nair RC, McDowell I, Reardon M, Stewart JP, Maloney J. Decision rules for the use of radiography in acute ankle injuries. Refinement and prospective validation. JAMA. 1993;269(9):1127–32. PMID: 8433468. https://doi.org/10.1001/jama.269.9.1127.
9. Egol KA, Amirtharajah M, Amirtharage M, et al. Ankle stress test for predicting the need for surgical fixation of isolated fibular fractures. J Bone Joint Surg Am. 2004;86-A(11):2393–8.
10. Aiyer AA, Zachwieja EC, Lawrie CM, Kaplan JRM. Management of isolated lateral malleolus fractures. J Am Acad Orthop Surg. 2019;27(2):50–9. PMID: 30278012. https://doi.org/10.5435/JAAOS-D-17-00417.
11. Schuberth JM, Collman DR, Rush SM, et al. Deltoid ligament integrity in lateral malleolar fractures: a comparative analysis of arthroscopic and radiographic assessments. J Foot Ankle Surg. 2004;43(1):20–9.

12. Bonness EK, Siebler JC, Reed LK, Lyden ER, Mormino MA. Immediate weight-bearing protocol for the determination of ankle stability in patients with isolated distal fibular fractures. J Orthop Trauma. 2018;32(10):534–7.

13. Michelson JD, Waldman B. An axially loaded model of the ankle after pronation external rotation injury. Clin Orthop Relat Res. 1996;328:285–93.

14. Bauer M, Jonsson K, Nilsson B. Thirty-year follow-up of ankle fractures. Acta Orthop Scand. 1985;56(2):103–6.

15. Stuart PR, Brumby C, Smith SR. Comparative study of functional bracing and plaster cast treatment of stable lateral malleolar fractures. Injury. 1989;20(6):323–6.

16. Port AM, McVie JL, Naylor G, et al. Comparison of two conservative methods of treating an isolated fracture of the lateral malleolus. J Bone Joint Surg Br. 1996;78(4):568–72.

17. Yde J, Kristensen KD. Ankle fractures. Supination-eversion fractures stage II. Primary and late results of operative and non-operative treatment. Acta Orthop Scand. 1980;51(4):695–702.

18. Koval KJ, Egol KA, Cheung Y, et al. Does a positive ankle stress test indicate the need for operative treatment after lateral malleolus fracture? A preliminary report. J Orthop Trauma. 2007;21(7):449–55.

19. Sagi HC, Shah AR, Sanders RW. The functional consequence of syndesmotic joint malreduction at a minimum 2-year follow-up. J Orthop Trauma. 2012;26(7):439–43. PMID: 22357084. https://doi.org/10.1097/BOT.0b013e31822a526a.

20. Schaffer JJ, Manoli A 2nd. The antiglide plate for distal fibular fixation. A biomechanical comparison with fixation with a lateral plate. J Bone Joint Surg Am. 1987;69(4):596–604. PMID: 3571317.

21. Monga P, Kumar A, Simons A, et al. Management of distal tibio-fibular syndesmotic injuries: a snapshot of current practice. Acta Orthop Belg. 2008;74(3):365–9.

22. Schepers T, Lieshout EMMV, Vries MRD, et al. Increased rates of wound complications with locking plates in distal fibular fractures. Injury. 2011;42(10):1125–9.

23. Brunner CF, Weber BG. The Antiglide plate. New York: Special Techniques in Internal Fixation; 1982. p. 115–33.

24. Ostrum RF. Posterior plating of displaced Weber B fibula fractures. J Orthop Trauma. 1996;10(3):199–203.

25. Redfern DJ, Sauvé PS, Sakellariou A. Investigation of incidence of superficial peroneal nerve injury following ankle fracture. Foot Ankle Int. 2003;24(10):771–4.

26. Weber M, Krause F. Peroneal tendon lesions caused by antiglide plates used for fixation of lateral malleolar fractures: the effect of plate and screw position. Foot Ankle Int. 2005;26(4):281–5.

27. Hess F, Sommer C. Minimally invasive plate osteosynthesis of the distal fibula with the locking compression plate: first experience of 20 cases. J Orthop Trauma. 2011;25(2):110–5.

28. Dunn WR, Easley ME, Parks BG, Trnka HJ, Schon LC. An augmented fixation method for distal fibular fractures in elderly patients: a biomechanical evaluation. Foot Ankle Int. 2004;25(3):128–31.

29. White TO, Bugler KE, Olsen L, Lundholm LH, Holck K, Madsen BL, Duckworth AD. A prospective, randomized, controlled, two-center, internationalq trial comparing the fibular nail with open reduction and internal fixation for unstable ankle fractures in younger patients. J Orthop Trauma. 2022;36(1):36–42.

30. Cosgrove CT, Putnam SM, Cherney SM, Ricci WM, Spraggs-Hughes A, McAndrew CM, Gardner MJ. Medial clamp tine positioning affects ankle syndesmosis malreduction. J Orthop Trauma. 2017;31(8):440–6. PMID: 28471914; PMCID: PMC5539925. https://doi.org/10.1097/BOT.0000000000000882.

31. Tornetta P 3rd, Yakavonis M, Veltre D, Shah A. Reducing the syndesmosis under direct vision: where should I look? J Orthop Trauma. 2019;33(9):450–4. PMID: 31259801. https://doi.org/10.1097/BOT.0000000000001552.

32. Høiness P, Strømsøe K. Tricortical versus quadricortical syndesmosis fixation in ankle fractures: a prospective, randomized study comparing two methods of syndesmosis fixation. J Orthop Trauma. 2004;18(6):331–7.

33. Sanders D, Schneider P, Taylor M, Tieszer C, Lawendy AR, Canadian Orthopaedic Trauma Society. Improved reduction of the tibiofibular syndesmosis with TightRope compared with screw fixation: results of a randomized controlled study. J Orthop Trauma. 2019;33(11):531–7. PMID: 31633643. https://doi.org/10.1097/BOT.0000000000001559.

34. Zhang P, et al. BMC musculoskeletal disorders 18, article 286, 2017; and Kortekangas T et al Injury. 2015;46(6):1119–26.

35. Herscovici D, Scaduto JM, Infante A. Conservative treatment of isolated fractures of the medial malleolus. J Bone Joint Surg Br. 2007;89(1):89–93.

36. Tornetta P 3rd. Competence of the deltoid ligament in bimalleolar ankle fractures after medial malleolar fixation. J Bone Joint Surg Am. 2000;82(6):843–8.

37. Ricci WM, Tornetta P, Borrelli J. Lag screw fixation of medial malleolar fractures: a biomechanical, radiographic, and clinical comparison of unicortical partially threaded lag screws and bicortical fully threaded lag screws. J Orthop Trauma. 2012;26(10):602–6.

38. Pollard JD, Deyhim A, Rigby RB, Dau N, King C, Fallat LM, Bir C. Comparison of pullout strength between 3.5-mm fully threaded, bicortical screws and 4.0-mm partially threaded, cancellous screws in the fixation of medial malleolar fractures. J Foot Ankle Surg. 2010;49(3):248–52. Epub 2010 Apr 2. PMID: 20362467. https://doi.org/10.1053/j.jfas.2010.02.006.

39. Buckley R, Kwek E, Duffy P, Korley R, Puloski S, Buckley A, Martin R, Rydberg Moller E, Schneider P. Single-screw fixation compared with double screw fixation for treatment of medial malleolar fractures: a prospective randomized trial. J Orthop Trauma. 2018;32(11):548–53. PMID: 30211788. https://doi.org/10.1097/BOT.0000000000001311.

40. Femino JE, Gruber BF, Karunakar MA. Safe zone for the placement of medial malleolar screws. J Bone Joint Surg Am. 2007;89(1):133–8. PMID: 17200320. https://doi.org/10.2106/JBJS.F.00689.

41. Fowler TT, Pugh KJ, Litsky AS, et al. Medial malleolar fractures: a biomechanical study of fixation techniques. Orthopedics. 2011;34(8):e349–55.

42. Johnson BA, Fallat LM. Comparison of tension band wire and cancellous bone screw fixation for medial malleolar fractures. J Foot Ankle Surg. 1997;36(4):284–9.

43. Ostrum RF, Litsky AS. Tension band fixation of medial malleolus fractures. J Orthop Trauma. 1992;6(4):464–8.

44. Cleak DK, Dawson MH, Phoenix OF. Tension band wiring of avulsion fractures of the medial malleolus: a modified technique minimizing soft tissue injury. Injury. 1982;13(6):519–20.

45. Lübbeke A, Salvo D, Stern R, et al. Risk factors for post-traumatic osteoarthritis of the ankle: an eighteen year follow-up study. Int Orthop. 2012;36(7):1403–10.

46. Tejwani NC, Pahk B, Egol KA. Effect of posterior malleolus fracture on outcome after unstable ankle fracture. J Trauma. 2010;69(3):666–9.

47. Fitzpatrick DC, Otto JK, McKinley TO, et al. Kinematic and contact stress analysis of posterior malleolus fractures of the ankle. J Orthop Trauma. 2004;18(5):271–8.

48. Harper MC. Posterior instability of the talus: an anatomic evaluation. Foot Ankle. 1989;10(1):36–9.

49. Raasch WG, Larkin JJ, Draganich LF. Assessment of the posterior malleolus as a restraint to posterior subluxation of the ankle. J Bone Joint Surg Am. 1992;74(8):1201–6.

50. Harper MC, Hardin G. Posterior malleolar fractures of the ankle associated with external rotation abduction injuries. Results with and without internal fixation. J Bone Joint Surg Am. 1988;70(9):1348–56.

51. McDaniel WJ, Wilson FC. Trimalleolar fractures of the ankle. An end result study. Clin Orthop Relat Res. 1977;122:37–45.

52. Haraguchi N, Haruyama H, Toga H, et al. Pathoanatomy of posterior malleolar fractures of the ankle. J Bone Joint Surg Am. 2006;88(5):1085–92.

53. Jaskulka RA, Ittner G, Schedl R. Fractures of the posterior tibial margin: their role in the prognosis of malleolar fractures. J Trauma. 1989;29(11):1565–70.

54. Gardner MJ, Brodsky A, Briggs SM, Nielson JH, Lorich DG. Fixation of posterior malleolar fractures provides greater syndesmotic stability. Clin Orthop Relat Res. 2006;447:165–71. PMID: 16467626.

55. Bois AJ, Dust W. Posterior fracture dislocation of the ankle: technique and clinical experience using a posteromedial surgical approach. J Orthop Trauma. 2008;22(9):629–36.

56. Tornetta P, Ricci W, Nork S, et al. The posterolateral approach to the tibia for displaced posterior malleolar injuries. J Orthop Trauma. 2011;25(2):123–6.

57. O'Connor TJ, Mueller B, Ly TV, Jacobson AR, Nelson ER, Cole PA. "A top" screw versus posterolateral plate for posterior malleolus fixation in trimalleolar ankle fractures. J Orthop Trauma. 2015;29(4):151.

Management of Bimalleolar Ankle Fractures

Amy Ford and Brian Mullis

1 Introduction

Bimalleolar ankle fractures are common musculoskeletal injuries that may emerge in a variety of different settings. While they may present similarly to unimalleolar injuries, they pose a greater threat to a patient's function than an unstable unimalleolar ankle fracture [1, 2]. As described in an earlier chapter, these injuries may result from direct or indirect trauma to the ankle, but most often they are the consequence of rotational or twisting mechanisms. Instability of the ankle joint causes translation of the talus and leads to marked changes in the biomechanics of the ankle [3]. Ultimately, the goal of treatment is to restore congruency between the talus and the mortise and to maintain this alignment during healing. This chapter will delve into the evaluation and treatment, both operatively and nonoperatively, of bimalleolar ankle fractures.

A. Ford (✉)
Orthopedics Northwest, Yakima, WA, USA

B. Mullis
Department of Orthopaedics, Indiana University, Bloomington, IN, USA
e-mail: bmullis@iu.edu

2 Evaluation-Physical Examination

As with any musculoskeletal injury, it is important to conduct a careful neurovascular examination as one of the initial steps in the evaluation of the patient. While neurovascular injuries are not common in the presentation of bimalleolar ankle fractures, it is important to note any abnormalities for comparison preoperatively and postoperatively (as well as before and after splinting). Additionally, the finding of baseline peripheral neuropathy on the initial examination may alter the surgeon's preoperative plan and expected postoperative protocol. More detail on the management of diabetic ankle fractures and the Charcot ankle may be found in Part IV: Chapters "Management of Acute Diabetic Ankle Fractures" and "The Neuropathic (Charcot) Ankle".

The most important determinant in the acute management of the bimalleolar ankle fracture is the soft tissue examination. Even unremarkable bony injuries may present with rapid swelling or fracture blisters that may affect the placement of surgical incisions or delay the timing of the procedure itself. Widely displaced fractures or dislocations are prone to open wounds or skin necrosis, which reflect the magnitude of injury. These complications may be exacerbated if the ankle is left unreduced long enough to compromise the vascularity of the surrounding soft tissue envelope and, depending on the degree of displacement, this can happen within hours. The state of the soft tissues is one of the most critical factors in deciding not only the urgency of a reduction or operation, but also the ankle's readiness for a surgical procedure. Skin than is blanched, tented or taut may have compromised vascularity, and should prompt a swift closed reduction in the acute setting, while an open wound would indicate the need for early antibiotic therapy and relatively urgent surgical intervention. In the closed fracture, excessive swelling at the time of surgery would increase the possibility of difficulty with wound closure and the resulting postoperative wound complications. The provider should evaluate the appearance of the skin (contused or abraded, tense or shiny, blanched or dusky, blistering), palpate for tension, mobility, skin wrinkling with gentle pinching around the surgical site before proceeding to the operating room for definitive fixation.

3 Evaluation-Studies

On the basis of history and physical examination, the physician may decide to order radiographs. The Ottawa ankle rules are used as standard of care for primary and emergency medicine providers to guide the ordering of diagnostic radiographs in patients presenting with ankle pain, in order to avoid unnecessary X-rays. These rules recommend radiographs when patients have pain and tenderness to palpation along the posterior border or tip of either malleolus or inability to bear weight for four steps, either at the time of injury or in the emergency department [4]. The first studies to order in the evaluation of bimalleolar ankle fractures are standard ankle radiographs: anteroposterior (AP), mortise, and lateral views. If there is an obvious deformity, a provisional reduction may be performed prior to imaging; however, it may be helpful to obtain radiographs first in order to identify the injury and be fully prepared for the reduction. In the instance of skin tenting or vascular compromise, a reduction maneuver should be performed without delay.

Standard radiographic parameters of normal ankles, as discussed earlier in chapter "Radiologic Imaging of the Ankle", should be assessed for disruption. Change in the talocrural angle (Fig. 1) or loss of parallelism of the lateral talus with the fibula may result from fibular shortening. Incongruity of the ankle mortise, talar tilt, or wid-

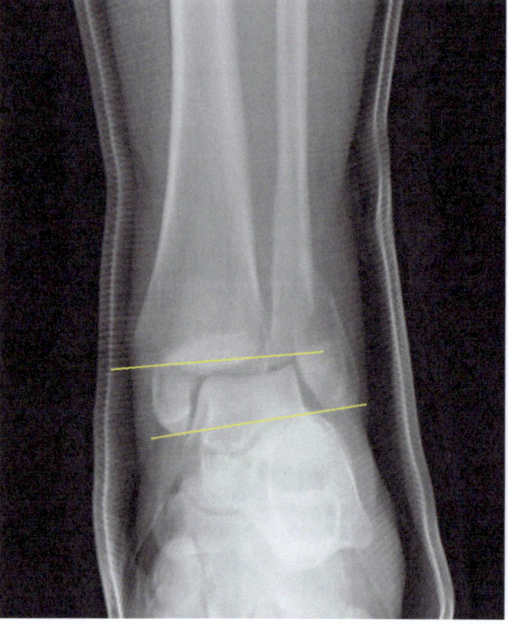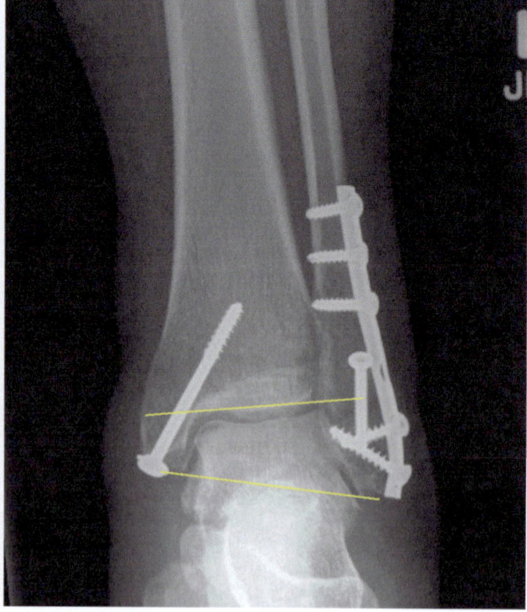

Fig. 1 Restoration of talocrural angle after ORIF. Talocrural angle is assessed with one line parallel to the tibial plafond and one line between the tips of each malleoli. Population normal range is 79–87°

ening of the medial ankle clear space (Fig. 2) are all indicators of displacement and instability. In addition to assessing for tibiotalar instability, providers should also look for syndesmotic instability. Classically, the relationship between the tibia and the fibula at the ankle is assessed radiographically by examining the tibiofibular overlap and the tibiofibular clear space (Fig. 3), although these may be difficult to evaluate in the setting of a displaced fracture. If these are not obviously disrupted, a stress exam should be performed after surgical fixation of the ankle. This will be further discussed later in this chapter.

Computed tomography (CT) scans, while not needed routinely, may be desired when the bimalleolar ankle fracture includes a posterior malleolus fragment, or when the fracture fragments appear complex or are not fully understood on radiographs. A CT scan may elucidate the orientation of fracture lines and dictate the necessary operative approach for fracture fixation. In ankle fractures with marginal impaction

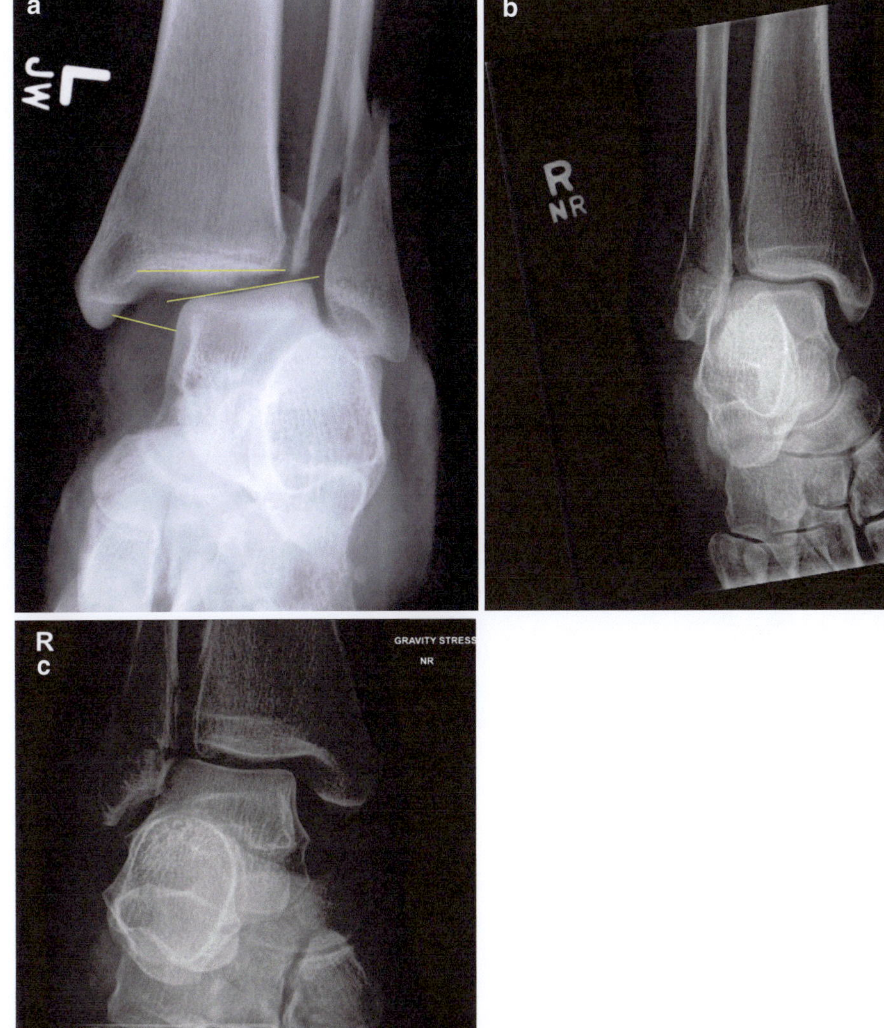

Fig. 2 Medial clear space widening and talar tilt as indicators of ankle instability. (**a**) shows obvious widening of the medial clear space and tilt of the talus relative to the plafond on injury films. (**b** and **c**) show a more subtle medial widening which increases on gravity stress testing. Radiographs courtesy of Jan Szatkowski, MD

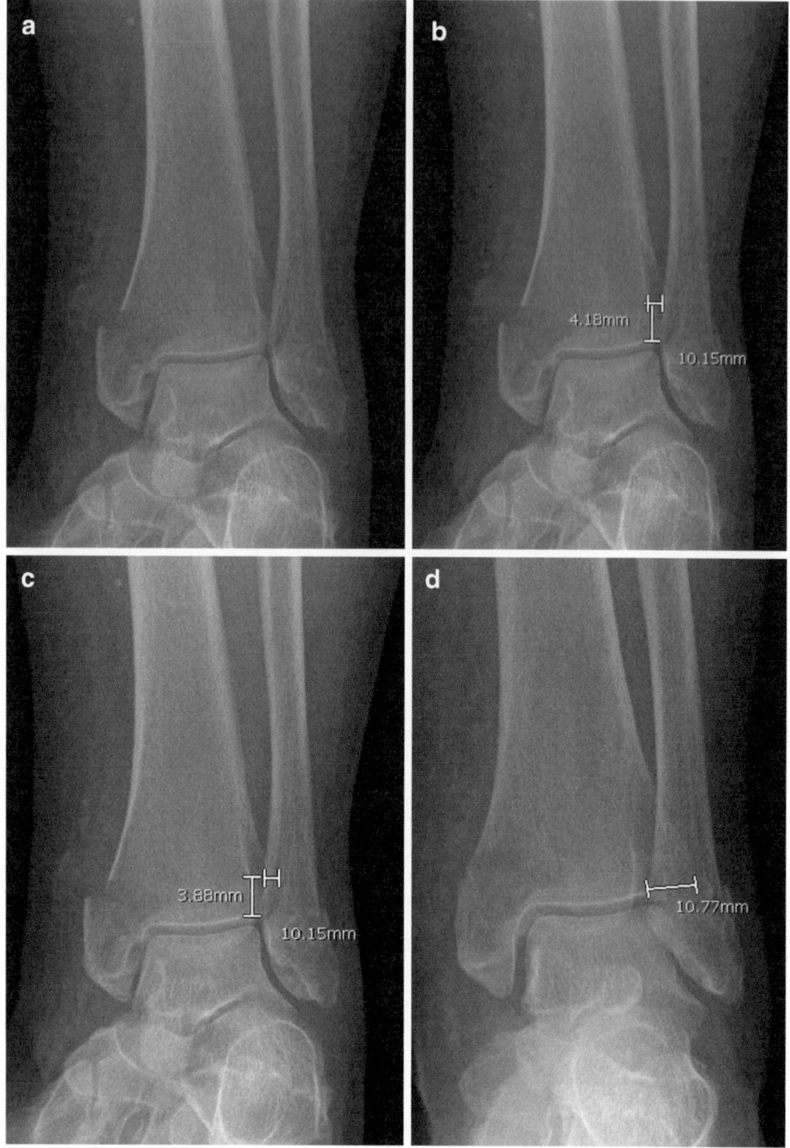

Fig. 3 Tibiofibular clear space and tibiofibular overlap to assess for syndesmotic instability. (**a**) Radiograph of an ankle with an intact syndesmosis. At 10mm above the joint line, tibiofibular clear space should be <6mm on a mortise view (4.18mm in **b**), and tibiofibular overlap should be >1mm (3.88mm in **c**). On an AP view, maximum tibiofibular overlap should be >10mm (10.77mm in **d**)

of the joint surface due to dislocation or subluxation, a CT scan can be helpful for quantifying the degree of articular injury. This is commonly seen in supination-adduction type fractures, where the talus impacts the anteromedial tibial plafond [5]. This particular fracture pattern, which is transitional between rotational fractures and pilon fractures, is discussed in more detail in chapter "Management of Fractures of the Tibial Plafond".

4 Closed Reduction Techniques

Closed reduction of an ankle fracture is a skill that any provider working in an urgent care or emergency room should attempt to master. While the primary goal is to center the talus under the tibial plafond, every effort should be put forth to obtain a reduction as near to anatomic as possible. The more anatomic the reduction, the less pressure is placed on the surrounding soft tissues. Post-reduction radiographs should be standard practice to ensure that an adequate reduction has been achieved.

The method for reducing any fracture is to apply longitudinal traction, then reverse the deforming force. It may be helpful to consider the Lauge Hansen classification of the ankle fracture (see chapter "Classification of Ankle Fractures") when planning the closed reduction maneuver. For example, the most common type is the supination/external rotation fracture. In these, the talus and foot are usually dislocated in a posterolateral direction with reference to the tibial plafond. In order to achieve a reduction, typically all that is needed is adequate analgesia (possibly intravenous sedation) with the patient supine on the gurney, flexing the knee, and then pulling traction with one hand on the great toe, and the other behind the heel while rotating the foot in an adduction and internal rotation maneuver. While an assistant holds the foot suspended by the great toe with the hip externally rotated, using gravity and the intact structures to maintain reduction, the splint is applied and molded firmly toward the medial side to hold the foot and talus in position. Since the classic 1959 article by Quigley, multiple technique articles have been published describing methods for immobilization, reduction, and splinting [6, 7]. Further detail as well as an illustration of the Quigley maneuver may be found in chapter "Emergency Management of Ankle Fractures".

Adequate analgesia can be obtained by doing a "fracture-hematoma" block prior to reduction. Typically, 20 mL of 1:1 ratio of short-acting and long-acting local anesthetic can be injected into the ankle joint. Letting this mixture sit in the hematoma/hemarthrosis for 5–10 min is required to achieve good pain control for the reduction, so be patient. Sodium bicarbonate (1 mL) can also be added to the block to reduce burning with injection. This may help reduce the need for systemic narcotics but does not address patient anxiety. A calm, relaxed, and patient demeanor, along with careful explanation of what is happening and a little bit of coaching on breathing techniques can go a long way in this setting, but some patients still might require conscious sedation.

Most patients will be more comfortable lying supine during the reduction, although, the patient can be sitting. Keep in mind, the sitting patient may have a vagal response during the reduction attempt and injure themselves if they lose consciousness and fall off the bed. For these reasons the senior author recommends the patient be supine during reduction.

A successful ankle reduction is only useful if the ankle can be immobilized in the reduced position. Learning to apply a splint is an invaluable skill for the emergency or urgent care provider, as well for as the orthopedist. The splint should consist of both a posterior slab to prevent anterior or posterior translation as well as a sugar-tong slab to immobilize the position and rotation of the foot. Care should be taken to avoid any wrinkles or focal points of pressure in the splint, and to ensure that the splint is of appropriate tightness to maintain the reduction but not be overly restrictive for the patient. The padding should be neither excessive nor deficient; 2–3 layers of webril are usually sufficient. When possible, Plaster of Paris should be used rather than pre-packaged fiberglass splinting material, due to its superior ability to be molded accurately. Ten layers of plaster per slab is a common thickness. The setting of the splint is an exothermic reaction and will heat up while setting. Lukewarm water is typically used as cold water will lead to prolonged time to set up and hot water can burn the patient. Post-reduction radiographs in the splint should be standard practice to ensure appropriate reduction has been maintained.

5 Indications for Surgery

Most bimalleolar ankle fractures are unstable, which means that they are likely to re-displace due to muscular forces after manipulative reduction and is an indication for operative intervention in the patient who can tolerate surgery. Exceptions may include the non-displaced fracture or the minimally displaced lateral malleolus fracture with a small associated medial anterior colliculus fracture, with a maintained medial clear space less than 4 mm due to an intact deep deltoid ligament. Furthermore, closed treatment has been described and may be a better option in elderly, low-demand patients. Other indications for nonoperative treatment with this injury pattern include patients who are too high risk for anesthesia, nonambulatory patients, or others for whom the risks of surgery outweigh the benefits. Closed treatment of bimalleolar ankle fractures requires great skill at reducing and casting a fracture in the reduced position, very close follow-up with weekly radiographs, and a prolonged time in immobilization: at least 4–6 weeks in a cast, many times requiring an above the knee cast followed by below the knee cast. At long-term follow-up, patients with unstable ankle fractures have been shown to do equally well with or without surgery, if tibiotalar congruity is maintained [8, 9]. However, surgical treatment is simpler, more reliable, and usually less disruptive to the patient's life [10].

The timing of surgery depends on multiple factors, including logistical considerations such as surgeon and operating room availability, and medical considerations such as optimizing the patient's medical readiness for undergoing anesthesia. If the ankle is adequately reduced and stabilized with a splint, there is low urgency to proceed to the operating room with closed injuries. However, as in all fractures, earlier intervention will likely afford an easier surgical dissection and fracture reduction.

As discussed in previous chapters, there are certain factors that require early intervention, and others that preclude it. An open fracture should be taken to the operating room with some urgency (within 24 h, possibly sooner or immediately if there is vascular occlusion, gross contamination, or gross deformity unable to be reduced with closed reduction). At minimum, an excisional debridement and irrigation of the open fracture wound should be performed, typically with at least minimal internal fixation or external fixation. During debridement, it is important to thoroughly examine and clean the wound, including careful extension of the laceration and gentle re-dislocation. Care should be taken to preserve skin during the debridement. No fracture should be left subluxated or dislocated because this threat-

ens not only the viability of the cartilage, but also the surrounding soft tissues. Soft tissue necrosis around the ankle may quickly lead to the need for a plastic surgery procedure or even amputation. Once in the operating room, treatment options include open or closed reduction and splinting, application of an external fixator, or definitive open reduction and internal fixation if the soft tissues allow. Even in the open fracture, if the wound is not grossly contaminated, definitive implants may be placed during the initial surgical encounter after a thorough irrigation and debridement. If there is too much swelling, blistering, or contaminated abrasion for surgical incisions, final fixation must be delayed until the soft tissues improve. Splinting and elevation can allow for soft tissue rest, but external fixation may be preferred to allow for easier examination of the skin while more reliably holding a reduction. External fixation may also help soft tissue swelling resolve faster as the external fixator acts to stabilize the soft tissues in addition to the bone injury. A staged surgery may then be performed once the soft tissues are appropriate.

6 Operative Techniques

Consider contralateral films preoperatively to help with surgical planning. This may also be done at the time of surgery, before the prep and drape, using fluoroscopy to obtain and save perfect lateral and mortise views of the uninjured ankle. These views can be particularly useful for judging fibular length and rotation and assessing the syndesmotic reduction. If the syndesmosis is found to be unstable after fixation of the malleoli, it must be addressed, and that issue will be discussed later in this chapter.

Bimalleolar fractures may include any two of the three malleoli, or a single malleolus fracture coupled with a disrupted ligament on the other side (usually deltoid), which is termed a "bimalleolar equivalent" ankle injury. When dealing with multiple injury sites around the ankle, it is important to plan the surgical incisions to allow access to each fracture while maintaining an appropriately sized skin bridge. While dogma has historically cited 7 cm as being the minimum acceptable distance between incisions, more recent literature has shown that a 5 to 6 cm skin bridge is typically well tolerated as long as the surgeon respects careful soft tissue handling, avoiding aggressive retracting, and placing the incisions within different angiosomes, which are areas of tissue that are supplied by different source blood vessels [11, 12]. Additionally, patient factors must be considered and, ideally, optimized, such as smoking, diabetes, and nutrition status. The surgical approaches to the ankle are numerous and include direct lateral, posterolateral, posteromedial, direct medial, anteromedial, direct anterior, and anterolateral.

For example, while a distal fibula fracture is commonly addressed through a direct lateral approach, a concomitant posterior malleolus fracture may also require surgical fixation. If an open approach to both is needed, the optimal route would be through a posterolateral incision. On the other hand, if the plan is to fix the fibula and supplement with syndesmotic screws as needed, with closed treatment of the posterior malleolus, then the surgeon may proceed with a direct lateral approach. If the orientation of the posterior malleolus is more medially based, the surgeon may plan to do a posteromedial approach instead. This is an example of when a CT scan may be very helpful for preoperative planning in more complex injuries.

Not every component of a bimalleolar ankle fracture must be repaired through a formal surgical approach. Any component that is nondisplaced may be treated in a percutaneous fashion, or without fixation if stable under stress views. However, if there is any concern for subtle displacement, an open reduction is preferred. Furthermore, once the fibula is stabilized, if the ankle and syndesmosis are found to be stable to stress exam, the surgeon may also choose to treat a medial or posterior malleolus in a closed manner, especially when these are small fragments. It is important to note the posterior malleolus fracture may be equivalent to a bony syndesmosis injury. In the setting of a posterior malleolus fracture, if the syndesmosis is found to be unstable after fixation of the fibula, stability may be

achieved with either fixation of the posterior malleolus or syndesmotic fixation traversing the fibula and tibia. Although it has been shown that fixing the posterior malleolus leads to increased syndesmotic stability when comparing the two techniques [13], sometimes a fragment of smaller size will lead a surgeon to favor syndesmotic fixation. Functional outcomes between the two techniques have been shown to be comparable [14].

Reduction and fixation techniques will be described here, followed by a few case scenarios to reinforce the topics discussed. The lateral malleolus is the key to ankle fracture reduction and stability and is usually approached first. The exceptions may be when the joint is irreducible due to interposed medial tissue, when the lateral side is relatively more complex with a simple tension-failure medial malleolus fracture, or when there is a posterior malleolus fracture and fibular hardware may obscure x-ray views of that reduction.

A lateral malleolus fracture may present in a variety of patterns, which in turn dictate the reduction and fixation methods used. The fibula usually shortens when it is fractured, and the sooner an operation can be performed the easier it is to regain the correct length. A simple oblique fracture, typically anterior-inferior to posterior-superior, may often be reduced with small clamps, which are usually either pointed "Weber" clamps or broad serrated "lobster claws". A pointed reduction clamp is used to regain length by placing the clamp tines closer to the apices of the fracture rather than perpendicular to the fracture plane, so that once the tines are engaged, the clamp may be rotated to bring the fracture out to length and then compressed to maintain that length. Remember that the fibula is often a quite fragile bone, particularly in older patients, and aggressive clamping may crush the bone and lead to comminution with loss of "keys" to reduction.

If length cannot be obtained with the gentle use of clamps, other techniques include attaching the chosen plate (based on pre-op planning) to the distal fragment with screws and clamping it loosely to the proximal fragment with a Verbrugge clamp. A lamina spreader is then used between the end of the plate and a 3.5 mm bicortical screw placed approximately 0.5 cm proximal to the end of the plate. The fibula is lengthened by opening the lamina spreader while watching the ankle joint on C-arm; when the fibula is at the correct length, the plate is more firmly clamped to the bone and screws applied. This is the "push-pull" technique. Another option is the use of the small distractor, an instrument that uses 2.5 mm threaded tip Schanz pins in each fragment and has a knurled knob on a threaded central bar.

Once the fracture is clamped, it may be stabilized with interfragmentary lag screw fixation, usually 2.0 to 3.5 mm depending on the size of the fragments, followed by a neutralization plate (Fig. 4), or it may be stabilized with a posterolateral antiglide plate, with or without interfragmentary fixation. Positioning the clamps out of the way of the definitive fixation may be tricky and may require an intermediate step with provisional fixation like Kirschner wires or a mini-fragment plate. A small fragment one-third tubular plate is often an appropriate size for the fibula, but patient factors such as diabetes, obesity, or osteoporosis may persuade the surgeon to opt for a plate of heavier stock, such as a small fragment lateral malleolus locking plate or transitional plate, which is more robust than a one third tubular plate. The senior author prefers a lateral malleo-

lus locking plate for comminuted fractures, but not because locking screws are needed. Rather, the pre-contoured locking plates are typically stronger plate stock with options for more screws distally. However, this comes at a cost (not just financially as these plates are more expensive). These pre-contoured plates may lead to more wound complications, so it is not advisable to use them for every fracture.

A fracture with a simple wedge intercalary fragment may still be anatomically reduced and fixed for primary bone healing as described above, but once the comminution becomes more extensive, bridge plating is typically utilized.

A transverse distal fibula fracture may require the surgeon to fashion a hook plate from a non-locking 1/3 tubular plate (Fig. 5) in order to increase fixation into the distal segment. Although, many vendors now have a pre-contoured hook plate which may save operative time. Sometimes, a percutaneously placed intramedullary fibular screw or rod may be sufficient fixation for well-reduced or transverse fractures, or when the skin condition precludes plate fixation. Special techniques may need to be employed for complex ankle fractures, such as in osteoporotic bone or diabetic ankle fractures. This may require multiple small plates or supplemental wire or screw fixation, or multiple screws

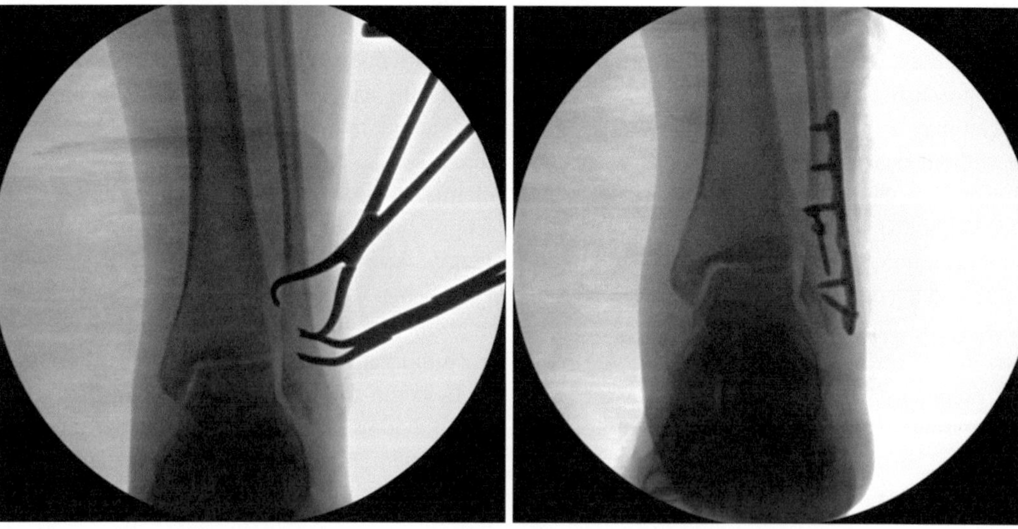

Fig. 4 Clamping of a lateral malleolus fracture and lag screw fixation followed by neutralization plating

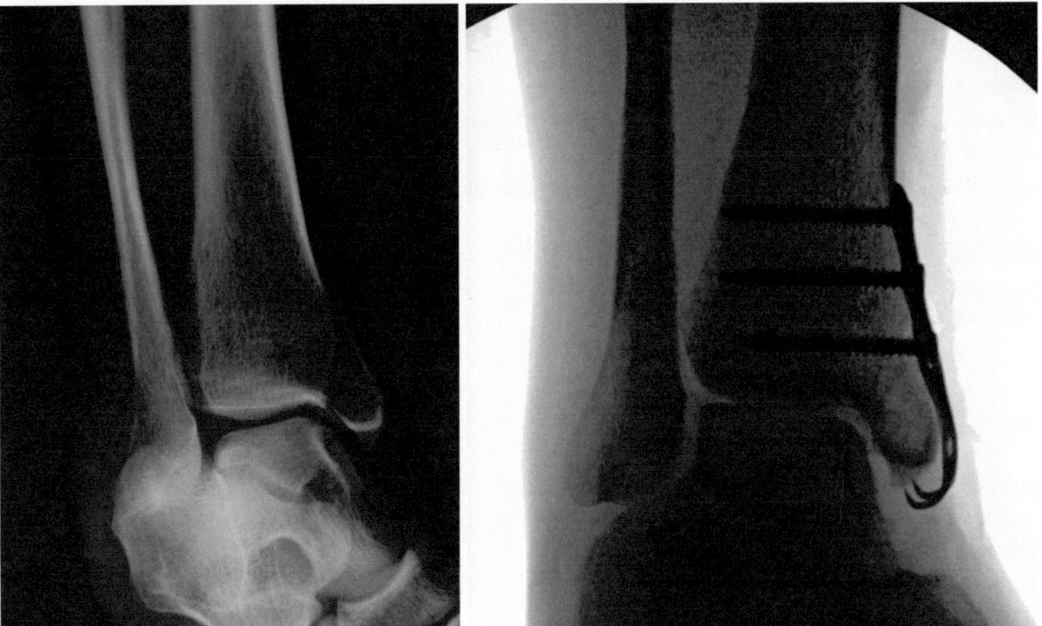

Fig. 5 Buttress plating of a vertical medial malleolus fracture with a hook plate. The most inferior screw is right at the apex of the fracture, providing optimal buttress function

through the plate and into the tibia. Ultimately, the goal in those patients is to maximize fixation of the distal fibular fragment, as failure of that segment will lead to failure of the entire construct. The importance of the lateral malleolus reduction becomes amplified in the presence of a syndesmotic injury, as a good reduction of the lateral malleolus is necessary for an anatomic reduction of the syndesmosis. This, in turn, is critical for the stability of the ankle and a good functional outcome [15–17].

Optimal fixation of the medial malleolus fragment may depend on the fracture pattern. While two screws are sufficient for most transverse medial malleolus fractures, a small fragment may only allow room for one screw, or a screw plus a Kirschner wire. Crowding fixation into a small medial malleolus fragment may cause comminution. Small medial malleolus fractures involving only the anterior colliculus may not need fixation if the ankle mortise is anatomic after fixation of the lateral malleolus and stable on stress exam. Very distal, small fragments or comminuted medial malleolar fractures can be fixed with K-wires and a figure 8 tension band construct

around a transversely placed screw. Vertically oriented fractures, such as those seen in supination-adduction type injuries, are best stabilized with a buttress plate (Fig. 5), as the deforming mechanism is a shearing force [18]. Comminuted fractures of the medial malleolus may require a combination of different techniques to stabilize the different fracture lines. It is important, also, to recognize that even after medial malleolar fixation, the deltoid ligament may still be incompetent, leading to medial instability [19]. The instability becomes evident after the bony reconstruction is completed and there is residual talar tilt with medial clear space widening, which may require additional ligamentous reconstruction. This can be achieved with direct repair, drill holes, or suture anchors depending on injury pattern and surgeon preference.

The surgeon should always be prepared to deal with a syndesmotic injury during ankle fracture fixation. A ligamentous syndesmotic injury in a bimalleolar fracture would be identified after fixation of the lateral and medial malleoli is completed. At this point, the surgeon should always stress the syndesmosis to identify instability.

Syndesmotic stress tests include the Cotton or hook test, which involves a maneuver that laterally translates the fibula, or a manual external rotation test. The external rotation stress method has been shown to be more sensitive than the lateral fibular stress method [20]. In addition to shifts in the mortise view, anterior or posterior translation of the fibula on the lateral view may be appreciated, and this may be an even more sensitive indicator of syndesmotic disruption [21]. There are several ways to assess a syndesmotic reduction, including direct open visualization at the level of the joint [22] and comparison to the saved fluoroscopic views of the uninjured side. On the lateral view, the position of the fibula relative to the tibia is particularly useful in assessing syndesmotic reduction [23]. Methods for reduction and fixation of the syndesmosis are topics of ongoing debate, with the only agreement being that accurate reduction of the syndesmosis is challenging. Historically, clamp placement followed by screw fixation from the fibula to the tibia was the standard of care. If a clamp is to be used, it must be "on-axis" with the syndesmosis in the sagittal plane. This has been shown to require one tine on the fibular ridge and the other on the anterior third of the medial distal tibia when evaluated on a lateral radiograph, although this is still subject to anatomic variability [24, 25]. However, some advocate against a clamp-based reduction, as the clamp can itself cause a malreduction in addition to over-compression of the syndesmosis. A manual digital reduction with direct visualization has been shown to improve reduction quality by comparison [26]. Similar to the trajectory of a clamp, the syndesmotic fixation should also aim posterior to anterior about 25–30°. While there is debate about whether the fixation should be trans-syndesmotic (0–2 cm above the joint line) or supra-syndesmotic (2–4 cm above the joint line), consensus shows that it should not be placed above 4 cm, as this was the only level resulting in a worsened functional outcome [27]. Multiple studies have sought to evaluate the required number of screws and cortices engaged for adequate syndesmotic stability, but there has been no clear difference found in radiologic or functional outcome between tricortical or quadricortical screw fixation, regardless of the number or size of screws [28–30]. Additionally, although some surgeons routinely remove syndesmotic screws after a period of at least 8 weeks, the need for and timing of this remains controversial [31–33]. Most recently, the suture button has become an established form of syndesmotic fixation. Though widespread adoption is slowed by implant cost and surgeon preference, multiple studies have shown it to produce lower malreduction rates, lower rates of symptomatic hardware, lower rates of hardware failure, and lower rates of reoperation [34, 35].

The posterior malleolus can vary greatly in morphology, and this should direct the surgeon's approach toward fixation [36]. The posterior malleolus fracture is indicative of a bony syndesmotic disruption, as it is the location of the insertion of the posterior inferior tibiofibular ligament. Small posterior malleolus fractures may be treated in a closed fashion, with syndesmotic fixation placed in the event of instability. However, large fragments involving >25% of the articular surface should be reduced and stabilized. Accurate evaluation of fragment size requires a CT scan. There is ongoing debate about whether smaller posterior malleolus fractures should be fixed. Fixation may improve stability in cases where the syndesmosis is unstable. If the fracture is nondisplaced or minimally displaced, it can be manipulated with a percutaneous 2.5 mm threaded tip K-wire joystick and a large Weber or peri-articular clamp can be placed percutaneously around the fibula posteriorly and on the anterior distal tibia. This can be followed by percutaneous lag screw fixation with washers. If an open approach to the fracture is needed, this should also incorporate the approach to either the lateral or medial malleolus, depending on the fracture orientation, with either a posterolateral or posteromedial approach. If necessary, the fracture can be booked open and any intercalary displacement or impaction can be reduced to the talar dome. A buttress plate utilizing a small or mini fragment or T plate works well for posterior malleolus fractures. Posterior malleolar fractures are discussed further in chapter "Trimalleolar Ankle Fractures".

Case 1: Medial and Lateral Malleoli

In the classic bimalleolar ankle fracture, both the medial and lateral malleoli are involved. The order of reduction and fixation is mostly based on surgeon preference and fracture pattern. Sometimes, with a particularly difficult reduction, both approaches need to be made and worked through simultaneously in order to remove interposed soft tissue within the medial or lateral gutters. The medial and lateral malleoli may then be fixed with the techniques described above. Before fixation of the fibula is completed, screw holes above the joint line should be left available for syndesmotic screws if placing a plate laterally. Once the syndesmosis is stressed, those holes may be filled appropriately.

Case 2: Lateral and Posterior Malleoli

If an open approach to both the lateral and posterior malleoli is planned, a posterolateral approach to the ankle is made. Generally, reduction of the fibula first can help with reduction of the posterior malleolus. However, implants on the fibula will obstruct the fluoroscopic view of the posterior malleolus. Therefore, a useful technique is to reduce the fibula and secure it with provisional fixation, such as small clamps, Kirschner wires, or even lag screws, and then move on to the posterior malleolus before completing fixation of the fibula. Again, the syndesmosis should be stressed, but if the posterior malleolus is secured, one would expect it to be stable.

Case 3: Medial and Posterior Malleoli

This scenario may require two separate approaches if the posterior malleolus is laterally based, or a single posteromedial approach if it is medially based. The surgeon should be thoughtful about patient positioning if needing to do a dual approach, as it can be difficult to work on the medial malleolus with the patient in the prone position. Options in this case are to work entirely prone, position in the lateral decubitus position and externally rotate at the hip to do the medial approach in a functionally supine position, or to start prone and then flip to supine.

Fixation may be performed with the techniques discussed above.

7 Rehabilitation Protocols

Weight bearing restrictions will vary depending on the treatment method employed. Closed treatment of a bimalleolar ankle fracture requires non-weightbearing on that extremity for at least 6 weeks to allow fracture healing. If there is syndesmotic injury involved, the time of restricted weight bearing may be increased to 12 weeks. For this reason and others, operative treatment of unstable ankle fractures is often preferred by patients.

With surgical fixation of the ankle, splint immobilization is usually maintained for 2 weeks or until the wounds have healed. At that point, immobilization continues in a boot, but patients are allowed to remove the boot and begin working on range of motion of their ankle to prevent stiffness. Allowing early range of motion with a removable brace after operative fixation of ankle fractures has been shown to lead to improved motion and increased functional outcome scores without increased complications compared to immobilization in a cast [37–39]; however, exceptions may be made for patients who are at high risk for wound complications [40]. Patients may typically begin early weight bearing at 2 weeks postoperatively without additional risk of wound complication or fixation failure [41, 42]. For patients with syndesmotic injuries, this topic becomes more controversial. Although there is evidence to show that they can safely be full weight bearing at 2 weeks [43], weight bearing is more typically begun at 6–8 weeks postoperatively. Diabetic or vasculopathic patients, or others with delayed healing, may require even longer periods of non-weightbearing. Physical therapy for an ankle fracture may be needed for special populations with gait difficulties, for patients who have developed ankle stiffness, or for those looking to return to high levels of activity. However, most patients who have undergone surgical fixation of an ankle fracture will not need physical therapy.

8 Conclusion

Surgical treatment of unstable bimalleolar ankle fractures is important for restoring ankle stability and preventing post-traumatic osteoarthritis. At 1 year postoperatively, most patients have little or no pain and few, if any, limitations in functional activity [44]. However, patients should be counseled that they should expect to see improvements in function through the first 2 years of recovery [45] and may have trouble in returning to sporting activity after their injury [46]. Syndesmotic injury further worsens outcomes, even after stabilization, and this should be emphasized to patients to set appropriate expectations [47].

References

1. Tejwani NC. Are outcomes of Bimalleolar fractures poorer than those of lateral malleolar fractures with medial ligamentous injury? J Bone Joint Surg. 2007;89(7):1438–4.
2. Stufkens SAS, Knupp M, Lampert C, van Dijk CN, Hintermann B. Long-term outcome after supination-external rotation type-4 fractures of the ankle. J Bone Joint Surg Br. 2009;91(12):1607–11.
3. Ramsey PL, Hamilton W. Changes in tibiotalar area of contact caused by lateral talar shift. J Bone Joint Surg. 1976;58(3):356–7.
4. Stiell IG, Greenberg GH, McKnight RD, Nair RC, McDowell I, Reardon M, Stewart JP, Maloney J. Decision rules for the use of radiography in acute ankle injuries: refinement and prospective validation. JAMA. 1993;269(9):1127–32.
5. McConnell T, Tornetta P. Marginal plafond impaction in association with supination-adduction ankle fractures: a report of eight cases. J Orthop Trauma. 2001;15(6):447–9.
6. Alton TB, Harnden E, Hagen J, Firoozabadi R. Single provider reduction and splinting of displaced ankle fractures: a modification of Quigley's classic technique. J Orthop Trauma. 2015;29:e166–71.
7. Skelley NW, Ricci WM. A single-person reduction and splinting technique for ankle injuries. J Orthop Trauma. 2015;29:e172–7.
8. Donken CCMA, Verhofstad MHJ, Edwards MJ, van Laarhoven CJHM. Twenty-one-year follow-up of supination-external rotation type II-IV (OTA type B) ankle fractures: a retrospective cohort study. J Orthop Trauma. 2012;26(8):e108–14.
9. Donken CCMA, Verhofstad MHJ, Edwards MJ, van Laarhoven CJHM. Twenty-two-year follow-up of pronation-external rotation type III-IV (OTA type C) ankle fractures: a retrospective cohort study. J Orthop Trauma. 2012;26(8):e115–22.
10. Makwana NK, Bhowal B, Harper WM, Hui AW. Conservative versus operative treatment for displaced ankle fractures in patients over 55 years of age. A prospective, randomised study. J Bone Joint Surg Br. 2001;83(4):525–9.
11. Howard JL, Agel J, Barei DP, Benirschke SK, Nork SE. A prospective study evaluating incision placement and wound healing for tibial plafond fractures. J Orthop Trauma. 2008;22:299–306.
12. Attinger CE, Evans KK, Bulan E, Blume P, Cooper P. Angiosomes of the foot and ankle and clinical implications for limb salvage: reconstruction, incisions, and revascularization. Plast Reconstr Surg. 2006;6:261S–93S.
13. Gardner MJ, Brodsky A, Briggs SM, Nielson JH, Lorich DG. Fixation of posterior malleolar fractures provides greater syndesmotic stability. Clin Orthop Relat Res. 2006;447:165–71.
14. Miller AN, Carroll EA, Parker RJ, Helfet DL, Lorich DG. Posterior malleolar stabilization of syndesmotic injuries is equivalent to screw fixation. Clin Orthop Relat Res. 2009;468(4):1129–35.
15. Leeds HC, Ehrlich MG. Instability of the distal tibiofibular syndesmosis after bimalleolar and trimalleolar ankle fractures. J Bone Joint Surg. 1984;66(4):490–503.
16. Sagi HC, Shah AR, Sanders RW. The functional consequence of syndesmotic joint malreduction at a minimum 2-year follow-up. J Orthop Trauma. 2012;26(7):439–43.
17. Andersen MR, Diep LM, Frihagen F, Castberg Hellund J, Madsen JE, Figved W. Importance of syndesmotic reduction on clinical outcome after syndesmosis injuries. J Orthop Trauma. 2019;33(8):397–403.
18. Dumigan RM, Bronson DG, Early JS. Analysis of fixation methods for vertical shear fractures of the medial malleolus. J Orthop Trauma. 2006;20(10):687–91.
19. Tornetta P. Competence of the deltoid ligament in bimalleolar ankle fractures after medial malleolar fixation. J Bone Joint Surg. 2000;82(6):843–8.
20. Matuszewski PE, Dombroski D, Lawrence JTR, Esterhai JLJ, Mehta S. Prospective intraoperative syndesmotic evaluation during ankle fracture fixation: stress external rotation versus lateral fibular stress. J Orthop Trauma. 2015;29(4):e157–60.
21. Candal-Couto JJ, Burrow D, Bromage S, Briggs PJ. Instability of the tibio-fibular syndesmosis: have we been pulling in the wrong direction? Injury. 2004;35(8):814–8.
22. Tornetta P III, Yakavonis M, Veltre D, Shah A. Reducing the syndesmosis under direct vision. J Orthop Trauma. 2019;33(9):450–4.
23. Summers HD, Sinclair MK, Stover MD. A reliable method for intraoperative evaluation of syndesmotic reduction. J Orthop Trauma. 2013;27(4):196–200.
24. Putnam SM, Linn MS, Spraggs-Hughes A, McAndrew CM, Ricci WM, Gardner MJ. Simulating clamp placement across the trans-syndesmotic angle of the

ankle to minimize malreduction: a radiological study. Injury. 2017;48(3):770–5.

25. Cosgrove CT, Putnam SM, Cherney SM, Ricci WM, Spraggs-Hughes A, McAndrew CM, Gardner MJ. Medial clamp tine positioning affects ankle syndesmosis malreduction. J Orthop Trauma. 2017;31(8):440–6.

26. Cosgrove CT, Spraggs-Hughes AG, Putnam SM, Ricci WM, Miller AN, McAndrew CM, Gardner MJ. A novel indirect reduction technique in ankle syndesmotic injuries: a cadaveric study. J Orthop Trauma. 2018;32(7):361–7.

27. Schepers T, van der Linden H, van Lieshout EMM, Niesten DD, van der Elst M. Technical aspects of the syndesmotic screw and their effect on functional outcome following acute distal tibiofibular syndesmosis injury. Injury. 2014;45(4):775–9.

28. Moore JA, Shank JR, Morgan SJ, Smith WR. Syndesmosis fixation: a comparison of three and four cortices of screw fixation without hardware removal. Foot Ankle Int. 2006;27(8):567–72.

29. Høiness P, Strømsøe K. Tricortical versus Quadricortical syndesmosis fixation in ankle fractures: a prospective, randomized study comparing two methods of syndesmosis fixation. J Orthop Trauma. 2004;18(6):331–7.

30. Wikerøy AKB, Høiness PR, Andreassen GS, Hellund JC, Madsen JE. No difference in functional and radiographic results 8.4 years after Quadricortical compared with Tricortical syndesmosis fixation in ankle fractures. J Orthop Trauma. 2010;24(1):17–23.

31. Manjoo A, Sanders DW, Tieszer C, MacLeod MD. Functional and radiographic results of patients with syndesmotic screw fixation: implications for screw removal. J Orthop Trauma. 2010;24(1):2–6.

32. Boyle MJ, Gao R, Frampton CMA, Coleman B. Removal of the syndesmotic screw after the surgical treatment of a fracture of the ankle in adult patients does not affect one-year outcomes: a randomized controlled trial. Bone Joint J. 2014;96-B(12):1699–705.

33. Walley KC, Hofmann KJ, Velasco BT, Kwon JY. Removal of hardware after syndesmotic screw fixation: a systematic literature review. Foot Ankle Spec. 2017;10(3):252–7.

34. Zhang P, Liang Y, He J, Fang Y, Chen P, Wang J. A systematic review of suture-button versus syndesmotic screw in the treatment of distal tibiofibular syndesmosis injury. BMC Musculoskelet Disord. 2017;18(286):286.

35. Ramadanov N, Bueschges S, Dimitrov D. Comparison of outcomes between suture button technique and screw fixation technique in patients with acute syndesmotic diastasis: a meta-analysis of randomized controlled trials. Foot Ankle Orthopaed. 2021;6(4):247301142110614.

36. Haraguchi N, Haruyama H, Toga H, Kato F. Pathoanatomy of posterior malleolar fractures of the ankle. J Bone Joint Surg. 2006;88(5):1085–92.

37. Dehghan N, McKee MD, Jenkinson RJ, et al. Early weightbearing and range of motion versus non-weightbearing and immobilization after open reduction and internal fixation of unstable ankle fractures: a randomized controlled trial. J Orthop Trauma. 2016;30(7):345–52.

38. Egol KA, Dolan R, Koval KJ. Functional outcome of surgery for fractures of the ankle. A prospective, randomised comparison of management in a cast or a functional brace. J Bone Joint Surg Br. 2000;82(2):246–9.

39. Simanski CJP, Maegele MG, Lefering R, et al. Functional treatment and early weightbearing after an ankle fracture: a prospective study. J Orthop Trauma. 2006;20(2):108–14.

40. Lehtonen H, Järvinen TLN, Honkonen S, Nyman M, Vihtonen K, Järvinen M. Use of a cast compared with a functional ankle brace after operative treatment of an ankle fracture. A prospective, randomized study. J Bone Joint Surg. 2003;85(2):205–11.

41. Firoozabadi R, Harnden E, Krieg JC. Immediate weight-bearing after ankle fracture fixation. Adv Orthopedics. 2015;2:491976.

42. Pyle C, Kim-Orden M, Hughes T, Schneiderman B, Kay R, Harris T. Reduction and internal fixation of unstable ankle fractures on wound complications or failures of fixation. Foot Ankle Int. 2019;40(12):1397–402.

43. Al-Hourani K, Stoddart M, Chesser TJS. Does early post-operative weight bearing affect radiographic outcomes? Injury. 2019;50(3):795.

44. Egol KA, Tejwani NC, Walsh MG, Capla EL, Koval KJ. Predictors of short-term functional outcome following ankle fracture surgery. J Bone Joint Surg. 2006;88(5):974–9.

45. Bhandari M, Sprague S, Hanson B, et al. Health-related quality of life following operative treatment of unstable ankle fractures: a prospective observational study. J Orthop Trauma. 2004;18(6):338–45.

46. Hong CC, Roy SP, Nashi N, Tan KJ. Functional outcome and limitation of sporting activities after Bimalleolar and Trimalleolar ankle fractures. Foot Ankle Int. 2013;34(6):805–10.

47. Egol KA, Pahk B, Walsh M, Tejwani NC, Davidovitch RI, Koval KJ. Outcome after unstable ankle fracture: effect of syndesmotic stabilization. J Orthop Trauma. 2010;24(1):7–11.

Trimalleolar Ankle Fractures

Alexander Crespo and Michael Gardner

1 Introduction

Ankle fractures are a common skeletal injury encountered by orthopedic surgeons. As a result, these injuries will be evaluated and treated by orthopedic surgeons across many subspecialties. While it is true that many of these injuries can be treated with an algorithmic approach, a spectrum of severity exists; there are subtleties in both patient and radiographic presentation that must be appreciated in order to ensure an optimal outcome. This chapter will discuss the spectrum of trimalleolar ankle fractures with particular emphasis on addressing the posterior malleolus (PM), as it is this structure that is often the defining feature of the "trimalleolar" pattern. The treatment of bimalleolar injuries and considerations regarding syndesmotic stability and fixation will be discussed in depth elsewhere.

2 Functional Anatomy and Biomechanics

The ankle is a ginglymoid (hinge) joint comprised of a generally concave distal tibial surface and corresponding convex talar dome surface, allowing for extensive uniaxial articulation. The posterior malleolus is a distal projection of the posterior tibial plafond. This bony prominence provides attachment for ligaments and comprises the posterior component of incisura fibularis, which provides stable tibio-fibular articulation [1]. Ankle stability is provided by static ligamentous attachments as well as the bony "mortise" arrangement of the tibia, fibula, and talus.

The posterior inferior tibio-fibular ligament (PITFL) anatomy and function is important to understand to appreciate the significance of posterior malleolus fractures to ankle function. The PITFL, comprised of superficial and deep components, originates from the posterior malleolus and runs obliquely and distally to its insertion on the posterior fibula [1, 2]. The ligament is often stronger in tension than the bony posterior malleolus and, thus, posterior injury may result in avulsion of the posterior malleolus. An intact PITFL-posterior malleolus complex provides approximately 42% of syndesmotic stability, with the remaining 58% attributed to the AITFL (36%) and interosseous ligament (22%) [1, 3].

Disruption of the PITFL-PM complex via either posterior malleolus fracture or ligament

A. Crespo
Orthopedic Surgeon, NorthShore Orthopaedic and Spine Institute, Chicago, IL, USA

M. Gardner (✉)
Orthopaedic Trauma Service, Stanford University School of Medicine, Palo Alto, CA, USA
e-mail: michaelgardner@stanford.edu

tear yields loss of tibio-talar constraint and pathologic change in the location, distribution, character, and intensity of peak forces in the ankle, leading to increased rate and severity of arthrosis. Our understanding of this pathophysiology has been primarily obtained from cadaveric studies demonstrating that posterior malleolar fragment size is a key determinate in the development of pathologic forces across the ankle. Increasing PM fragment size results in decreased total joint contact area and reciprocal increased load concentration with alterations in pressure distribution [4, 5]. A posterior malleolus fragment that is larger than 25% of the total tibial articular surface causes significant instability to rotational and translational stresses and increases shear forces—a particularly damaging force to articular cartilage [6]. Biomechanical cadaver studies have shown alteration in magnitude, location, distribution, or vector of peak forces following posterior malleolus fracture [7]. These changes may lead to development of arthritis and functional loss. However, because these alterations in biomechanics may occur with smaller fragments as well, modern treatment of posterior malleolus fractures does not rely solely on the size of the fracture fragment.

## 3	Pre-Operative Workup

### 3.1	History

As with all skeletal injuries, the surgeon must appreciate the character of the injury as well as the patient's functional demands in order to formulate a successful treatment plan. Low energy mechanisms are commonly a result of torsion; this mechanism yields simple fracture patterns and less frequently associated with significant soft tissue injury. Conversely, high energy mechanisms may be characterized by axial loading patterns distinguished by metaphyseal comminution and are associated with substantial soft tissue injury.

An understanding of the patient is equally important to ensure optimal outcome. The surgeon must identify concomitant comorbidities that may compromise soft tissue healing or construct stability, particularly: neuropathy, osteopenia, vasculopathy, tobacco use, or a threatened soft-tissue envelope. Furthermore, patients at risk for noncompliance (i.e., psychiatric conditions, substance abuse) may be at increased risk of failure. The treatment decision should be individually tailored to each patient depending on the presence or absence of such factors.

### 3.2	Physical Exam

The examination begins with inspection of the ankle. Open wounds and obvious deformity are noted. All dislocations should be immediately reduced to prevent further soft tissue insult and unkink any tethered vessels that may result in vascular compromise. Any fracture with a wound or break in the skin is an open fracture, and immediate antibiotic administration is essential. The dorsalis pedis and posterior tibial arteries are palpated, and capillary refill time is noted. All bony prominences about the ankle are palpated for tenderness. It is also important to palpate the fibular neck for tenderness as this may help to identify a syndesmotic injury (Maisonneuve fracture). Finally, the neurologic examination should assess protective sensation as its absence is indicative of underlying neuropathy.

### 3.3	Imaging

AP, lateral and mortise radiographs are obtained when evaluating ankle injuries that meet the Ottawa rules, as outlined in see chapter "Management of Bimalleolar Ankle Fractures". A manual external rotation stress view is indicated in cases where occult instability or syndesmotic injury is suspected. To obtain the manual external rotation stress view, a mortise view is obtained, and the foot is then externally rotated and tibiotalar stability evaluated. Tibiotalar congruency and medial clear space widening is evaluated and compared with the uninjured side. Greater than 4 mm of medial widening indicates deltoid ligament injury and tibiotalar instability.

Classification of ankle fractures is covered in see chapter "Classification of Ankle Fractures". There are two system classifications for posterior malleolus fractures, the Mason-Molloy system and the Haraguchi system. All current classification systems for the posterior malleolus are purely descriptive and have not been shown to correlate with outcomes nor guide treatment. The most commonly utilized is the Haraguchi system which describes three patterns: posterolateral oblique (Type 1), medial extension (Type 2), and small-shell (Type 3).

Computed-tomography (CT) scanning is useful in evaluating the posterior malleolus. Plain radiographs consistently lead to underestimating the size of the posterior fragment. Managing posterior malleolus fractures based on size alone oversimplifies the decision-making process. A CT scan reveals clinically relevant fracture details including size, obliquity, marginal impaction, incarcerated fragments within the fracture, and evidence of associated syndesmosis injury.

4 Surgical Management of Medial and Lateral Malleolar Injuries

4.1 Surgical Approaches

The surgical approaches to the lateral malleolus and medial malleolus are discussed in see chapter "Management of Bimalleolar Ankle Fractures". If all three fractures in a trimalleolar pattern are indicated for reduction and fixation, we most commonly utilize the posterolateral and medial approaches. The patient is positioned prone with the operative ankle placed on a radiolucent bump to allow maximum dorsiflexion of the ankle. The posterolateral approach is utilized first to allow for reduction and fixation of the posterior malleolus and fibula. Fixation of the posterior malleolus prior to fixation of the fibula allows radiographic assessment of the posterior malleolar reduction; when the fibula is fixed first, the fibular plate will often obscure the posterior malleolar fracture line when obtaining an intraoperative lateral of the ankle. The medial malleolus is addressed follow-

ing reduction and fixation of the posterior and lateral malleoli. This is typically done by internally rotating the hip, allowing the medial aspect of the ankle to face the surgeon. The C-arm can then be rotated "over-the-top" to obtain a mortise view without manipulating the position of the foot. Some surgeons may opt to flex the knee, operating "upside-down" with foot pointing to the ceiling. This allows full view of the leg but inverts the anatomy and requires an assistant to maintain the position of the leg. Alternatively, the patient may be repositioned supine with a new prep and drape to allow for the most familiar surgical orientation, positioning, and imaging. The medial malleolus may then be approached, reduced, and fixed in typical fashion.

4.2 Posterolateral Approach

The posterolateral approach is very useful for the combined treatment of fibular and posterior malleolar fracture patterns and is the preferred method for trimalleolar patterns in which the posterior malleolus will be treated surgically. An incision is made midway between the lateral border of the Achilles and the posterior border of the fibula. The sural nerve courses in the medial distal aspect of the incision and must be preserved during the approach. The crural fascia is identified and incised. Immediately deep to this fascial layer lies an interval between the peroneal fascia and the fascia of the flexor hallucis longus (FHL). Identifying and developing this potential space allows the dissection to remain in an intermuscular plane. The FHL is elevated off the posterior malleolus by sliding a small Hohman retractor over the medial malleolus. The peroneal fascia is incised and the peroneals retracted posteriorly, giving direct access to the fibula (Fig. 1).

4.3 Posteromedial Approach

The posteromedial approach is an acceptable option for reduction of posterior malleolus fractures with medial extension. A curvilinear incision is made along the posterior border of the tibia and curving anteriorly at the level of the medial malleolus. If direct access to the medial malleolus is required, the incision can be placed centered over the medial malleolus. It may need to be lengthened to comfortably work in the posteromedial interval described below, avoiding tension on the skin. The posterior tibial tendon sheath is incised, and the posterior tibial tendon retracted anteriorly, while the flexor tendons and neurovascular bundle are retracted posteriorly. The posterior malleolus fracture is accessed through this interval (Fig. 2).

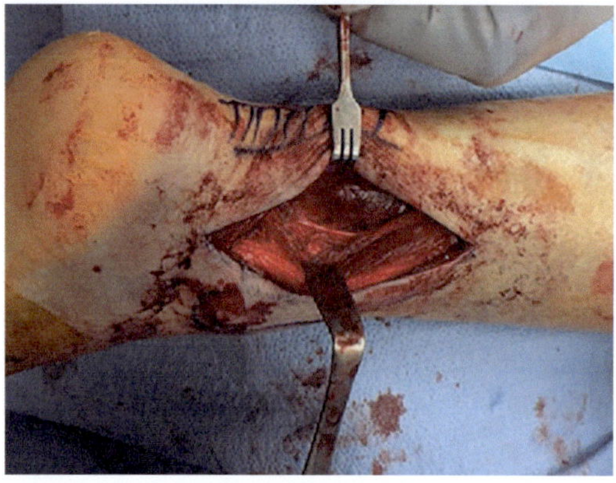

Fig. 1 The peroneals are retracted laterally and the deep posterior compartment is elevated to expose the posterior malleolus

4.4 Fibular Reduction and Fixation

4.4.1 Spiral Pattern

These simple fracture patterns are the most common. The fracture hematoma is debrided, and the periosteum adjacent to the fracture is elevated to clearly define the fracture edges. The axilla of the fracture is most commonly posterolateral and should be clearly visualized. A small-pointed reduction clamp is applied transversely to the fracture and the posterior tine is rotated distally to restore length. Once reduction is obtained, it can be maintained with either lag-screw and laterally based neutralization plating or with posterolateral anti-glide plating. Although a 3.5 mm lag screw is commonly employed, we find a 2.0 mm or 2.4 mm screw to be more optimally sized for this application. A 1/3rd tubular plate or precountoured fibular plate may be placed in neutralization mode. Posterolateral antiglide plating may be less familiar but avoids subcutaneous implant placement, is biomechanically optimal, and allows the surgeon to use the plate to assist with the fracture reduction. An undercontoured 1/3rd tubular plate is applied to the posterolateral fibula with a screw placed in the axilla of the fracture so that plate functions in antiglide mode. Keeping the plate 1 cm from the tip of the fibula avoids peroneal irritation. An additional screw is

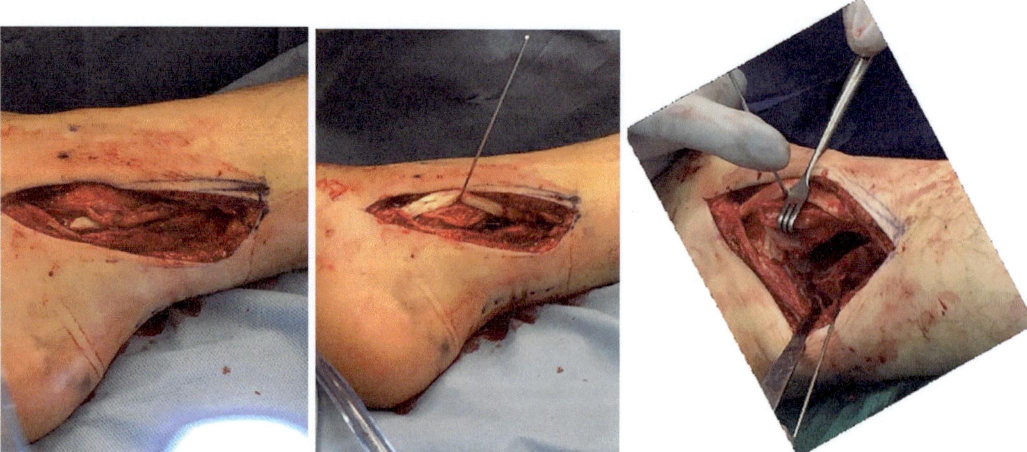

Fig. 2 The posterior tibial tendon sheath is incised and the tendon retracted anteriorly. The posterior malleolus is accessed through this interval

placed into the proximal segment to control plate rotation. This provides sufficient fixation although a supplemental lag screw or screws into the distal segment can be placed at the surgeon's discretion.

4.4.2 Transverse

This simple fracture pattern typically occurs in an infrasyndesmotic location (Weber A) and infrequently contributes to tibiotalar instability. If fracture displacement or other variables are felt to merit reduction and fixation, tension band plating and intramedullary screw fixation are viable options. For intramedullary fixation, a long 3.5 mm fully threaded screw can be used. An incision is made 2 cm distal to the tip of the fibula, in line with its longitudinal axis. The start point must be in line with the medullary canal on mortise, and lateral views otherwise eccentric drilling and iatrogenic deformity can occur. Over-drilling the distal fibula with a 3.5 mm drill often facilitates screw insertion and allows the screw to function in a lag-by-technique fashion.

The drill is advanced to the fracture site, and a 2.5 mm drill is used to enter the fibular shaft. The screw is then placed in retrograde fashion; often, the screw will be noted to bend due to interference fit within the isthmus of the fibula.

4.4.3 Comminuted

Accurate fibular reduction is more complicated in comminuted patterns. Bridge plating of the comminuted fibula is generally preferred and a "push" technique is often utilized to restore fibular length (Fig. 3). In these circumstances, a precontoured lateral locking plate may be useful as this is stout, optimizes distal fixation, and provides the best vector for restoring length when pushed on. The plate is affixed to the distal segment and a bicortical screw is placed 1 cm proximal to the plate. The plate is held to the proximal segment with a gently applied Verbrugge clamp. A lamina spreader is placed between the screw and the proximal plate and expanded to push the distal fibula distally. Appropriate length is judged using a combination of the talocrural angle, fibu-

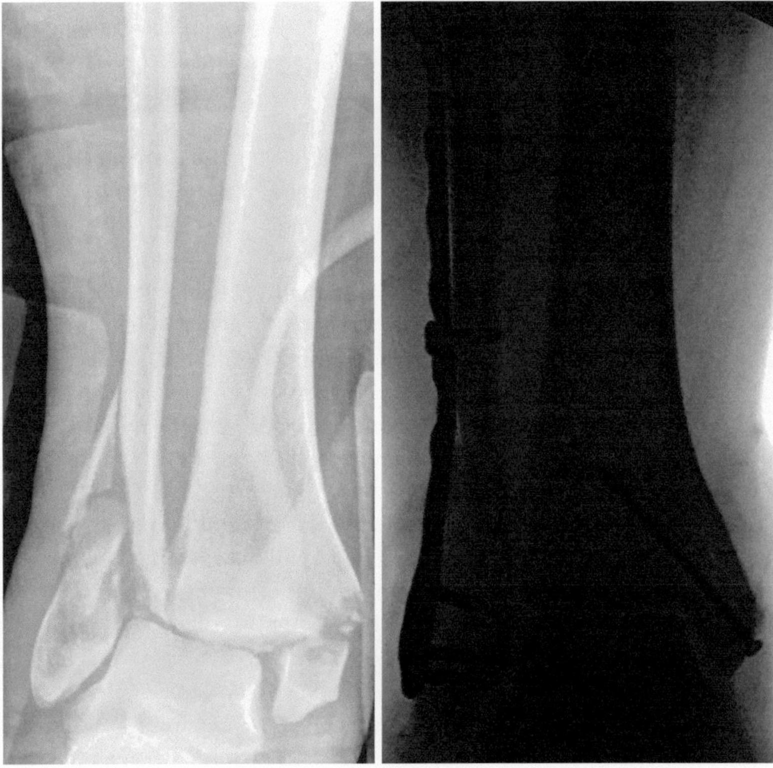

Fig. 3 A pronation-abduction injury pattern with a comminuted fibula. The fibula was treated with a precontoured locking plate placed in bridge mode

lar "dime sign" (defined by an unbroken curve, or "Shenton line", between the inferior fibula and the arc of the lateral process of the talus), and anatomic articulation of the lateral talar facet and distal fibula. Once length is achieved, screws are placed proximally in the plate to create a length stable construct.

4.5 Medial Malleolar Reduction and Fixation

4.5.1 Transverse

Transverse medial malleolus fractures are the most commonly encountered pattern. The anteromedial shoulder should be visualized as it provides the best reduction key; this is best performed with an apex-anterior incision that curves around the anterior aspect of the medial malleolus. Temporary reduction can be performed with a small pointed reduction clamp with one tine in a proximal 2.5 mm drill hole, or by use of a K-wire joystick placed centrally in the distal fragment. Definitive fixation is usually obtained with one or two lag screws placed perpendicular to the fracture line.

4.5.2 Vertical Shear

This injury pattern is seen in supination-adduction injuries and merits separate discussion for two reasons: the fracture line is vertical and cannot be adequately stabilized with the retrograde lag-screw construct, and it is associated with anteromedial impaction of the tibial plafond. Visualization of the medial gutter and anteromedial plafond is essential, as well as proximal access to the apex of the fracture line. The fracture is "booked-open" to allow access to anteromedial impaction of the plafond. The articular injury is fully disimpacted using the intact plafond and talar dome to template reduction. Care is taken to preserve as much cancellous bone with the subchondral shelf as possible; we often use a freer or periosteal elevator to find the "fault line" of impaction within cancellous bone. The reduction is held with k-wires and the void can be backfilled with calcium phosphate or cancellous allograft if required. The medial malleolar frag-

ment is then reduced and fixed with an antiglide buttress plate, as discussed in previous chapters.

5 The Posterior Malleolus

5.1 Decision Making: To Fix or Not to Fix?

Historically, the indication for fixing the posterior malleolus has been based largely on the size of the fragment, with those that are greater than 25% of the articular surface being indicated for operative fixation [8, 9]. However, more recent studies have demonstrated that the decision making should be more nuanced. Articular incongruity with greater than 2 mm step-off [10], syndesmotic-associated instability [11, 12], and persistent posterior subluxation despite fibular fixation [13] should also be considered as indications for open reduction and internal fixation (ORIF).

The goal of operative fixation of ankle fractures is to restore a stable and congruent tibiotalar articulation. If fixation of the posterior malleolar fragment aids in obtaining this goal, then it should be reduced and fixed anatomically. Provided the PITFL is intact, which is almost universally the case, reduction and fixation of the posterior malleolar fragment will aid in stabilizing the syndesmosis by restoring PITFL function. It will also prevent posterior fibular translation by restoring congruity of the incisura [1, 11]. This has been demonstrated in a cadaver study which showed that, in the presence of PM fracture, syndesmotic stability is restored to 70% with isolated plating of the posterior malleolus versus only 40% with isolated syndesmotic fixation [12]. Furthermore, ORIF of the posterior malleolus yields improved restoration of the tibiofibular clear space compared to isolated syndesmotic screw fixation [14].

In practice, clinical decision making regarding posterior malleolus fixation is variable. A survey of surgeon practices demonstrated that approximately 1/3rd of orthopedic surgeons indicate PM fractures for operative fixation based on the "25% rule" whereas the remaining 2/3rds of surgeons reported the indication depends on ankle stability and "other factors." Size did appear to play some role in decision making, as 97% of respondents would indicate fragments larger than 50% of the articular surface and 9% of respondents would indicate fragments less than 10% of the articular surface for internal fixation. The presence of comminution and posteromedial extension were also considered indications for surgery by approximately 50% of respondents [15].

A systematic review of this topic was unable to determine evidence-based guidelines for the treatment of PM fractures due to a lack of standardized functional outcomes in the available literature [7]. As such, the decision to proceed with operative fixation of the posterior malleolus must be made on a case-to-case basis after considering its implications on tibiotalar stability and syndesmotic reduction.

5.2 Reduction and Fixation

Both posterolateral and posteromedial approaches to the posterior ankle may be utilized, as discussed earlier in this chapter. We find the posterolateral approach to be most applicable because it allows fixation of the posterior malleolar fragment as well as the fibula through a single inci-

sion [13, 16]. The surgical dissection proceeds as previously described. The posterior malleolar fracture is identified and mobilized from medial to lateral and proximal to distal to maintain PITFL attachment to the fragment [13]. The fracture site is booked open and inspected for any incarcerated fragments, which are often present; scrutinizing the preoperative CT scan will help the surgeon to anticipate these fragments. The articular fragment may then be reduced through the distracted posterior malleolar fracture line. The posterior malleolus is then reduced using a ball spike pusher (Fig. 4). In cases where it is difficult to restore distal position, a 2.5 mm pilot hole may be drilled in the fragment and a hook or dental pick is used to pull the fragment distally with more force. The fragment is provisionally fixed with K-wires and articular reduction is confirmed with fluoroscopy.

Posterior malleolus fixation may be obtained with either buttress plating versus posterior to anterior screw fixation. While evidence comparing these methods is sparse, studies suggest that an open reduction with buttress plating provides optimal biomechanical strength and may improve clinical outcomes [17]. The clinical results of buttress plating versus screw fixation are limited and varied, with one study showing superior clinical outcomes with buttress plating [18] and

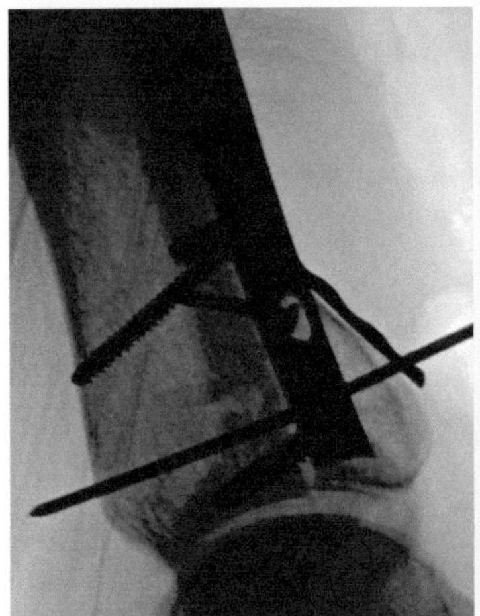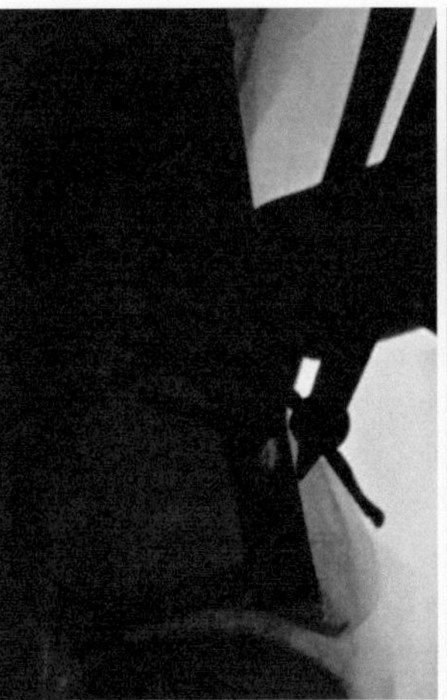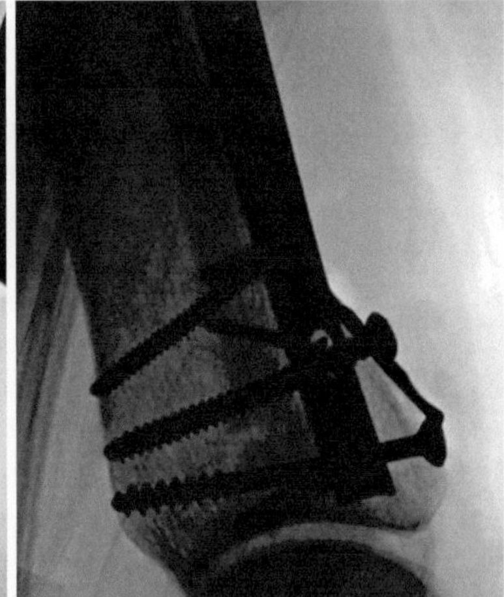

Fig. 4 Note the proximal position of the posterior malleolus with diastasis and incongruity of the joint surface. A ball spike pusher is used to push the fragment distally and the articular surface is compressed using a posterior to anterior lag screw outside of the buttress plate

another demonstrating no significant difference between the two constructs [19]. In practice, choice of construct is likely of little significance provided that syndesmotic stability and articular congruity are securely restored.

6 Outcomes

In general, the presence of a posterior malleolus fracture and/or trimalleolar patterns portend a worse functional outcome compared to unimalleolar and bimalleolar patterns regardless of whether the fragment is fixed [20–22]. This was further demonstrated in a study comparing patients with PM fracture to those with unstable ankle fractures lacking a PM component. The authors used American Orthopaedic Foot and Ankle Society (AOFAS), Short Musculoskeletal Function Assessment (SMFA) and Short Form-36 (SF-36) scores to compare 54 patients with PM fracture to 255 patients without PM fracture. The results showed patients with a posterior malleolar component had significantly worse pain and lower ankle scores at 1-year post-op, although this difference did not maintain significance at 2-years post-op [23]. A systematic review of long-term outcomes in surgically managed ankle fractures showed only 58% of patients with trimalleolar ankle fractures achieved "good or excellent" results at 4-years post-op compared to 92.2% in those with uni- or bimalleolar ankle fractures [24].

The effect of posterior malleolus fragment size has been well studied, and there is modest agreement that increasing size is associated with worse outcome. One study shows that fixing PM fragments ≥25% in size results in better AOFAS scores, although this was not statistically significant [25]. In a separate study, improved function was demonstrated with fixation of the PM fragment compared to those which were indirectly reduced by fixation of the fibula, but without PM fixation. The average size of those which were fixed was 25.2% while those which were unfixed were about 16.1% of the articular surface, suggesting that fragments smaller than 25% may still impart a deleterious effect [23]. Several

studies show that fixing fragments as small as 5–10% of articular surface results in improved long-term outcomes [14, 20, 26–28], which has led some authors to recommend fixing all PM fragments, regardless of size, except small posterior lip avulsions [14, 28]. These clinical findings regarding fragment size are supported by biomechanical studies discussed earlier in this chapter [4–7].

When there is persistent posterior subluxation of the talus, instability of the syndesmosis, or loss of articular reduction despite adequate bimalleolar reduction and fixation, then reduction and fixation of the posterior malleolus fragment may lead to better reduction of the articular surface and restoration of syndesmotic stability. Miller et al. compared the following three constructs in trimalleolar ankle fractures: fibular plating with syndesmotic screws, PM fixation with fibular plating, and PM fixation with fibular plating and syndesmotic screws. There was no significant difference in functional outcomes, although PM fixation with fibular plating (no syndesmotic screws) more accurately restored the articular surface and syndesmotic stability than those constructs including syndesmotic screw fixation. The authors concluded that posterior malleolus fixation without syndesmotic screws was noninferior to constructs utilizing syndesmotic screws and avoided the complications and morbidity associated with syndesmotic screws (malreduction, breakage, screw removal) [14]. This is supported by a biomechanical study showing improved syndesmotic stability with PM fixation [11]. Finally, fixation of the posterior malleolus was shown to yield articular reduction with less than 1 mm step off in 90% of cases [29].

Literature investigating the effect of posterior malleolus fixation on long-term function is difficult to critically evaluate due to lack of consistent functional outcome measures. A retrospective review of 38 patients demonstrated "good to excellent" AOFAS scores (> 80 points) when the PM fragment was fixed, and only one patient developed clinically significant post-traumatic ankle arthritis. Unfortunately, this study did not include a "no-fixation" cohort for comparison [29]. A large, albeit dated, study of 306 ankle fractures, 64 of which included PM fractures, showed a high (14%) incidence of post-traumatic ankle arthritis and decreased function regardless of fracture pattern. All posterior malleolus fragments were fixed. Interestingly, functionally limiting post-traumatic arthritis was significantly more common among cases with surface-bearing posterior fragments (34%) than in cases with small posterior fragments (17%) and without posterior fragments (4%) despite fixation of all posterior fragments [30]. This finding was reproduced in a later study demonstrating worse functional outcome with PM fragments >33% despite "perfect" reduction and fixation [31]. Overall, no studies demonstrate profound functional improvement with plate fixation of posterior malleolus fractures despite literature supporting superior biomechanical and radiographic results.

References

1. Hermans JJ, Beumer A, de Jong TA, et al. Anatomy of the distal tibiofibular syndesmosis in adults: a pictorial essay with a multimodality approach. J Anat. 2010;216(6):633–45.
2. Sarrfian SK, Kelikian AS: Osteology, in Kelikian AS, Sarrafian SK: Sarrafian's anatomy of the foot and ankle: descriptive, topographic and functional. Philadelphia, PA. Lippincott Williams & Wilkins, 2011; p 40–48.
3. Ogilvie-Harris DJ, Reed SC, Hedman TP. Disruption of the ankle syndesmosis: biomechanical study of ligamentous restraints. Arthroscopy. 1994;10(5):558–60.
4. Macko VW, Matthews LS, Zwirkoski P, Goldstein SA. The joint-contact area of the ankle: the contribution of the posterior malleolus. J Bone Joint Surg Am. 1991;73(3):347–51.
5. Hartford JM, Gorczyca JT, McNamara JL, Mayor MB. Tibiotalar contact area: contribution of the posterior malleolus and deltoid ligament. Clin Orthop Relat Res. 1995;320:182–7.
6. Scheidt KB, Stiehl JB, Skrade DA, Barnhardt T. Posterior malleolar ankle fractures: an in vitro biomechanical analysis of stability in the loaded and unloaded states. J Orthop Trauma. 1992;6(1):96–101.
7. van den Bekerom MP, Haverkamp D, Kloen P. Biomechanical and clinical evaluation of posterior malleolar fractures. A systematic review of the literature. J Trauma. 2009;66(1):279–84.
8. De Vries JS, Wijgman AJ, Sierevelt IN, Schaap GR. Long-term results of ankle fractures with a posterior malleolar fragment. J Foot Ankle Surg. 2005;44(3):211–7.
9. White TO, Bugler KE. Ankle fractures. In: Court-Brown CM, Heckman JD, MM MQ, et al., editors. Rockwood and Green's fractures in adults. Philadelphia, PA: Wolters Kluwer Health; 2014. p. 2542–91.
10. Berkes MB, Little MT, Lazaro LE. Articular congruity is associated with short-term clinical outcomes of operatively treated SER IV ankle fractures. J Bone Joint Surg Am. 2013;95(19):1769–75.
11. Gardner MJ, Brodsky A, Briggs SM, Nielson JH, Lorich DG. Fixation of posterior malleolar fractures provides greater syndesmotic stability. Clin Orthop Relat Res. 2006;447:165–71.
12. Gardner MJ, Demetrakopoulos D, Briggs SM, et al. Malreduction of the tibiofibular syndesmosis in ankle fractures. Foot Ankle Int. 2006;27(10):788–92.
13. Irwin TA, Lien J, Kadakia AR. Posterior malleolus fracture. J Am Acad Orthop Surg. 2013;21(1):32–40.
14. Miller AN, Carroll EA, Parker RJ, et al. Posterior malleolar stabilization of syndesmotic injuries is equivalent to screw fixation. Clin Orthop Relat Res. 2010;468(4):1129–35.
15. Gardner MJ, Streubel PN, McCormick JJ, et al. Surgeon practices regarding operative treatment of posterior malleolus fractures. Foot Ankle Int. 2001;32(4):385–93.
16. Abdelgawad AA, Kadous A, Kanlic E. Posterolateral approach for treatment of posterior malleolus fracture of the ankle. Foot Ankle Int. 2001;50:607–11.
17. Huber M, Stutz PM, Gerber C. Open reduction and internal fixation of the posterior malleolus with a posterior antiglide plate using a postero-lateral approach—a preliminary report. J Foot Ankle Surg. 1996;2:95–103.
18. TJ OC, Mueller B, Ly TV, et al. "A to P" screw versus posterolateral plate for posterior malleolus fixation in trimalleolar ankle fractures. J Orthop Trauma. 2015;29(4):151–6.
19. Erdem MN, Erken HY, Burc H, et al. Comparison of lag screw versus buttress plate fixation of posterior malleolar fractures. Foot Ankle Int. 2014;35(10):1022–30.
20. Jaskulka RA, Ittner G, Schedl R. Fractures of the posterior tibial margin: their role in the prognosis of malleolar fractures. J Trauma. 1989;29(11):1565–70.
21. McDaniel WJ, Wilson FC. Trimalleolar fractures of the ankle. An end result study. Clin Orthop Relat Res. 1977;122:37–45.
22. Mingo-Robinet J, Lopez-Duran L, Galeote JE, et al. Ankle fractures with posterior malleolar fragment: management and results. J Foot Ankle Surg. 2011;50(2):141–5.
23. Tejwani NC, Pahk B, Egol KA. Effect of posterior malleolus fractures on outcome after unstable ankle fracture. J Trauma. 2010;69(3):666–9.
24. Stufkens SA, van den Bekerom MP, Kerkhoffs GM, et al. Long-term outcome after 1822 operatively treated ankle fractures: a systematic review of the literature. Injury. 2011;42(2):119–27.
25. Evers J, Barz L, Wähnert D, et al. Size matters: the influence of the posterior fragment on patient

outcomes in trimalleolar ankle fractures. Injury. 2015;S109-113:S109.

26. Harper MC, Hardin G. Posterior malleolar fractures of the ankle associated with external rotation-abduction injuries: results with and without internal fixation. J Bone Joint Surg Am. 1988;70(9):1348–56.

27. Langenhuijsen JF, Heetveld MJ, Ultee JM, et al. Results of ankle fractures with involvement of the posterior tibial margin. J Trauma. 2002;53(1):55–60.

28. Heim UP. Trimalleolar fractures: late results after fixation of the posterior tibial margin. Orthopedics. 1989;12(8):1053–9.

29. Roukun H, Ming X, Zhihong X, et al. Postoperative radiographic and clinical assessment of the treatment of posterior Tibial plafond fractures using a posterior lateral incisional approach. J Foot Ankle Surg. 2014;53(6):678–82.

30. Lindsjo U. Operative treatment of ankle fracture dislocations. A follow-up study of 306/321 consecutive cases. Clin Orthop Relat Res. 1985;199:28–38.

31. Broos PL, Bisschop AP. Operative treatment of ankle fractures in adults: correlation between types of fracture and final results. Injury. 1991;22:403–6.

Management of Fractures of the Tibial Plafond

Florence Unno and Sean E. Nork

1 Introduction

Fractures involving the weight-bearing surface of the distal tibia are among the most challenging injuries treated by orthopedic surgeons. The combination of soft tissue swelling, limited access for visualization during reduction, and intolerance of the joint to malreduction conspire to challenge the surgeon. There is no consistent algorithm which can be globally applied to these injuries; a thorough understanding of the injury pattern and astute choice of surgical tactics are required to minimize complications. This chapter will discuss the evaluation of the injury, common injury patterns, surgical strategies, and outcomes associated with fractures of the tibial plafond.

2 Anatomy and Mechanism of Injury

Fractures of the ankle and the associated anatomy have been studied in previous chapters. Many of the described principles can be applied to pilon fractures. In particular, the importance of ligamentous attachments and their contribution to the stability of the ankle are applicable to articular fractures of the distal tibia. Additionally, several ankle fracture injuries represent transitional patterns: their overall treatment may relate to pilon fractures rather than malleolar injuries.

This chapter is dedicated to details pertaining to specific pilon injury patterns. However, an understanding of the common mechanisms and applied forces resulting in all pilon fractures is important for overall planning. *Grosso modo*, pilon fractures are the result of a rotational force or an axial load, with or without an associated bending stress. Rotational forces are commonly associated with lower energy patterns, with milder soft tissue compromise and articular impaction; they are generally easier to manage. They are often observed to occur in sporting activities. A spiral distal tibial diaphyseal or metaphyseal fracture with an articular extension is typical. An associated spiral fracture of the fibula, at variable levels of the bone, is commonly observed.

Axial loading injuries are often associated with significant soft tissue swelling or open wounds, articular impaction, shortening, and comminution, both at the articular surface and at the distal tibial metaphysis. These are often complete articular injuries (OTA/AO type C) and present numerous challenges to the treating physician. Axial injuries are most often due to falls from height or motor vehicle crashes [1].

Supination adduction ankle injuries represent a transitional pattern between a typical bimalleo-

F. Unno · S. E. Nork (✉)
University of Washington, Seattle, WA, USA
e-mail: unno@uw.edu; nork@uw.edu

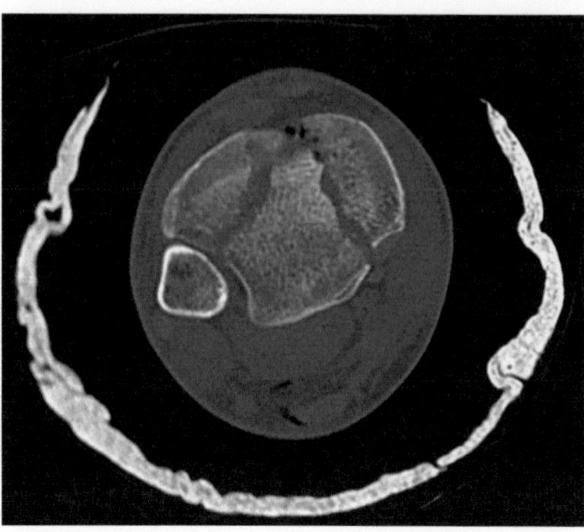

Fig. 1 The "classic" articular patterns of a complete articular injury are demonstrated on this axial CT image of a right pilon. The primary ligamentous attachments to these fragments are the deltoid (medial segment), anterior tibiofibular ligament (Chaput fragment), and the posterior inferior tibio-fibular ligament (Volkmann's fragment). Accurate and stable restoration of these fragments often results in overall ankle joint and syndesmotic stability

lar ankle fracture and a partial articular pilon fracture.

The ankle joint presents very little inherent osseus stability given the relatively unconstrained relationship between the talus, the tibia, and the fibula. Understanding the ligamentous attachments between these structures is essential in order to restore stability. Interestingly, the deltoid, anterior tibiofibular and postero-inferior tibiofibular ligaments are rarely torn in complete articular fractures. Instead, their tibial osseous attachments typically displace. Consequently, reestablishing the anatomy of these specific fracture fragments restores ankle joint stability (See Fig. 1).

3　History, Physical Examination, and Imaging

3.1　History

The mechanism of injury as well as the patient history and co-morbidities are important when formulating a plan of care. Rotational and lower energy fractures, which are commonly associated with mild soft-tissue swelling and simple fracture patterns for both tibia and fibula, may be amenable to early definitive fixation. Higher energy injuries, associated with articular and metaphyseal comminution, soft tissue swelling and possibly open wounds, may require a staged approach, intensive planning, and complex fixation strategies.

Patients' comorbidities such as osteoporosis, diabetes, nicotine use, and peripheral vascular disease may significantly impact prognosis by affecting fracture fixation and soft tissue healing. Patients' compliance with extended periods of protected weight-bearing and intense rehabilitation is key in the treatment of these difficult injuries. Goals and expectations should be discussed and adjusted to each patient.

3.2　Physical Examination

Circumferential inspection is necessary to appreciate open wounds and deformities in all planes. Sites of pressure on the skin due to fracture displacement or angular deformity should be expeditiously relieved with limb repositioning and appropriate splinting. Fracture blisters are a common finding, especially in fractures due to high energy mechanisms and those presenting significant swelling. They potentially affect the choice of surgical approaches. A careful neurological and vascular evaluation is important, with documentation of distal pulses, capillary refill time, and sensorimotor function in all nerve distributions.

3.3　Imaging

Initial evaluation consists of biplanar tibial radiographs and three views of the ankle. These images help understanding the vector of displacement in the coronal and sagittal planes, the coronal plane angular deformity and the amount of shortening. Postreduction radiographs demonstrate the position of the talus relative to the tibia. Fractures patterns which fail in varus tend to be associated with a transverse fibular fracture, while comminuted fibular fractures are seen in injuries presenting a valgus deformity [2]. This has significant implications for surgical planning, as the location of plating is dictated by the need to resist the angular deformity. Fracture patterns liable to fail into varus require a medial buttress plate. In the OTA/AO classification, pilon fractures are typically classified as partial articular (43B) or complete articular (43C) fractures; this is relevant for preoperative planning. The fibular bone presents many anatomic variants, and contralateral (uninjured) ankle radiographs may be useful. AP views furthermore help in evaluating the articular contour as well as the anterior distal tibial angle.

Computed tomography scans are necessary in virtually all pilon fractures. The axial, sagittal, and coronal images identify articular and metaphyseal comminution, zones of articular impaction, articular displacement, osseous fragments which may block reduction, entrapped structures, and bone loss. Identifying the classically seen fracture fragments features help surgical planning [3, 4]. The timing for obtaining CT scan imaging depends on the overall treatment strategy. In some patterns, especially those with proximal metaphyseal or diaphyseal extension where an early proximal posteromedial approach may be part of a staged surgical plan, a post reduction injury CT is helpful to ensure that the fracture extension proximally allows early reduction through a limited approach [5]. Similarly, if early total operative care of the pilon is planned, an injury CT is critical. If a staged approach is planned, CT is typically obtained after placement of the external fixator to minimize cost and radiation exposure for the patient. While entrapment of the posteromedial neurovascular structures is uncommon, early advanced imaging may be necessary [6].

4 Timing and Initial Management

The following is the most important statement of the chapter: *treatment decisions made initially affect all subsequent aspects of the strategy for surgical care of a pilon fracture.*

Several key decisions must be considered on day 1. This itemized list should be addressed:

- Will the patient be referred to another institution for definitive operative care.
- Do the soft tissues allow early definitive fixation.
- Is staged management with a temporizing external fixator necessary for resolution of soft tissue swelling.
- What surgical approach(es) can be used considering the fracture pattern, the state of soft tissues and possible complicating factors (previous surgeries, traumatic open wounds, medical co-morbidities etc.).
- Should the fibula be fixed initially? Should it be fixed at all.
- Does the pattern lend itself to early partial fixation.
- In the presence of an open injury, can some part of the fixation be completed through the traumatic wound, which the intention to obtain primary wound healing and avoid reopening the traumatized skin in the future.

Proper realignment and splinting of the leg and the ankle are an essential step of the initial management. Failure to promptly relieve pressure exerted by osseous displacement or joint dislocation on the tenuous soft-tissue envelope of the leg and ankle results in exacerbation of swelling, fracture blisters, skin necrosis, neurological or vascular compromise, with potentially disastrous consequences. Radiographic confirmation of an adequate reduction is imperative. The decision to surgically manage any portion of a pilon fracture depends on the surgeon's overall expertise and comfort. According to prior reviews, some component of the primary procedure is revised in the majority of cases by the receiving surgeon when a pilon fracture is referred for definitive management after some partial surgical treatment was performed. This leads to a higher rate of overall complication when compared to injuries treated from start to finish by a single experienced surgeon. Referring physicians should communicate early with the receiving surgeon about the initial plan of care. For instance, if fixation of the fibula and/or placement of an ankle spanning external fixator are performed prior to referring the patient to another institution, site of incisions and pin placement should be discussed.

The majority of high-energy pilon fractures are managed in a staged fashion with early restoration of length followed by definitive fixation performed when the appropriate surgical approach can be safely performed [7, 8]. However, many low-energy and length-stable patterns can be definitively managed with open reduction and internal fixation within 24 to 48 h of the injury, with a low complication rate [9, 10]. Reduction is typically easier to obtain in the setting of early total care (See Fig. 2). Discomfort as well as logistical issues related to

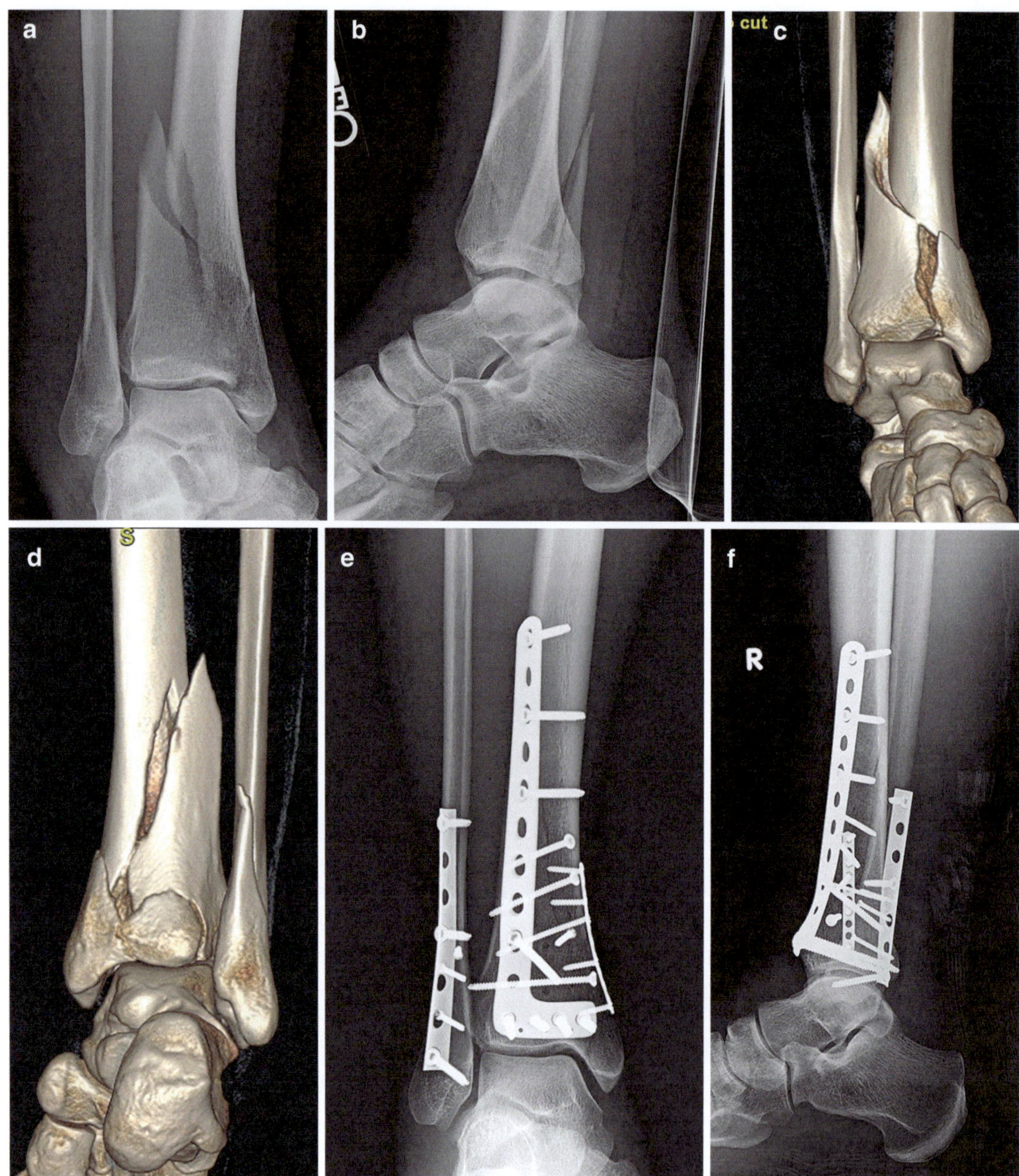

Fig. 2 This young female with no associated comorbidities sustained this low energy pilon fracture skateboarding (**a**, **b**). The 3-D CT scans demonstrate the simple torsional pilon pattern with an associated posterior malleolus fracture (**c**, **d**). The soft tissue envelope allowed definitive fixation within 24 h of injury through an extensile anteromedial approach (**e**, **f**)

external fixation and delayed treatment can be avoided.

For the length-unstable fracture patterns where soft tissues injury preclude early definitive fixation, controversy exists regarding fixation of the fibula. Although some authors have advocated against it [11], we strongly believe that the fibula can be approached in the vast majority of cases at the time of external fixation, even when soft tissues are compromised on the anterior and anteromedial leg. Early fixation of the fibula, in appropriate fracture patterns, provides precious help for anatomic reduction of the distal tibia by restoring the precise length of the fibula, improving evaluation of tibial length when applying an external fixator, restoring the position of the posterolateral fragment via the attachments of the PITFL and aligning the center the talus with the anatomic axis of the tibia. As a bonus, in complex patterns where definitive tibial fixation will likely require a significant amount of time and attention, prior completion of part of the treatment is valuable.

The choice of the surgical approach depends on several factors including fracture patterns, soft tissue compromise, associated open traumatic wounds, and comfort level of the surgeon. While the vast majority of pilon fractures can be addressed through a single surgical incision, some patterns may require multiple approaches. The surgeon must balance the benefits associated with additional strategic buttressing with the possible biological cost. We recommend envisaging all possible surgical approaches at the time of initial management, as the final choice might change after CT imaging brings further understanding of the fracture pattern.

Some fractures are optimally treated by addressing the extra-articular components early and anatomically reduce the proximal metaphyseal or diaphyseal fracture extensions. Early partial fixation is particularly useful when fractures of the articular surface extend proximally with a long spiral or oblique noncomminuted fracture. In this circumstance, a proximal posteromedial or anterolateral approach can allow anatomic reduction and fixation, accurately restoring one of the columns of the pilon [5].

This strategy further assists realignment of the talus beneath the anatomic axis of the tibia when placing the external fixator, helps to minimize skin swelling by controlling fracture fragments and eliminates the need to revisit the proximal fracture line at the time of definitive fixation See Fig. 3.

Traumatic open wounds associated with pilon fractures represent a significant complicating factor. They also can be viewed as an opportunity. The open wound typically represents a tension failure of the skin which mirrors the tension failure of the bone: reduction of the fracture at that site will likely decrease stress on the compromised soft tissues. Since exposure of the open wound is necessary for the initial surgical debridement, the underlying fragment may be reduced and stabilized using low-profile implants which present small surface areas for bacterial adhesion. Implants should be placed over the periosteum to minimize the biological footprint. This avoids the need for future exposure of the traumatized skin. Careful soft tissue management often is a powerful tool and even in open pilon fractures, the requirement of plastic surgery intervention for coverage should remain an exception.

In summary, the principles guiding initial surgical management are:

- Definitive immediate fixation by an experience surgeon in low energy patterns.
- Temporizing external fixation when early definitive treatment is not possible, keeping in mind that the initial goals in a staged approach are restoration of length, centering of the talus beneath the anatomic axis of the tibia and resolution of swelling by minimizing pressure on the skin.
- Planning all anticipated surgical approaches.
- Fixation of proximal extensions of fracture lines when appropriate (preferably using an approach which can be extended at the time of definitive surgery).
- Accurate reduction and fixation of the fibula when appropriate.
- Use of open traumatic wounds for reduction when possible.

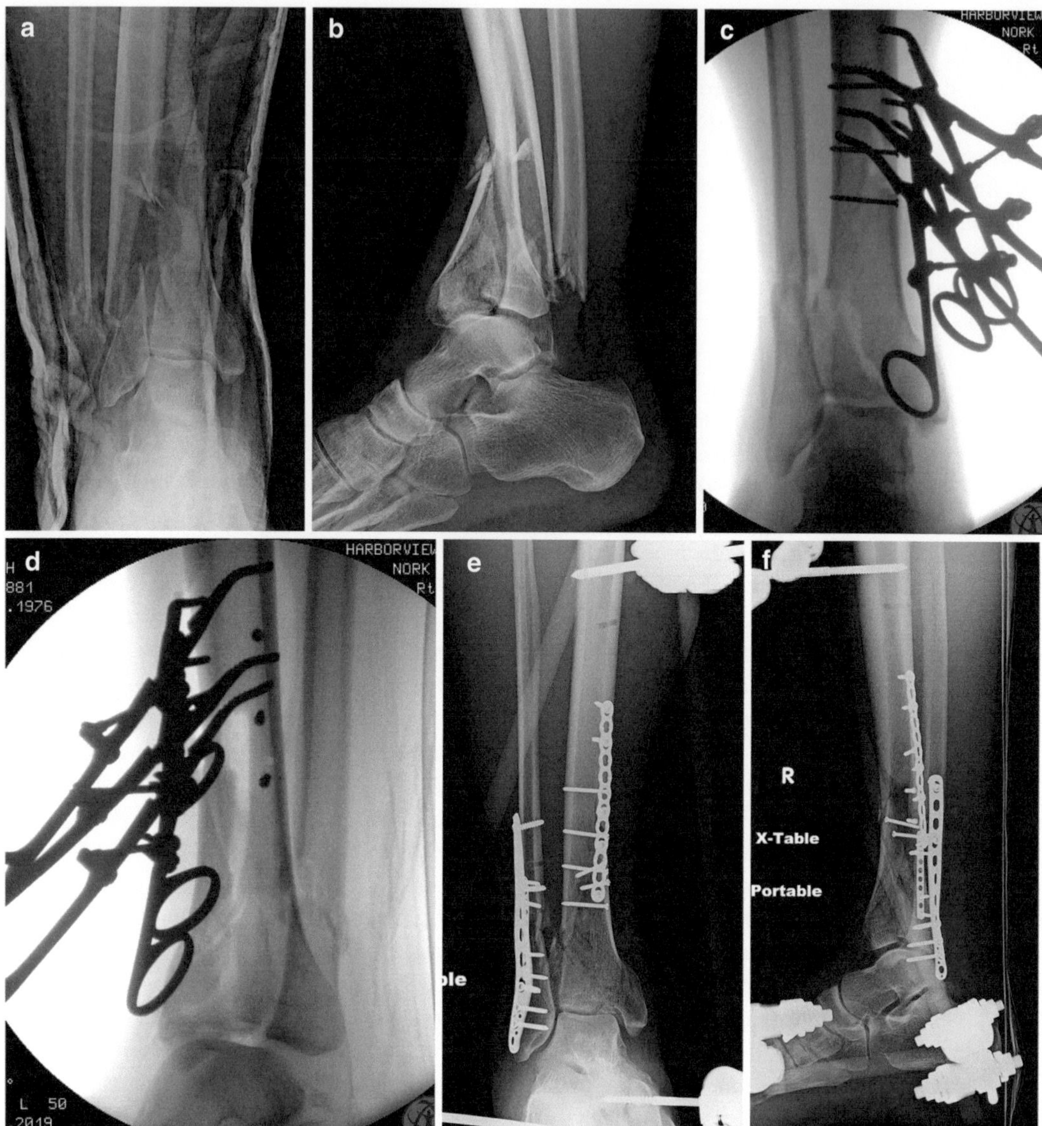

Fig. 3 Injury radiographs of a complete articular pilon with proximal extension of the fracture (**a**, **b**). On the date of injury, a posteromedial approach was performed to allow fixation of the diaphyseal extension (**c**, **d**), followed by fibular fixation through a posterolateral approach and placement of an ankle spanning external fixator (**e**, **f**). Several weeks later the soft tissue swelling had resolved to allow definitive fixation of the remaining (now) partial articular pilon through an anteromedial approach (**g**, **h**)

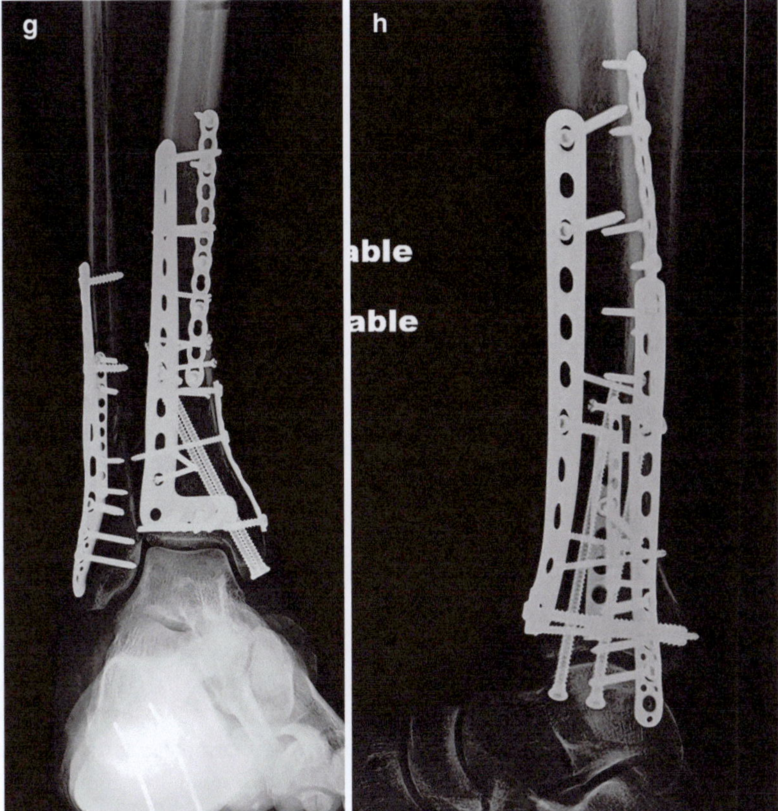

Fig. 3 (continued)

5 Surgical Details

5.1 Fixation of Fibula

The surgical approach for fibular fixation should be posterior to the posterolateral border of the fibula, in order to minimize soft tissue complications and to maximize the skin bridge between this approach and a potential anterolateral or anteromedial approach. In the rare circumstance where the surgeon needs to approach the pilon through a posterolateral approach, the fibular approach can be extended proximally to expose the interval between the peroneal tendons and flexor hallucis longus.

The size and location of the implant for fibular fixation are variable. Tension failure patterns of the fibula (varus patterns and supination adduction ankle injuries resulting in transverse fracture lines) can be addressed with a retrograde medullary screw which compresses the fracture plane [12]. Plating is also an option. It offers a more accurate reduction and enhanced rotational stability. For rotational pilon fractures with an associated spiral Weber B fibular fracture, low profile nonlocking implants using the principles described for ankle fractures apply. For higher fibular fractures and those presenting significant comminution, precontoured or stiffer implants may offer some advantages. Locking implants are rarely required but can be considered in patients with compromised bone quality or in the presence of segmental comminution with a short distal segment.

5.2 External Fixation

Some basic tenets applicable to pilon fractures deserve mention. The external fixator pins should be placed out of the "zone of injury." Although a recent study failed to demonstrate an increased rate of infection when placement of pins overlapped with the location of future plating [13], logic dictates that this practice certainly doesn't lower infection rates, and the pins should be placed at a distance from the anticipated location of implants. Furthermore, placing the pins in proximity to the ankle joint with the goal to optimize the biomechanics of the joint is likely superfluous when providing a temporary stabilization. External fixator pins into the talar neck should be avoided as future surgical approaches are likely to include the neck of the talus. Pins in the calcaneus should be located posterior and inferior to an imaginary line drawn between the Achilles insertion and the plantar tuberosity in order to avoid injury to the calcaneal branches of the tibial nerve. As the delay between placement of the external fixator and definitive fixation is unpredictable, the surgeon must decide how to best avoid an equinus contraction of the ankle or of the forefoot. To maintain the foot in a neutral plantigrade position, pins at the first and fifth metatarsal bones or a transverse pin at the midfoot should be considered. Alternatively, a well-padded posterior plaster splint can be used.

5.3 Surgical Approaches

Numerous surgical approaches are available for fixation of pilon fractures. The optimal access is dictated by the fracture pattern, the planned location of the implants, and the condition of the soft tissues [14]. The ideal surgical approach cannot always be safely performed due to open traumatic rounds, resolving blisters, or previous surgical approaches. The ultimate choice of approach(es) aims to optimize reduction of the fracture and strategic buttressing, whilst minimizing insult to the soft tissues. This decision requires significant experience on the part of the surgeon. The main surgical approaches include the direct anterior, anteromedial, anterolateral, posterolateral, posteromedial, and direct lateral approaches. While small incisions can be placed medially and distally to allow for placement of a buttressing implant, an extensile direct medial approach should be avoided. The majority of pilon fractures can be addressed through a single approach. However, the judicious use of simultaneous or sequential incisions might be necessary in more complex patterns. If a lateral or, preferably a posterolateral approach is used for early fixation of an associated fibular fracture, a definitive anterolateral or anteromedial approach can be safely added, even if the arbitrary 7 cm skin bridge is not available [15].

The anteromedial approach has been well described: it is extensile and allows for visualization of both the extra-articular cortical reduction reads and the articular surface [16]. The vast majority of complete articular, anterior partial articular, and medial partial articular (supination adduction ankle variants) patterns can be approached through this exposure. The incision is placed approximately 1 cm lateral to the crest of the tibia over the anterior compartment and extends distally past the ankle joint. At the ankle joint, the incision can be curved medially at a 110° angle and terminates 1 cm distal to the tip of the medial malleolus. Alternatively, it can be more gently curved toward the medial cuneiform. Undermining the medial skin flap over the anteromedial face of the tibia should be avoided. The tibialis anterior tendon sheath should not be violated throughout the surgical procedure. An arthrotomy medial to the anterior tibialis tendon can be performed to allow direct access to the articular surface for reduction. This approach allows reduction and plating on the anterolateral, anterior, and medial distal tibia. Whenever possible, maintain periosteal layers on the bone fragments by not using elevators directly on the bone, and by placing implants extra-perioteally. Closure is a critical step and must include repair of the arthrotomy, the extensor retinaculum and the anterior compartment fascia along the length of the incision. The skin closure should avoid any tension to the skin: a modified Allgower-Donati suture technique has been shown to be potentially beneficial in animal and clinical studies [17, 18] See Fig. 4.

The anterolateral approach has been well described [19–21]. It allows exposure and fixation of most anterior and anterolateral pilons as well as many complete articular patterns. The

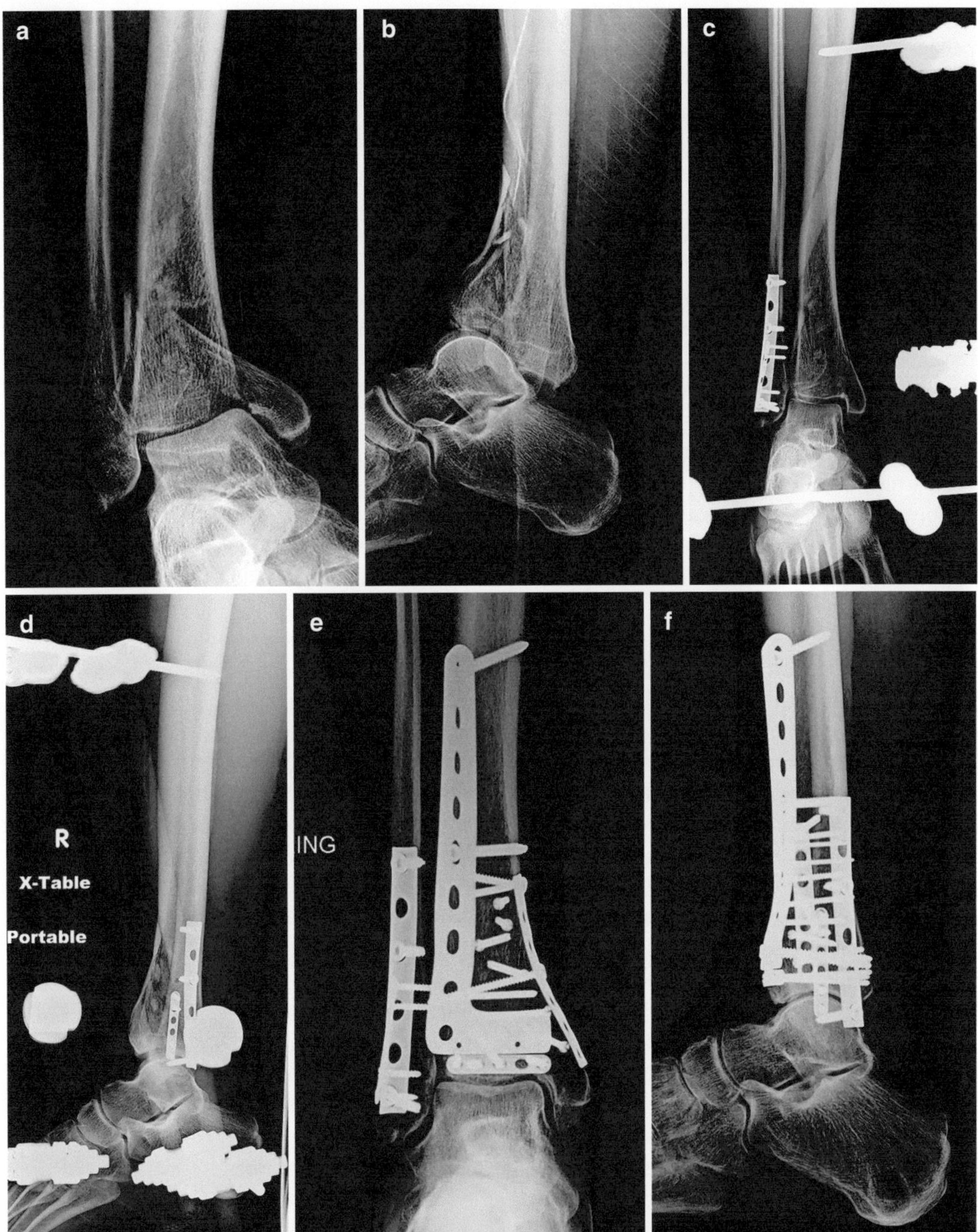

Fig. 4 These injury radiographs demonstrate an anterior and medial partial articular injury with significant shortening and varus (**a**, **b**). Given the associated soft tissue swelling, the patient underwent early fibular fixation combined with external fixation (**c**, **d**) followed by definitive fixation 11 days later. Healing progressed and is confirmed at 1 year (**e**, **f**)

visualization of the medial shoulder joint impaction is limited. This surgical exposure does not permit medial buttressing in varus patterns, although a medial implant can be placed through a small additional incision over the medial malleolus and slid subcutaneously. For valgus patterns with tension failure of the medial tibia, fixation with smaller implants (medial column screws, low profile plates) may be appropriate. This can be safely performed through a separate and limited direct medial approach. The anterolateral approach is typically placed in line with the fourth metatarsal bone. The incision is placed approximately 7 cm proximal to the ankle joint and extends distally lateral to the talo-navicular joint. Branches of the superficial peroneal nerve travel from lateral proximally to dorsal distally; they are invariably encountered and must be protected. The distal extensor retinaculum can be incised to allow medial retraction of the anterior compartment. Alternatively, deep exposure is performed lateral to the extensor retinaculum, avoiding violation of the anterior compartment tendons. The location of the arthrotomy is dictated by the level of the fracture into the joint. Closure must include repair of the extensor retinaculum to avoid bow-stringing of the tendons.

The posterolateral approach is identical to the one used for fixation of the posterior malleolus in complex ankle fracture patterns and has been described in previous chapters. An isolated posterolateral approach is rarely used for complete articular pilon patterns given the high rate of complications observed with this strategy [22]. The posterolateral approach is useful for partial articular posterior pilon patterns [23]. It can also be used to address the posterolateral component of some complete articular patterns [24–26]. A posterolateral approach is more forgiving for soft tissues: if combined exposures are planned, it can often be performed in the initial phase of care, while the remaining components of the pilon might be addressed later through an anterior exposure. The incision can be placed slightly posterior to the posterolateral border of the fibula, closer towards the Achilles tendon, whether or not fibular fixation is planned through the same surgical approach. The sural nerve is potentially

at risk and should be protected. Deep dissection exploits the interval between the peroneal muscles and the flexor hallucis longus. The location of the peroneal vessels and the associated branches has been well described, and a careful deep dissection can protect them [27]. Since direct visualization of the articular surface is not typically possible through a posterior arthrotomy, reduction is guided by the extra-articular cortical reduction reads and the judicious use of C-arm. Access to impaction and free osseus fragments is possible through the fracture of the posterior malleolus and should be performed cranial to caudal.

The posteromedial approach is typically used as an adjunct to other surgical approaches for some complete articular patterns and posterior partial articular fractures [23, 24, 28, 29]. The skin incision is longitudinal and is placed between the posterior border of the tibia and the Achilles tendon. Deep dissection is dictated by the location of the fracture: it can exploit the interval between the tibia and the posterior tibial tendon (limited distally due to the tendon sheath attachments to the tibia behind the medial malleolus); between the posterior tibial tendon and the tendon of flexor digitorum longus; between the latter and the neurovascular bundle or between the bundle and the tendon of flexor hallucis longus. The modified posteromedial approach using an incision just medial to Achilles has been shown to allow for wide exposure of the posterior tibia, with less traction on the flap and the neurovascular bundle [28]. Multiple deep intervals can be used for reduction and fixation through a single skin incision in the posteromedial approach. Similar to the posterolateral approach, direct articular visualization is typically not performed through this approach. More proximally, the interval between the posteromedial border of the tibia and the tibial posterior tendon can be used in patterns including proximal extensions of the posterior articular segment. This more proximal but limited posteromedial exposure can be combined with other anterior exposures, either simultaneously or sequentially.

The direct lateral approach has been well described. It is extensile and allows for visualization, reduction, and fixation of anterior pilon and complete articular pilon patterns [30]. The incision is placed along the anterior border of the fibula. The superficial peroneal nerve must be protected. The anterior compartment is carefully dissected off the anterior fibula, the interosseus membrane, and the anterior tibia, taking care to protect the anterior tibio-fibular ligaments distally. This approach allows for simultaneous access to the fibula and the tibia and can be combined with percutaneous medial plating techniques.

5.4 Reduction Techniques

The need to concurrently perform the reduction of both the extra-articular components of the fracture as well as their extensions into the joint and address articular impaction represents the true challenge in the surgical management of tibia pilon fractures. Visualization is critical and should include articular fragments through an arthrotomy if an anteromedial or anterolateral surgical exposure is used. Length and alignment can be obtained with distraction using either the external fixator or a femoral distractor. Distraction helps visualize the joint and reestablish proper length as well as coronal and sagittal alignment. The previously placed external fixator can be safely prepped at the time of definitive surgery and used intraoperatively [31]. The external fixation is also useful if acute definitive fixation is performed. Typically, building from "knowns" to "less knowns" is used. In complete articular injuries, reduction of one of the columns (posterior, medial, or anterior) is typically performed first, and the remaining portions of the articular reduction are sequentially built on the restored column. The order of reduction is variable and depends on the fracture pattern, surgical approach, and complexity of the articular injury [14, 20]. In general, for complete articular injuries approached through an anterior exposure (either anterolateral or anteromedial), the posterior and/or posterolateral fragments are reduced first relative to the intact distal tibial diaphysis or metaphysis. The medial column is then reduced before the articular impaction is addressed. Finally, the anterior or anterolateral articular segments are reduced. This allows for sequential visualization from the posterior articular segments to the anterior segments. In complex patterns, the surgeon should be prepared to revise the order of sequence and repeat reduction maneuvers.

In partial articular pilon patterns, one of the columns is by definition intact. The remaining joint fragments can be reduced to this intact column. However, impaction on the leading edge of the "intact" column is frequently seen, particularly in anterior and medial partial articular injuries. They require reduction prior to building back the remaining displaced articular fragments, using techniques with osteotomes and Freer elevators to elevate the displaced impacted fragments with bone grafting (autograft or a bone graft substitute) which have been well described [32–34].

In simple patterns, reduction and fixation can be tightly linked. In more complex patterns, sequential reduction and provisional fixation with clamps and smooth Kirschner wires is often necessary prior to committing to definitive fixation.

5.5 Fixation Strategies

As a general rule, the fixation of a pilon fracture should accomplish several goals simultaneously: compression of the reduced articular surface and stable fixation of the columns of the tibial pilon to avoid future angular deformity. In most patterns, the reduced articular segment can be accurately reduced to the intact tibia using direct visual and/or radiographic assessments. However, in fracture patterns with cortical bone loss, segmentally comminuted fractures and fractures with metaphyseal impaction, bridge plating may be necessary. Regardless, the goal is to accurately reduce any angulation or translation in the axial, coronal, and sagittal planes. Direct visualization of the articular surface is necessary given the inaccuracy of intraoperative lateral radiographs when appreciating articular reduction [35].

Once reduced, the articular segments are ideally compressed with independent lag screws placed through a small plate functioning as a washer or through the definitive plating construct. Plates are intelligently placed to prevent shortening or angulation. Frequently, these plates function as a buttress. In general, varus failure pilons benefit from medial buttress plating and valgus failure pilons benefit from anterolateral buttress plating [2] See Fig. 5. A combination of low-profile medial and anterolateral plates placed with minimal soft tissue dissection can be used to prevent future displacement. Currently available medial and anterolateral plates do not adequately stabilize all components of the articular injury in complete articular fractures [36]. In most cases, non-locking implants can be used and have been shown to have a lower rate of nonunion [1, 37, 38]. Importantly, medial column fixation, either with medial column screws [39] or strategic buttress plating, is associated with fewer complications [1, 38]. Although single plates are associated with more callus formation, dual plating have been shown to allow better healing at 6 months in complete articular patterns [40]. Furthermore, the use of stiffer implants, with decreased callus formation, have been associated with better maintenance of the coronal plane reduction [41].

5.6 Complicating Factors

Numerous factors complicate the management of fractures of the tibial plafond. They include, but are not limited to, associated open traumatic wounds, bone loss, associated syndesmotic injuries, articular impaction, metaphyseal or diaphyseal comminution, articular comminution, poor bone quality, and small articular fragments.

Open traumatic wounds are associated with a higher risk of infection and may hinder the ideal surgical approach. Transverse medial open wounds might violate the surgical approaches, constraining the choices for definitive reduction and fixation. As previously mentioned, in order to minimize the need for secondary soft tissue coverage, fixation using low-profile implants through the open wound can be considered during the initial debridement. Gustillo type III-B open injuries, while quite rare in pilon fractures, are difficult to manage and require a multidisciplinary coordinated approach.

Bone loss in open injuries can make an accurate reduction daunting. Fibular fixation can be used to guide restoration of the overall length and assessment of an intact column when present. Non-segmental bone loss can be managed with an antibiotic cement spacer (in addition to plate fixation) followed by delayed bone grafting. Segmental bone loss often requires a similar approach but assessing the reduction in multiple planes is difficult [42].

Associated syndesmotic injuries requiring fixation are observed in approximately 15% of pilon fractures [38]. Given the ligamentous attachments of the anterior and posterior tibiofibular ligaments to the Chaput and Volkmann's fragments respectively, an accurate reconstruction of these articular segments is important not only to restore the joint surface but also to secure the stability of the syndesmosis. Small articular fragments can be particularly problematic but are equally important in these locations.

Articular impaction and comminution require a careful appreciation of the fracture pattern, direct visualization of the joint and infinite patience. Joint impaction is typically addressed prior to reduction of other fragments that may later obscure visualization. Again, the surgical tactic typically involves sequential reduction, starting with least visible components of the joint and working from deep to superficial layers.

Metaphyseal and diaphyseal comminution often complicates reduction of the articular components. In a minority of pilon patterns, bridge plating may be required if accurate cortical reductions along the columns of the pilon cannot be accurately assessed. Fixation of multiple columns with independent implants may be necessary [1, 38].

Poor bone quality is problematic and frustrating. However, results of ORIF reported in the literature suggest that elderly patients can be treated similarly to younger patients with better bone

Fig. 5 The coronal plane angular deformity at the time of maximum displacement is revealing and highlights the optimal plate location and function to prevent future displacement. In (**a**), the valgus pattern has a medial malleolar avulsion fracture and a comminute fibular fracture pattern. Fixation was accomplished with an anterolateral plate with minimal medial fixation (**b**). In (**c**), the varus pattern (with an open traumatic wound and bone loss) has the typical medial tibial metaphyseal comminution associated with a simple fibular fracture pattern. Medial buttress plating was used to prevent varus and healing progressed (**d**)

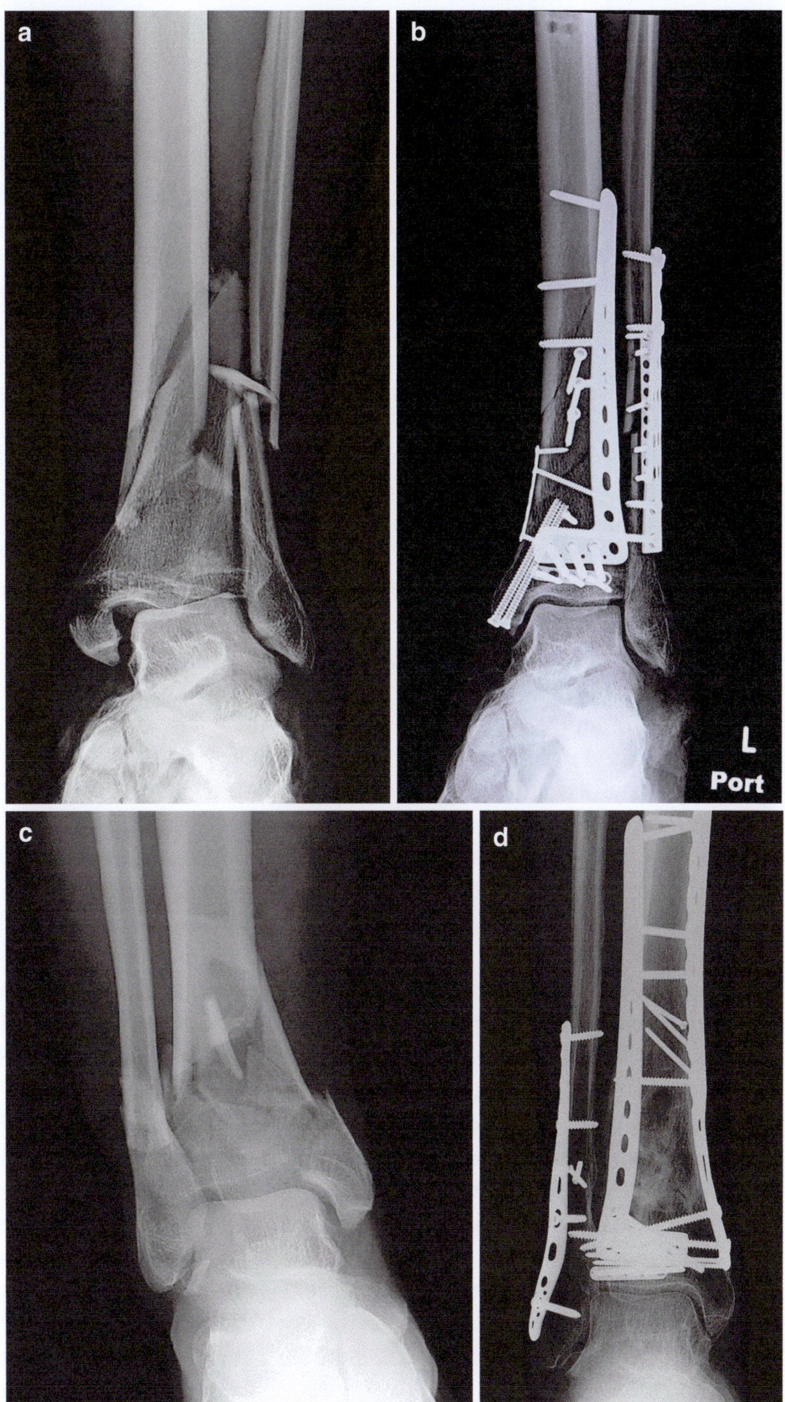

quality [33]. Overall, a strategy centered on accurate articular reduction with stable fixation can be employed in elderly patients with pilon fractures.

5.7 Specific Patterns: Supination-Adduction Ankle Injuries

Supination-adduction ankle injuries deserve a specific mention as these injury patterns represent a transitional pattern between rotational ankle injuries and partial articular pilon fractures [33, 43]. These injury patterns are characterized by combination of a transverse fibular fracture representing a tension failure with a vertical medial malleolus fracture. The latter component is associated with articular impaction and/or articular comminution at the medial distal tibia [32]. These patterns can present associated soft tissue compromise laterally over the fibula given the typical deformity in varus. Impaction of the medial tibial articular surface is often seen on the intact pillar of the distal tibia. This requires elevation of the depressed fragment in order to accurately reduce the joint. Medial buttressing with low profile implants appears to yield predictable early results, with a low incidence of infection or nonunion ([32, 38, 44, 45]).

In general, supination-adduction ankle injuries result from high energy mechanisms and are associated with a high incidence of articular impaction [32, 33, 43, 44]). The quality of fracture reduction, including the articular reduction, has been shown to be somewhat protective of osteoarthrosis [32, 33, 43]. However, the incidence of ankle degenerative disease, at relatively short follow-ups, ranges from 20 to 80% depending on the definition used for arthrosis. Despite commonly observed ankle joint arthrosis, secondary procedures in the short term are relatively uncommon.

Interestingly, the concept that supination-adduction ankle injuries represent a transitional pattern has been investigated in several recent studies [33, 43–45]. The authors observed that post-traumatic arthrosis is approximately twice as likely to occur in supination-adduction ankle injuries compared to torsional ankle injury patterns, with worse functional outcomes [44]. Another slightly larger review confirmed a high incidence of ankle arthrosis, with however a much smaller incidence of significant arthritis requiring a secondary procedure. Overall, the reported 6% incidence of failure (defined as the need for an ankle arthrodesis or arthroplasty) associated with supination-adduction ankle injuries is higher than the rate described in rotational ankle injuries (<2%) but substantially lower than the one observed in partial articular pilon fractures (12%) [33, 43]. In summary, supination-adduction ankle fractures represent a higher energy injury with overall worse results when compared with rotational ankle fractures, but an accurate articular reduction matters and can influence prognosis.

5.8 Outcomes

The outcome after surgical treatment of tibial plafond fractures is extremely variable and depends on numerous elements including patient-related factors, fracture patterns, zones of comminution, timing of fixation, fixation technique, associated soft tissue injury, presence of open wounds, bone loss, and others (1, 9, 25, 33, 43, 46–51]). Ankle joint stiffness, swelling, persistent discomfort, the need for activity modification, loss or change of employment, and ankle joint arthrosis are relatively common after these injuries. An understanding of the injury mechanism and careful planning including management of bone loss and open traumatic wounds can help minimize complications and improve outcome. Most studies have focused on relatively short-term outcomes and complications such as infection, loss of reduction, nonunion, early arthrosis. A two-decade old study by Pollak et al. still provides useful information for patient outcomes at 3 years or more after treatment of high energy tibial plafond fractures [47]. Ankle stiffness (35%), persistent pain (33%), swelling (29%), and loss of employment were reported.

Interestingly, poor overall result was associated with definitive treatment with external fixation, with or without limited internal fixation of the articular surface, as opposed to formal open reduction and internal fixation. Since this is a controlled variable, this chapter focuses on techniques and details of internal fixation.

Timing of fixation for pilon fracture remains controversial and may affect patient outcome. Decades ago, a staged approach allowing resolution of soft tissue swelling before definitive fixation [7], was shown to significantly decrease short-term rate of infection, soft tissue complications, and amputation. Other studies have suggested that early definitive fixation was possible in most fractures when evaluated and treated within a safe operative window by experienced surgeons [10]. Furthermore, a retrospective comparison study at a mean follow-up of 6 years showed improved results with primary open reduction compared to a staged approach [9]. It is our conviction that some injury patterns mostly resulting from low-energy injuries, are optimally treated with early definitive fixation, while others are best treated in a staged fashion; both the experience and expertise of the surgeon likely impact prognosis significantly.

Avoidance of complications is the "motto" when treating pilon fractures with surgery. Despite improvements in surgical techniques, the overall risk of infection in the hands of experienced surgeons remains at a dire rate of 5 to 17% [1, 9, 49]. Superficial infection may be related to surgical timing, local swelling, choice of approach, and soft tissue handling. The risk for deep infection is increased in open fractures and bone loss; in these scenarios the choice of surgical approach(es) as well as the proximity of open traumatic wounds to the incisions are determinant [49]. Nonunions have been shown to be associated with complex fracture patterns, open injuries, and bone loss [1]. Locked plates are associated with an increased risk for loss of reduction [37] and nonunion [1]. Some medial column fixation (independent column screws or plates) appears to be necessary in most complete articular pilon patterns [1]. While most studies

fail to show a relationship between surgical approach and union, Chan and co-authors reported a 40% nonunion rate when an early posterior approach to the posterior malleolus was followed by a delayed anterior approach for definitive fixation. The source of this striking nonunion rate is unclear but the study certainly underscores the importance of soft tissue handling and the possible dangers associated with multiple approaches [51].

Associated soft tissue injuries including open wounds impact outcome of pilon fractures. The incidence of compartment syndrome is surprisingly low (approximately 3%) [1] but can significantly complicate early and late management. Associated traumatic open wounds increase the complications rate [1, 9, 49]. However, good results have been reported with patient specific approaches and meticulous soft tissue handling associated with experience [1, 9, 46]. Bone loss represents a unique challenge. With defined protocols, soft tissue coverage, and delayed bone grafting good results can however be achieved [1, 9, 42, 46, 49].

Syndesmosis injuries have been reported in 15% of pilon fractures and are associated with post-traumatic arthrosis in half of the cases. A missed syndesmosis injury however, while rare, results in post-traumatic arthrosis in nearly all patients. Careful preoperative and intraoperative assessment is mandatory to minimize complications associated with syndesmotic instability [38].

In addition to avoiding early complications such as infection and nonunion, one essential goal of surgery is to minimize post-traumatic arthrosis. Once again, the quality of the reduction matters [25, 48]. Sadly however, despite efforts to optimize the reduction of the joint surface and the anatomical alignment of the distal tibia, weight-bearing CT scan imaging at 6 months demonstrate significant early joint space narrowing, especially in the lateral and central zones of the distal tibia [50]. This study did not describe the correlation between these findings and functional scores, and surgeons should strive to achieve good reduction in these difficult injuries.

References

1. Haller JM, Githens M, Rothberg D, Higgins T, Nork S, Barei D. Risk factors for Tibial plafond nonunion: medial column fixation may reduce nonunion rates. J Orthop Trauma. 2019b;33(9):443–9. https://doi.org/10.1097/BOT.0000000000001500; PMID: 31094937.
2. Busel GA, Watson JT, Israel H. Evaluation of fibular fracture type vs location of Tibial fixation of Pilon fractures. Foot Ankle Int. 2017;38(6):650–5. https://doi.org/10.1177/1071100717695348; Epub 2017 Mar 13. PMID: 28288519.
3. Cole PA, Mehrle RK, Bhandari M, Zlowodzki M. The Pilon map: fracture lines and comminution zones in OTA/AO type 43C3 Pilon fractures. J Orthop Trauma. 2013;27(7):e152–6. https://doi.org/10.1097/BOT.0b013e318288a7e9; PMID: 23360909.
4. Topliss CJ, Jackson M, Atkins RM. Anatomy of Pilon fractures of the distal tibia. J Bone Joint Surg Br. 2005;87(5):692–7. https://doi.org/10.1302/0301-620X.87B5.15982; PMID: 15855374.
5. Dunbar RP, Barei DP, Kubiak EN, Nork SE, Henley MB. Early limited internal fixation of Diaphyseal extensions in select Pilon fractures: upgrading AO/OTA type C fractures to AO/OTA type B. J Orthop Trauma. 2008;22(6):426–9. https://doi.org/10.1097/BOT.0b013e31817e49b8; PMID: 18594309.
6. Eastman JG, Firoozabadi R, Benirschke SK, Barei DP, Dunbar RP. Entrapped posteromedial structures in Pilon fractures. J Orthop Trauma. 2014;28(9):528–33. https://doi.org/10.1097/BOT.0000000000000046; PMID: 24343256.
7. Patterson MJ, Cole JD. Two-staged delayed open reduction and internal fixation of severe Pilon fractures. J Orthop Trauma. 1999;13(2):85–91. https://doi.org/10.1097/00005131-199902000-00003; PMID: 10052781.
8. Sirkin M, Sanders R, DiPasquale T, Herscovici D Jr. A staged protocol for soft tissue management in the treatment of complex Pilon fractures. J Orthop Trauma. 1999;13(2):78–84. https://doi.org/10.1097/00005131-199902000-00002; PMID: 10052780.
9. Duckworth AD, Jefferies JG, Clement ND, White TO. Type C Tibial Pilon fractures: short- and long-term outcome following operative intervention. Bone Joint J. 2016;98-B(8):1106–11. https://doi.org/10.1302/0301-620X.98B8.36400; PMID: 27482025.
10. White TO, Guy P, Cooke CJ, Kennedy SA, Droll KP, Blachut PA, O'Brien PJ. The results of early primary open reduction and internal fixation for treatment of OTA 43.C-type Tibial Pilon fractures: a cohort study. J Orthop Trauma. 2010;24(12):757–63. https://doi.org/10.1097/BOT.0b013e3181d04bc0; PMID: 21076248.
11. Kurylo JC, Datta N, Iskander KN, Tornetta P 3rd. Does the fibula need to be fixed in complex Pilon fractures? J Orthop Trauma. 2015;29(9):424–7. https://doi.org/10.1097/BOT.0000000000000304; PMID: 26295736.
12. Evans JM, Gardner MJ, Brennan ML, Phillips CJ, Henley MB, Dunbar RP. Intramedullary fixation of fibular fractures associated with Pilon fractures. J Orthop Trauma. 2010;24(8):491–4. https://doi.org/10.1097/BOT.0b013e3181eb5c4f; PMID: 20657258.
13. Dombrowsky A, Abyar E, McGwin G, Johnson M. Is definitive plate fixation overlap with external fixator pin sites a risk factor for infection in Pilon fractures? J Orthop Trauma. 2021;35(1):e7–e12. https://doi.org/10.1097/BOT.0000000000001884; PMID: 32618814.
14. Assal M, Ray A, Stern R. Strategies for surgical approaches in open reduction internal fixation of Pilon fractures. J Orthop Trauma. 2015;29(2):69–79. https://doi.org/10.1097/BOT.0000000000000218; PMID: 25072286.
15. Howard JL, Agel J, Barei DP, Benirschke SK, Nork SE. A prospective study evaluating incision placement and wound healing for Tibial plafond fractures. J Orthop Trauma. 2008;22(5):299–305. https://doi.org/10.1097/BOT.0b013e318172c811; ; discussion 305-6. PMID: 18448981.
16. Assal M, Ray A, Stern R. The extensile approach for the operative treatment of high-energy Pilon fractures: surgical technique and soft-tissue healing. J Orthop Trauma. 2007;21(3):198–206. https://doi.org/10.1097/BOT.0b013e3180316780; PMID: 17473757.
17. Sagi HC, Papp S, Dipasquale T. The effect of suture pattern and tension on cutaneous blood flow as assessed by laser Doppler Flowmetry in a pig model. J Orthop Trauma. 2008;22(3):171–5. https://doi.org/10.1097/BOT.0b013e318169074c; PMID: 18317050.
18. Shannon SF, Houdek MT, Wyles CC, Yuan BJ, Cross WW 3rd, Cass JR, Sems SA. Allgöwer-Donati versus vertical mattress suture technique impact on perfusion in ankle fracture surgery: a randomized clinical trial using intraoperative angiography. J Orthop Trauma. 2017;31(2):97–102. https://doi.org/10.1097/BOT.0000000000000731; PMID: 28129268.
19. Herscovici D Jr, Sanders RW, Infante A, DiPasquale T. Bohler incision: an extensile anterolateral approach to the foot and ankle. J Orthop Trauma. 2000;14(6):429–32. https://doi.org/10.1097/00005131-200008000-00009; PMID: 11001418.
20. Mehta S, Gardner MJ, Barei DP, Benirschke SK, Nork SE. Reduction strategies through the anterolateral exposure for fixation of type B and C Pilon fractures. J Orthop Trauma. 2011;25(2):116–22. https://

doi.org/10.1097/BOT.0b013e3181cf00f3; PMID: 21245716.

21. Nork SE, Barei DP, Gardner MJ, Mehta S, Benirschke SK. Anterolateral approach for Pilon fractures. Tech F&A Surg. 2009;8(2):53–9. https://doi.org/10.1097/BTF.0b013e3181a77e45.

22. Bhattacharyya T, Crichlow R, Gobezie R, Kim E, Vrahas MS. Complications associated with the posterolateral approach for Pilon fractures. J Orthop Trauma. 2006;20(2):104–7. https://doi.org/10.1097/01.bot.0000201084.48037.5d; PMID: 16462562.

23. Campbell ST, DeBaun MR, Kleweno CP, Nork SE. Simultaneous posterolateral and posteromedial approaches for fractures of the entire posterior Tibial plafond: a safe technique for effective reduction and fixation. J Orthop Trauma. 2022;36(1):49–53. https://doi.org/10.1097/BOT.0000000000002144; PMID: 34924545.

24. Assal M, Dalmau-Pastor M, Ray A, Stern R. How to get to the distal posterior Tibial malleolus? A cadaveric anatomic study defining the access corridors through 3 different approaches. J Orthop Trauma. 2017;31(4):e127–9. https://doi.org/10.1097/BOT.0000000000000774; PMID: 28323767.

25. Ketz J, Sanders R. Staged posterior Tibial plating for the treatment of Orthopaedic trauma association 43C2 and 43C3 Tibial Pilon fractures. J Orthop Trauma. 2012;26(6):341–7. https://doi.org/10.1097/BOT.0b013e318225881a; PMID: 22207206.

26. Tornetta P 3rd, Ricci W, Nork S, Collinge C, Steen B. The posterolateral approach to the tibia for displaced posterior malleolar injuries. J Orthop Trauma. 2011;25(2):123–6. https://doi.org/10.1097/BOT.0b013e3181e47d29; PMID: 21245717.

27. Lidder S, Masterson S, Dreu M, Clement H, Grechenig S. The risk of injury to the peroneal artery in the posterolateral approach to the distal tibia: a cadaver study. J Orthop Trauma. 2014;28(9):534–7. https://doi.org/10.1097/BOT.0000000000000089; PMID: 24662988.

28. Assal M, Ray A, Fasel JH, Stern R. A modified posteromedial approach combined with extensile anterior for the treatment of complex Tibial Pilon fractures (AO/OTA 43-C). J Orthop Trauma. 2014;28(6):e138–45. https://doi.org/10.1097/01.bot.0000435628.79017.c5; PMID: 24857906.

29. Hoekstra H, Rosseels W, Rammelt S, Nijs S. Direct fixation of fractures of the posterior Pilon via a posteromedial approach. Injury. 2017;48(6):1269–74. https://doi.org/10.1016/j.injury.2017.03.016; Epub 2017 Mar 19. PMID: 28336099.

30. Grose A, Gardner MJ, Hettrich C, Fishman F, Lorich DG, Asprinio DE, Helfet DL. Open reduction and internal fixation of Tibial Pilon fractures using a lateral approach. J Orthop Trauma. 2007;21(8):530–7. https://doi.org/10.1097/BOT.0b013e318145a227; PMID: 17805019.

31. Nielsen PJ, Grossman LS, Siebler JC, Lyden ER, Reed LK, Mormino MA. Is it safe to prep the external fixator in situ during second-stage Pilon surgical treatment? J Orthop Trauma. 2018;32(3):e102–5. https://doi.org/10.1097/BOT.0000000000001050; PMID: 29065036.

32. Githens MF, DeBaun MR, Jacobsen KA, Ross H, Firoozabadi R, Haller J. Plafond malreduction and talar dome impaction accelerates arthrosis after supination-adduction ankle fracture. Foot Ankle Int. 2021;42(10):1245–53. https://doi.org/10.1177/10711007211006032; Epub 2021 May 21. PMID: 34018419.

33. Haller JM, Githens M, Rothberg D, Higgins T, Nork S, Barei D. Pilon fractures in patients older than 60 years of age: should we be fixing these? J Orthop Trauma. 2020a;34(3):121–5. https://doi.org/10.1097/BOT.0000000000001661; PMID: 31842187.

34. Hebert-Davies J, Kleweno CP, Nork SE. Contemporary strategies in Pilon fixation. J Orthop Trauma. 2020;34(Suppl 1):S14–20. https://doi.org/10.1097/BOT.0000000000001698; PMID: 31939775.

35. Graves ML, Kosko J, Barei DP, Taitsman LA, Tarquinio TA, Russell GV, Woodall J Jr, Porter SE. Lateral ankle radiographs: do we really understand what we are seeing? J Orthop Trauma. 2011;25(2):106–9. https://doi.org/10.1097/BOT.0b013e3181e52ec5; PMID: 21245714.

36. Penny P, Swords M, Heisler J, Cien A, Sands A, Cole P. Ability of modern distal tibia plates to stabilize comminuted Pilon fracture fragments: is dual plate fixation necessary? Injury. 2016;47(8):1761–9. https://doi.org/10.1016/j.injury.2016.05.026; Epub 2016 May 20. PMID: 27264277.

37. d'Heurle A, Kazemi N, Connelly C, Wyrick JD, Archdeacon MT, Le TT. Prospective randomized comparison of locked plates versus nonlocked plates for the treatment of high-energy Pilon fractures. J Orthop Trauma. 2015;29(9):420–3. https://doi.org/10.1097/BOT.0000000000000386; PMID: 26165256.

38. Haller JM, Githens M, Rothberg D, Higgins T, Barei D, Nork S. Syndesmosis and syndesmotic equivalent injuries in Tibial plafond fractures. J Orthop Trauma. 2019a;33(3):e74–8. https://doi.org/10.1097/BOT.0000000000001363; PMID: 30768532.

39. Goodnough LH, Tigchelaar SS, Van Rysselberghe NL, DeBaun MR, Gardner MJ, Hecht GG, Lucas JF. Medial column support in Pilon fractures using percutaneous intramedullary large fragment fixation. J Orthop Trauma. 2021;35(12):e502–6. https://doi.org/10.1097/BOT.0000000000002073; PMID: 33675625.

40. Campbell ST, Goodnough LH, Salazar B, Lucas JF, Bishop JA, Gardner MJ. How do Pilon fractures heal? An analysis of dual plating and bridging callus formation. Injury. 2020;51(7):1655–61. https://doi.org/10.1016/j.injury.2020.04.023; Epub 2020 May 12. PMID: 32434713.

41. Van Rysselberghe NL, Campbell ST, Goodnough LH, Salazar BP, Bishop JA, Bellino MJ, Lucas JF, Gardner MJ. Metaphyseal callus formation in Pilon fractures

is associated with loss of alignment: is Siffer better? Injury. 2021;52(4):977–81. https://doi.org/10.1016/j.injury.2020.10.080; Epub 2020 Oct 17. PMID: 33097204.

42. Gardner MJ, Mehta S, Barei DP, Nork SE. Treatment protocol for open AO/OTA type C3 Pilon fractures with segmental bone loss. J Orthop Trauma. 2008;22(7):451–7. https://doi.org/10.1097/BOT.0b013e318176b8d9; PMID: 18670284.

43. Haller JM, Ross H, Jacobson K, Ou Z, Rothberg D, Githens M. Supination adduction ankle fractures: ankle fracture or Pilon variant? Injury. 2020b;51(3):759–63. https://doi.org/10.1016/j.injury.2020.01.008; Epub 2020 Jan 8. PMID: 31932039.

44. Benedick A, Kavanagh M, Audet M, Simske NM, Vallier HA. Supination adduction ankle fractures are associated with arthritis and poor outcomes. J Orthop Trauma. 2021;35(6):e195–201. https://doi.org/10.1097/BOT.0000000000001992; PMID: 33105458.

45. Carney J, Ton A, Alluri RK, Grisdela P, Marecek GS. Complications following operative treatment of supination-adduction type II (AO/OTA 44A2.3) ankle fractures. Injury. 2020;51(6):1387–91. https://doi.org/10.1016/j.injury.2020.03.032; Epub 2020 Mar 13. PMID: 32197830.

46. Boraiah S, Kemp TJ, Erwteman A, Lucas PA, Asprinio DE. Outcome following open reduction and internal fixation of open Pilon fractures. J Bone Joint Surg Am. 2010;92(2):346–52. https://doi.org/10.2106/JBJS.H.01678; PMID: 20124061.

47. Pollak AN, McCarthy ML, Bess RS, Agel J, Swiontkowski MF. Outcomes after treatment of high-energy Tibial plafond fractures. J Bone Joint Surg Am. 2003;85(10):1893–900. https://doi.org/10.2106/00004623-200310000-00005; PMID: 14563795.

48. Sommer C, Nork SE, Graves M, Blauth M, Rudin M, Stoffel K. Quality of fracture reduction assessed by radiological parameters and its influence on functional results in patients with Pilon fractures-A prospective multicentre study. Injury. 2017;48(12):2853–63. https://doi.org/10.1016/j.injury.2017.10.031; Epub 2017 Oct 20. PMID: 29079366.

49. Spitler CA, Hulick RM, Weldy J, Howell K, Bergin PF, Graves ML. What are the risk factors for deep infection in OTA/AO 43C Pilon fractures? J Orthop Trauma. 2020;34(6):e189–94. https://doi.org/10.1097/BOT.0000000000001726; PMID: 31868764.

50. Willey MC, Compton JT, Marsh JL, Kleweno CP, Agel J, Scott EJ, Bui G, Davison J, Anderson DD. Weight-bearing CT scan after Tibial Pilon fracture demonstrates significant early joint-space narrowing. J Bone Joint Surg Am. 2020;102(9):796–803. https://doi.org/10.2106/JBJS.19.00816; PMID: 32379120.

51. Chan DS, Balthrop PM, White B, Glassman D, Sanders RW. Does a staged posterior approach have a negative effect on OTA 43C fracture outcomes? J Orthop Trauma. 2017;31(2):90–4. https://doi.org/10.1097/BOT.0000000000000728; PMID: 27763960.

Management of Talus Fractures

Heather A. Vallier

1   Introduction

Fractures of the talus are rare injuries and generally result from high energy mechanisms. Historically, talus neck and body fractures have portended poor prognoses due to high rates of associated osteonecrosis and post-traumatic arthrosis. Expeditious initial management of dislocations, timely surgical care, and accurate reduction with rigid fixation will provide the best chances for a functional outcome [1].

The talus has unique, fundamental functions during the gait cycle, as it articulates with the distal tibia and fibula at the ankle and the calcaneus via three facets of the subtalar joint, along with the navicular at the midfoot. Over 70% of the surface of the bone is articular cartilage, allowing for the essential mobility and purpose during the gait cycle through ankle dorsiflexion and plantarflexion, subtalar inversion and eversion, and midfoot pronation and supination [2]. With the array of mobility and function of the peritalar joints, fractures and dislocations of the talus often have profound impact on ambulation [2, 3]. Even when anatomic reduction is possible, post-traumatic stiffness is expected, and risks of osteonecrosis due to damage to the blood supply during the injury and/or post-traumatic arthrosis may result in functional limitations [1, 4].

The blood supply to the talus is furnished via all three arteries from the lower leg. Because of the extensive chondral coverage, few areas exist for vessels to enter the bone, and these areas are commonly fractured—directly damaging the arterial flow [5–8]. The arterial supplies may also be damaged due to the injury event, which affects the surrounding soft tissues. The tarsal canal is a groove between the medial talar neck and the calcaneus. This exits laterally into the tarsal sinus. The arteries of the tarsal canal and tarsal sinus anastomose within the tarsal canal. The artery of the tarsal canal originates from the deltoid branch of the posterior tibial artery, and it provides the primary blood supply to the talar body, flowing retrograde via the inferior talar neck. The artery of the tarsal sinus originates from the anterior tibial artery, and it provides blood supply to the talar head and neck. The peroneal artery supplies posterior portions of the talar body and may also contribute to the artery of the tarsal sinus. Fractures and dislocations are apt to injure the talar blood supply. However, anastomoses among the main arterial branches may continue to provide blood flow to the talus after injury [8, 9]. Revascularization may also occur [10, 11].

H. A. Vallier (✉)
Department of Orthopaedic Surgery, MetroHealth
Medical Center affiliated with Case Western Reserve
University, Cleveland, OH, USA
e-mail: hvallier@metrohealth.org

2 Pathogenesis and Classification

High energy mechanisms of injury account for the majority of displaced talus neck and body fractures, and peritalar dislocations. Motorized collisions or falls from height generate axial load, which causes these injuries. Fractures are described by location and orientation. Lateral or posterior process fractures may occur in isolation or in combination with other fracture elements. Talar head fractures occur infrequently and may be associated with talonavicular dislocation. More commonly talar neck and/or body fractures occur. Fractures of the body are most often described based on orientation and comminution. Many occur in the sagittal plane, while some are coronal, and most have some comminution [12]. Fractures within the coronal plane are considered talar body fractures when the primary fracture line is within the anterior margin of the talar dome cartilage or posterior to it, and the inferior fracture extent is posterior to the lateral process [13].

Fractures of the talar neck were described by Hawkins in 1970, with a classification based on initial fracture displacement and with risk of osteonecrosis [14]. Group 1 fractures are truly nondisplaced and often difficult to see with plain radiography, potentially requiring a CT scan to delineate. All peritalar articulations remain congruent. Fractures with any displacement should be classified as Hawkins Group 2, which was defined as a talar neck fracture with subtalar subluxation or dislocation (Fig. 1). When the subtalar joint is dislocated, the risk of osteonecrosis increases, thus the Hawkins system was modified to differentiate between those injuries without subtalar dislocation (2A) and those with associated subtalar dislocation (2B) [11]. The third group described by Hawkins included talar neck fracture with associated tibiotalar dislocation [14]. Canale and Kelly later modified Hawkins classification by adding a fourth type, which further includes dislocation of the talonavicular joint (Fig. 1) [15].

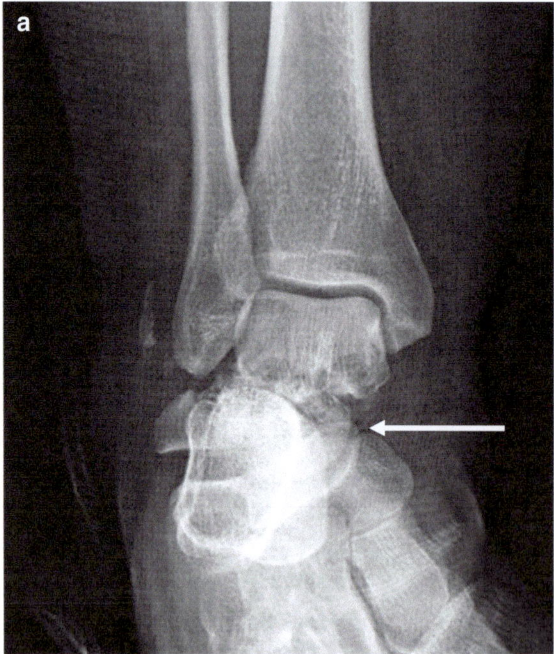

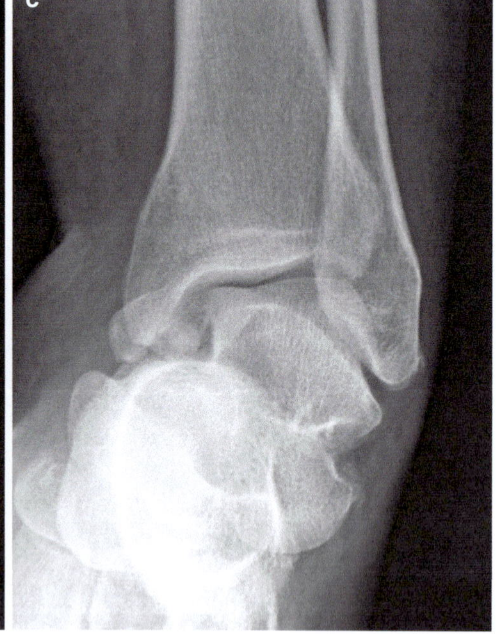

Fig. 1 Injury plain radiographs demonstrate initial fracture displacement described by Hawkins' classification. Anteroposterior view of the ankle shows dislocation of the subtalar joint, Hawkins 2B (**a**). An arrow denotes the fracture line of the talar neck. Further dislocation of the ankle joint defines Hawkins 3 (**b**), and Hawkins 4 is associated with dislocation of the talonavicular joint (**c, d**)

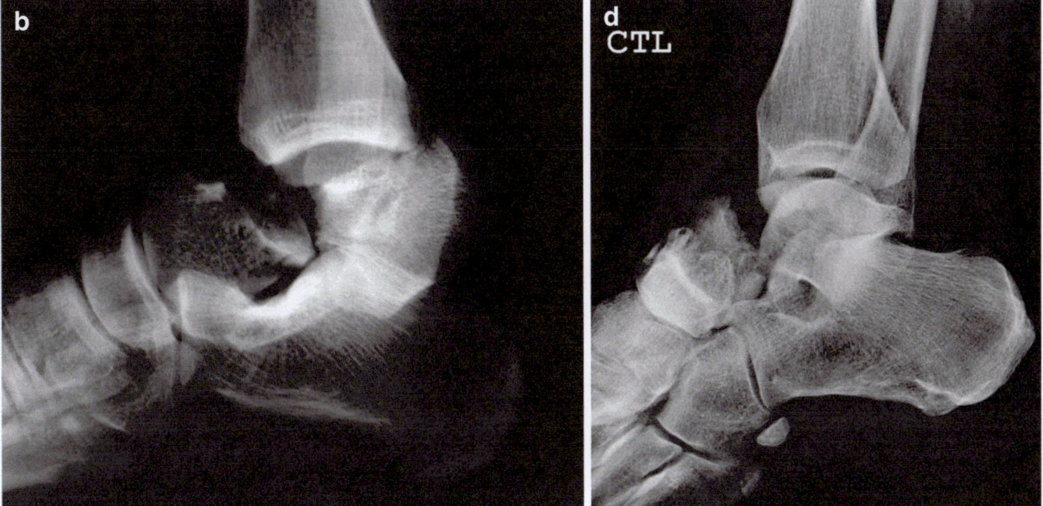

Fig. 1 (continued)

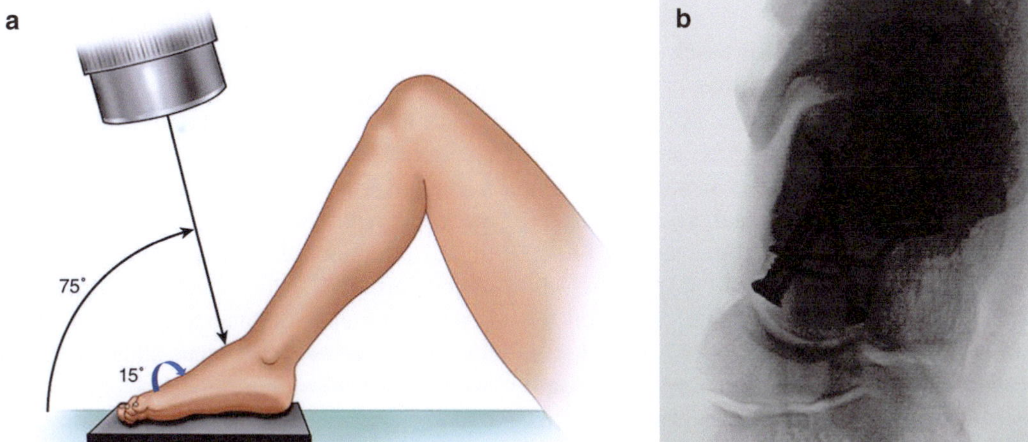

Fig. 2 (**a**, **b**) Intraoperative Canale view of the talus demonstrates axial alignment of the talar neck fracture following open reduction and internal fixation

3 Diagnosis and Imaging

Initial assessment includes physical examination, which may reveal soft tissue swelling and open wounds. Closed dislocations will be associated with palpable bony prominences, often in combination with plantar paresthesias due to neuropraxia [16]. Plain radiographs of the ankle and foot should be obtained. These images will demonstrate displaced fractures of the neck and body and any subluxation or dislocation of associated joints. A Canale view portrays the axial alignment of the talus and may be obtained by pronating the foot on the radiograph plate with the radiographic beam at an angle of 15° from perpendicular to the cartridge [15, 17]. This is helpful during fixation of talar neck fractures (Fig. 2). CT scans with reconstructions may be helpful in planning surgery for comminuted articular fractures of the talus. MRI scan is rarely indicated in the acute setting but may offer benefit during recovery to assess healing and vascularity [9].

4   Treatment

4.1   Nonoperative

Rarely, nondisplaced fractures of the talar neck or talar body are identified. Nonoperative management is only indicated for nondisplaced fractures or patients who are nonambulatory or unable to medically tolerate surgery. Initial immobilization in a splint will provide stability and comfort. Non-weightbearing and elevation should be encouraged. Once the initial soft tissue swelling has diminished, the splint may be replaced by a removable boot or a cast, depending on whether range of motion should be permitted. Approximately 6 to 8 weeks following the injury the fracture will likely be healed to permit progressive weightbearing [1].

4.2   Operative: Talar Neck and Body Fractures

Displaced fractures should be managed with open reduction and internal fixation to restore both articular alignment and axial alignment. Surgical timing depends on the severity of soft tissue swelling, where delay of several days to a few weeks may be appropriate, based on the energy of the initial injury [1, 10, 11, 18, 19]. Irreducible dislocations and open fractures should be managed urgently, however (Fig. 3). Intravenous antibiotics are indicated urgently for open fractures and dislocations, followed by surgical debridement. In cases where the patient's systemic status and the soft tissue injury can tolerate definitive management acutely, open reduction and internal fixation can be undertaken (Fig. 4).

Displaced talar neck and talar body fractures are treated with reduction and fixation. Both fracture types and combined injuries are best addressed through dual anteromedial and anterolateral surgical approaches with the patient in the supine position [10, 20–22]. An exception would be simple talar body fractures in the sagittal plane, which may be successfully visualized and stabilized via a single anteromedial, anterolateral, or posteromedial incision. Combined anteromedial and anterolateral exposures are recommended to accurately reduce and stabilize talar neck fractures under direct view. Attempting to perform this through a single anteromedial approach may result in failure to accurately reduce and stabilize subtle dorsal and medial impaction and/or comminution within the talar neck. Untreated, this would result in malalignment of the longitudinal axis of the talus in extension and varus [1, 23]. The anterolateral approach usually affords a more reliable reduction assessment and also promotes placement of additional implants. Purely percutaneous reduction and fixation should be avoided, as subtle malalignment will not be evident on fluoroscopic imaging, and would promote fixation of a yet, displaced fracture.

The anteromedial approach extends from the anterior aspect of the medial malleolus to the medial aspect of the medial cuneiform and navicular joint. This incision is just medial to the tibialis anterior tendon, providing exposure directly over the medial talar neck. Sharp dissection is preferred to elevate the capsule of the tibiotalar and talonavicular joints, although care is taken to avoid dissection and retractor placement into the tarsal canal, so as not to jeopardize arterial supply. The anterolateral approach extends from the tip of the distal fibula along the axis of the fourth metatarsal. The extensor digitorum brevis origin is elevated to expose the lateral aspect of the talar neck, providing visualization to the lateral neck, lateral process, and anterolateral body (Fig. 5). On occasion, access to the talar body may be obstructed by the malleoli, in which case a malleolar osteotomy may improve visualization.

Medial malleolar osteotomy affords excellent visualization of the medial aspect of the talar body. When a medial malleolus fracture is pres-

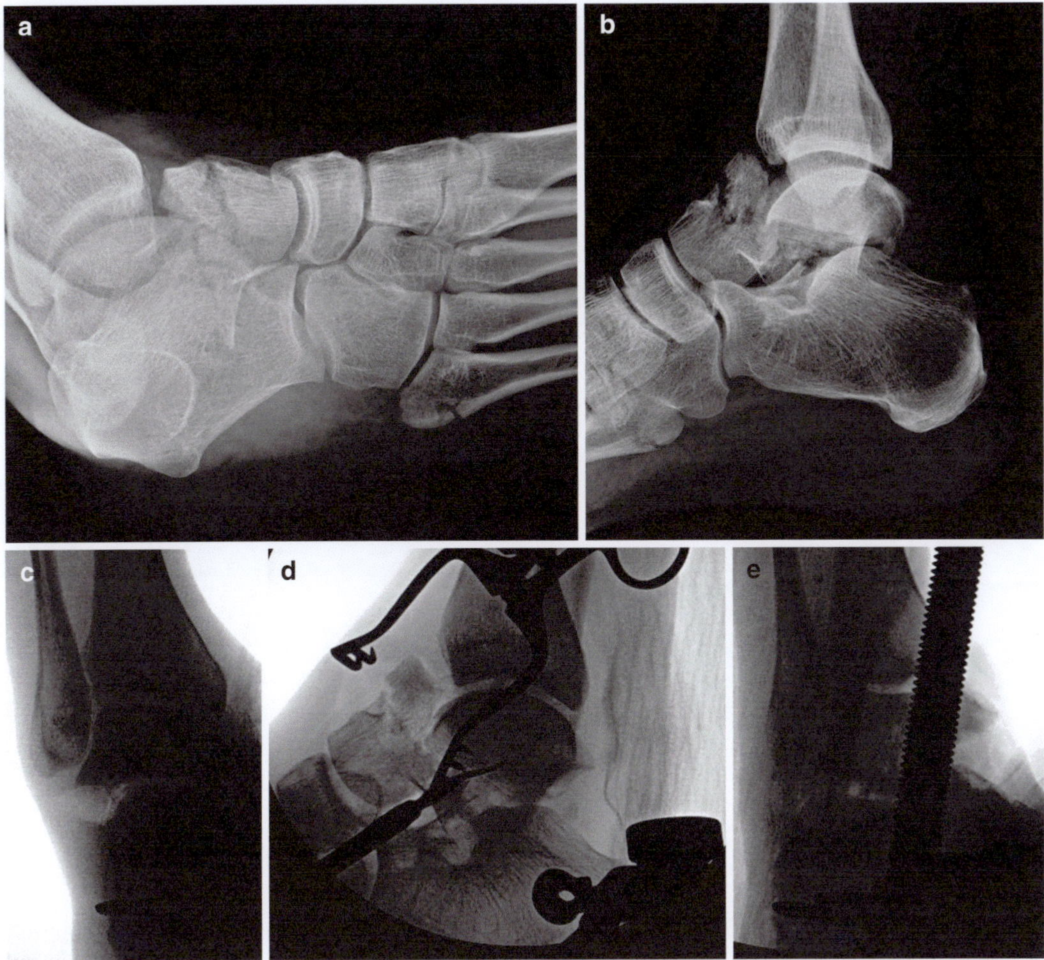

Fig. 3 A 40 year-old man sustained irreducible closed talar neck fracture with associated subtalar dislocation, shown on oblique and lateral views of the foot (**a, b**). A percutaneous Schanz pin was placed into the calcaneus to facilitate reduction with longitudinal traction on the leg with the knee flexed and the ankle plantarflexed. Concurrent torsion and translation of the talus were also attempted with the Schanz pin, but these maneuvers were not successful (**c**). Thus, anteromedial exposure was developed for open reduction of the dislocation. A universal distractor was placed to distract the subtalar joint, and posterior capsule was released using a #15 blade and fluoroscopic guidance. The talar body was reduced with aid of a freer elevator (**d, e**)

ent, it may be exploited to provide a similar exposure (Fig. 6). Care is taken to preserve the deltoid ligament, thus protecting any remaining arterial supply. Osteotomy should be performed after predrilling for the planned (later) screw fixation of the osteotomy. An oscillating saw and irrigation are utilized, but the osteotomy is completed with an osteotome to prevent articular injury and to provide interdigitating surfaces to facilitate

reduction and repair of the osteotomy after talus fixation is completed [21, 24–27].

Reduction is undertaken under muscular paralysis, and may require manual traction and percutaneous or direct manipulation, using Schanz pins or clamps. Provisional Kirschner wires and clamps permit careful direct visualization and multiplanar radiography to verify restoration of anatomic alignment. Intraoperative

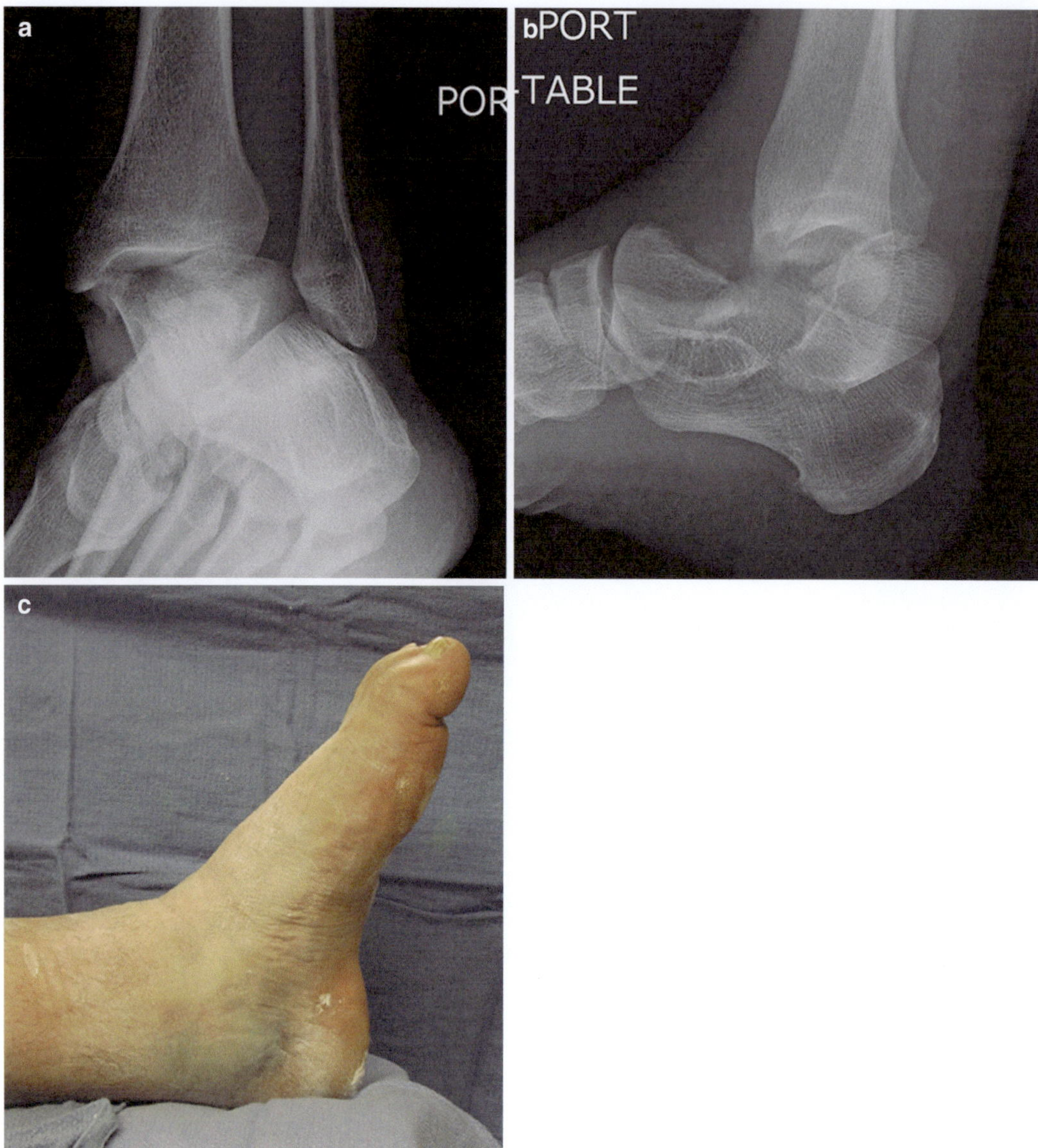

Fig. 4 A young man sustained talar neck fracture with associated closed subtalar and tibiotalar dislocations (**a**, **b**). After transfer to our hospital from another facility, now 12 h after injury, he had profound soft tissue swelling and plantar paresthesias, though compartments were compressible (**c**). He underwent closed reduction and splinting (**d**, **e**), then returned for open reduction and internal fixation in 15 days when swelling had subsided

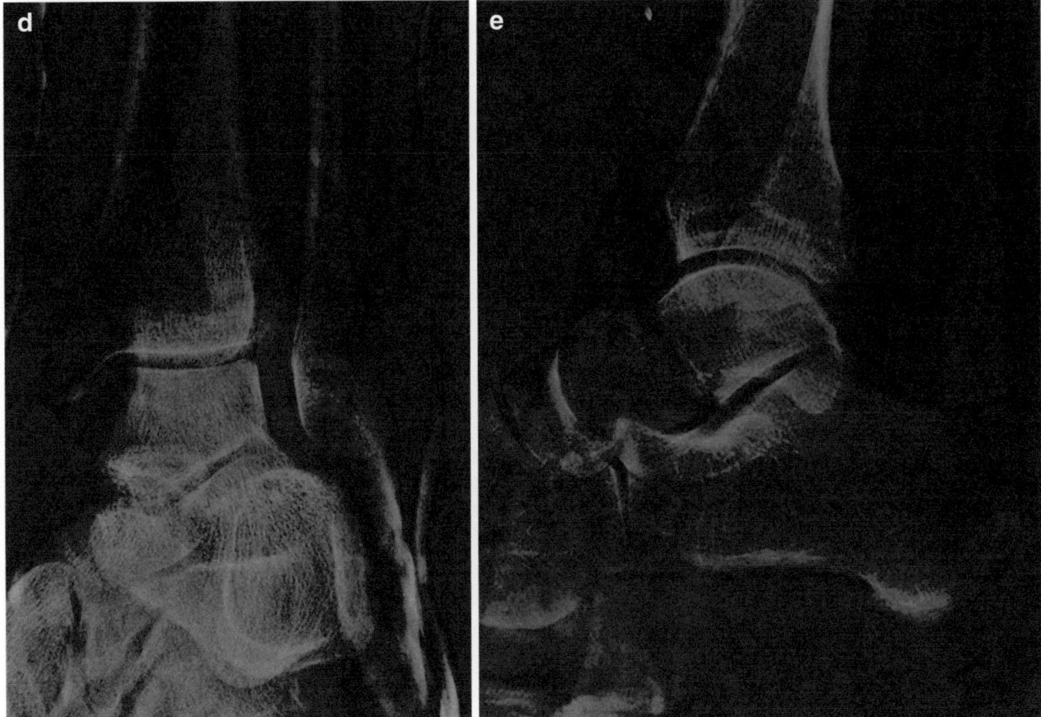

Fig. 4 (continued)

Canale view is routinely obtained to demonstrate the axial alignment of the talus, averting varus malalignment (Fig. 5c).

Fixation is accomplished with small fragment and mini fragment implants [1, 21, 28]. Stainless steel or titanium implants are acceptable. Titanium permits MRI imaging with less artifact, but MRI is rarely indicated postoperatively. The fixation construct is dependent on the fracture pattern. One common configuration involves a lag screw countersunk within or just adjacent to the articular cartilage of the medial side of the talar head with a mini fragment plate contoured to conform to the lateral talar neck and extending along the lateral process as indicated. Positional screws placed axially down the neck of the talus are used when neck comminution precludes interfragmentary screw compression. Most high energy fractures have neck comminution and/or impaction of the fracture margins there, prohibiting compression of the neck fracture. Occasionally mini fragment plates may be placed medially to bridge comminution. Care must be taken to prevent impingement of the implants on the articular surfaces of the medial malleolus and talar head (Fig. 7). Headless screws may also be employed to prevent chondral irritation.

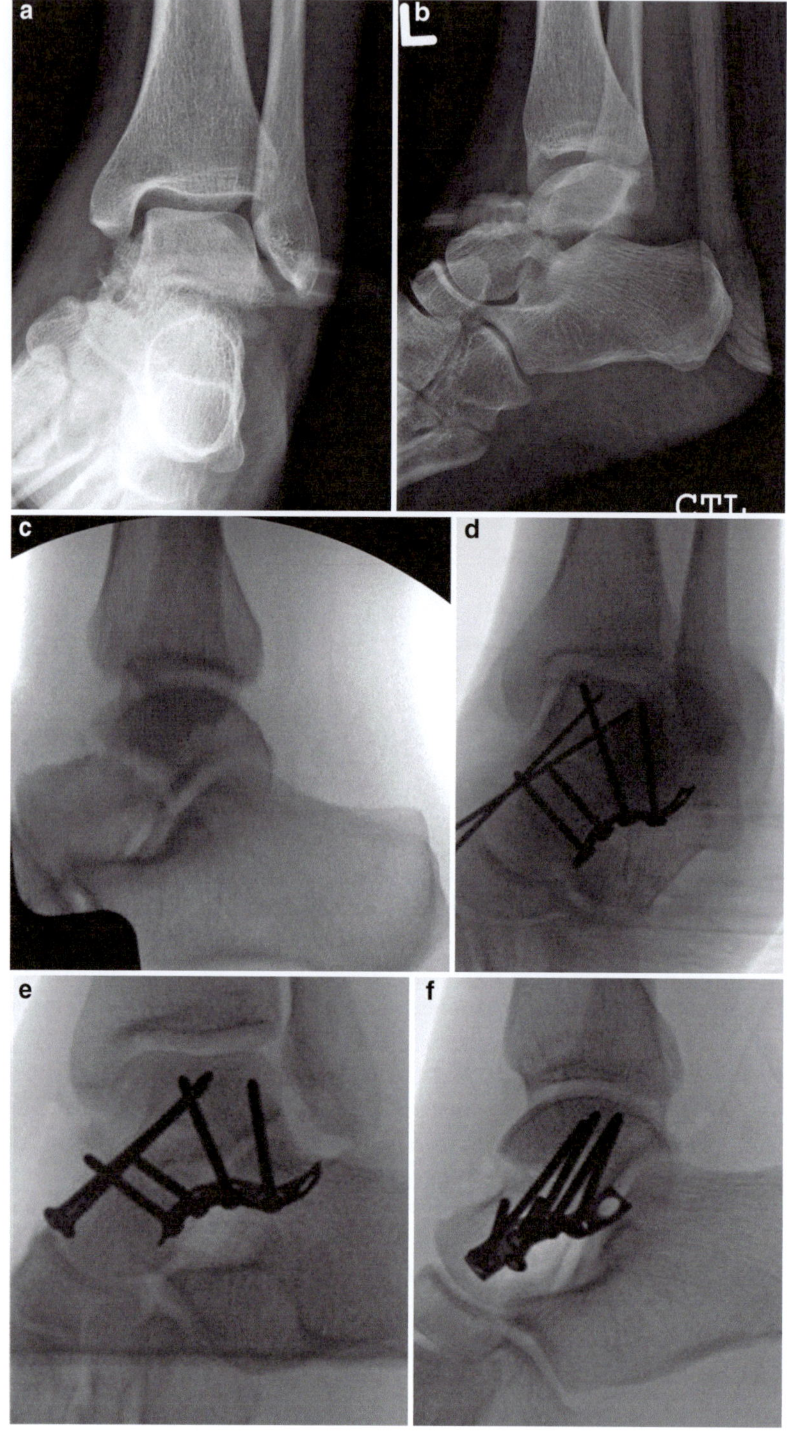

Fig. 5 A 45 year-old woman sustained multiple injuries in motorized collision. She presented with a comminuted fracture dislocation of the talar neck, including coronal plane fracture into the talar body and the lateral process. Anteroposterior and lateral views demonstrate initial fracture displacement (**a**, **b**). She went to the operating room where other procedures were performed and a closed reduction of the dislocation was possible (**c**). Two weeks later she returned to surgery for ORIF via anteromedial and anterolateral exposures. Intraoperative images show the accuracy of the reduction on Canale view, with provisional wires in place (**d**). Small and mini fragment implants provide definitive fixation (**e**, **f**)

Local autogenous bone graft may be obtained from the medial edge of the navicular, which debulks the pathway for instrumentation directed down the long axis of the talus. The bone may then be placed into deficiencies within the dorsal and medial neck, when present. Additional autograft may be harvested from the calcaneus in small amounts. Supplemental external fixation may be placed to augment the internal fixation in very comminuted fractures and/or those with poor bone quality or patients with limited potential to adhere to postoperative non-weightbearing recommendations.

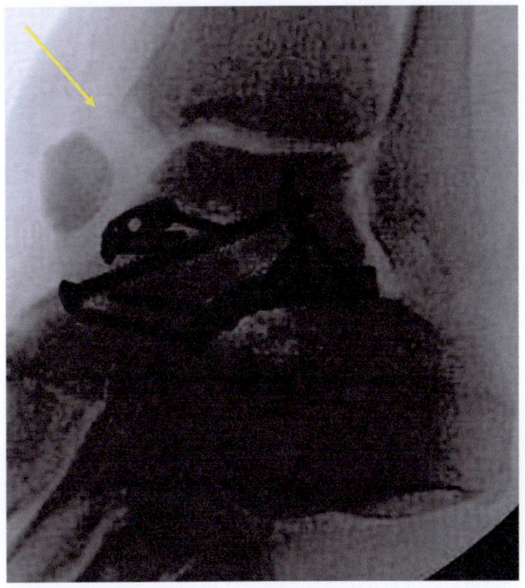

Fig. 6 Intraoperative visualization and access is facilitated with a medial malleolar osteotomy

4.3 Lateral Process Fractures

Large lateral process fractures occurring in isolation or in combination with talar neck fracture are addressed via the anterolateral approach [21]. Displaced fragments too small for reduction and fixation are excised [29–31]. Frequently, very small, impacted fragments on the plantar aspect of the lateral process must either be maintained in that position or removed altogether, as there is often not ability to reduce and stabilize them due to the very limited amount of subchondral bone. When interstitial bone of the lateral process is impacted and/or not reconstructable, the peripheral portion of the lateral process may be advanced medially to achieve bony contact with the intact talar body, providing congruous articular alignment along the posterior facet [1]. When stabilized in that position, the lateral process will remain functional, although with less width than prior to the injury.

4.4 Posterior Process Fractures

Nondisplaced or minimally displaced posterior process fractures may be treated nonoperatively (Fig. 8). Displaced posterior process are best addressed via a posteromedial approach [32]. This is best performed with the patient positioned supine using a bump underneath the contralateral hip, which externally rotates the injured leg to direct the hindfoot toward the surgeon. The posteromedial approach may also be performed with

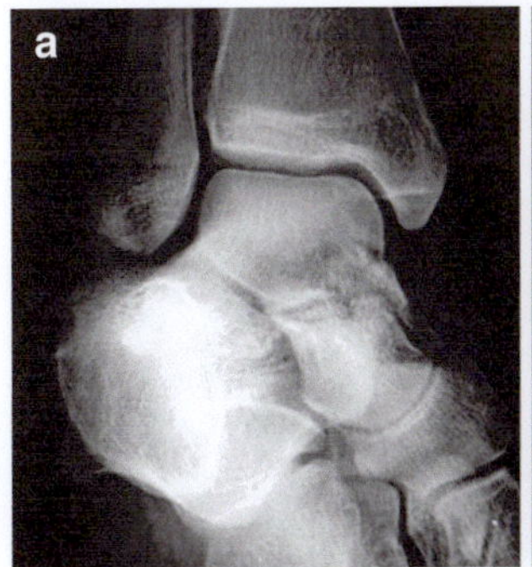
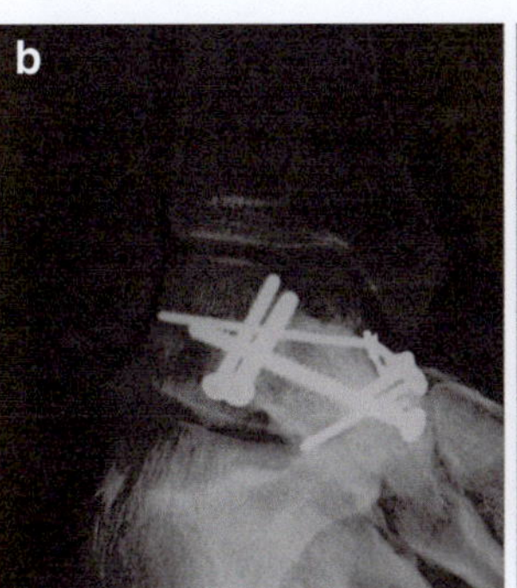
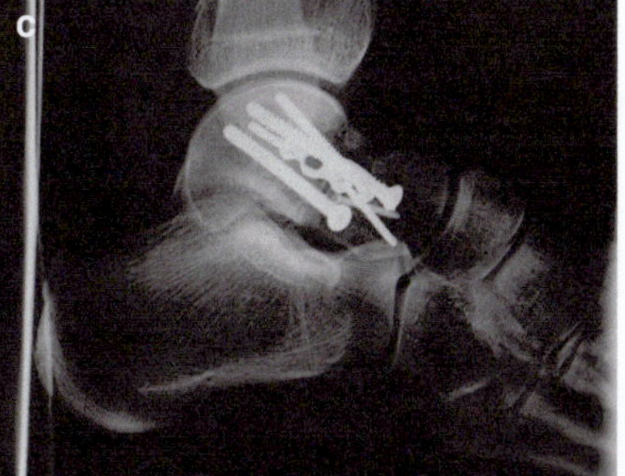

Fig. 7 Injury ankle mortise view (**a**) demonstrates a comminuted talar neck fracture. Open reduction and internal fixation included a medial plate to bridge the medial neck comminution (**b**, **c**)

the patient in the prone position. Care should be taken to position the injured limb slightly higher than the other side, so that lateral imaging will not be obscured. The surgical approach is between the posterior edge of the medial malleolus and the medial border of the Achilles tendon [21, 32, 33]. Sharp dissection without undermining of subcutaneous tissue is recommended to minimize trauma to the soft tissues. The deep interval extends either anterior or posterior to the flexor digitorum longus tendon, depending on the fracture location. The adjacent neurovascular bundle should be identified and protected. The fracture will be visualized once the thick poste-

rior capsule is incised, and screw fixation can be directed in the posterior to anterior direction (Fig. 9).

4.5 Postoperative Management

Splints are placed in the operating room and rest, elevation and non-weightbearing are recommended. Between 2 and 3 weeks postoperatively sutures may be removed and range of motion exercises may be initiated. Non-weightbearing should be continued for 12 weeks or until adequate fracture union. Ankle mortise and lateral projections with plain radiography are the most useful views to assess this. Often some of the fracture lines are still present around the 12-week visit, but progressive weightbearing can be safely recommended when healing is present on sequential plain radiographs. Within several weeks postoperatively, disuse osteopenia occurs within the talar dome, seen as subchondral lucency, best depicted within the medial shoulder of the talar body on the mortise radiograph (Fig. 10). This plain radiographic finding is also known as Hawkins' sign, denoting functional blood supply to the talar body [14]. In the absence of Hawkins' sign, the density of the talar dome will be increased relative to adjacent structures, consistent with osteonecrosis. In the presence of early osteonecrosis, weightbearing may also be advanced [1, 10, 11, 18].

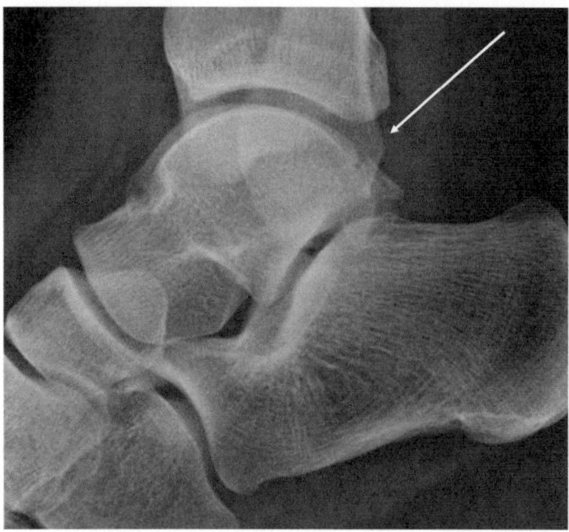

Fig. 8 Ankle mortise and lateral views demonstrate a minimally displaced fracture of the posterior process

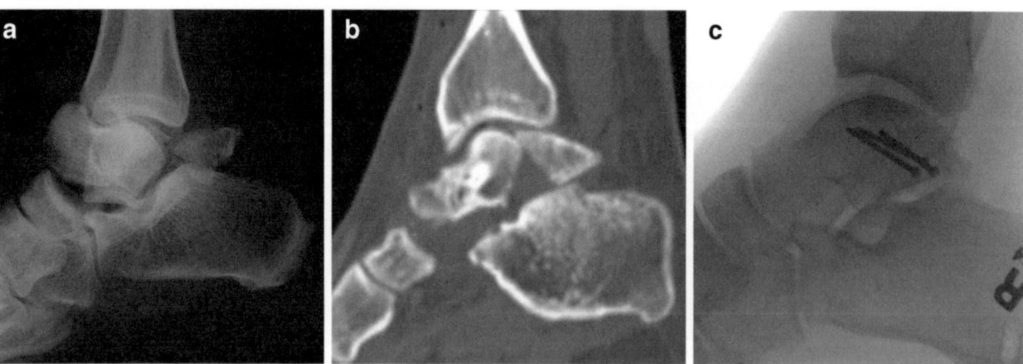

Fig. 9 Displaced posterior process fracture with associated talonavicular dislocation shown on plain radiographs and CT scan (**a**, **b**) is treated with open reduction and internal fixation via a posteromedial approach (**c**)

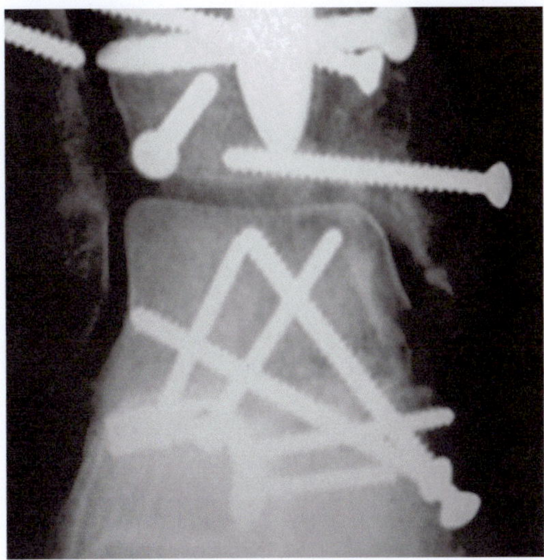

Fig. 10 Ankle mortise view demonstrates a healed talar neck fracture with disuse osteopenia in the medial talar dome, consistent with revascularization after this Hawkins 3 injury

5 Complications

The most common complication following talus fractures is stiffness of the ankle and subtalar joints. Even when the fracture pattern is simple, reduction is anatomic, and early motion is initiated, some residual stiffness will be present [3]. Ankle stiffness is most noticeable when attempting to walk quickly, as the hip must externally rotate to accommodate limited tibiotalar excursion. Subtalar stiffness is most noticeable when ambulating on uneven surfaces. Immobility of the subtalar joint may cause foot pain when standing and walking on uneven surfaces.

5.1 Post-Traumatic Arthrosis

Most patients also develop some radiographical findings of post-traumatic arthrosis following fractures of the talar body and neck. While arthrosis may result from damage sustained to the cartilage at the time of injury, it is also produced by imperfect reduction and malunion [1]. Ankle arthrosis is more likely following talar body fractures, while subtalar arthrosis is more common following talar neck fractures, although many patients experience some symptoms in both locations [19, 34]. Recent studies have reported tibiotalar arthrosis in 18–61% and subtalar arthrosis in 15–100% following talar neck fracture [4, 10, 11, 18, 22, 35, 36]. Mild activity-related pain and stiffness may be the only symptoms. However, some patients experience debilitating pain, preventing vocational activities and activities of daily living. Arthritis that becomes symptomatic can be treated with arthrodesis of the subtalar joint or the ankle joint. Tibiotalar arthrosis may potentially be treated with ankle arthroplasty when arthrosis is isolated to the tibiotalar joint without substantial subchondral collapse of the talar dome from osteonecrosis.

5.2 Osteonecrosis

Osteonecrosis occurs less frequently than arthrosis after talar body or neck fractures. The risk is directly related to initial fracture displacement, which may have damaged the talar blood supply, thus risk is associated with the Hawkins classification for talar neck fractures [1, 11, 14, 22, 35, 36]. Fractures with associated subtalar dislocation (Hawkins 2B) develop osteonecrosis in up to 30%, while it rarely occurs following type 2A [1, 11]. Osteonecrosis occurs in 41–91% following Hawkins 3 and up to 100% following Hawkins 4 displacement [10, 11, 18, 22, 35]. Approximately 40% of patients with talar body fractures will develop osteonecrosis, more likely with open fractures or with comminuted patterns [19, 34, 37]. Risk for osteonecrosis does not increase with prolonged time to definitive fixation, once dislocations have been reduced [1, 11, 38, 39]. Over several months, the talar body will usually revascularize without collapse in about half of patients who initially exhibit some increased radiodensity of the talar body (Fig. 10) [1, 10, 11, 40]. When collapse occurs a salvage procedure may be considered (Fig. 11).

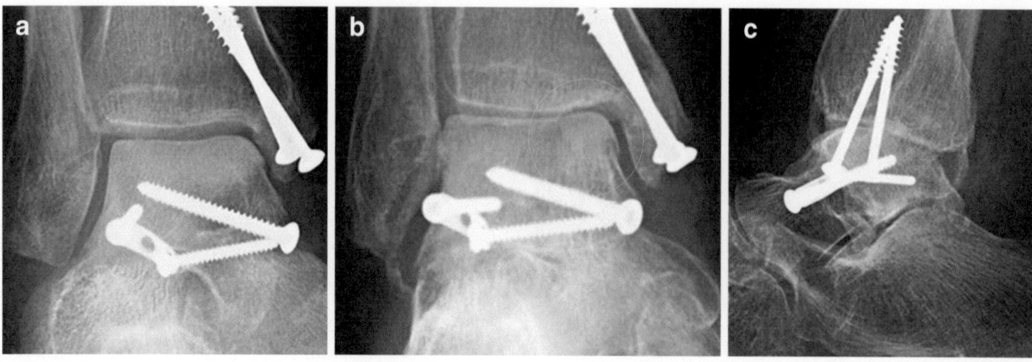

Fig. 11 Ankle mortise view 3 months after ORIF of a talar neck fracture shows increased density of the talar body, suggesting osteonecrosis (**a**). Over 12 months later mortise and lateral ankle radiographs show collapse of the talar dome (**b, c**)

5.3 Infections

Despite the high energy nature of many of these injuries and the frequency of open fractures, wound healing complications and infections are minimized with careful soft tissue handling, including meticulous surgical dissection and staged definitive fixation based on timing to permit diminution of swelling. Wound complications and deep infections occur in up to several percent of cases, based on summary of modern literature [10, 11, 18, 22, 35, 36].

5.4 Nonunion and Malunion

In general, nonunion is rare after talar neck or body fractures, occurring in several percent. Nonunion occurs more often after open fractures versus closed fractures. Malunion occurs in up to 40%, depending on the definition of malunion [4, 10, 11, 19, 34, 35]. However, malunion is likely underestimated in published reports, as it is difficult to adequately evaluate talar alignment based on plain radiographs.

References

1. Vallier HA. Fractures of the talus: state of the art. J Orthop Trauma. 2015;29:385–92.
2. Daniels TR, Smith JW, Ross TI. Varus malalignment of the talar neck: its effect on the position of the foot and on subtalar motion. J Bone Joint Surg Am. 1996;78-A:1559–67.
3. Sangeorzan BJ, Wagner UA, Harrington RM, et al. Contact characteristics of the subtalar joint: the effect of talar neck misalignment. J Orthop Res. 1992;10:544–3.
4. Fournier A, Barba N, Steiger V, et al. Total talar fracture—long-term results of internal fixation of talar fractures. A multicentric study of 114 cases. Orthop Traumatol Surg Res. 2012;98:S48–55.
5. Gelberman RH, Mortensen WW. The arterial anatomy of the talus. Foot Ankle. 1983;4:64–72.
6. Haliburton R, Sullivan R, Kelly P, et al. The extra-osseous and intra-osseous blood supply of the talus. J Bone Joint Surg Am. 1958;40-A:1115–20.
7. Mulfinger GL, Trueta J. The blood supply to the talus. J Bone Joint Surg Br. 1970;52-B:160–7.
8. Prasarn ML, Miller AN, Dyke JP, et al. Arterial anatomy if the talus: a cadaver and gadolinium-enhanced MRI study. Foot Ankle Int. 2010;31:987–93.
9. Miller AN, Prasarn ML, Dyke JP, et al. Quantitative assessment of the vascularity of the talus with gadolinium-enhanced magnetic resonance imaging. J Bone Joint Surg Am. 2011;93:1116–21.
10. Vallier HA, Nork SE, Barei DP, et al. Talar neck fractures: results and outcomes. J Bone Joint Surg Am. 2004;86-A:1616–24.
11. Vallier HA, Reichard SG, Boyd AJ, et al. A new look at the Hawkins classification for talar neck fractures: which features of injury and treatment are predictive of osteonecrosis? J Bone Joint Surg Am. 2014; 96:192–7.
12. Sneppen O, Christensen SB, Krogsoe O, et al. Fracture of the body of the talus. Acta Orthop Scand. 1977;48:317–24.
13. Inokuchi S, Ogawa K, Usami N, et al. Long-term follow up of talus fractures. Orthopedics. 1996;19:477–81.
14. Hawkins LG. Fractures of the neck of the talus. J Bone Joint Surg Am. 1970;52-A:991–1002.

15. Canale ST, Kelly FB. Fractures of the neck of the talus: long term evaluation of 71 cases. J Bone Joint Surg Am. 1978;60-A:143–56.
16. Huynh T, Staley C, Singer A, Schenker M, Moore T Jr. Tibial nerve dysfunction associated with operatively treated talar neck fractures. J Orthop Trauma. 2020;34:488–91.
17. Thomas JL, Boyce BM. Radiographic analysis of the Canale view for displaced talar neck fractures. J Foot Ankle Surg. 2012;51:187–90.
18. Lindvall E, Haidukewych G, DiPasquale T, et al. Open reduction and stable fixation of isolated, displaced talar neck and body fractures. J Bone Joint Surg Am. 2004;86-A:2229–34.
19. Vallier HA, Nork SE, Benirschke SK, et al. Surgical treatment of talar body fractures. J Bone Joint Surg Am. 2003;85-A:1716–24.
20. Mayo KA. Fractures of the talus: principles of management and techniques of treatment. Tech Orthop. 1987;2:42–7.
21. Vallier HA, Nork SE, Benirschke SK, et al. Surgical treatment of talar body fractures. J Bone Joint Surg Am. 2004;86-A Suppl 1(Pt 2):180–92.
22. Xue Y, Zhang H, Pei F, et al. Treatment of displaced talar neck fractures using delayed procedures of plate fixation through dual approaches. Int Orthop. 2014;38:149–54.
23. Sproule JA, Glazebrook MA, Younger AS. Varus hindfoot deformity after talar fracture. Foot Ankle Clin. 2012;17:117–25.
24. Gonzalez A, Stern R, Assal M. Reduction of irreducible Hawkins III talar neck fracture by means of a medial malleolar osteotomy: a report of three cases with a 4-year mean follow up. J Orthop Trauma. 2011;25:47–50.
25. Smith PN, Ziran BH. Fractures of the talus. Operative Tech Orthop. 1999;9:229–38.
26. van Bergen CJ, Tuijthof GJ, Sierevent IN, et al. Direction of the oblique medial malleolar osteotomy for exposure of the talus. Arch Orthop Trauma Surg. 2011;131:893–901.
27. Ziran BH, Abidi NA, Scheel MJ. Medial malleolar osteotomy for exposure of complex talar body fractures. J Orthop Trauma. 2001;15:513–8.
28. Fleuriau Chateau PB, Brokow DS, Jelen BA, et al. Plate fixation of talar neck fractures: preliminary review of a new technique in twenty-three patients. J Orthop Trauma. 2002;16:213–9.
29. Lunebourg A, Zermatten P. Fracture of the lateral process of the talus: a report of two cases. J Foot Ankle Surg. 2014;53:316–9.
30. Perera A, Baker JF, Lui DF, et al. The management and outcome of lateral process fracture of the talus. J Foot Ankle Surg. 2010;16:15–20.
31. Shakked RJ, Tejwani NC. Surgical treatment of talus fractures. Orthop Clin North Am. 2013;44:521–8.
32. Shi Z, Zou J, Yi X. Posteromedial approach in treatment of talar posterior process fractures. J Investig Surg. 2013;26:204–9.
33. Ziran NM. Associated lateral process and posteromedial tubercle talus fractures: a case report and literature review. Am J Orthop. 2011;40:179–82.
34. Thordarson DB. Talar body fractures. Orthop Clin North Am. 2001;32:65–77.
35. Sanders DW, Busam M, Hattwick E, et al. Functional outcomes following displaced talar neck fractures. J Orthop Trauma. 2004;18:265–70.
36. Schulze W, Richter J, Russe O, et al. Surgical treatment of talus fractures: a retrospective study of 80 cases followed for 1-15 years. Acta Orthop Scand. 2002;73:344–51.
37. Thordarson DB, Triffon MJ, Terk MR. Magnetic resonance imaging to detect avascular necrosis after open reduction and internal fixation of talar neck fractures. Foot Ankle Int. 1996;17:742–7.
38. Bellamy JL, Keeling JJ, Wenke J, et al. Does a longer delay in fixation of talus fractures cause osteonecrosis? J Surg Orthop Adv. 2011;20:34–7.
39. Patel R, Van Bergeyk A, Pinney S. Are displaced talar neck fractures surgical emergencies? A survey of orthopaedic trauma experts. Foot Ankle Int. 2005;26:378–81.
40. Babu N, Schuberth JM. Partial avascular necrosis after talar neck fracture. Foot Ankle Int. 2010;31:777–80.

Management of Acute Diabetic Ankle Fractures

Dolfi Herscovici Jr. and Julia M. Scaduto

Ankle fractures are common skeletal injuries and are one of the most managed joint injuries in orthopedic surgery. Surgical fixation is well-established as the treatment of choice for displaced fractures with an anatomic reduction of the mortise decreasing instability and lessening the development of post-traumatic arthrosis. Even in the diabetic patient, acute, displaced fractures are routinely managed with surgical intervention [1]. Although the use of nonoperative care for some fractures have demonstrated good outcomes, nonsurgical treatment is usually reserved for patients presenting with non-displaced fractures, those whose medical co-morbidities that preclude any surgical intervention, patients who refuse surgery or most often as an intermediate step to allow the soft tissue envelope to improve. This then allow surgeons to proceed with surgical intervention of the ankle. After an anatomic reduction and stable fixation, and excluding any skin or wound complications, the postoperative care of the nondiabetic often results in reproducible and good outcomes.

So why then is there a different concern in managing the diabetic patient? One large prob-lem is that because ankle fractures are so routinely treated, there is often a certain disregard for the seriousness and potential complications that can occur in the diabetic population. Due to their hyperglycemia, the preoperative diabetic can already have impaired healing of the wound and bone, a decrease in their immune response, vascular insufficiency, terrible skin problems, and peripheral neuropathy. Although these are all significant factors, it is their peripheral neuropathy, of sensory, motor and autonomic dysfunction, which may result in patients failing to recognize that they have sustained an injury and have them seek medical attention in a timely manner. This may result in a late presentation of the fracture, a deformity and contracture of the ankle, and potentially ulceration and compromise of the soft tissue envelope, all of which may lead to the development of Charcot arthropathy, even after undergoing surgery [1, 2].

How then, do we manage the acute diabetic ankle fracture? Do we withhold certain treatments because they will be too expensive? Or do we withhold treatments, due to expectations that they will have poorer outcomes than the nondiabetic patient? This comes with the understanding that withholding treatment can produce avoidable complications, result in significant disabilities, and create chronic conditions that can lead to socio-economic burdens to the patient, their families, and to payer systems. Given the advancements in techniques, implants, and the

D. HerscoviciJr. (✉)
Foot and Ankle Service, Center for Bone and Joint Disease, Hudson, FL, USA

J. M. Scaduto
Foot and Ankle Service, Center for Bone and Joint Disease, Hudson, FL, USA

management of diabetes, this chapter will hopefully provide a rational approach for physicians tasked with managing acute ankle fractures in the diabetic patient.

1 Epidemiology

Current estimates report that there are more than 34 million people in the United States diagnosed with diabetes mellitus, with greater than eight million who are undiagnosed [3–5]. This represents about 13% of adults, affects more than 25% of people greater than 65 years of age and is the seventh leading cause of death in the United States [4, 5]. Worldwide diabetes has increased from 108 million in 1980 to 463 million in 2019 [6–8]. This equates to one of every 11 people and current projections indicate that this number will exceed 700 million people (1 in 10) by the year 2045 [6–8]. In addition, two studies have reported that the lifetime risk of developing diabetes in the United States [9] and India [10] for males was 32.5% (55.5% India) and 38.5% for females (64.6% India), with the results of both studies reporting that the diagnosis of diabetes produced a dramatic decrease in life-years for both males and females.

Although complications are often related to poor glucose control, hypertension, and dyslipidemia, only 36% to 57% of patients achieve adequate glycemic or blood pressure levels, while only 13.2% of all patients achieve all three target levels [11]. Approximately 89% have one additional comorbidity and 15% have four or more [12]. Contributing to problems, patients often smoke and have sedentary lifestyles that often lead them to being overweight or obese [12]. Additionally, 10% of patients in the United States present with some degree of neuropathy at initial diagnosis, 40% will develop neuropathy within the first decade following that diagnosis and > 50% of patients over age sixty have some degree of neuropathy [13, 14]. The combination of neuropathy and at least one other comorbidity produces higher rates of complications (47% vs. 14%) compared to diabetics without neuropathy or another comorbidity [15]. All of which has

resulted in an increase in medical expenditures for the care of these patients. This has been borne out with studies demonstrating that in the United States $302 billion (USD) is spent annually managing diabetes with an additional $102 billion (USD) lost in revenue due to a reduced labor force, early mortality and lower productivity. The result is an economic burden of $1240 (USD) for each American with an annual medical expenditure of $13,240 (USD) for the medical care of each diabetic patient [12, 16, 17].

Specifically addressing adult ankle fractures, the incidence has been reported to be 100.8/100,000/per year. The ratio of men to women is 47:53, with bi- and trimalleolar fractures increasing in incidence, more so in women, as patients get older. In the United States, it has been estimated that approximately 260,000 Americans per year sustain an ankle fracture, with about 25% undergoing surgical management [18]. Within this population nearly 6%, or almost 16,000 patients per year, are diabetics who sustain an ankle fracture [19]. If the 25% needing surgery is extrapolated into the diabetic population, one would expect that annually approximately 4000 diabetics sustain an ankle fracture requiring surgery. Thus, less than 2% of all patients who sustain an ankle fracture in the United States are diabetics who are managed surgically for their injury.

2 Pathophysiology

Diabetes mellitus, and its resulting hyperglycemia, can lead to neuropathy, retinopathy, nephropathy, and cardiovascular damage [20, 21]. Chronic hyperglycemia results in increased blood viscosity, it impairs the ability of the red blood cell to deliver oxygen, it affects nitric oxide, which functions as an antioxidant and neurotransmitter, and it leads to microvascular compromise. The last of which can lead to coronary artery disease, stroke, peripheral artery disease, and produce nerve ischemia [22, 23]. In addition, hyperglycemia also decreases the ability of immune cells, specifically fibroblasts, from migrating and attaching to wounds, resulting in healing stagnation that may last for up to 8 weeks [24].

Chronic hyperglycemia also affects bone physiology with the hallmarks being a decrease in bone turnover, a functionally weaker bone and an increased fracture risk [25]. Accumulation of advanced glycation end products (AGEs) disrupts cellular biology and the bony microarchitecture producing inflammation. This results in its binding to the receptor for AGEs (RAGE) [25, 26]. RAGE increases osteoclastic activity, i.e., bone loss, leading to osteoporosis and demineralization. In addition, AGEs also interfere with osteoblastic development, collagen, and osteocalcin production and increases osteoblast apoptosis [27]. The result is a decrease in osteon formation and the ability of the bone to remodel. Hyperglycemia also impairs proliferation and migration of the osteocytes primarily by increasing adipogenesis of mesenchymal stem cells to preferentially differentiate into adipocytes rather than osteocytes [28].

The results of this fatty tissue formation, combined with hemoglobin A1c levels $\geq 6.5\%$, decreases callus formation, tensile strength, bone stiffness, and fracture healing [29], resulting in poorer radiographic restoration. Studies have reported union times to increase to 163%, compared to nondiabetic patients, which is further increased to 187% when the fractures are displaced [30]. This abnormal bony pathology also increases the chances of sustaining a more severe ankle fracture, along with increasing mortality rates, postoperative complications, lengths of hospital stays, and costs, than in the nondiabetic patient [30, 31]. It is, perhaps, for all of these reasons that the use of nonoperative care is more often considered for management of the diabetic patient who presents with an ankle fracture.

3 Preoperative Evaluations

Unless the patient presents with an open fracture or an irreducible dislocation, there is no need for emergency surgery. It is important that one understands that both *medical and surgical* treatment will be needed to manage these patients, rather than placing them conveniently onto the surgical schedule.

3.1 History

The management begins with a thorough history, specifically asking about the mechanisms and the timing of the injury. Up to 74% of diabetic patients have scores less than the threshold for osteopenia and 39% below the threshold for osteoporosis [32]. Therefore, a low (ground level fall) mechanism of energy resulting in a complex fracture pattern may indicate poor bone quality. Additionally, how long they have been a diabetic and questions about when the injury occurred are also important. Because neuropathy is present in 10% of diabetics, 40% within the first decade following that diagnosis and > 50% of patients over age 60 [13, 14], neuropathy can be inferred for any patient continuing to ambulate on the injured extremity and presenting more than 24 h after the injury occurred.

The history should also include questions about the presence of comorbidities since these have also been shown to increase the rates of complications. With approximately 89% of diabetics presenting with one additional comorbidity and 15% have four or more [12], this means that all medical and vascular evaluations should be performed prior to any surgical intervention. Additional questions should also include whether ambulatory aids were used prior to their injury, whether they smoke, their use of insulin or other medications, and whether they have a history of previous ulcers, amputations, or infections.

3.2 Physical Examination

The examination should begin by inspecting the soft tissue envelope of the limb. Any wounds or lacerations should be evaluated for an open fracture. Look and palpate for changes in skin color, temperature changes, or any bony prominences, all of which may be an indication of impending skin necrosis. Additionally, fracture blisters or the presence of any tense compartments may indicate that the extremity is not ready for operative fixation.

The neurologic examination begins with an observation of the extremity. Motor dysfunction, indicating intrinsic atrophy, is often manifested as clawing of the toes while autonomic dysfunction is suspected in patients presenting with dry, cracking, hyperemic skin (Fig. 1a, b). Of greatest concern is the loss of protective sensation due to neuropathy. Loss of vibratory sensation, pinprick, sense of position, or absence of deep tendon reflexes at the ankle (difficult to perform in the presence of a fracture) may indicate neuropathy but have only a fair agreement amongst evaluators [33]. Although the gold standard for identifying peripheral neuropathy is a nerve conduction study, the accepted method for detecting the loss of protective sensation is the use of a 5.07 (10-g) Semmes-Weinstein monofilament. This simple exam has a sensitivity and specificity of 91% and 86%, respectively [34], which increases with a minimum testing of four plantar sites (great toe, first, third, and fifth metatarsal heads) [33]. Detecting peripheral neuropathy is important since it contributes to poor protective sensation, physiologically inappropriate weight-bearing, noncompliance, and postoperative infections by a factor of four [35].

The last part of the physical exam should include a vascular evaluation. This is important since more than 40% of diabetics present with peripheral arterial disease [36]. The popliteal trifurcation is most affected however, vessel calcification in the ankle and the foot are also suggestive of vascular compromise (Fig. 2a, b). Visual signs suggestive of peripheral artery disease include dependent rubor, pallor with elevation of the extremity, dystrophic toenails, and hair loss [37]. The evaluation should continue with an attempt to palpate pulses and comparing it with the contralateral extremity. If pulses are still absent or diminished, after reducing the dislocation or improving the fracture alignment, the aid of Doppler ultrasound can be used to identify the vessels. Further evaluations can be made with the use of the ankle-brachial (ABI) index, which is often described as a more sensitive, noninvasive test for evaluating the patient's vascular status. A value of 0.91 to 1.3 is considered normal. In the diabetic, an ABI $\geq$ 1.1 is suggestive of arterial calcinosis and an ABI > 1.3 indicates poor compressibility of the vessel [37, 38]. However, in patients with acute ankle fractures an ABI may be difficult to perform, so for these patients one should pursue additional testing.

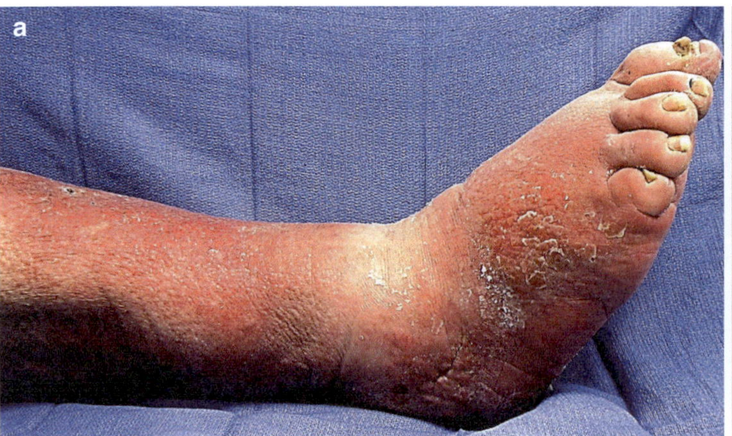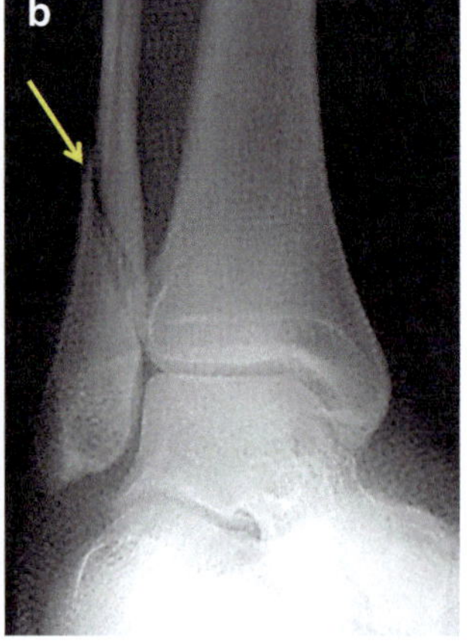

Fig. 1 (**a**) Picture of hyperemic skin in a 68-year-old male presenting with significant autonomic neuropathy and a fracture of the right ankle. Note the thick, stiff, dry, scaly and inflexible appearance of the skin that can crack easily and become an entry for infection. (**b**) Mortise view of the patient's ankle demonstrating a non-displaced fracture of the fibula (arrow) with no talar shift, treated successfully nonoperatively

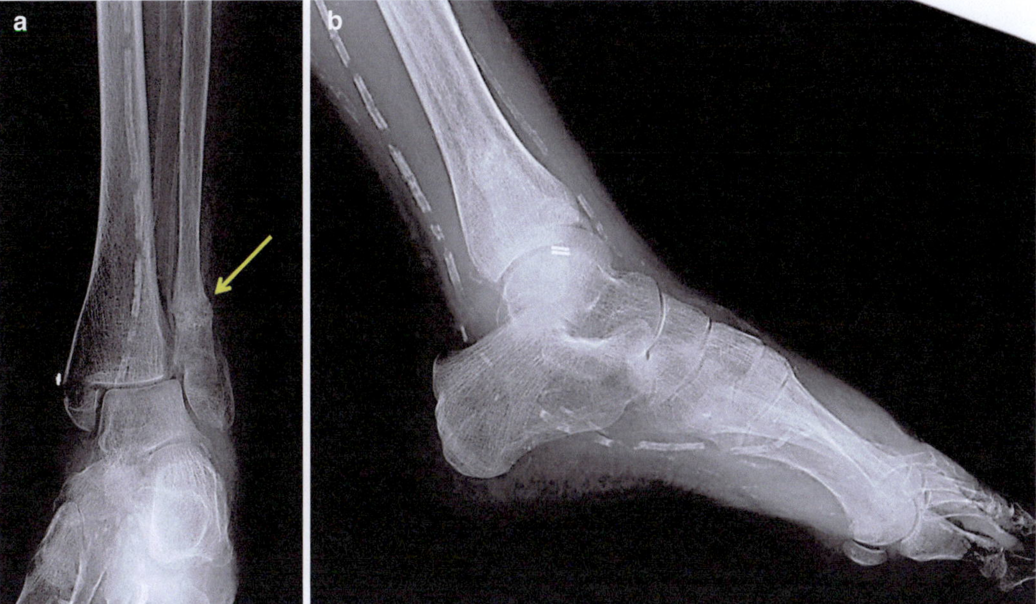

Fig. 2 (**a**) Mortise view of left ankle demonstrating a displaced left bimalleolar ankle fracture (and a healing stress fracture of the fibula, arrow) with calcification of the vessels. (**b**) Lateral view demonstrating that the calcification of the vessels extends into the foot

Currently, three noninvasive vascular tests are available. These consist of measuring transcutaneous oxygen pressures (T_cPO_2), toe pressures (TP), and the toe-brachial index (TBI). The T_cPO_2 measures oxygen level beneath the skin. Pressures >70 mmHg are normal, < 40 mmHg the minimum indicate impaired wound healing [36]. The TP test places small blood pressure cuffs around each toe and measures the systolic pressure of each toe. A toe pressure of ≥68 mmHg is predictive of good wound healing [37, 38]. The TBI is calculated by dividing the toe pressure by the highest obtained ankle pressure. Currently a value >0.7 has been reported as the cutoff for a normal value [39]. The problem with the TBI is that in the presence of a fracture the patient may not tolerate a cuff placed around the ankle. If there is any question about the patient's vascular supply, they should be referred to a vascular surgeon for further workup. Currently, the authors' preferred method of vascular evaluation is to obtain toe pressures on all patients.

3.3 Laboratory Evaluations/ Radiologic Evaluations

As discussed, uncontrolled hyperglycemia results in pathophysiologic dysfunctions and can produce an increased rate of complications not seen in the nondiabetic population or in well-controlled diabetics [20, 21, 35, 40–43]. Therefore, in addition to standard preoperative laboratory studies, all patients should also have their glycated hemoglobin A_{1c} (HgA_{1c}) levels evaluated. Levels >6.5 have been shown to increase the risk of complications, produce longer hospital stays, and result in poor radiologic outcomes [44]. Those with HgA_{1c} values >8 have a 2.5 times greater risk of developing an infection and poor surgical outcomes [45, 46]. However, for every 1% reduction in HgA_{1c}, there is approximately a 25–30% reduction in the rate of complications [47]. Patients should not be excluded from surgery, due to an elevated HgA_{1c}, but this information may help manage their diabetes during their postoperative care. In addition, during routine laboratory evaluations, the authors also evaluate preoperative albumin levels. Studies have shown that low levels of serum albumin may denote malnutrition, which may be an indicator for developing postoperative complications [48, 49]. As with HgA$_{1c}$ values, evaluating these values preoperatively will help during the postoperative management of these patients. The radiologic examination should begin with standard anteropsterior (AP), lateral and mortise views of the ankle. X-rays of the foot can also be performed to determine if there are any injuries to the foot. Advanced imaging studies, consisting of a computed tomographic (CT) scans and magnetic resonance imaging (MRI) images can also be performed to improve accuracy in diagnosing the patient's injuries. A CT scan helps to identify occult fractures and evaluate the incisura for syndesmotic injuries. An MRI scan can help diagnosis bony injuries not identified on plain films and help in diagnosing ligamentous, tendon and chondral injuries.

4 Fracture Management

Whether managed operatively or nonoperatively, the goals of treatment are to achieve a stable and congruent joint, restore function, and to prevent complications. Surgical goals should include obtaining an anatomic reduction of the mortise, providing stable fixation to maintain the reduction until adequate healing has occurred, avoiding the production of pressure areas to the ankle, and avoiding complications that can lead to loss of limb or death. An additional goal, not often noted in nondiabetic patients, is to prevent instability or an early loss of the reduction that leads to the development of a Charcot joint. Regardless of whether the patient is treated operatively or nonoperatively, a discussion should also include whether prolonged immobilization and non-weight bearing of the patient will be needed as well as whether supplementary (nonoperative) forms of treatment will be necessary to obtain adequate healing. These can include the use of calcium, vitamin D and protein supplements, ambulatory aids, wheelchairs, and appliances such as a Charcot Restraint Orthotic Walker (CROW) boot. The decision driving treatment should be based on the injury pattern and the patient's physiology. Unfortunately, there is no clear algorithm to guide the treatment, based on fracture displacement, for this population. The timing of surgery is important to consider for patient management. Within 8–12 hours after the injury there is interstitial edema that may last 7–21 days. Here, the use of an external fixator, using fine wire/circular fixation or standard transarticular external fixation, will allow one to improve the alignment of the fracture, delay definitive fixation until there is improvement of the soft tissue envelope and allow for medical optimization of the patient before undergoing definitive fixation. Looking for wrinkling of the skin can indicate that tissues can now undergo fixation safely.

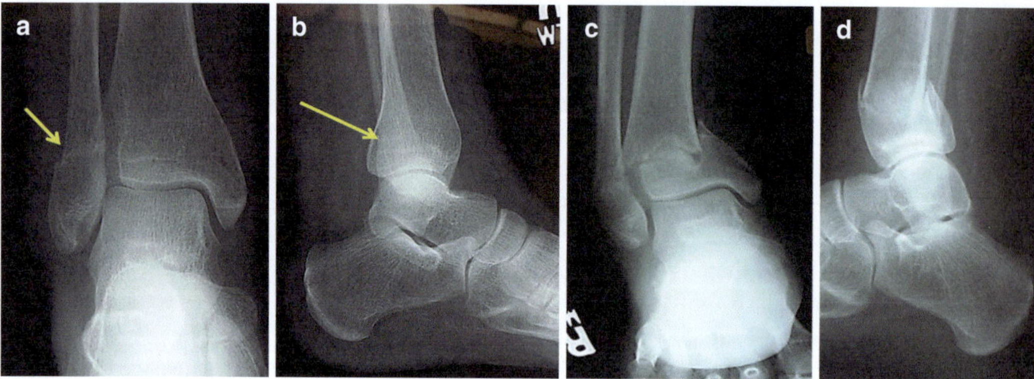

Fig. 3 (**a**, **b**) An AP and lateral views of a 52-year-old female, renal transplant, insulin dependent diabetes, who presented with a stress fracture (arrow) of the fibula demonstrating no displacement of the fracture. (**c**, **d**) Patient was treated conservatively in a walking boot and returned 1 month later. AP and lateral radiographs demonstrate displacement of both the fibula as well as a tibia fracture. The patient underwent surgical management

4.1 Nonoperative Treatment

The nonsurgical management can be controversial because of the concern for displacement however, these patients can be treated successfully. Nonsurgical care is offered to patients presenting with nondisplaced fractures, with a good rule of thumb being to double or triple the treatment offered to nondiabetic patients. Therefore, the nonoperative treatment consists of placing patients into a short leg, non-weight bearing cast for 10–12 weeks. Weekly or biweekly radiographs along with inspection of the soft tissue envelope to ensure that there has been no displacement of the mortise, and no problems to the soft tissue envelope have developed (Fig. 3a–d). After the casting period, patients are placed into a period of protective weight bearing, using a brace or boot, for an additional 2–3 months.

Very few studies discuss the nonsurgical management of diabetic ankle fractures. Most contain small numbers of patients and are often discussed as one of the arms of treatment, *in-lieu* of surgical management [18, 31, 40–43]. The complications reported in these studies have included malunions, due to a loss in the initial reduction; nonunions; the development of Charcot neuroarthropathy; infections; and the development of ulcers. Risk factors for developing a complication include seeing patients infrequently, early weight bearing or noncompliance, having a long duration of diabetes, the presence of neuropathy, insulin dependence, and patients with a history of Charcot neuroarthropathy. All these factors have been shown to contribute to a significantly increased mortality rate, postoperative complications, lengths of hospital stay, rate of nonroutine hospital discharge, and costs, when compared to nondiabetic patients with ankle fractures [19]. Risk factors not associated with complications include age, gender, and type of fracture [18, 31].

4.2 Operative Treatment

4.2.1 Preoperative Care and Planning

Prior to surgery, a discussion with the patient and their family should include the need for preoperative medical evaluations, whether a preoperative vascular evaluation should be performed, whether any adjunctive fixation will be needed to augment and hold the reduction until adequate healing has occurred and whether placement into a rehab or skilled-nursing facility will be needed

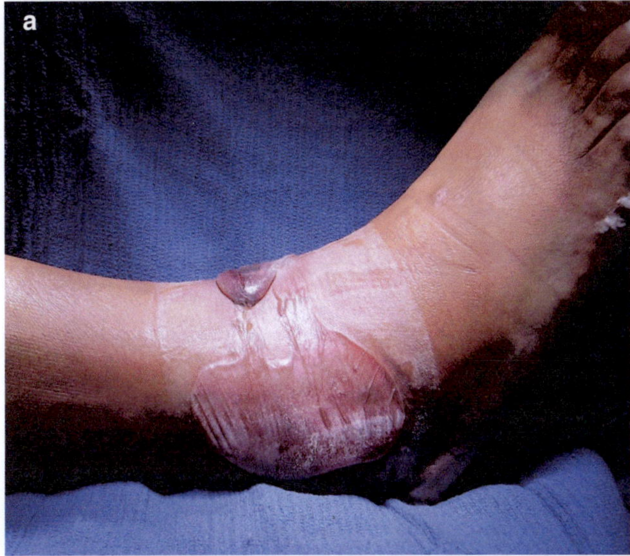
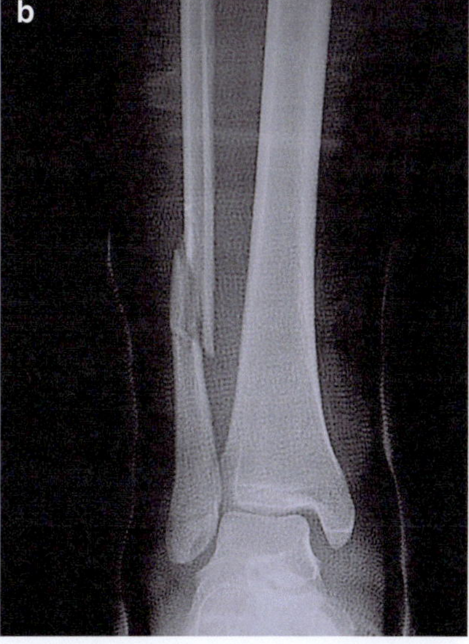

Fig. 4 (**a**) A 49-year-old male missed a step at home twisting his right ankle when he fell. The patient was transferred from an outlying hospital and on presentation demonstrated near circumferential fracture blisters about the ankle. (**b**) The mortise radiograph demonstrates the displaced fracture of the ankle. The patient was initially placed into an external fixator until the soft tissue improved allowing definitive fixation

until the patient and their family can be safely cared for at home.

The indication for surgical management is an unstable ankle fracture. However, before fixation is performed it is important to stabilize the soft tissue envelope. This includes a prompt reduction and splinting of the extremity, especially if fracture blisters have occurred. Immobilization can be achieved using a well-padded, nonremovable splint, or with the use of an external fixator if the reduction cannot be maintained by using the splint alone. The patient is instructed to keep the leg elevated as much as possible and is evaluated at weekly intervals. The ability to wrinkle the skin and a reepithelialization of the skin, after fracture blisters have resolved, indicates that the soft tissues have stabilized and are ready for surgical management (Fig. 4a, b). This may take anywhere between 10 to 21 days and during this period the preoperative evaluations previously discussed should be undertaken as part of the preoperative planning.

A large part of the preoperative planning should be to ensure that all the equipment and implants needed for surgery will be present. This equipment includes small, large and periarticular bone clamps, extra-long drill bits, extra-long screws, with lengths reaching 90–110 mm in length and in sizes ranging from 2.7-mm to 4.5-mm, Steinman pins, and extra-long k-wires. In addition, having a locking mini-fragment set, along with extra-long, small, and large fragment locking plates, should also be readily accessible. Simple rules of thumb are to extend the plates beyond the zone of injury and to use the strongest device that can be tolerated by the soft tissue envelope. The authors prefer the use of a 3.5-mm or 4.5-mm locking plates, or even the use of a plate designed for use in tibial plating, of at least ten holes in length, for fixation of the fibula while avoiding the use of semi-tubular or easily deformable (malleable) plates. Lamina spreaders or distractors should also be on hand if distraction of the fractures to achieve length, especially in the fibula, is anticipated. Lastly, an external fixator should also be ready for use if the ankle construct will need external augmentation.

4.2.2 Operative Management

There are five approaches that can be used to manage the diabetic ankle fracture: *standard*, *trans-syndesmotic*, circular (thin wire) external fixation, *trans-articular,* and a hybrid or *combination* of these techniques. Standard fixation, with expected good outcomes, can be considered for any patient presenting with an HgA_{1c} less than 7.0, a body-mass index (BMI) less than 30, able to sense a 5.07 or smaller Semmes-Weinstein monofilament, good vibratory sensation with a 128-hertz tuning fork, the presence of palpable pulses, nonosteoporotic bone, and those without any manifestations of autonomic dysfunction. Postoperatively, these patients can be managed like nondiabetic patients.

For patients who do not meet these criteria, three methods of fixation are available. These three techniques are different than standard methods of ankle fixation but have been developed to maintain an anatomic mortise and decrease the risk that failure of fixation will occur prior to adequate healing, leading to the development of a Charcot joint. In addition to prolonged immobilization and non-weight bearing, the operative principles for these three techniques include the use of long, rigid, locking plate fixation with long bicortical or quadricortical screw placement, using adjunctive fixation, considering the addition of a bone graft, and contemplating the use a bone stimulator (Table 1). Because of the patient's abnormal bony metabolism, the authors' current treatment of choice is to try (if insurance approval can be obtained) to add a bone stimulator to all patients when using one of these three alternative techniques. Small, prospective studies have described benefit of using a bone stimulator among diabetics undergoing foot and ankle surgery [50, 51]. Additional adjunctive fixation also includes bone graft or bone cement, inserting Steinman pins and leaving them in position until adequate healing has occurred, using calcium, vitamin D, and protein supplementation, and the use of a Strayer or Vulpius procedure to lengthen the Achilles tendon.

The *trans-syndesmotic fixation technique* uses the tibia to help stabilize the fibular fixation. This

Table 1 Authors preferences for the operative management and postoperative care of the acute diabetic ankle fracture

Rigid Fixation

Longer and Thicker Plates (Minimum 10 holes)
Locking Plate Technology
More and Longer Screws
    Multiple tetracortical screws used for trans-syndesmotic fixation through plate
    Bicortical screws for medial/posterior malleolar fixation, 4.0mm or larger
Possible use of an Intramedullary nail

Adjunctive Fixation

External Fixation
K-wires across ankle joint
Steinman Pins antegrade across ankle or retrograde through ankle/subtalar joints
Combinations of these techniques
Cement (Calcium Sulfate/Phosphate or polymethyl methacrylate)

Bone Graft/Supplements

Consider using bone for fracture. Add calcium, Vitamin D, protein supplements

Bone Stimulator

Recommend for use in these patients due to pathologic bone

Post-operative Care

Week 1: Well-padded post-operative splint
Week 2: Apply short leg non-weightbearing cast
Week 3: Remove sutures
Week 12: Remove Steinman pins, casting completed
Month 4-5: Boot or brace, therapy, advance to WBAT*
Month 6: Unrestricted activity

*WBAT: Weight bearing as tolerated

method consists of getting the fibula out to length, reducing the fracture and applying at least a 10-hole 3.5-mm or larger locking plate onto the fibula. The surgeon then inserts as many quadricortical (crossing four cortices), locking screws as possible through the fibula and into the tibia [52]. The advantage of using a locking plate is that it provides angular stability, which increases its load-carrying capacity and allows locking plates to be four times stronger than load-sharing constructs. This means that for failure of fixation to occur it requires that all points of fixation fail as opposed to the loosening of individual screws, as seen with traditional compression plating techniques. To complete the fixation of the ankle, long, 4.0-mm bicortical screws should be used to stabilize the medial and posterior malleolar fractures (Fig. 5). This construct improves fixation stiffness without relying solely on the screw's purchase in the fibula. Although there is concern that this technique may alter the biomechanics of the syndesmosis, this has not been demonstrated clinically.

The *trans-articular (nonfusion)* method of fixation and can be approached in one of two ways. The first is to treat the patient using standard reduction techniques, which is then augmented using two or three large, smooth, Steinmann pins, placed ante- or retrograde through the tibia, talus, and calcaneus [53, 54]. Although this is an older, described technique, its use can augment fixation in cases where tibiotalar instability may occur (Fig. 6a–d). This technique produces some stiffness of ankle and the hindfoot, but the advantage is it does not rely solely on standard fixation techniques to maintain the reduction. The second approach is the use of a retrograde tibio-talar-calcaneal intramedullary nail [55]. Although some calcification or arthrodesis of the ankle or subtalar joints is possible, the difference between this method and an arthrodesis technique is that neither the subtalar nor the ankle joint is exposed and prepared as when performing a formal arthrodesis. This approach works well in patients presenting with

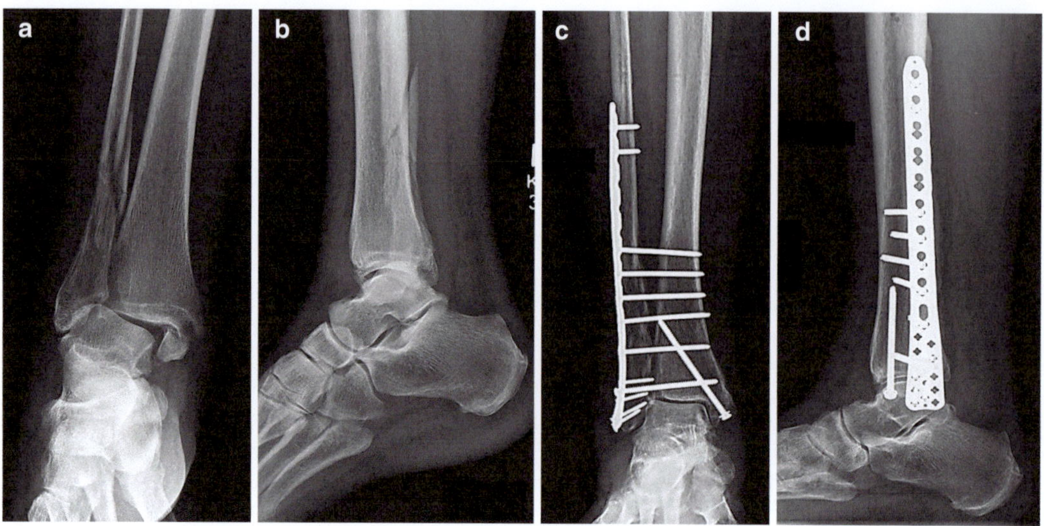

Fig. 5 (**a**, **b**) AP and lateral injury radiographs of the right ankle of a 48-year-old neuropathic, insulin dependent female who sustained a grand level fall at home. Patient's BMI was 28. A closed reduction and a splint were performed in the emergency department. (**c**, **d**) Postreduction AP and lateral radiographs at 11 months demonstrating a *trans-syndesmotic* technique, using a tibial plate that was used to manage the fracture. Note the bicortical screw used to fix the medial malleolar fracture

pilon fractures but can also be used in certain unstable bi- or trimalleolar ankle fractures, especially in patients with morbid obesity (Fig. 7a–c). Once the fracture is healed a decision regarding nail removal can be made. To complete the discussion of trans-articular methods of fixation, immediate arthrodesis of the ankle has also been described for non-reconstructable fractures [56] but has rarely been performed for an acute diabetic ankle fracture. However, in the setting of poor bone quality, a poorly controlled diabetic with neuropathy, autonomic changes, and poor potential to heal the fracture, an immediate arthrodesis may be considered to improve the outcome of that patient.

The third technique is *a combined technique*. In this approach the trans-syndesmotic technique is augmented using two or three large, smooth Steinman pins, which are placed ante- or retrograde through the tibia, talus, and calcaneus (Fig. 8a–c). This approach provides significant stiffness to the construct and is currently the authors' treatment of choice for the management of acute diabetic ankle fractures that are unable to be managed with standard fixation, especially in the morbidly obese patient. Like other methods described, the resulting stiffness acquired by the ankle with this approach does not seem to be a problem clinically because ambulation progressively restores motion between the tibia and fibula. The authors' preference is to leave the Steinman pins for either the trans-articular or combined technique in place for at least 2 (and possibly) 3 months before they are removed.

Fig. 6 (**a**, **b**) An AP and lateral views demonstrating a displaced ankle fracture in a 60-year-old insulin dependent diabetic female, status post renal transplant who sustained a ground level fall at home. (**c**, **d**) An AP and lateral views demonstrating a *trans-articular fixation* technique consisting of standard fixation augmented with two vertically placed Steinman pins. Pins were pulled at 3 months

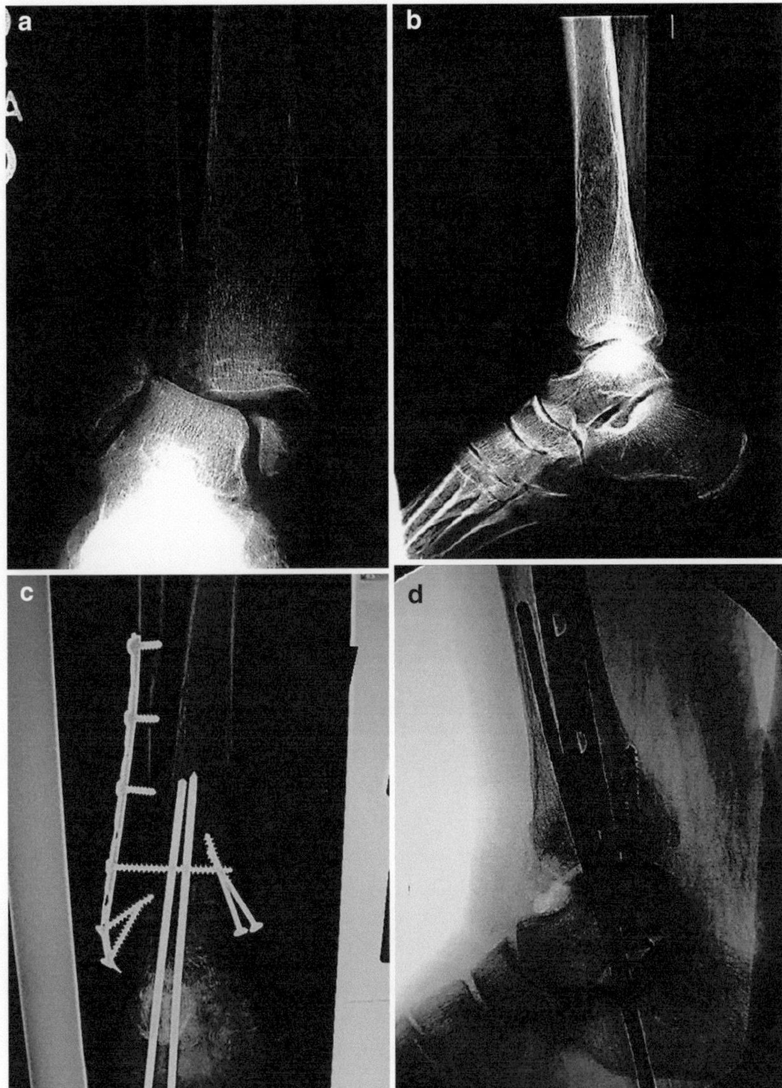

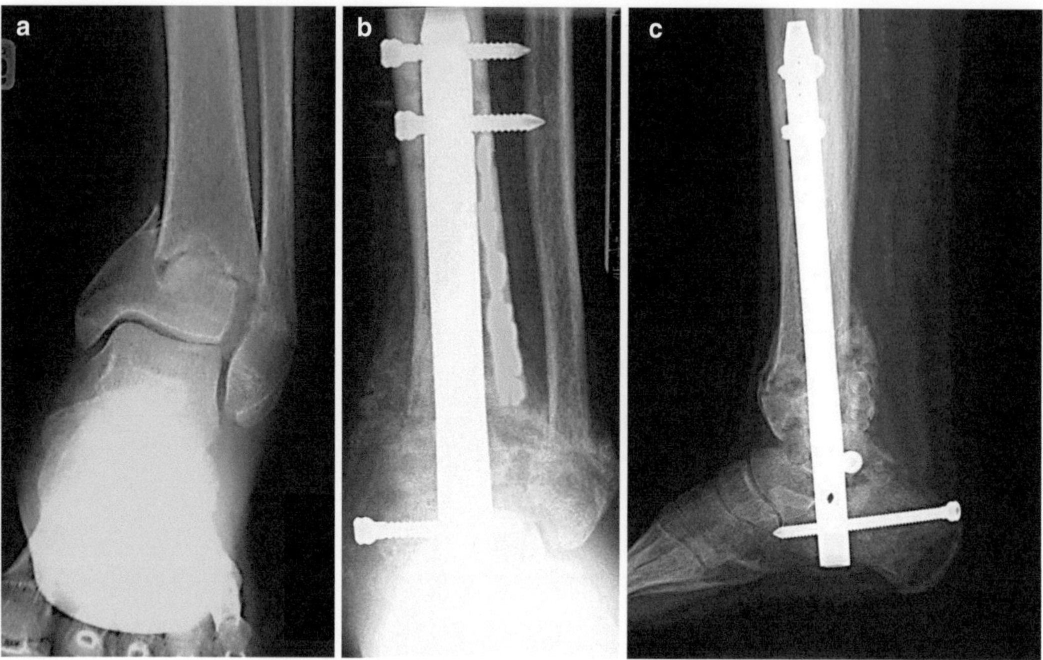

Fig. 7 (**a**) An AP view of the left ankle in a morbidly obese male who tripped walking downstairs demonstrating a displaced extra-articular pilon fracture. (**b, c**) An AP and lateral views demonstrating fixation using an intra-medullary hindfoot nail. Note that the preoperative varus positioning has been corrected. No takedown of the ankle or subtalar joints were performed

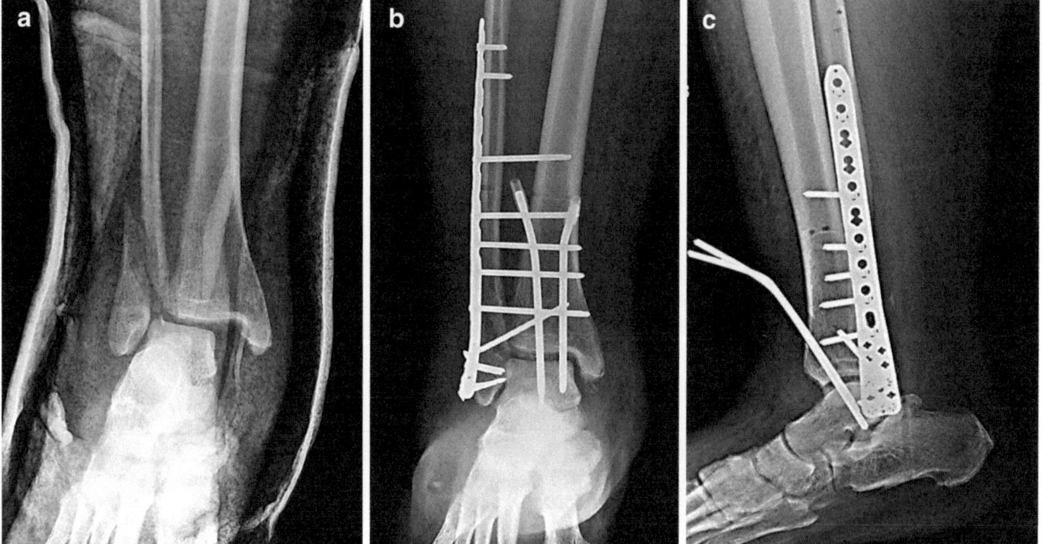

Fig. 8 (**a**) A 68-year-old morbidly obese female fell while getting out of her car, twisting her right ankle. The AP view demonstrates an unstable ankle fracture with a displaced fibula fracture and a lateral talar shift. The patient was neuropathic and was a poorly controlled type II diabetic. (**b, c**) Postoperative AP and lateral views demonstrating the use of a *combination* technique in which a tibial plate was used for fixation of the fibula showing the placement of multiple trans-syndesmotic screws augmented with two vertical Steinman pins placed antegrade

5 Complications and Salvage

Complications are more common in diabetics than nondiabetics, occurring in 26% of patients [57, 58] but can range from 3.6% to 43% [19, 31, 35, 40–43, 45, 58–61] and can occur individually or in any combination. Using multivariable regression analysis, African American race, obesity, tobacco use, and neuropathy were found to be significant independent predictors of worse functional outcomes, with an unplanned secondary operation rate over two times that of nondiabetic patients [57]. The four major complications associated with managing these patients consist of *failure of fixation* leading to malunions or nonunions, *skin and wound problems*, *infections,* and the *development of Charcot neuroarthropathy*. It should not be surprising that the rates of complications are higher in poorly controlled diabetics [42, 60]. The question is, after operating on these high-risk patients, can their complication(s) be treated without necessitating an amputation as the only salvageable option?

5.1 Failure of Fixation

In this context, failure of fixation is empirically defined as a loss of the reduction early in the postoperative period (within the first 2–4 weeks), without the development of a Charcot joint (Fig. 9a, b). The most common reasons for this complication are often a combination of the patient's neuropathy, their inability to avoid weight bearing on the extremity, and an inadequate fixation performed at the time of the index procedure. By far the biggest mistake is in trying to manage these patients like a well-controlled or nondiabetic patient. More than 60% of patients are obese or morbidly obese [48] and have little or no upper body strength. Thus, immobility and non-weight bearing becomes a significant issue for these patients. Either because of their central nervous system (CNS) neuropathy or because they are seeking independence, they will often begin full weight bearing within hours or days after their surgery. To decrease failure of fixation, leading to nonunions or malunions (2–5%) [58], patients may need to be placed into a skilled nursing or rehabilitation facility where they can be supervised. If they are going home, they should be placed into wheelchairs to help them maintain a non-weight bearing attitude. In addition, a discussion should be made with their caregivers about the importance of non-weight bearing, with weekly visits necessary if noncompliance persists, to make sure that displacement or failure of fixation has not occurred.

The salvage of a failed fixation is via one of the three previously discussed alternative approaches, with the timing dependent on the health of the soft tissue envelope. Continued conservative treatment of the misaligned extremity will often result in malunions, nonunions, the development of contractures, and skin breakdown and/or ulcerations. In some cases, the addition of trans-articular external fixation can improve the overall alignment, but it may not always produce an anatomic reduction of the mortise (Fig. 10a–d). If a revision of the fixation is unable to be performed, then a salvage using an ankle or double hindfoot arthrodesis (ankle and subtalar joint), may be necessary to salvage the extremity.

5.2 Skin and Wound Problems

Wound edge necrosis and dehiscence, without the presence of infection, are always concerns when managing these patients. Even without surgery, there is already a considerable challenge in trying to get things to heal in this population [42, 43, 62]. It has already been noted that hyperglycemia decreases blood flow to both small and large vessels [63], increases blood viscosity, impairs the ability of the red blood cells to flow, and decreases the amount of oxygen reaching the tissues. This hypoxia inhibits fibroblasts from migrating to the wound and causes them to lose their ability to proliferate, which may last for up to 8 weeks [19, 42, 62, 64]. The addition of smoking, hypertension, dyslipidemia, increased body mass index and advanced age, have also been shown to have a negative effect on wound healing [19, 30, 31, 38, 41, 45, 64].

The combination of hyperglycemia, fracture edema, and hypoxia create a poor environment for diabetic wound healing [38, 58, 59, 62], even in patients managed nonoperatively. Early salvage requires frequent (weekly) clinic visits since these

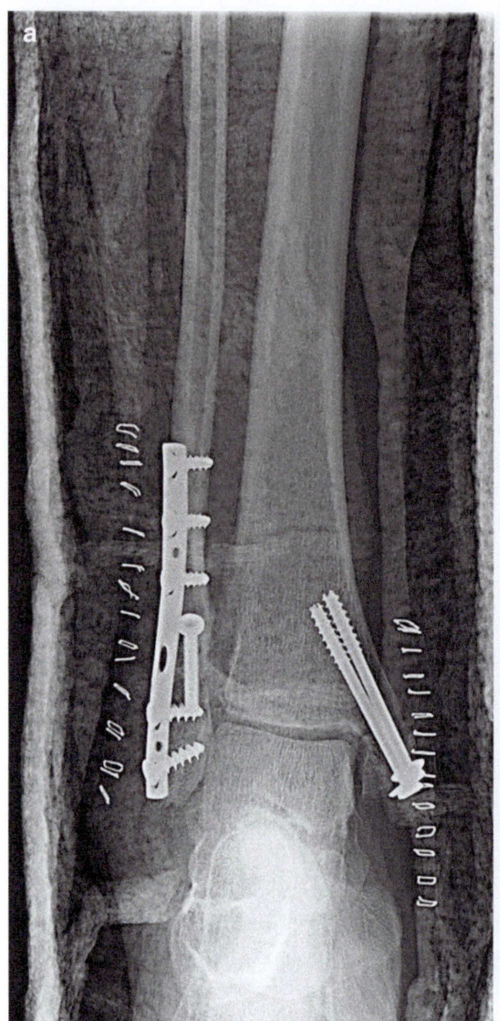
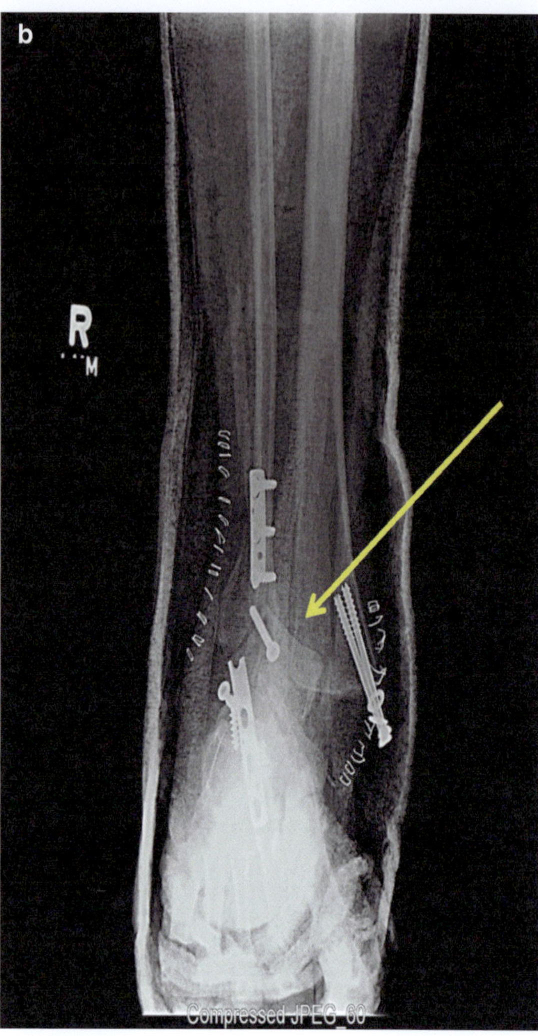

Fig. 9 (**a**) Immediate postoperative AP view of a supination-external rotation injury that was managed using standard fixation technique in an obese, neuropathic 51-year-old male. (**b**) At the first postoperative visit 2 weeks later, the AP radiograph demonstrates failure of fixation with a broken fibular plate and displacement of the fracture. Note the dislocation of the tibiotalar joint (arrow). Salvage was achieved using a hindfoot nail

problems may be identified early during routine cast changes. During these visits, encouraging good control of their diabetes, discussing the need for elevating the extremity, and placing them into wheelchairs may all help with healing, compliance, and edema. In addition, reapplying a well-padded splint, *in-lieu* of the cast, may help avoid pressure to the compromised skin. When skin or wound problems are identified, the authors' preference is for weekly office visits, daily wound care (e.g., wet-to dry-dressings) [65], through a windowed cast, and the empiric use of a broad-spectrum oral antibiotic. If the wound fails to improve, the formal use of irrigation and debridement and negative pressure wound therapy may be necessary. If after 4–6 weeks of negative pressure therapy, worsening or no improvement is noted, a plastic surgery consultation may be needed.

5.3 Infection

A major concern in managing these patients is the development of an infection. Both superficial and deep infections can occur with rates ranging from 6% to 43% [41, 57]. Risk factors for the development of an infection include, the presence of peripheral arterial disease, neuropathy, diabetes

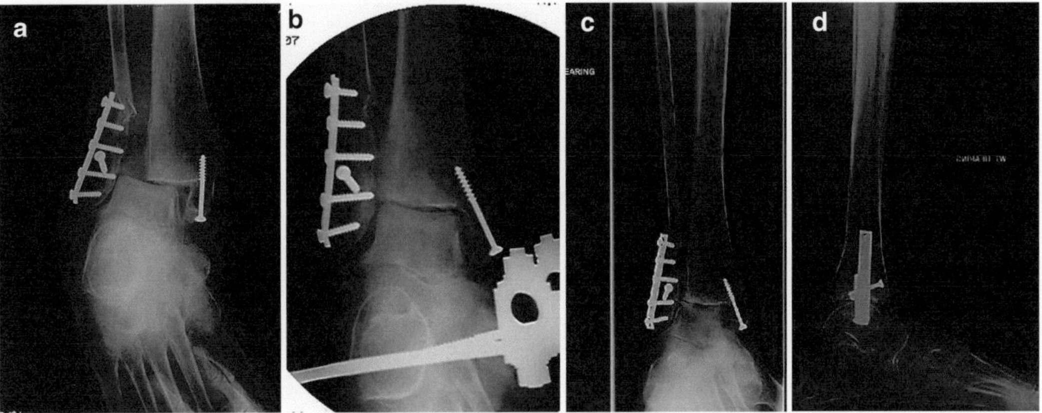

Fig. 10 (**a**) Use of a standard fixation technique demonstrating failure of fixation in an obese, neuropathic female seen on postoperative day 16. (**b**) The patient underwent the placement of a trans-articular external fixator. The mortise view demonstrates an anatomic reduction of the mortise. The fixator was left in position for 3 months. (**c, d**) At 3.6 years, AP and lateral radiographs demonstrate an anatomic mortise of the ankle joint. Note that the patient does have some post-traumatic arthritis of the tibiotalar joint but did not develop a Charcot joint

of long duration, poor glucose control (especially a $HgA_{1c} > 8$), the presence of a Charcot joint, the presence of edema and ecchymosis, older patients, obesity, a history of rheumatoid arthritis, a history of a previous ulcer, and in patients presenting with an open fracture [18, 31, 35, 40, 45]. The presence of neuropathy is biggest risk factor. Patients lose their ability to sense an infection, which is why even patients treated nonoperatively have been identified with an infection [18]. Factors that do not increase the risk of infection include tobacco use, gender, type of fracture, American Society of Anesthesiologists (ASA) classification, and whether the surgery was performed as an inpatient or an outpatient [31, 35]. Consistent with current literature, diabetes on admission has a 2–3 times greater risk of infection and a seven times risk of amputation after an ankle fracture [57, 59].

Frequent visits may not decrease this complication from occurring but can offer earlier treatment when they are identified. As with wound complications, the infection is often identified during a routine change of the patient's cast. For superficial infections, windowing the cast, to allow local, daily wound care, providing oral antibiotics, and weekly office visits may be sufficient to manage the problem. In contrast, all deep infections should be managed with irrigation and debridement, a minimum 6-week course of intravenous antibiotics, and removal of all loose implants. Avoid the urge to perform a local swab of the area. Rather, deep cultures or even a bone biopsy may be necessary to identify the organism(s) if osteomyelitis is suspected. Once the infection has been controlled, the use of a local flap or a free tissue transfer may be necessary if the wound is not able to be managed with secondary closures. If after bony debridement significant bone has been removed or the articular surfaces have been lost, then an ankle or double hindfoot arthrodesis may be needed to salvage the extremity. If the extremity is not salvageable then an amputation may be necessary.

5.4 Charcot Neuroarthropathy

The incidence, in diabetic ankle fractures, has been reported to occur between 6% and 47% [31, 43, 45, 61, 64, 66]. It is challenging to manage, especially when it presents after the surgical care of an ankle fracture, because it is often confused with infection. On initial presentation, patients often present with erythema, edema and warmth to palpation. The differential diagnosis can include gout, cellulitis, abscess, and osteomyelitis however, the diagnosis of a Charcot joint should be considered in any compliant patient, who had an anatomic reduction of the mortise and presents with failure of fixation. Careful physical, laboratory, and radiographic examinations will identify whether the patient has developed a Charcot neuroarthropathy or has a postoperative infection (Table 2).

Table 2 Differentiation of charcot and charcot with infection

	Charcot	**Infected Charcot**
Physical Findings		
Skin	Edema, Erythema, Warm	Edema, Erythema, Warm
Leg Elevation	Resolves edema/erythema	Edema/erythema persist
Ulcer	Non-draining	Draining, extends to bone
Temperature	Afebrile	Febrile
Discomfort	Painless	Painful
Lab Findings		
Glucose	No change	Out of Control
WBC**	Normal	Elevated
CRP,ESR+	Normal	Elevated
X-ray Exam	Fracture/Dislocation, periosteal reaction	Same, *Air Present*
99m-TC^ Bone Scan	Positive	Positive
Indium-111 Bone Scan	Negative (usually)	Positive
MRI* Scan	Soft tissue & bony edema, joint destruction	Fluid Collections; Air

White blood cells**
C-reactive protein, E Sed Rate+
Technetium-99m^
Magnetic Resonance Imaging*

The salvage of these patients can be difficult because they often present late with malunions, nonunions, and contractures of the extremities. Reconstruction should be considered when the extremity is in the subacute or chronic stages. Indications for surgery should include failure of conservative care, chronic deformity, instability not amenable to bracing, and evidence of abnormal plantar pressures, despite the use of an orthoses and special shoes. Reconstructions often involve the combination of bony and soft tissue procedures to improve the alignment and obtain a viable extremity. Further discussions on reconstructions can be found in the chapter on the Management of the Charcot Ankle.

In conclusion, if the patient is neuropathic, obese, has peripheral arterial disease and an elevated HgA_{1c}, avoid managing the acute diabetic ankle fracture like those treated in the nondiabetic population. These patients have increased rates of complications and infections and are usually noncompliant due to their neuropathy. Patients should be advised about higher risks of complications as related to ankle surgery. Careful preoperative evaluations and postoperative vigilance can improve outcomes. These patients require very rigid fixation, often with adjunctive fixation, with extended periods of immobilization and protective weight bearing. Significant deformities can produce abnormal plantar pressure, irritability with shoewear and malalignment of the extremity. However, good outcomes can be expected with alternative techniques and even some mild residual deformity does not seem to produce much disability.

References

1. Bibbo C, Lin SS, Beam HA, Behrens FF. Complications of ankle fractures in diabetic patients. Orthop Clin N Am. 2001;32:113–33.
2. Vaudreuil NJ, Fourman MS, Wukich DK. Limb salvage after failed initial operative management of bimalleolar ankle fractures in diabetic neuropathy. Foot Ankle Int. 2016;38:248–54.
3. U.S. Diabetes Surveillance System. https://gis.cdc.gov/grasp/diabetes/DiabetesAtlas/html. Accessed 16 Aug 2021.
4. Centers for Disease Control and Prevention. National diabetes statistics report, 2020. Atlanta, GA: Centers

for Disease Control and Prevention, US Department of Health and Human Services; 2020.

5. Heron M. Deaths: leading causes for 2017. Natl Vital Stat Rep. 2019;68:1–77.

6. Cheng H-T, Xu X, Lim PS, Hung K-Y. Worldwide epidemiology of diabetes-related end-stage renal disease, 2000–2015. Diabetes Care. 2021;44:89–97.

7. International Diabetes Federation. IDF Diabetes Atlas. 9th ed. Brussels: International Diabetes Federation; 2019.

8. Cho NH, Shaw JE, Karuranga S, Huang Y, da Rocha Fernandes JD, Ohlrogge AW, Malanda B. IDF diabetes atlas: global estimates of diabetes prevalence for 2017 and projections for 2045. Diabetes Res Clin Pract. 2018;138:271–81.

9. Venkat Narayan KM, Boyle JP, Thompson TJ, Sorenson SW, Williamson DF. Lifetime risk for diabetes mellitus in the United States. JAMA. 2003;290:1884–90.

10. Luhar S, Kondal D, Jones R, Anjana RM, Patel SA, Kinra S, Clarke L, Ali MK, Prabhakaran D, Kadir MM, Tandon N, Mohan V, Venkat Narayan KM. Lifetime risk of diabetes in metropolitan cities in India. Diabetologia. 2021;64:521–9.

11. Ong KL, Cheung BM, Wong LY, Wat NM, Tan KC, Lam KS. Prevalence, treatment, and control of diagnosed diabetes in the U.S. National Health and Nutrition Examination Survey 199–2004. Ann Epidemiol. 2008;18:222–9.

12. O'Connell JM, Manson SP. Understanding the economic costs of diabetes and prediabetes and what we may learn about reducing the health and economic burden of these conditions. Diabetes Care. 2019;42:1609–11.

13. Prisk VR, Wukich DK. Ankle fractures in diabetics. Foot Ankle Clin. 2006;11:849–63.

14. Singh N, Armstrong DG, Lipsky BA. Preventing foot ulcers in patients with diabetes. JAMA. 2005;293:217–28.

15. Zhang Y, Lazzarini PA, McPhail SM, van Netten JJ, Armstrong DG, Pacella RE. Global disability burdens of diabetes-related lower-extremity complications in 1990 and 2016. Diabetes Care. 2020;43:964–74.

16. Centers for Disease Control and Prevention. National Diabetes Statistics Report: Estimates of Diabetes and Its Burden in the United States, 2014. Atlanta, GA: U.S. Department of Health and Human Services; 2014; http://www.cdc.gov/diabetes/pubs/statsreport14/national-diabetes-report-web.pdf.

17. Dall TM, Yang W, Gillespie K, Mocarski M, Byrne E, Cintina I, Beronja K, Semilla AP, Iacobucci W, Hogan PF. The economic burden of elevated blood glucose levels in 2017: diagnosed and undiagnosed diabetes, gestational diabetes mellitus, and prediabetes. Diabetes Care. 2019;42:1661–8.

18. Court-Brown CM, Caesar B. Epidemiology of adult fractures: a review. Injury. 2006;37:691–7.

19. Flynn JM, Rodriguez-del Río F, Pizá PA. Closed ankle fractures in the diabetic patient. Foot Ankle Int. 2000;21:311–9.

20. Ganesh SP, Pietrobon R, Cecílio WAC, Pan D, Lightdale N, Nunley JA. The impact of diabetes on patient outcomes after ankle fracture. J Bone Joint Surg Am. 2005;87:1712–8.

21. American Diabetes Association. Standards of medical care in diabetes-2022. Diabetes Care. 2022;45(suppl 1):S113–94.

22. Emanuelsson F, Marott S, Tybjærg-Hansen A, Nordestgaard BG, Benn M. Impact of glucose level on micro- and macrovascular disease in the general population: a mendalian randomization study. Diabetes Care. 2020;43:894–902.

23. Vincent AM, Russell JW, Low P, Feldman EL. Oxidative stress in the pathogenesis of diabetic neuropathy. Endocr Rev. 2004;25:612–28.

24. Paraskevas KI, Baker DM, Pompella A, Mikhailidis DP. Does diabetes mellitus play a role in restenosis and patency rates following lower extremity peripheral arterial revascularization? A critical overview. Ann Vasc Surg. 2008;22:481–91.

25. Stadelmann WK, Digenis AG, Tobin GR. Impediments to wound healing. Am J Surg. 1998;176(2A Suppl):39S–47S.

26. Sellmeyer DE, Civitelli R, Hofbauer LC, Khosla S, Lecka-Czernik B, Schwartz AV. Skeletal metabolism, fracture risk, and fracture outcomes in type 1 and type 2 diabetes. Diabetes. 2016;65:57–66.

27. Yao D, Brownlee M. Hyperglycemia-induced reactive oxygen species increases expression of the receptor for advanced glycation end products (RAGE) and RAGE ligands. Diabetes. 2010;59:249–55.

28. Fong Y, Edelstein D, Wand E, Brownlee M. Inhibition of matrix-induced bone differentiation by advanced glycation end-products in rats. Diabetologia. 1993;36:802–7.

29. Sundararaghavan V, Mazur MM, Evans B, Liu J, Ebraheim NA. Diabetes and bone health: latest evidence and clinical implications. Ther Adv Musculoskelet Dis. 2017;9:67–74.

30. Weinberg E, Maymon T, Moses O, Weinreb M. Streptozotocin-induced diabetes in rats diminishes the size of the osteoprogenitor pool in bone marrow. Diabetes Res Clin Pract. 2014;103:35–41.

31. Boddenberg U. Healing time of foot and ankle fractures in patients with diabetes mellitus: literature review and report on own cases. Zentralbl Chir. 2004;129:453–9.

32. Jones KB, Maiers-Yeldon KA, Marsh JL, Zimmerman MB, Estin M, Saltzman CL. Ankle fractures in patients with diabetes mellitus. J Bone Joint Surg Br. 2005;87:489–95.

33. Herbst SA, Jones KB, Saltzman CL. Pattern of diabetic neuropathic arthropathy associated with peripheral bone mineral density. J Bone Joint Surg Br. 2004;86:378–83.

34. Smieja M, Hunt DL, Edelman D, Etchells E, Cornuz J, Simel DL. Clinical examination for the detection of protective sensation in the feet of diabetic patients. International cooperative group for clinical examination research. J Gen Intern Med. 1999;14:418–24.

35. Pham H, Armstrong DG, Harvey C, Harkless LB, Giurini JM, Veves A. Screening techniques to identify people at high risk for diabetic foot ulceration: a prospective multicenter trial. Diabetes Care. 2000;23:606–11.

36. Wukich DK, Lowery NJ, McMillen RI, Fryberg RG. Postoperative infection rates in foot and ankle surgery: a comparison of patients with and without diabetes mellitus. J Bone Joint Surg Am. 2010;92:287–95.

37. Novo S. Classification, epidemiology, risk factors, and natural history of peripheral artery disease. Diabetes Obes Metab. 2002;4(Suppl 2):S1–6.

38. American Diabetes Association. Peripheral arterial disease in people with diabetes. Diabetic Care. 2003;26:3333–41.

39. Vitti MJ, Robinson DV, Hauer-Jensen M, et al. Wound healing in forefoot amputations: the predictive value of toe pressures. Ann Vasc Surg. 1994;8:99–106.

40. Høyer C, Sandermann J, Petersen LJ. The toe-brachial index in the diagnosis of peripheral artery disease. J Vasc Surg. 2013;58:231–8.

41. Wukich DK, Joseph A, Ryan M, Ramirez C, Irrgang JJ. Outcomes of ankle fractures in patients with uncomplicated versus complicated diabetes. Foot Ankle Int. 2011;32:120–30.

42. SooHoo NF, Krenek L, Eagan M, Zingmond DS. Elevated risks of ankle fractures surgery in patients with diabetes. Clin Diabetes. 2010;28:166–70.

43. Henderson S, Izuchukwu I, Cahill S, Chung Y-H, Lee FY. Bone quality and fracture-healing in type-1 and type-2 diabetes mellitus. J Bone Joint Surg Am. 2019;101:1399–410.

44. Chaudhary SB, Liporace FA, Gandhi A, Donley BG, Pinzur MS, Lin SS. Complications of ankle fracture inpatients with diabetes. J Am Acad Orthop Surg. 2008;16:159–70.

45. Liu J, Ludwig T, Ebraheim NA. Effect of the blood HbA1c level on surgical treatment outcomes of diabetics with ankle fractures. Orthop Surg. 2013;5:203–8.

46. Wukich DK, Crim BE, Frykberg RG, Rosario BL. Neuropathy and poorly controlled diabetes increase the rate of surgical site infection after foot and ankle surgery. J Bone Joint Surg Am. 2014;96:832–9.

47. Underwood P, Askari R, Hurwitz S, Chamarthi B, Garg R. Preoperative A1C and clinical outcomes in patients with diabetes undergoing major noncardiac surgical procedures. Diabetes Care. 2014;37:611–6.

48. Hoogwerf BJ, Sferra J, Bonley BG. Diabetes mellitus-overview. Foot Ankle Clin N Am. 2006;11:703–15.

49. Shaoguang L, Zhang J, Zheng H, Wang X, Lih Z, Sun T. Prognostic role of serum albumin, total lymphocyte count, and mini nutritional assessment on outcomes after geriatric hip fracture surgery: a meta-analysis and systemic review. J Arthroplasty. 2019;34:1287–96.

50. Ernst A, Wilson JM, Ahn J, Shapiro M, Schenker ML. Malnutrition and the orthopaedic patient: a systematic review of the literature. J Orthop Trauma. 2018;32:491–9.

51. Busse JW, Bhandari M, Einhorn TA, Schemitsch E, Heckman JD, Tornetta P III, Leung KS, Heels-Ansdell D, Makosso-Kallyth S, Della Rocca GJ, Jones CB, Guyatt GH, TRUST Investigators Writing Group. Re-evaluation of low pulsed ultrasound in treatment of tibial fractures (TRUST): randomized clinical trial. BMJ. 2016;355:i5351.

52. Saxena A, DiDomenico LA, Widtfeldt A, Adams T, Kim W. Implantable electrical bone stimulation for arthrodesis of the foot and ankle in high-risk patients: a multicenter study. J Foot Ankle Surg. 2005;44:450–4.

53. Jani MM, Ricci WM, Borrelli J Jr, Barrett SE, Johnson JE. A protocol for treatment of unstable ankle fractures using transarticular fixation in patients with diabetes mellitus and loss of protective sensation. Foot Ankle Int. 2003;24:838–44.

54. Childress HM. Vertical transarticular pin fixation for unstable ankle fractures. Impressions after 16 years of experience. Clin Orthop Rel Res. 1976;120:164–71.

55. Scioscia TN, Ziran BH. Use of a vertical transarticular pin for stabilization of severe ankle fractures. Am J Orthop. 2003;32:46–8.

56. Ebaugh MP, Umbel B, Goss D, Taylor BC. Outcomes of primary tibiotalocalcaneal nailing for complicated diabetic ankle fractures. Foot Ankle Int. 2019;40:1382–7.

57. Bozic V, Thordarson DB, Hertz J. Ankle fusion for definitive management of non-reconstructable pilon fractures. Foot Ankle Int. 2008;29:914–8.

58. Schmidt T, Simske NM, Audet MA, Benecick A, Kim C-Y, Vallier HA. Effects of diabetes mellitus on functional outcomes and complications after torsional ankle fracture. J Am Acad Orthop Surg. 2020;28:661–70.

59. Olsen LL, Møller AM, Brorson S, Hasselager RB, Sort R. The impact of lifestyle risk factors on the rate of infection after surgery for a fracture of the ankle. Bone Joint J. 2017;99-B:225–30.

60. McCormack RG, Leith JM. Ankle fractures in diabetics. Complications of surgical management. J Bone Joint Surg Br. 1998;80:689–92.

61. Blotter RH, Connolly E, Wasan A, Chapman MW. Acute complications in the operative treatment of isolated ankle fractures in patients with diabetes mellitus. Foot Ankle Int. 1999;20:687–94.

62. Centers for Disease Control and Prevention: National health and nutrition examination survery. Questionaires, datasets, and related documentation. NHANES, 2015–2016. https://www.cdc.gov/nchs/nhanes/default.aspx. Accessed 12 May 2019.

63. Forslund JM, Archdeacon MT. The pathobiology of diabetes mellitus in bone metabolism, fracture healing and complications. Am J Orthop. 2015;44:453–7.

64. Gotler H, Godbout C, Chahal J, Schemitsch EH, Nauth A. Diabetes and healing outcomes in lower extremity fractures: a systematic review. Injury. 2018;49:177–83.

65. Wukich DK, Kline AJ. The management of ankle fractures in patients with diabetes. J Bone Joint Surg-Am. 2008;90:1570–8.

66. Ahmad J. The diabetic foot. Diabetes Metab Syndr. 2016;10:48–60.

The Neuropathic (Charcot) Ankle

Michael S. Pinzur

There is a growing consensus on both surgical indications and clinical outcome expectations for the treatment of diabetes-associated neuropathic (Charcot Foot) arthropathy at the midfoot level [1–5]. The historical metrics for measuring successful clinical outcomes were simply resolution of infection and limb salvage. There was no reported metric associated with brace use or ambulatory activity. It is currently appreciated that successful treatment is associated with the ability to walk using commercially-available therapeutic footwear and avoid the need for cumbersome orthotic devices [6–8]. These goals are generally achieved by correcting the acquired deformity and achieving a stable plantigrade foot. Treatment guidelines are not as well understood, nor are outcome expectations as favorable, when the ankle joint is involved [9]. The goals of this chapter are to explain the impediments to achieving favorable clinical outcomes in the treatment of Charcot Foot arthropathy when the ankle joint is involved in the neuropathic process, and describe the current strategies for achieving a stable plantigrade foot capable of walking with commercially-available therapeutic footwear.

1 Why Is the Ankle Different

The human foot is a unique organ that is adapted for weight bearing on both level and nonlevel surfaces. It is composed of approximately 28 to 32 bones that pre-position the very durable plantar tissue to accept the forces associated with weight bearing. The individuals most prone to develop Charcot Foot Arthropathy are long-standing morbidly obese diabetics with peripheral neuropathy. In order to fully comprehend the pathophysiology associated with this disorder, one must appreciate that during the period of development of peripheral neuropathy, affected individuals also develop osteoporosis [1]. Eichenholtz Stage I Charcot Foot Arthropathy actually behaves similar to a "stress fracture" associated with either a single episode of trauma, or repetitive loading of biomechanically poor quality bone. Most patients heal after a period of immobilization and do not progress to either the "nonunion," or malunion deformity associated with Eichenholtz Stage III disease. The best observational study associated with Charcot Foot Arthropathy would suggest that

M. S. Pinzur (✉)
Orthopaedic Surgery and Rehabilitation, Loyola
University Health System, Maywood, IL, USA
e-mail: mpinzu1@lumc.edu

© The Author(s), under exclusive license to Springer Nature Switzerland AG 2023
D. Herscovici Jr. et al. (eds.), *Evaluation and Surgical Management of the Ankle*,
https://doi.org/10.1007/978-3-031-33537-2_17

the incidence is actually approximately 0.3 per 1000 per year [10]. The initial presentation of Charcot Foot is often wrongly diagnosed as gout, cellulitis, tendonitis, or other maladies, with the actual diagnosis of Charcot Foot not being appreciated until much later when x-rays are taken for various reasons [11]. If the "stress fracture" does not progress to union, the deformity will likely progress [12, 13]. If the deformity progresses to the point where the foot is not clinically or radiographically plantigrade, tissue breakdown with subsequent infection is likely [14, 15].

The difference in biomechanical loading of the ankle joint is likely responsible for the increased potential for a poor clinical outcome when the ankle joint is involved in the neuropathic process. The foot is normally loaded in a plantigrade fashion, whereas the ankle is loaded in valgus (Fig. 1). If an ankle fracture does not progress to union, the weight bearing vector will displace laterally, accentuating valgus loading, thus increasing the deforming forces [12, 13] (Fig. 2). This explains the observation that, while the development of Charcot Foot Arthropathy at the midfoot level be attritional, the neuropathic (Charcot) ankle almost always develops following a fracture [9].

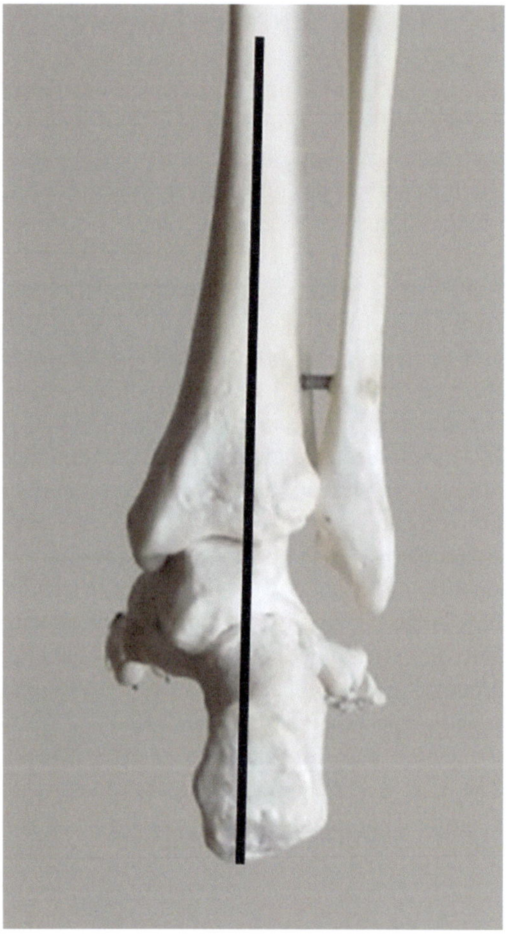

Fig. 1 The normal weight bearing line passes through the middle of the ankle, with a vector that interacts with the floor through the heel

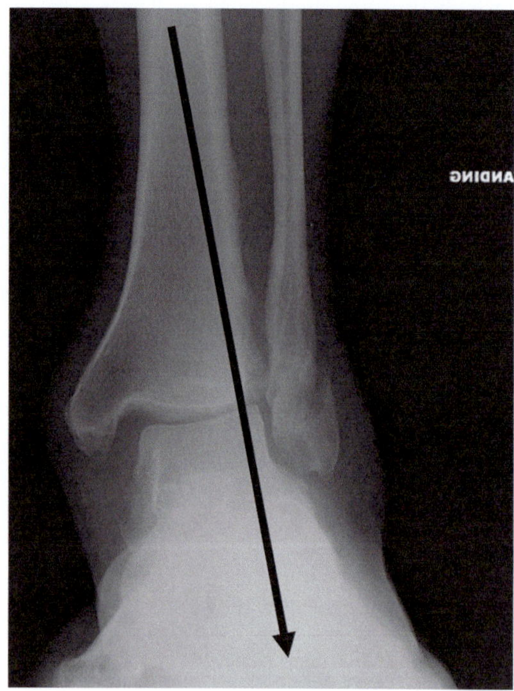

Fig. 2 An unstable ankle fracture with widening of the ankle displaces the weight-bearing vector laterally. The biomechanical loading applied to the unstable ankle tends to accentuate the deforming forces

2 Treatment of Unstable Ankle Fractures in Neuropathic Diabetics

Connally first observed the risk for amputation in diabetics following an ankle fracture [16]. Multiple subsequent authors have demonstrated the high risk for the development of complications following ankle fracture in diabetics with peripheral neuropathy [13, 17–23]. The logical explanation for the increased rate of complications in diabetics is the associated comorbidities of osteoporosis and immunodeficiency. The common development of mechanical failure following internal fixation of ankle fractures in diabetics is likely associated with the inability of standard orthopaedic implants to maintain mechanical construct stability in severely poor quality bone. The increased rate of postoperative infection is, likewise associated, with the known impaired immunity in this patient population [2]. This combination of factors influenced Johnson to advise "doubling down" on diabetic ankle fractures by *doubling* the magnitude of surgical fixation and *doubling* the period of immobilization [19–21, 24, 25].

The first step in decision-making in diabetic patients with an ankle fracture is the decision of which ankle fractures require surgery. The insensate diabetic patient in Fig. 3 has what appears to be a stable ankle fracture. This was confirmed with a weight-bearing radiograph taken 1 week later, demonstrating no loss of alignment. The decision was made to continue nonoperative treatment. Radiographs at both 6 and 12 weeks demonstrated delayed healing without loss of alignment. Nonoperative treatment was continued. Radiographs taken at 6 months following injury demonstrate eventual radiographic union (Fig. 3). A similar diabetic patient with peripheral neuropathy presented with the radiographs demonstrated in Fig. 4. A weight-bearing radiograph at 1 week demonstrated instability, leading to treatment with augmented internal fixation. *Augmented* internal fixation can be accomplished via a large transarticular pin crossing the ankle joint, or multiple syndesmotic screws, using the fibular plate as a "washer" for the screws (Fig. 5) [19–21].

The use of closed reduction and stabilization with a percutaneous retrograde locked intramedullary nail without arthrodesis has recently been advocated for complex ankle fractures in high risk patients or patients with a questionable soft tissue envelope (Fig. 6) [26].

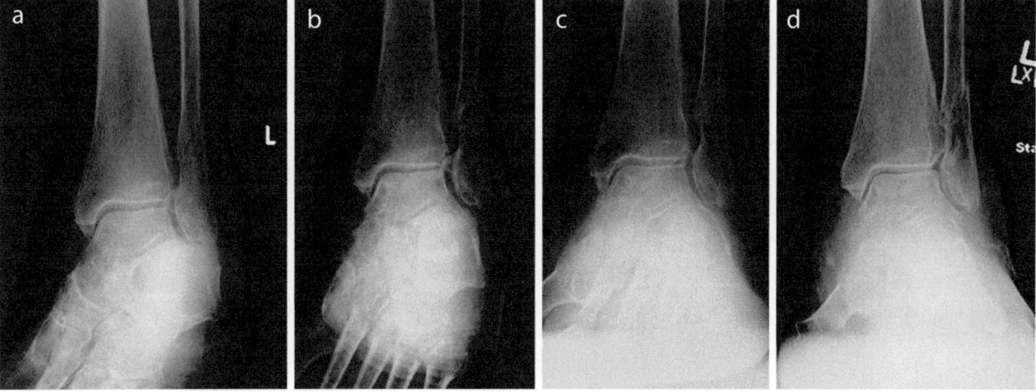

Fig. 3 This diabetic patient with peripheral neuropathy presented to the Emergency Room with ankle pain following a twisting injury (**a**). She was treated with a fracture boot and still had discomfort at 6 weeks following injury (**b**). A 12-week radiograph did not demonstrate bony union in spite of her not being symptomatic (**c**). Radiographs at 6 months demonstrate bony union (**d**). (Used with permission of Jeremy McCormack)

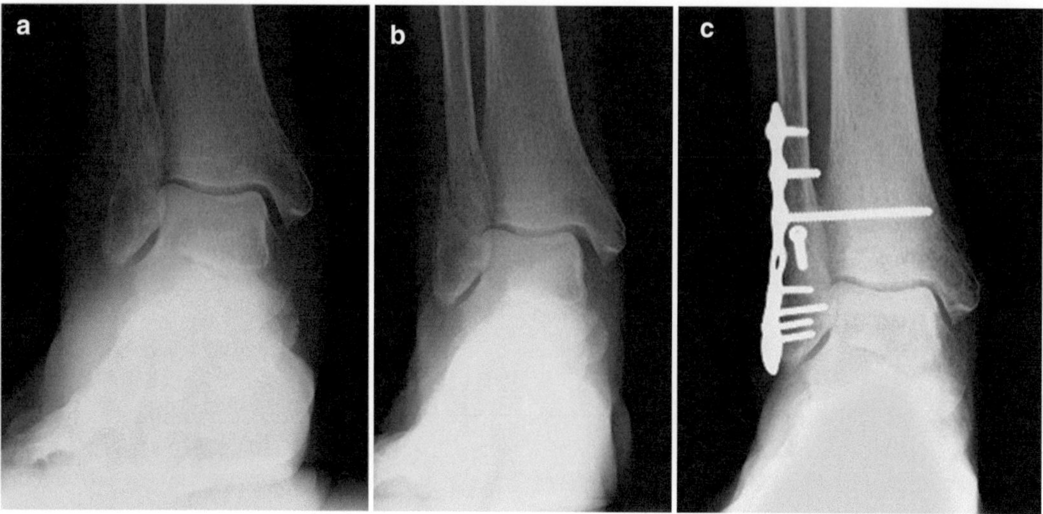

Fig. 4 Emergency Room radiographs of a similar patient with ankle pain following an injury (**a**). Weight-bearing radiograph at 1 week demonstrating unstable ankle fracture (**b**). Radiograph following successful open reduction internal fixation (**c**). (Used with permission of Jeremy McCormack)

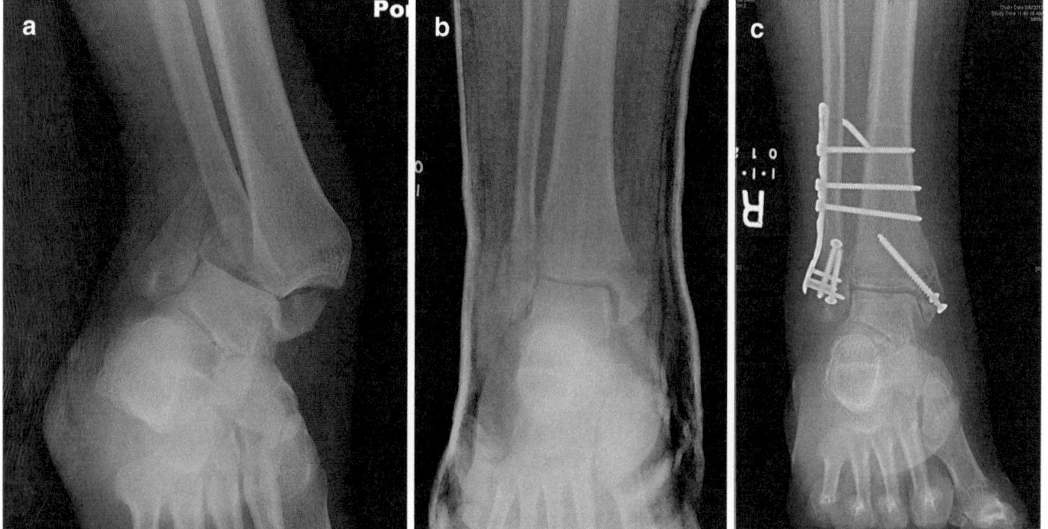

Fig. 5 Unstable ankle fracture following a low energy injury in an insensate diabetic patient (**a**). Radiographs following closed reduction reveal the low energy nature of the injury (**b**). Radiographs following open reduction internal fixation with augmented internal fixation (**c**). The lateral plate is used as a *washer* for the syndesmotic screws that are used for augmented internal fixation

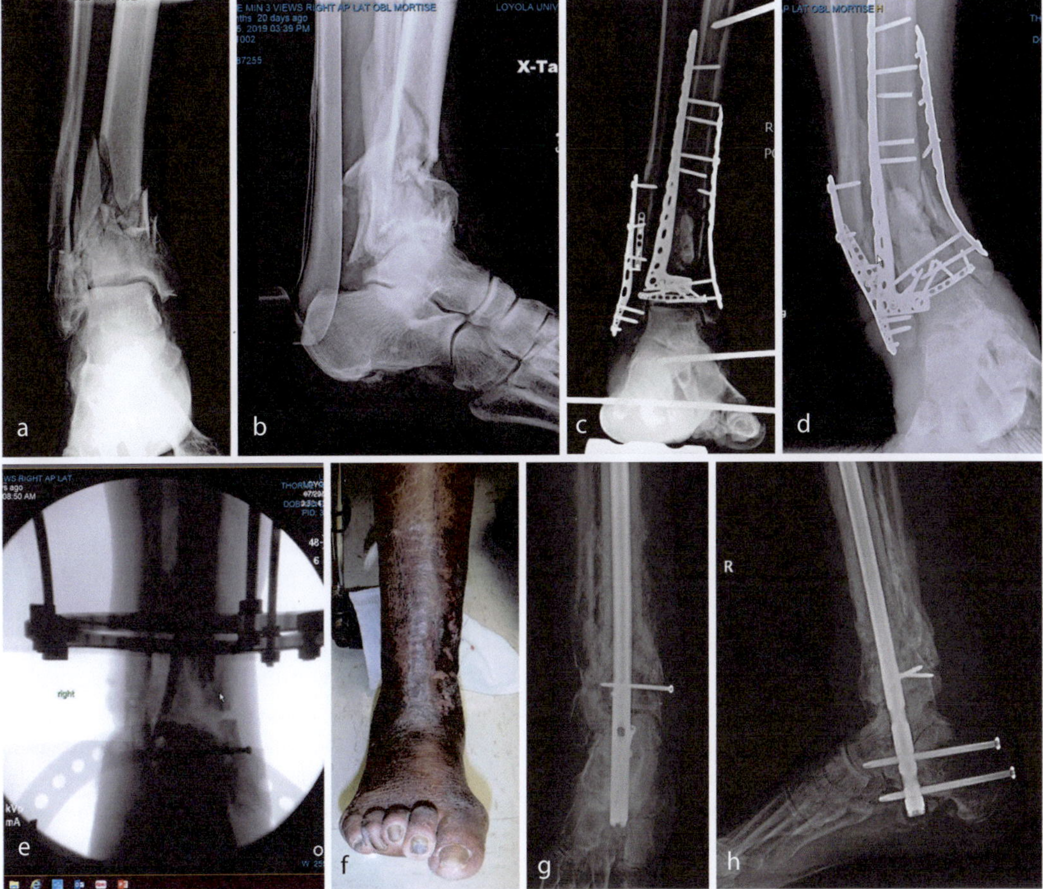

Fig. 6 This 72-year old neuropathic male sustained this unstable distal tibia fracture (**a, b**). He was initially treated with closed reduction and application of a damage control external fixator. This was followed by open reduction with standard orthopaedic implants (**c**). The patient was strictly non-weight bearing, but had this radiograph 2 weeks later (**d**). The failed implants were removed, and an external fixator was placed until the articular component of the fracture healed (**e**). A percutaneous locked nail and bone grafting led to eventual painless union at 2 years (**f, g, h**)

3 Arthrodesis in the Neuropathic Patient with No Infection

Neuropathic arthropathy can develop in a diabetic patient with long standing peripheral neuropathy following fracture or recurrent ankle sprains. Ankle replacement is generally not advised in diabetics with peripheral neuropathy due to the high risk for failure. Plate and screw constructs to achieve ankle or tibiotalocalcaneal arthrodesis is probably best avoided due to the potential for mechanical failure in patients with known osteoporosis and poor bone quality. The most reliable mechanical construct for achieving tibiotalocalcaneal arthrodesis is a retrograde locked intramedullary nail [9, 27]. Augmentation with one or two transarticular large fragment screws increases the likelihood of achieving a successful arthrodesis (Fig. 7) [28].

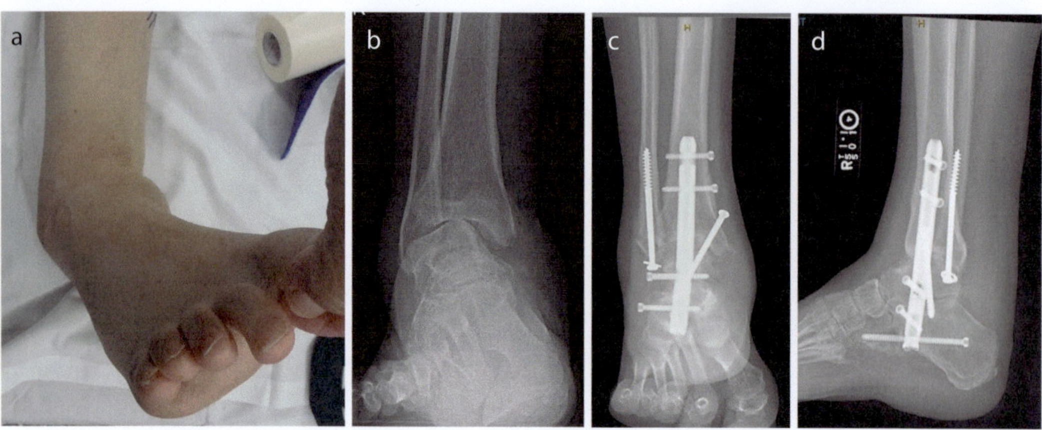

Fig. 7 This 63-year old neuropathic diabetic male developed this deformity after multiple ankle "sprains" (**a**, **b**). Radiographs at 1.5 years following ankle fusion with retrograde locked intramedullary nail and augmented fixation (**c**)

4 Arthrodesis in the Neuropathic Patient with Infection

Obtaining and maintaining a stable ankle reduction is essential to achieve a favorable clinical outcome following treatment of an ankle fracture in the neuropathic diabetic. Failure to achieve and maintain a stable reduction increases the mechanical load on the fixation construct, leading to mechanical failure, tissue break down, and deep infection (Figs. 1 and 2).

Accommodative bracing is generally inadequate longitudinally. The patient in Fig. 8 sustained a fracture of the medial malleolus that was initially determined to be stable. The instability was not appreciated until she presented with a limb threatening infection. Treatment required resolution of the infection and stabilization afforded by arthrodesis. This was accomplished by a single stage debridement of the infected bone, and ankle fusion with a circular external fixation construct [9, 29]. A similar situation presented with the patient in Fig. 9 following failure of internal fixation.

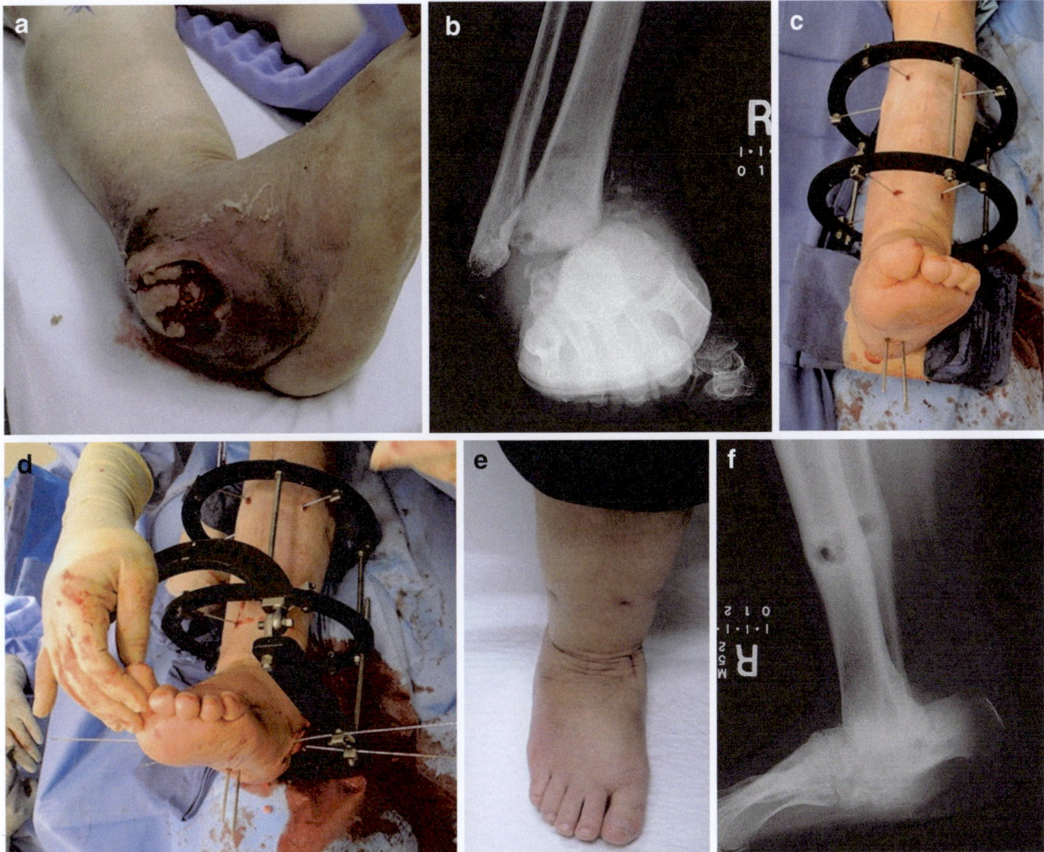

Fig. 8 This 61-year old neuropathic female sustained an unstable fracture of the medial malleolus that was treated nonoperatively in a fracture boot. Photograph and image 6 weeks later when she was referred for amputation (**a, b**). The first step in surgery was a debridement of the infected wound, followed by preparation of the ankle joint for arthrodesis. Provisional fixation was accomplished with two transarticular smooth pins. A tibial ring block was applied to the tibia to be used as the "reference" segment (**c**). A closed foot ring was then applied to the foot. The "moving segment" is then attached to the reference segment with either threaded rods of adjustable struts. Compression of the "moving" segment to the "reference" segment creates a stable construct (**d**). Photo and image at 2 years demonstrating successful limb salvage (**e, f**)

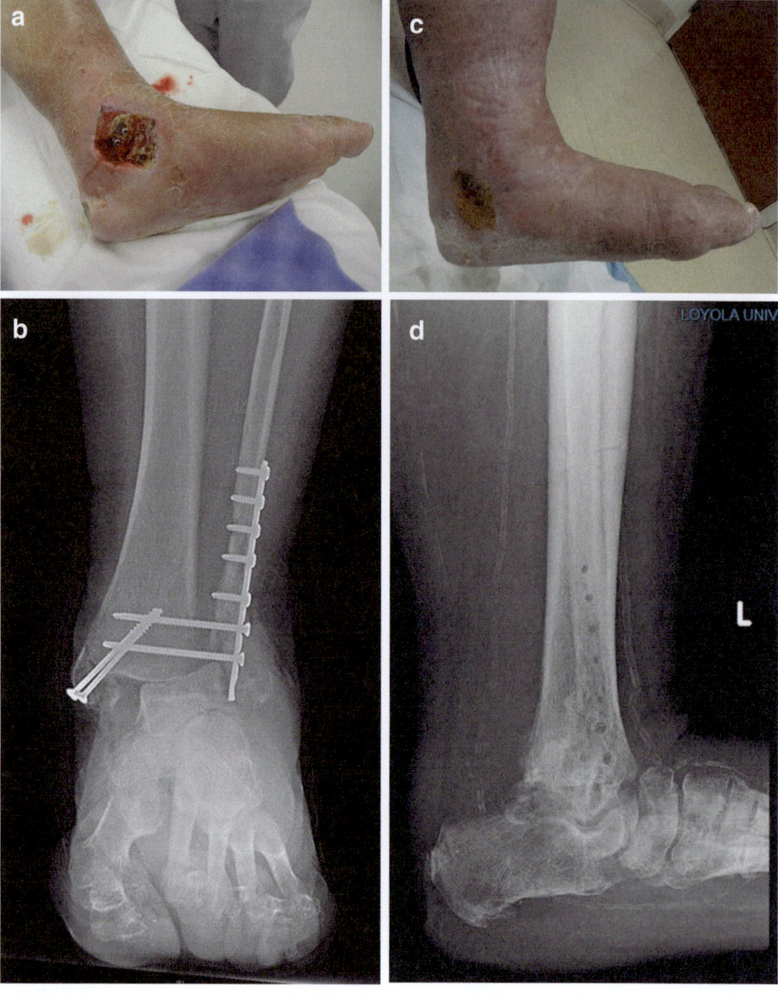

Fig. 9 This 61-year old neuropathic female presented 6 weeks after a failed attempt at surgical stabilization of an unstable ankle fracture (**a**, **b**). Photo and radiograph at 1.5 years following successful single stage removal of implants, debridement of osteomyelitis, and application of an ankle fusion construct circular external fixator (**c**, **d**)

5　Circular External Fixation to Accomplish Ankle Fusion

Circular external fixation is an excellent surgical technique to accomplish ankle fusion. The basic principles of deformity corrected are employed. In Fig. 8, the tibial mounting block segment is considered the *reference* segment, and the closed foot ring is considered the *moving* segment. Note that percutaneous K-wires were used to achieve provisional fixation. Either threaded rods or compressible struts are used to connect the moving segment to the reference segment. Compression between these two segments provides rigid internal fixation; a conduit to achieve successful bony union. Unique to the diabetic patient population with accepted osteoporosis, threaded half-pins should be avoided due to the high risk for developing a tibial stress fracture [30]. All bony fixation should be accomplished with tensioned wires, following the techniques of Illizarov.

6　Hybrid Fixation

The most recent innovation in the treatment of the neuropathic ankle is the use of hybrid fixation that combines elements of internal and external fixation in the treatment of complex ankle deformity patterns. Various combinations of retrograde locked intramedullary nails, transarticular screws, and circular external fixation have been employed to accomplish this task in the most complex patients (Fig. 10) [31].

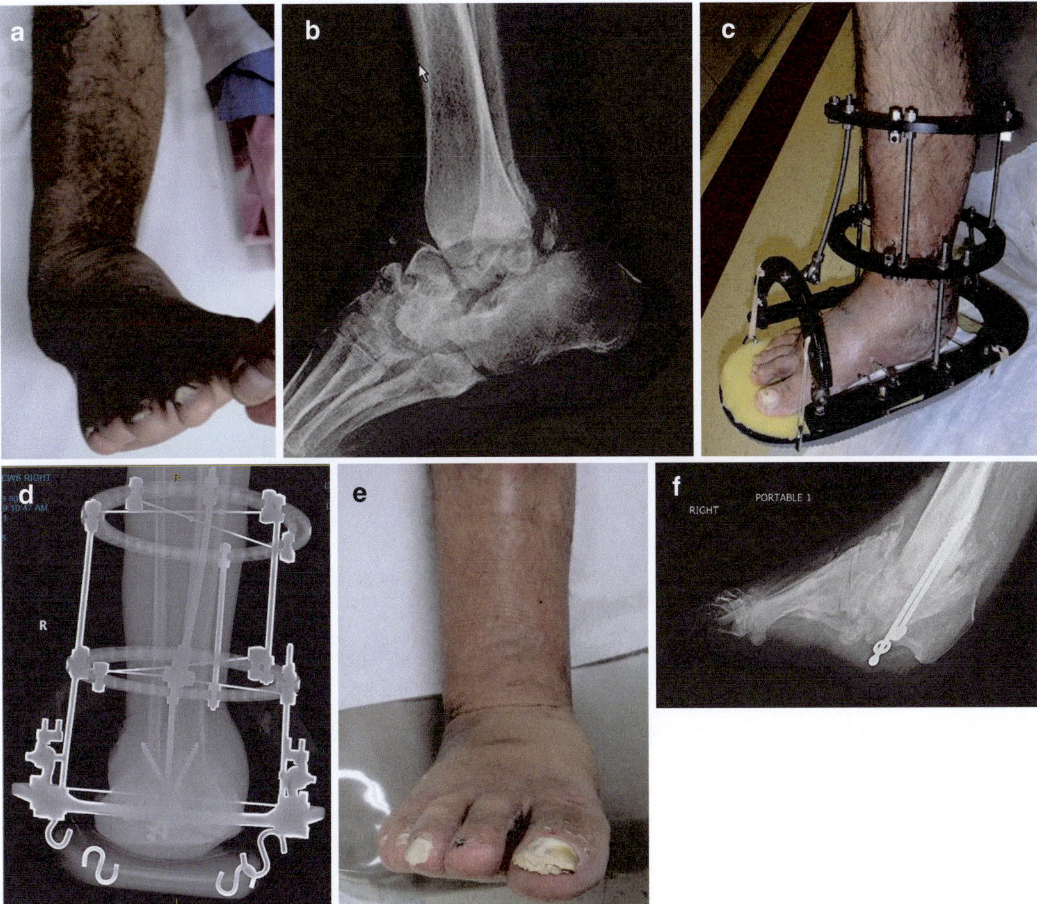

Fig. 10 This 41-year old diabetic male with renal transplant developed gross ankle instability following resorption of the body of the talus (**a**, **b**). He underwent tibiocalcaneal arthrodesis. Due to the high risk of failure with either internal or external fixation methods, he underwent "hybrid" fixation with crossed compression screws and neutralization with a circular external fixator (**c**, **d**). This has also been accomplished with a retrograde intramedullary nail combined with circular external fixation [31]. Photograph and radiograph at 2 years (**e**, **f**)

References

1. Rogers LC, Frykberg RG, Armstrong DG, Boulton AJM, Edmonds M, Ha Van G, Hartemann A, Game F, Jeffcoate W, Jirkovska A, Jude E, Morbach S, Morrison W, Pinzur M, Pitocco D, Sanders L, Wukich DK, Uccioli L. The diabetic Charcot foot syndrome: a report of the joint task force on the Charcot foot by the American Diabetes Association and the American podiatric medical association. Diabetes Care. 2011;34:2123–9.
2. Jones C, McCormick J, Pinzur MS. Surgical treatment of Charcot foot. In: instructional course lectures of the American Academy of Orthopaedic Surgeons. 67: 255–267, 2018.
3. Pinzur MS, Schiff AP. Deformity and clinical outcomes following surgical correction of Charcot foot: a new classification with implications for treatment. Foot Ankle Int. 2018;39(3):265–70.
4. Sammarco VJ, Sammarco GJ, Walker EW, Guiao RP. Midtarsal arthrodesis in treatment of Charcot midfoot arthropathy. J Bone Joint Surg. 2009;91(1):80–91.
5. Ford SE, Cohen BE, Davis WH, Jones CP. Clinical outcomes and complications of midfoot Charcot reconstruction with intramedullary beaming. Foot Ankle Int. 2019;40(1):18–23.
6. Dhawan V, Spratt KF, Pinzur MS, Baumhauer J, Rudicel S, Saltzman CL. Reliability of AOFAS diabetic foot questionnaire in Charcot arthropathy: stability, internal con-sistency and measurable difference. Foot Ankle Int. 2005;26(9):717–31.
7. Kroin E, Schiff AP, Pinzur MS, Davis ES, Chaharbakhshi E, FA DS Jr. Functional impairment of patients undergoing surgical correction for Charcot foot Arthropathy. Foot Ankle Int. 2017;38(7):705–9.

8. Kroin E, Chaharbakhshi EO, Schiff A, Pinzur MS. Improvement in quality of life following surgical correction of midtarsal Charcot foot deformity. Foot Ankle Int. 2018;39(7):808–11.

9. Harkins E, Murphy M, Schneider A, Schiff A, Pinzur MS. Deformity and clinical outcomes following surgical correction of Charcot ankle. Foot Ankle Int. 2019;40(2):145–51.

10. Fabrin J, Larsen K, Holstein PE. Long-term follow-up in diabetic Charcot feet with spontaneous onset. Diabetes Care. 2000;23:796–800.

11. Pinzur MS, Kernan-Schroeder D, Emmanuele NV, Emmanuele MA. Development of a nurse-provided health system strategy for diabetic foot care. Foot Ankle Int. 2001;22:744–6.

12. Hastings MK, Johnson JE, Strube MJ, Hildebolt CF, Bohnert KL, Pryor FW, Sinacore DR. Progression of foot deformity in Charcot neuropathic osteoarthropathy. J Bone Joint Surg. 2013;95A:1206–13.

13. Wukich DK, Raspovic KM, Hobizal KB, Rosario B. Radiographic analysis of diabetic midfoot Charcot neuroarthropathy with and without midfoot ulceration. Foot Ankle Int. 2014;35(11):1108–15.

14. Bevan WP, Tomlinson MP. Radiographic measure as a predictor of ulcer formation in diabetic Charcot midfoot. Foot Ankle Int. 2008;29:568–73.

15. Pinzur MS. Surgical vs. accommodative treatment for Charcot arthropathy of the midfoot. Foot Ankle Int. 2004;25:545–9; PMID: 15363375.

16. Connolly JF, Csencsitz TA. Limb threatening neuropathic complications from ankle fractures in patients with diabetes. Clin Orthop. 1998;348:212–9.

17. Strotman P, Reif TJ, Pinzur MS. Current concepts: Charcot arthropathy of the foot and ankle. Foot Ankle Int. 2016;37(11):1255–63.

18. Bibbo C, Lin SS, Beam HA, Behrens FF. Complications of ankle fractures in diabetic patients. Orthop Clin North Am. 2001;32:113–33.

19. Jani MM, Ricci WM, Borrelli J Jr, Barrett SE, Johnson JE. A protocol for treatment of unstable ankle fractures using transarticular fixation in patients with diabetes mellitus and loss of protective sensibility. Foot Ankle Int. 2003;24(11):838–44.

20. Koval KJ, Petraco DM, Kummer FJ, Bharam S. A new technique for complex fibula fracture fixation in the elderly: a clinical and biomechanical evaluation. J Orthop Trauma. 1997;11(1):28–33.

21. Perry MD, Taranow WS, Manoli A II, Carr JB. Salvage of failed neuropathic ankle fractures: use of large fragment fibular plating and multiple syndesmotic screws. Foot Ankle Int. 2005;14(2):85–91.

22. Ganesh SP, Pietrobon R, Cecílio WA, Pan D, Lightdale N, Nunley JA. The impact of diabetes on patient outcomes after ankle fracture. J Bone Joint Surg Am. 2005;87(8):1712–8.

23. Wukich DK, Kline AJ. The management of ankle fractures in patients with diabetes. J Bone Joint Surg Am. 2008;90(7):1570–8.

24. Johnson JE. Surgical reconstruction of the diabetic foot and ankle. Foot Ankle Clin. 1997;2:37–55.

25. Johnson JE. Operative treatment of neuropathic arthropathy of the foot and ankle. J Bone Joint Surg. 1998;80A(11):1700–9.

26. Ebaugh MP, Umbel B, Goss D, Taylor BC. Outcomes of primary tibiotalocalcaneal nailing for complicated diabetic ankle fractures. Foot Ankle Int. 2019;40(12):1382–7.

27. Muckley T, Eichorn S, Hoffmeier C, von Oldenburg G, Speitling A, Hoffman GO, Buhren V. Biomechanical evaluation of primary stiffness of tibiotalocalcaneal fusion with intramedullary nail. Foot Ankle Int. 2007;28(2):224–31.

28. Santangelo JR, Glisson RR, Garras DN, Easley ME. Tibiocalcaneal arthrodesis: a biomechanical comparison of multiplanar external fixation with intramedullary fixation. Foot Ankle Int. 2009;29(9):936–41.

29. Easley ME, Montijo HE, Wilson JB, Fitch RD, Nunley JA. Revision tibiotalar arthrodesis. J Bone Joint Surg. 2008;90(6):1212–23.

30. Finkler ES, Kasia C, Kroin E, Davidson-Bell V, Schiff AP, Pinzur MS. Pin tract infection following correction of Charcot foot with static circular fixation. Foot Ankle Int. 2015;36:1310–5.

31. El-Mowafi H, Abulsaad M, Kandil Y, El-Hawary A, Ali S. Hybrid fixation for ankle fusion in diabetic Charcot arthropathy. Foot Ankle Int. 2018;39(1):93–8.

Part V

Chronic Ankle Problems

Management of Malunions, Nonunions, and Late Syndesmotic Injuries of the Ankle

Stefan Rammelt ⓘ and Choon Chiet Hong ⓘ

1 Etiology and Pathomechanics

Although commonly seen in orthopaedic practice, ankle fractures are often complex and underestimated during primary treatment, leading to poor outcomes due to inadequate reduction or fixation with secondary loss of reduction [1–4]. Malunion and/or nonunion then occurs affecting the articular congruency and anatomical axis of the joint. This leads to asymmetrical loading and abnormally high load stresses on the articular contact surfaces [5–9]. The alteration in load distribution, often with talar subluxation, can progress to posttraumatic ankle osteoarthritis [8, 9]. In addition, intra-articular malunion of the tibial plafond can also occur due to residual step-offs on the articular surface of the distal tibia from improperly reduced pilon fractures or neglected partial impactions of the tibial plafond in malleolar fractures [6, 7].

Posttraumatic deformities of the ankle are not uncommon with reported malreduction rates of up to 44% following operative treatment [10–12].

Besides bony deformities, chronic ligamentous instabilities are frequent findings that may occur in isolation or in combination with bony malunion [4, 12]. On the contrary, malleolar nonunions are only seen rarely with the advancement in stabilization of displaced malleolar fractures [4, 5].

A deviation of $\geq 10°$ from the anatomical axis leads to significantly decreased tibiotalar contact area [13, 14]. Lateral translation of the talus by 1 mm decreases the articular contact surface by 42% in a static biomechanical model [8]. In other clinical and biomechanical studies, fibular shortening or translation of ≥ 2 mm was associated with eccentric load shift in the ankle joint and inferior outcome [9, 10, 12]. This alteration is reversible with a corrective osteotomy of the fibula [15]. Besides, intra-articular step-off of ≥ 2 mm in posterior malleolar malunion has also been shown to be an independent risk factor for inferior outcomes and development of posttraumatic arthritis irrespective of the fragment size [16]. The impact of fibular malrotation is less clear. Although a fibular rotation of 5° can result in significant weight shift at the ankle joint in a biomechanical setting, the patients in a clinical study did still tolerate up to 15° of fibular rotation [9, 10]. Besides inadequate assessment and treatment at initial presentation, patient-related factors leading to malunions and nonunions such as noncompliance, smoking, substance abuse, and comorbidities like diabetes mellitus or osteoporosis have to be considered.

S. Rammelt (✉)
University Center for Orthopaedics, Trauma and Plastic Surgery, University Hospital Carl Gustav Carus at the TU Dresden, Dresden, Germany
e-mail: stefan.rammelt@uniklinikum-dresden.de

C. C. Hong
Department of Orthopaedic Surgery, National University Hospital, Singapore, Singapore

Numerous studies have demonstrated poorer clinical outcome following malreduced ankle fractures when compared to patients with anatomically reduced fractures at the time of initial surgery [10, 12, 16–18]. Similarly, inaccurate articular reduction of the tibial plafond has also been shown to be negative prognostic factor [6, 11]. Reasons include overlooked marginal plafond impaction in malleolar fractures or definite treatment of AO/OTA type C pilon fractures with external fixation, leading to improper joint reduction which is reported in up to 25% [11, 16]. Finally, malreduction of the distal fibula into the tibial incisura (notch) following syndesmotic injury has been identified as an independent negative prognostic factor in several studies [10, 12, 19, 20]. This can occur in isolation or in combination with bony deformities and will be addressed in section 5 of this chapter.

2 Preoperative Planning

A complete assessment of the patient with residual complaints after ankle fractures is vital to achieve a successful outcome. Clinical examination includes gross deformities, callosities, swelling, soft tissue condition including previous surgical scars, ulcers and skin defects, neurovascular status, residual range of motion, and joint stability. The uninjured leg should always be evaluated, too, because it serves as a reference for the patient's physiological status. Comorbidities such as diabetes mellitus, peripheral vascular disease, osteoporosis, rheumatoid arthritis, neuropathy, and risk factors such as smoking or substance abuse must be noted. The patient's primary complaint and functional deficits in terms of impairment of activities of daily living, work, and sports should be ascertained. Ambulatory status, walking aids, orthotics, and regularly worn shoes are reviewed preoperatively. The patient must be counselled about possible complications and the chance of residual deformity that cannot be corrected due to soft tissue contracture and scarring as well as functional deficits due to swelling, stiffness, and pain.

It is important to obtain bilateral weight-bearing anteroposterior and lateral radiographs of the foot and ankle prior to any corrective surgery [4]. In addition, a special projection showing the hindfoot alignment with respect to the tibial axis with the patient standing is important to distinguish the true level of deformity at the hindfoot and compensatory deformities. These special views are commonly referred to as hindfoot alignment view or long axial view [21]. If the clinical examination raises the suspicion of an additional deformity at the knee or a limb length discrepancy, standing long leg alignment radiographs should be taken from the hip to the heel.

Computerized tomography (CT) imaging is very useful in demonstrating the three-dimensional (3D) outline of complex malunions, extent of bone loss and nonunion, avascular necrosis, subchondral cysts, and severity of arthritis of both the ankle and adjacent joints. The use of weight-bearing CT imaging improves the visualization of the ankle and hindfoot alignment under physiologic loading. This is helpful if additional or compensatory deformities at the hindfoot are suspected in the presence of ankle deformities [4, 22]. A 3D printed reconstruction of the deformity can also be produced to help aid preoperative planning for complex deformities in terms of planning the level of osteotomy and optimal implant placement [22]. However, these resources may not be widely available at present and can be costly. Magnetic resonance imaging (MRI) is often used for evaluation of osteochondral defects, ligamentous, and tendon injuries as well as determining the presence and extent of AVN within the tibial plafond or talus. Nonetheless, it is in the authors' experience that MRIs produce many false-positive pathologic diagnoses in the foot and ankle and tend to overread AVN and cartilage damage [4]. Cartilage mapping with T2 weighted MRI may provide a more sensitive information about cartilage quality [23].

At the time of surgery, it is important to assess the status of the joint cartilage visually and mechanically by probing the cartilage over the tibial plafond and talus [4]. This is because the primary cartilage damage at the time of trauma and the secondary damage from eccentric loading due to malalignment and/or instability will almost always lead to radiographic evidence of posttraumatic arthritis. Therefore, examination of the cartilage status during reconstructive surgery will in many instances provide the definitive decision to preserve or fuse/replace the ankle joint. If the joint surface cartilage is of good quality and has reasonably good covering on more than 50% of the joint surface, a joint preserving reconstruction may still be possible [1, 2, 4, 6, 14, 24]. This aspect of the surgery should be discussed with the patient preoperatively.

3 Indications for Joint-Preserving Procedures

Joint preserving osteotomies to manage intra- and/or extra-articular deformities of the ankle are usually indicated in the following cases [1, 2, 4–7, 13, 14, 24]:

1. Young, active patients.
2. Good bone stock.
3. Sufficient cartilage coverage over the weight bearing areas (first to second degree chondromalacia and at more than 50% of the ankle joint articular surface should be preserved in asymmetric ankle arthritis more commonly in the coronal plane and less so in the sagittal plane).
4. Compliant patient.

Conversely, contraindications to joint preserving osteotomies include:

1. Poor bone stock with extensive AVN of the tibial plafond or talus.
2. Loss of cartilage at 50% or more of the ankle joint surface.
3. Poor soft tissue coverage from initial trauma/open fracture.
4. Chronic bone infection (osteomyelitis).

5. Poor patient compliance (smoking, substance abuse, severe mental impairment).
6. Comorbidities such as recalcitrant, poorly controlled diabetes mellitus, severe peripheral vascular disease not amenable to revascularization or systemic disorders that can cause threat to life such as those with ASA $\geq$ 3.

In patients contraindicated for ankle joint preserving osteotomies, ankle arthrodesis is an acceptable alternative as it is a definitive surgery that will correct deformity, reduce pain, and improve function [25]. Ankle arthroplasty is also a good alternative for those patients with good functional ankle range of motion without significant AVN or bone loss of the tibial plafond [4]. These alternative treatment options will be discussed in detail in other chapters.

If joint-preserving reconstruction is pursued, the prospect of progressive arthritis despite deformity correction and realignment of the weight-bearing forces should be discussed at length with the patient. On the other hand, with joint-preserving procedures, no bridges are burnt, and if ankle fusion or replacement become necessary at a later stage, it can be performed on a well-aligned ankle, which is technically less demanding and less prone to complications. Finally, any late consequences of ankle arthrodesis or ankle arthroplasty like adjacent joint arthritis and loosening of the prosthesis are further delayed into the future, thus "buying time" for the predominately young patient with posttraumatic ankle arthritis.

4 Malunions and Nonunions of the Ankle

4.1 Types of Deformities and Reconstructive Options

Pathoanatomy of malleolar malunion usually follows the initial mechanism of injury with its resultant bony and ligamentous lesions. When considering reconstructive options, the surgical approaches can be guided according to the location of the malpositioned malleoli. Acute ankle fractures (AO/OTA 44) are classified as unimalleolar, bimalleolar, trimalleolar, and quadrimalleolar fractures [3, 26], Thus, **malleolar malunions and nonunions** (Fig. 1) can be divided in posttraumatic deformities of the:

1. Lateral malleolus.
2. Medial malleolus.
3. Posterior malleolus.
4. Anterior malleolus.

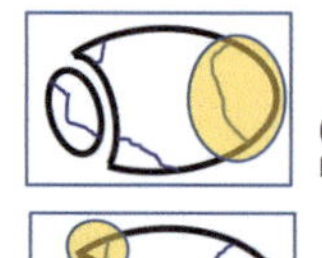
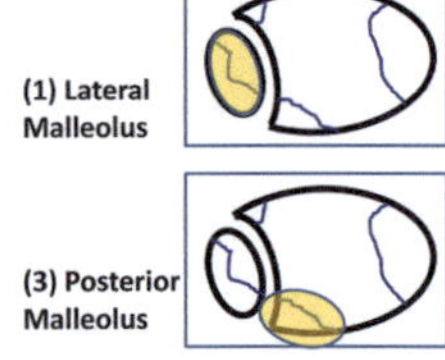

Fig. 1 Ankle malunions may be easily characterized like acute ankle fractures with respect to the affected malleoli. Malunions of the tibial pilon (supramalleolar and intra-articular) and talus are of distinct etiologies

As with acute malleolar fractures, all **combinations** of bony injuries can be observed and may be further combined with **ligamentous instability** (most frequently syndesmotic and medial instability which will be dealt with in detail in the last part of this chapter), and **partial impactions of the tibial plafond**.

Malunions following tibial **pilon fractures** can be supramalleolar or intra-articular [7] depending on the initial type of injury (AO/OTA 43A vs. B or C). The latter are rarely amenable to joint-preserving corrections due to the amount of initial cartilage damage from axial impaction and the typically rapid progression to symptomatic osteoarthritis [6, 11]. Finally, **malunions and nonunions of the talus** [4] will in many cases also affect ankle joint but are beyond the scope of this chapter.

4.2 Lateral Malleolar Malunion

The typical pathoanatomy of the lateral malleolar malunion (Fig. 2) illustrates an inadequately treated ankle fracture with fibular shortening that is often accompanied by external rotation, lateral

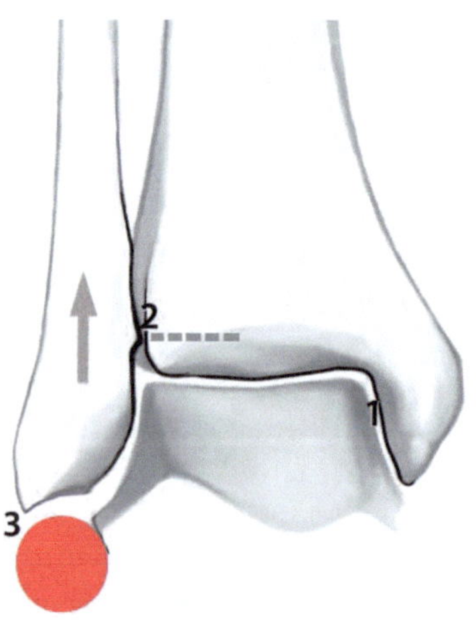
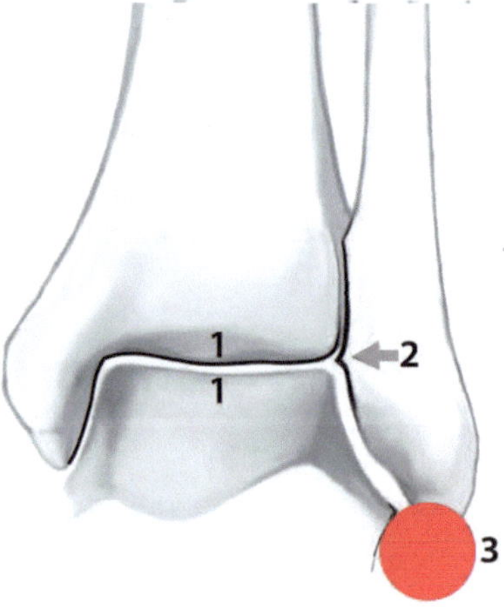
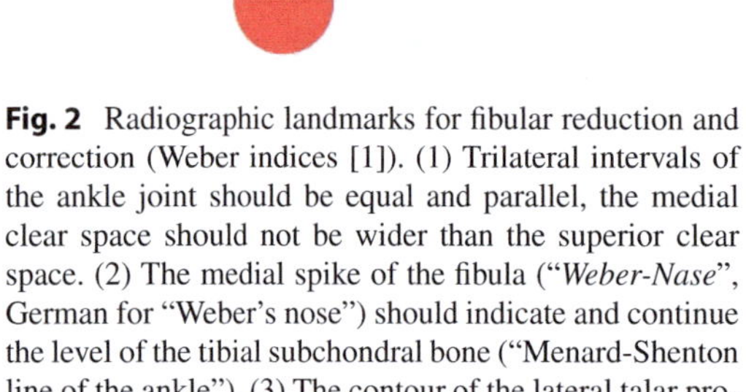

Fig. 2 Radiographic landmarks for fibular reduction and correction (Weber indices [1]). (1) Trilateral intervals of the ankle joint should be equal and parallel, the medial clear space should not be wider than the superior clear space. (2) The medial spike of the fibula ("*Weber-Nase*", German for "Weber's nose") should indicate and continue the level of the tibial subchondral bone ("Menard-Shenton line of the ankle"). (3) The contour of the lateral talar process continues as an unbroken curve to the peroneal recess in the distal fibula ("*Weber–Kreis*", German for "Weber circle" or "dime sign"). [From: Rammelt S, Zwipp H. *Korrektur fehlverheilter Fibulafrakturen*. In: Hamel, J, Zwipp H (eds.): Meistertechniken in der operativen Orthopädie und Unfallchirurgie. Sprunggelenk und Rückfuß. Berlin, Springer, 2016, S. 83–92, with permission]

and posterior displacement of the distal fragment [1]. This results in increased lateral tibiatalar contact forces [27]. In the presence of a medial malleolar malunion, nonunion, or deltoid ligament instability (Fig. 3), the talus will rotate externally and shift laterally following the displaced fibula [1, 4, 28]. This will decrease the superior tibiotalar contact [8, 27]. In addition, the medial malleolus may be malunited following a bimalleolar fracture where the deltoid ligament is intact pulling the medial malleolar fragment laterally as well [1, 4, 28]. Occasionally, an additional malunited posterior malleolus and/or the anterolateral tibial tubercle (anterior malleolus/ Chaput fragment) can be present as well [30]. Because both are attached to the tibiofibular syndesmosis, this may manifest as syndesmotic instability with widening of the mortise and tibiofibular clear space due to bony displacement and malunion [29, 30].

The treatment of choice is a fibular osteotomy (Fig. 4) which is primarily aimed at lengthening the shortened fibula while correcting any accompanying valgus or rotational deformity [1]. This technique uses a lateral approach to the fibula while protecting the superficial peroneal nerve especially at the proximal portion of the incision. An oblique or Z-shaped fibular osteotomy (see Fig. 16) is sufficient for lengthening up to 5 mm without the need for bone grafting [7, 28]. However, if further lengthening is required, a transverse osteotomy with corticocancellous bone graft from the tibia or iliac crest would be more reliable [1]. Once the osteotomy is completed, a rigid straight plate is first fixed to the distal fragment of the fibula. A single cortical

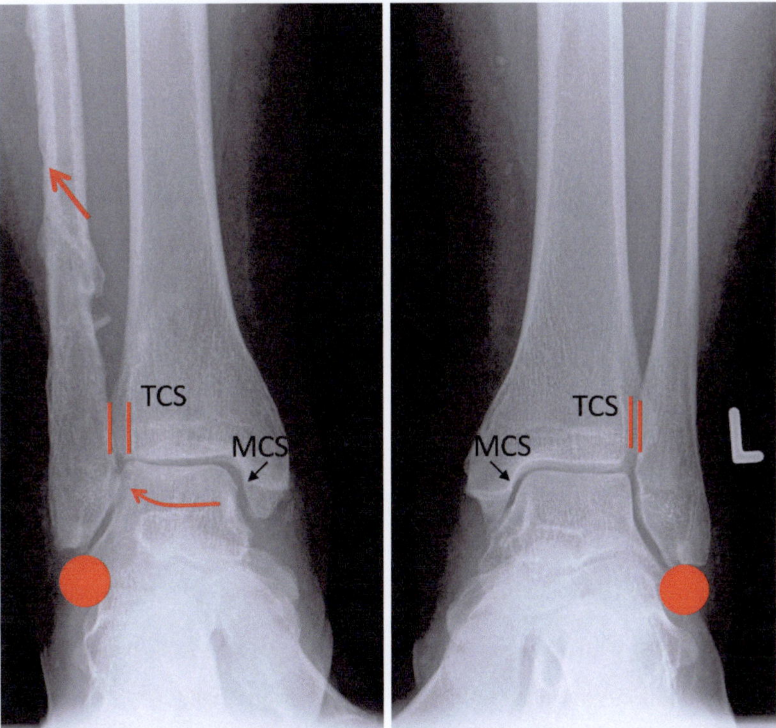

Fig. 3 Bilateral standing radiographs (mortise view) of a patient with painful fibular malunion. Note the mismatch of the Weber circle, widening of the tibiofibular clear space (TCS) and medial clear space (MCS) when compared to the superior clear space and to the uninjured side. The former oblique line of the high fibular fracture with shortening can still be delineated (red arrow). Frequently, as in this case, the fibular spike cannot be clearly seen in malunions. [Adapted from: Rammelt S, Zwipp H. *Korrektur fehlverheilter Fibulafrakturen.* In: Hamel, J, Zwipp H (eds.): Meistertechniken in der operativen Orthopädie und Unfallchirurgie. Sprunggelenk und Rückfuß. Berlin, Springer, 2016, S. 83–92, with permission]

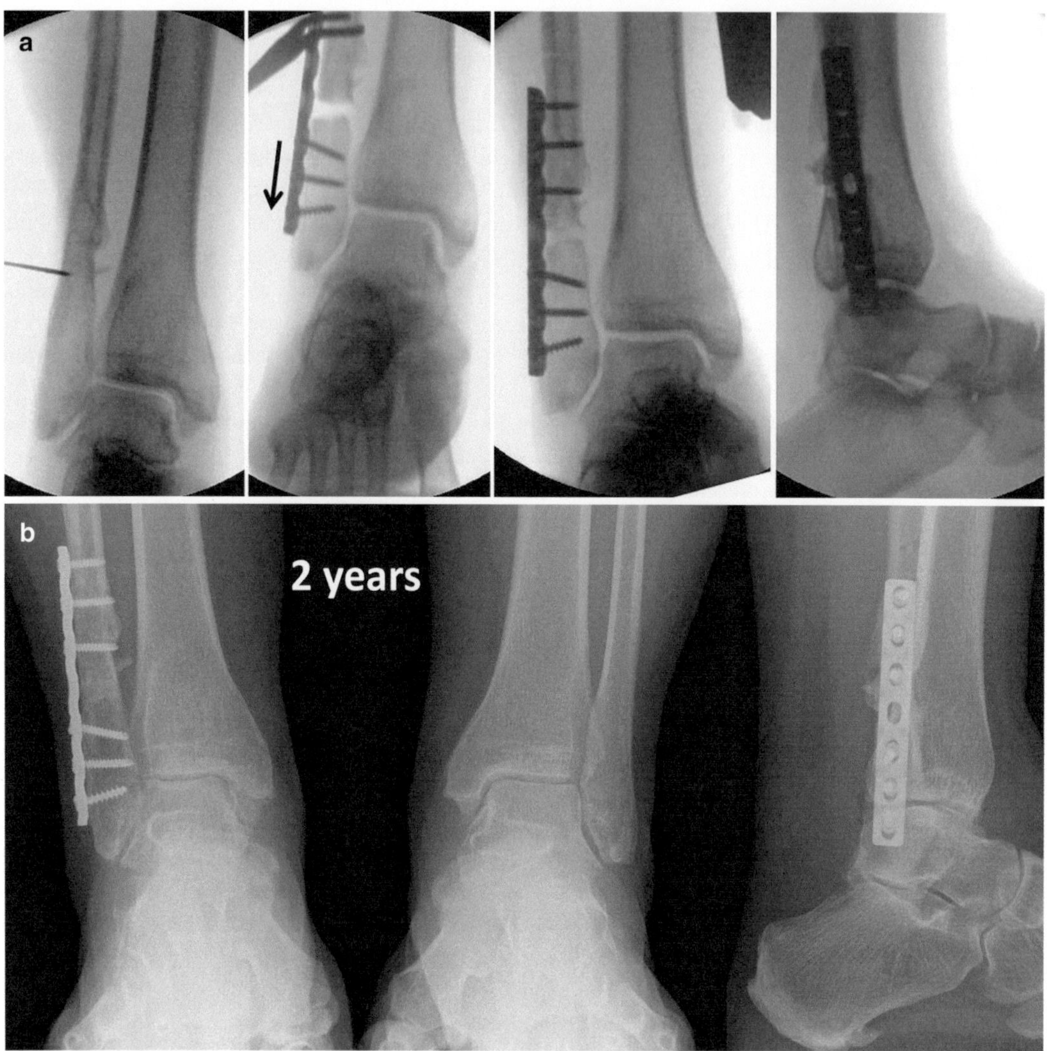

Fig. 4 Classical technique of fibular lengthening (same patient as in Fig. 3). (**a**) The horizontal osteotomy is marked with a K-wire and the plate fixed in the distal fragment. With a laminar spreader introduced between the proximal end of the plate and a separately placed screw, the correct fibular length can be fine-tuned under fluoroscopy. Then the plate is fixed proximally and the gap is filled with a bicortical bone graft from the iliac crest. Note the correction of the Weber indices. With fibular lengthen-ing, the syndesmotic fibres are stretched and the TCS is normalized so that no separate syndesmotic stabilization is needed. (**b**) At 2 years follow-up the patient has a congruent and stable mortise without functional restrictions. [Adapted from: Rammelt S, Zwipp H. *Korrektur fehlverheilter Fibulafrakturen.* In: Hamel, J, Zwipp H (eds.): Meistertechniken in der operativen Orthopädie und Unfallchirurgie. Sprunggelenk und Rückfuß. Berlin, Springer, 2016, S. 83–92, with permission]

screw is inserted proximal to the plate and with the use of a lamina spreader or plate tensioner, the distal fragment of the fibula is lengthened accordingly. Image-intensifier can be used here to ascertain congruency of the ankle mortise after lengthening using the Weber indices [1]. Once the desired length is achieved and deformity has been corrected, the plate is fixed proximally.

Mild residual valgus will be corrected once the rigid straight plate is tightened as the straightened fibula would push the talus medially. The accompanying rotational deformity of the distal fibular fragment will correct as it glides distally along the curved lateral facet of the talus through lengthening of the fibula with the foot in neutral position [7]. Alternatively, rotational correction can be controlled using K-wires introduced into the distal and proximal fragments at the exact angle of malrotation as measured with the preoperative CT scan. These K-wires should be parallel after completion of reconstruction [7]. Using the K-wire method in a cadaver study, experimental fibular malrotation could be restored within 1.6° of the values of the uninjured side as judged with CT scanning [31].

In the event of an additional medial malleolus malunion, the correction via fibula osteotomy should only be attempted once medial malleolar malunion has been osteotomized and freed from intervening scar tissues. Even if there is no medial malleolar malunion, the medial clear space has to be debrided to remove scar tissues if it does not close with fibular correction. Any remaining deltoid ligament instability as evident from residual valgus tilt of the talus in the ankle mortise, can be reconstructed simultaneously once the fibular lengthening is completed.

In case of **fibular nonunion**, the fibrous pseudarthrosis and any sclerotic bone is removed until viable bone becomes visible at both ends. Typically, nonunions will be accompanied by malposition of the fragments necessitating correction as outlined above [5, 6]. The resulting gap is filled with bone graft and fixation is typically achieved with a plate (Fig. 5). Adjunct treatments like bone morphogenic protein or bone stimulation should be considered. Any underlying comorbidities potentially leading to nonunion must be addressed. In particular, blood glucose levels should be controlled tightly and smoking strongly discouraged. Blood supply to the foot and ankle should be optimized preoperatively in case of peripheral vascular disease [5]. The few available studies on fibular nonunions uniformly report favourable mid-term results with this treatment regimen [5, 7, 32].

Multiple authors have shown good results and outcomes from fibular lengthening as treatment of malunited ankle fractures [1, 2, 4, 6, 7, 24, 28]. Reidsma et al. reported good or excellent results obtained in 85% of patients lasting up to 27 years with secondary ankle fusion in less than 15% of

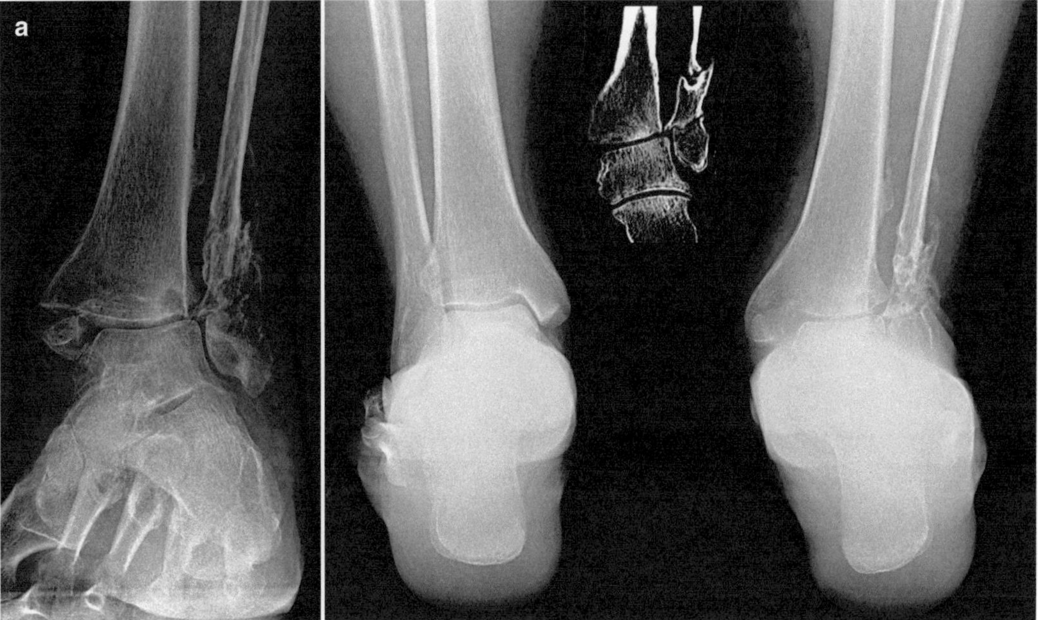

Fig. 5 (**a**) Anteroposterior radiographs, hindfoot alignment views and CT image of a nonunion of the distal tibia and fibula following a bimalleolar fracture. The ankle and hindfoot are in valgus because of fibular shortening and lateral shift of the talus. (**b**) Intraoperative aspect of the two-level nonunion of the distal fibula. (**c**) Treatment consisted of debridement of the fibrous pseudarthrosis, bone grafting, correction of the malposition and internal fixation. All former nonunions were solidly healed at 10 weeks post correction

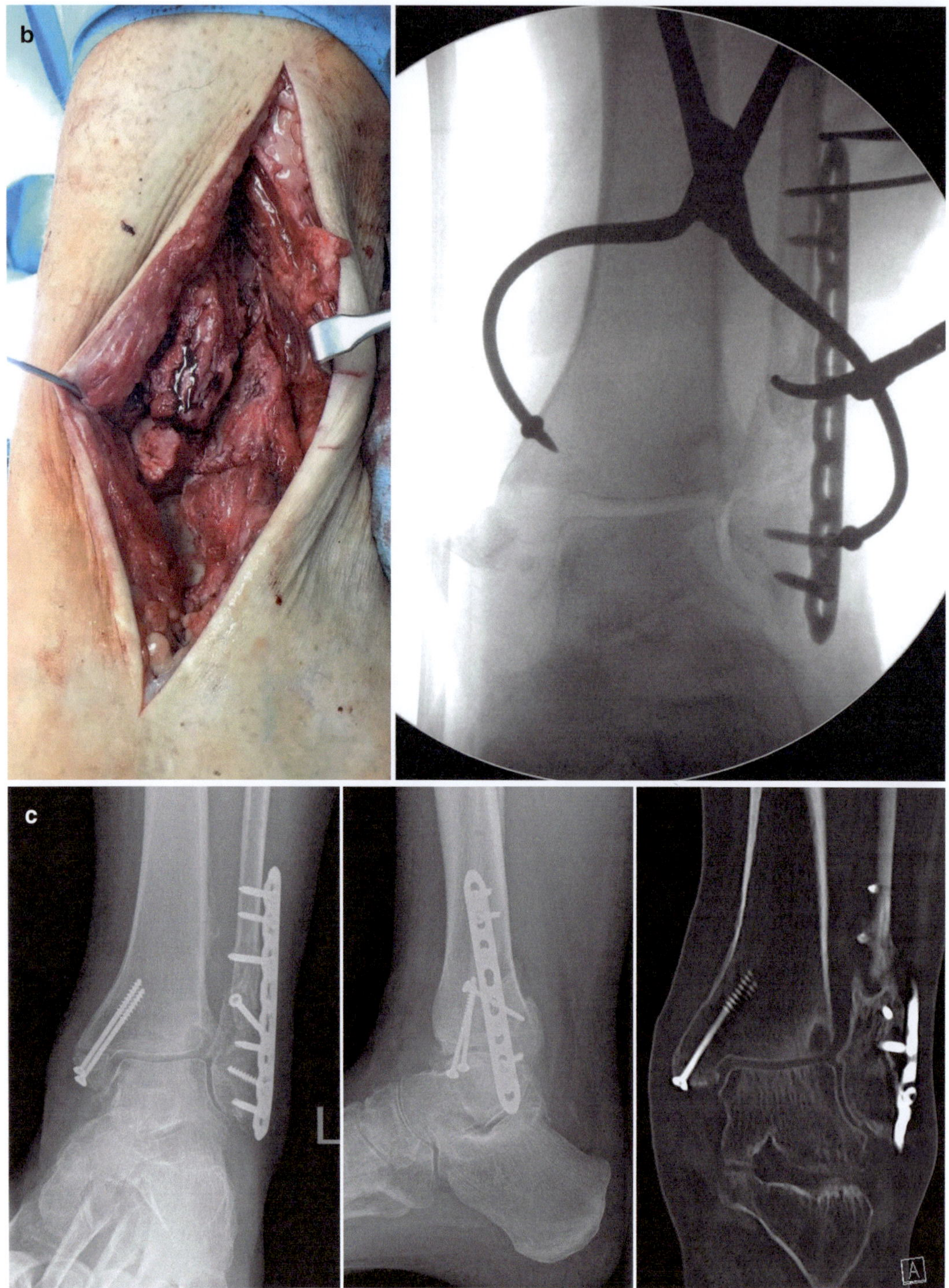

Fig. 18.5 (continued)

patients despite radiographic progression of arthritis in 52% of cases [2]. Recently, Mosca and colleagues also reported ankle joint rebalancing by fibular lengthening was effective in cases with fibular malunion in 33 patients leading to good functional and quality of life scores at 36 months [24]. Although the rates of secondary fusion are low throughout the studies, pre-existing arthritis has been shown to correlate with inferior outcome [1, 2, 28].

4.3 Medial Malleolar Malunion

Isolated malunion of the medial malleolus is uncommon. It is usually part of a more complex deformity with malunion superiorly, laterally, posteriorly or intra-articularly [7, 28]. Less frequently, a supination-adduction mechanism will result to shortening of the medial malleolus due to malunion of the typical vertical shear fracture coupled with the medial displacement of the distal fibular fragment creating the medial talar shift [4]. If there is an additional varus tilt to the talus, it is important to look for accompanying intra-articular impaction of the medial tibia plafond and be ready to correct the intra-articular malunited fragments if necessary. Because in supination-adduction fractures the lateral side gets injured first, there will be either associated lateral ligament instability, an avulsion fracture of the lateral ligament complex, or an inframalleolar fibular fracture malunion as well (Fig. 6). Much rarer, abduction injuries can lead to a transverse avulsion fracture of the medial malleolus and lateral tibial plafond impaction. This can result in avascular necrosis (AVN) of the anterolateral tibial fragment due to injury to the lateral branch of the anterior tibial artery especially in high energy trauma and open fractures [33]. Nonunions of the medial malleolus are rare and are thought to result from technical errors in fixation or non-operative treatment of medial malleolar fractures [34].

For correction, a direct medial approach is used with care taken to protect the greater saphenous vein and saphenous nerve anteriorly, the posterior tibial tendon and posterior tibial neuro-vascular bundle posteriorly. In the case of malunited supination-adduction injury where the medial malleolus is shortened, a lengthening osteotomy (Fig. 7) is performed via the more vertical former fracture line [4]. In cases of malunited bimalleolar fracture such as pronation-external rotation injury, the medial malleolus is osteotomized along the more oblique former fracture line. The osteotomy is aimed towards the medial edge of the ankle joint at the notch of Harty. In case of additional malunion of the lateral malleolus, it has to be osteotomized also to allow medial malleolar correction.

After the medial malleolar osteotomy is completed, any intra-articular impaction at the medial tibial plafond should be addressed. Any small, loose, or nonviable fragments are removed. Depressed osteochondral fragments can be reduced and congruency of the tibial plafond visually ascertained before fixation with screws. If the fragment is too small, K wires can be used as definitive fixation with the ends cut flush with the edge of the fracture to improve fixation of the osteochondral fragments. Following that, the correct length of the medial malleolus is restored while controlling for congruency of the ankle mortise with direct visualization and image-intensifier. The medial malleolus can be fixed with a medial antiglide plate following a vertical osteotomy and screws or tension-band wiring following a more horizontal osteotomy.

If the distal fibula was simultaneously osteotomized for varus deformity, it can then be shifted laterally and fixed with a lateral plate. Small fragments are alternatively fixed with screws or tension-band wiring. Small avulsed fragments are resected. Lateral ligament reconstruction is performed at this stage, typically with a Brostrøm/Gould repair. This can include reefing of the elongated ligaments, reinsertion into the fibula, and/or talus with suture anchors and augmentation with the inferior peroneal retinaculum [4].

Symptomatic nonunion of the medial malleolus is treated at the same time with debridement of the fibrous pseudarthrosis, drilling of the fragments, and cancellous bone grafting. To fill original screw holes, bone dowels can be

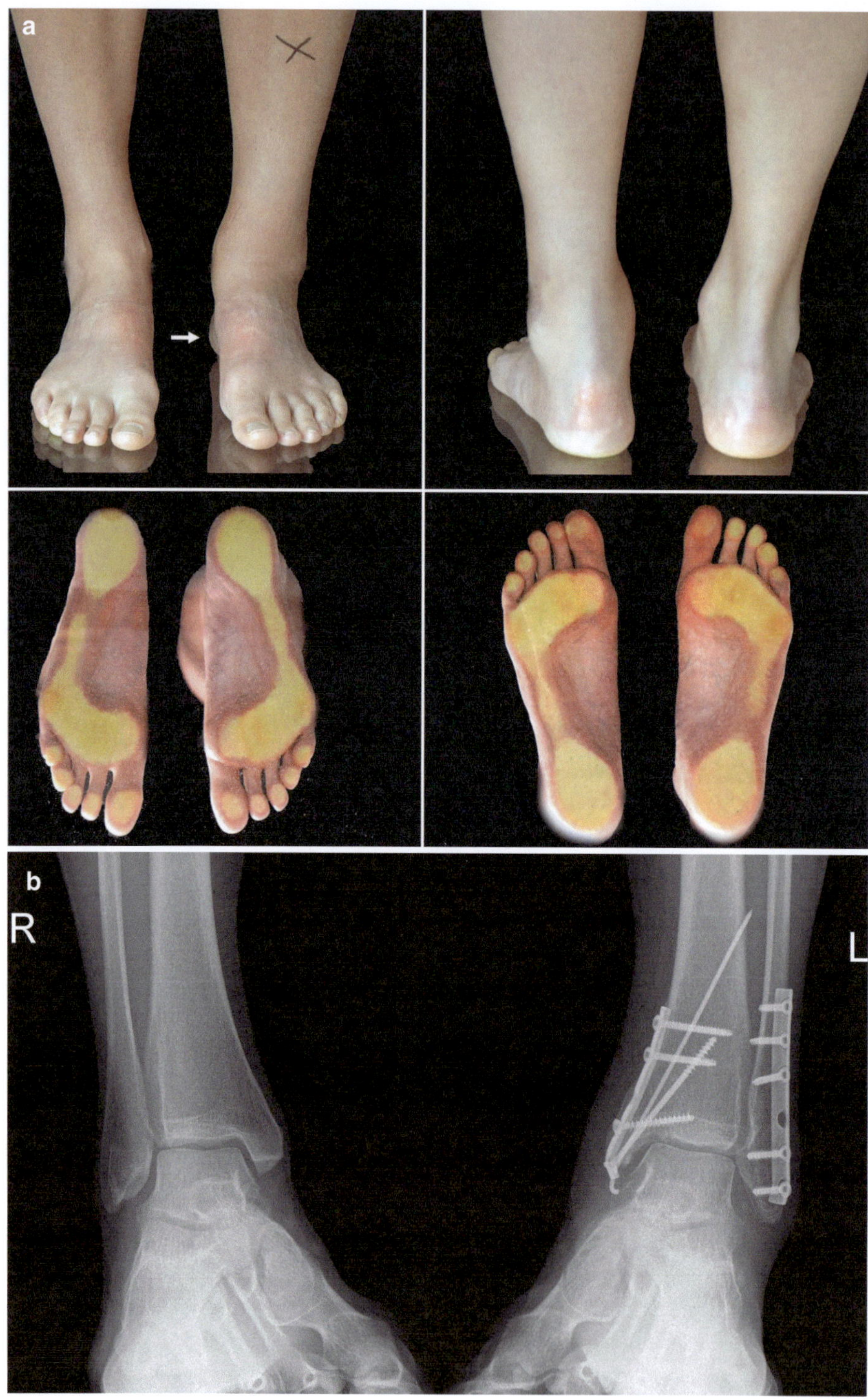

Fig. 6 (**a**) Clinical aspect of a patient with varus malalignment because of medial malleolar malunion following a delayed union of a supination-adduction injury. Note the protruding medial aspect of the heel seen from the front ("peak-a-boo-heel" according to A. Manoli). (**b**) The standing radiographs show shortening and varus malposition of the medial malleolus and widening of the ankle mortise. The lateral malleolus displays a plastic deformity following a low (Weber Type A) fibular fracture but no shortening or medial shift. [Adapted from Ochman S, Rammelt S. Sprunggelenkfrakturen und Korrektur von Fehlheilungen. In: Sabo D, Rammelt S (eds.): Rückfußchirurgie. Berlin, Springer, 2017, S. 236–255, with permission]

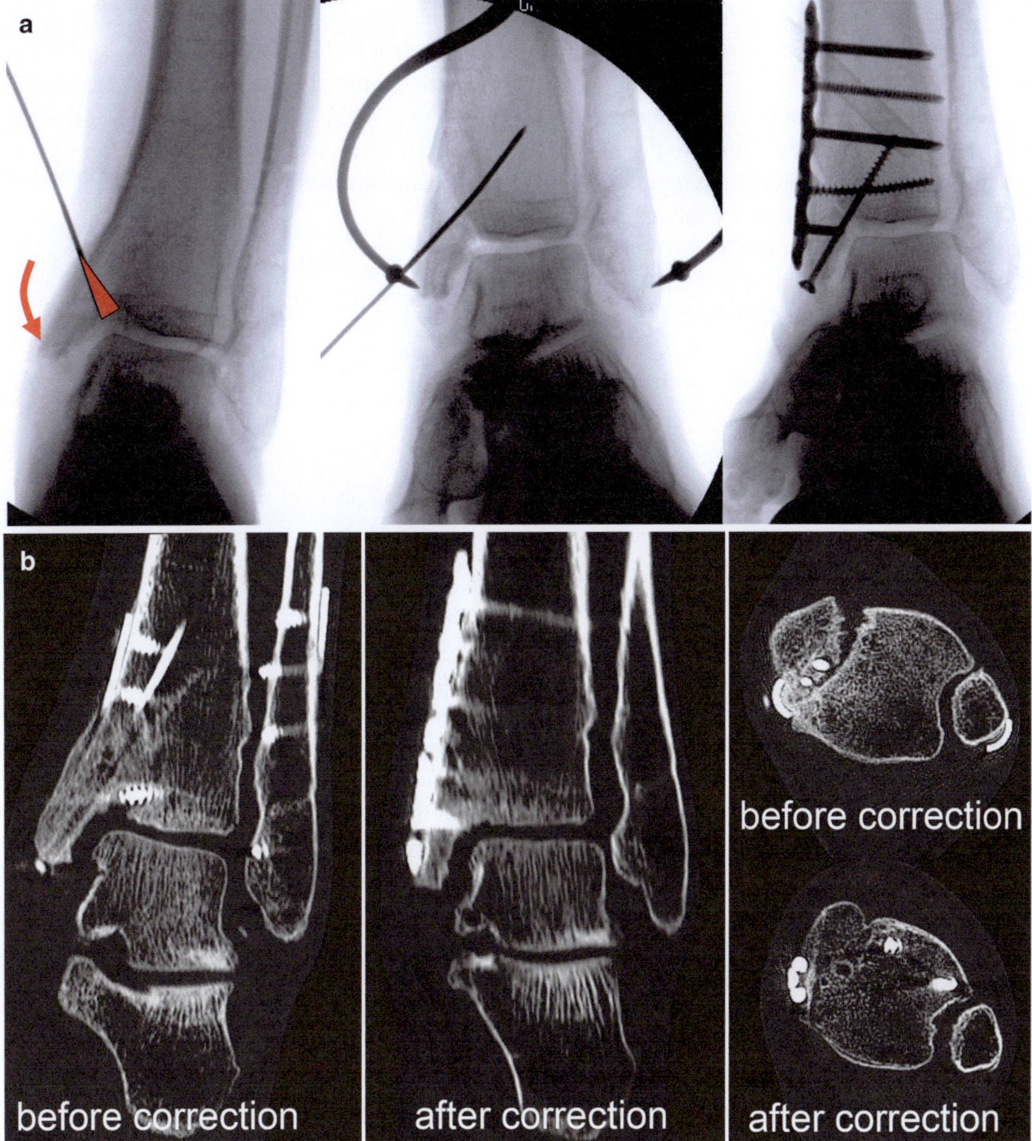

Fig. 7 (**a**) Correction of medial malleolar malunion (same patient as in Fig. 6). A vertical osteotomy is performed together with a wedge resection in order to close the ankle mortise. The medial malleolus is then lengthened, moved laterally, derotated and fixed with a lag screw and medial buttress plate. (**b**) CT scanning at 1 year (prior to implant removal) demonstrates correction of medial malleolar length varus and malrotation in the coronal plane with a stable ankle mortise and correction of hindfoot varus. [Adapted from Ochman S, Rammelt S. *Sprunggelenkfrakturen und Korrektur von Fehlheilungen*. In: Sabo D, Rammelt S (eds.): Rückfußchirurgie. Berlin, Springer, 2017, S. 236–255, with permission]

inserted, press fit, into the former screw holes [4]. Internal fixation can be achieved with a medial plate.

Data on outcome following medial malleolar malunion and nonunion correction are scarce. Sneppen et al. [32] reported a union rate of just 50% after revision surgery for medial malleolar nonunions. Others only anecdotally reported successful revision fixation with bone grafting or excision for small fragments [4, 5, 7]. In the authors' experience, the outcomes of medial malleolar correction are favourable without the need for secondary fusion.

4.4   Posterior Malleolar Malunion

Malunions and nonunions of the posterior malleolus are common as up to 50% of ankle fractures have posterior malleolar involvement that is not always adequately addressed [16, 29, 35, 36]. Malunited posterior malleolar fragments can present as an isolated deformity or in combination with lateral, medial, or intra-articular malunion of the ankle according to the original pathomechanism. Smaller fragments (Bartoníček and Rammelt Types 1 and 2) are most likely caused by ligamentous avulsion in a rotational injury [37]. Two-part and multifragmentary fractures with medial extension and large triangular fractures (Bartoníček and Rammelt Types 3 and 4) usually arise from combination mechanisms of rotational, abduction, and axial compression forces which is associated with pronation injuries [37]. Intercalary fragments and plafond impaction point to an additional axial force resulting in "partial" or "posterior" pilon fractures [16, 38]. Notably, posterior malleolar malunion can be associated with bony syndesmotic instability as it carries the attachment of the posterior inferior tibiofibular ligament (PiTFL). With increasing fragment size, it also affects the integrity of the

tibial incisura leading to fibular malposition and syndesmotic incongruity [16, 29]. Irrespective of the size of the fragment, articular incongruity with a step-off ≥2 mm is an independent risk factor for inferior outcomes and development of posttraumatic arthritis [35, 38].

Depending on the individual original pathoanatomy, correction of posterior malleolar malalignment aims at restoring:

1. Articular congruency.
2. Posterior ankle stability and talar containment.
3. The shape of the tibial incisura to enable correct positioning of the distal fibula.
4. Bone-to-bone syndesmotic stability.

Typically, the posterior malleolar fragment malunites in a superiorly displaced position with a posterior articular step-off (Fig. 8). This can be associated with a shortened fibula as illustrated earlier in combination injuries. These deformities can be treated with corrective osteotomies and/or debridement with bone grafting along the former fracture line and fixed with screws or plates [4, 7, 29]. The malunited posterior fragment can be accessed like an acute posterior malleolar fracture via a posterolateral or posteromedial approach. Alternatively, a transfibular approach can be used if a fibular osteotomy is needed for complete correction.

In the authors' preference, the patient is placed prone and a posterolateral approach is utilized. The sural nerve has to be identified and protected in the subcutaneous tissue. Dissection is carried down through the superficial and deep crural fascia in the interval between the peroneal and flexor hallucis longus muscles to the posterior distal tibia surfaces. The posterior ankle joint capsule

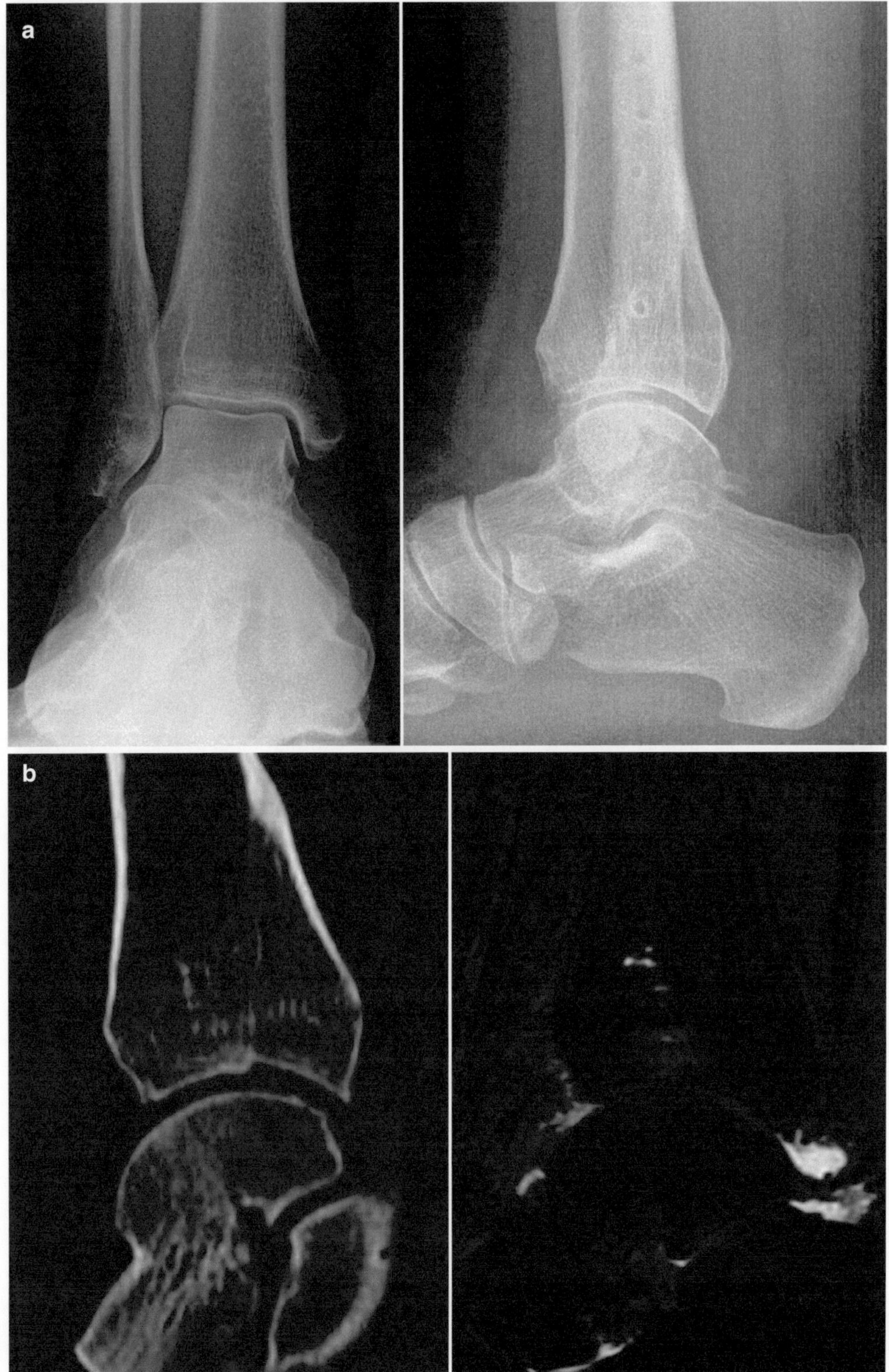

Fig. 8 (a) Malunion of a large posterior malleolar fragment (Bartoníček & Rammelt Type 4) following a trimalleolar ankle fracture. The medial and lateral malleolus are healed in a physiological position. (b) Sagittal CT shows a 2-mm step and MRI reveals bone marrow edema in the distal tibia adjacent to the step-off indicating pathologic pressure distribution at the joint. [Adapted from Ochman S, Rammelt S. *Sprunggelenkfrakturen und Korrektur von Fehlheilungen.* In: Sabo D, Rammelt S (eds.): Rückfußchirurgie. Berlin, Springer, 2017, S. 236–255, with permission]

can be dissected to visualize the joint while the PiTFL must remain intact. Using fluoroscopy, the former fracture line is marked with 1 or 2 K-wires, and an osteotomy is performed with a chisel carefully along this line to the articular step-off (Fig. 9). As mentioned earlier, a transfibular approach can be performed for direct visualization of the posterior lateral joint surface if a fibular osteotomy has to be carried out as part of a more complex correction [7].

Occasionally, a separate posteromedial incision may be necessary for those with medial extension in malunited Bartoníček and Rammelt Type-3 fractures [29].

The posterior malunited fragment is reduced flush to the anterior articular surface of the tibia together with some coronal plane adjustment. This adjustment is typically medial because the posterior tibial fragments follow the fibula via the pull of the PiTFL. Fixation can be performed with interfragmentary screws alone or a dorsal antiglide plating with compression screws through the plate [7, 36, 47]. Once the posterior tibial fragment has been fixed in the correct position, syndesmosis stability will be restored in most cases without the need for additional tibiofibular fixation [17].

While there is a large body of literature dealing with the results of malleolar fractures involving the posterior malleolus, only a few studies report the results of posterior malleolar correction. However, they exclusively report favourable results with pain relief and joint-preservation over several years [7, 9, 29, 36].

4.5 Anterior Malleolar Malunion

Malunions of the anterolateral tibia tubercle (anterior malleolus, Tillaux/Chaput fragment)—like acute fractures—are rarely seen in isolation [39]. Acute anterior malleolar fractures are thought to occur during the first stage of SER injuries, representing avulsions of the anterior inferior tibiofibular ligament (AiTFL) [39, 40]. In pronation injuries, the anterolateral distal tibia fracture is thought to occur in a second stage [40]. An additional abduction mechanism may lead to marginal impaction of the anterolateral tibial plafond [33, 39]. Consequently, anterior malleolar fractures have recently been characterized using CT imaging into 3 types [39];

Type 1—extra-articular avulsion of the AiTFL.
Type 2—fracture involving the joint surface and tibial incisura.
Type 3—fracture with impaction of the anterolateral tibial plafond.

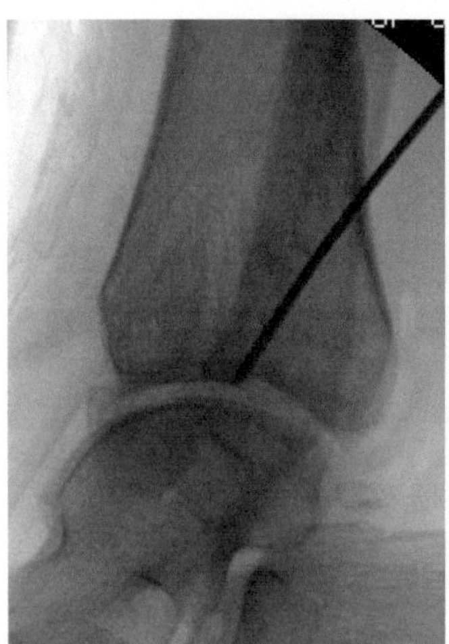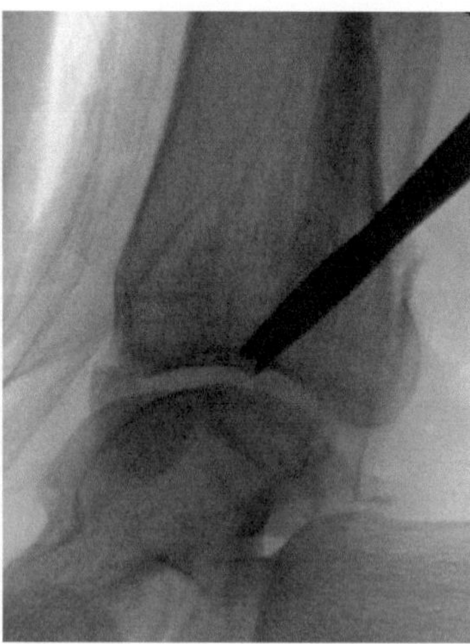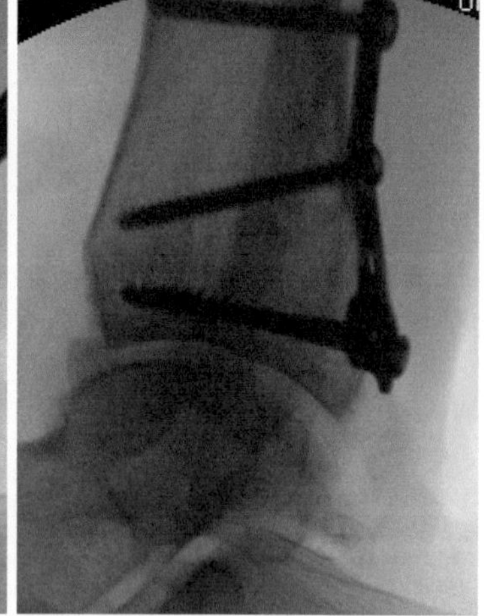

Fig. 9 Correction of a posterior malleolar malunion (same patient as in Fig. 8). The patient is placed prone and a posterolateral approach is employed. The osteotomy is marked with a K-wire and carried out with a chisel under fluoroscopy. The fragment is reduced flush to the anterior part of the tibia and fixed with a posterior antiglide plate

Similar to the posterior malleolus injury, with medial extension, the impaction fracture may involve the whole anterior tibial plafond, resulting in an **anterior pilon** fracture and malunion if not treated adequately [39, 41].

The anterior malleolus shares many analogies with the posterior malleolus with regard to potential consequences in case of malunion and nonunion. Anterior malleolar malunion can lead to bony **syndesmotic instability** due to the attachment of the AiTFL, **malpositioning of the distal fibula** because of malunion of the anterior incisura and **joint incongruity** in the case of residual step-off or marginal plafond impaction [20, 30, 39]. Typically, there is superior and anterior displacement of the plafond fragment that pulls the distal fibula due to the AiTFL and loss of the anterior tibial incisura. The talus shifts anteriorly because of the loss of anterior containment (Fig. 10). A specific late complication is avascular necrosis of the (antero-) lateral tibial plafond [33].

Correction of the anterior malleolar malalignment aims at recreating

1. The articular surface of the anterolateral tibial plafond.
2. The shape of the incisura.
3. The position of the distal fibula.
4. Bone-to-bone syndesmotic stability
5. Anterior talar containment.

Malunited fractures of the anterolateral distal tibia are typically accessed via a direct anterolateral approach [30, 41–43]. Approaches may vary due to additional procedures, e.g. fibular or supramalleolar osteotomy (Fig. 11). Existing scars from previous surgery are respected. Dissection is carried down to the scarred anterior joint capsule which is resected. This exposes the anterior tibial plafond, the syndesmotic attachments at the anterior tibial and fibular tubercle, the anterior talar dome and lateral compartment

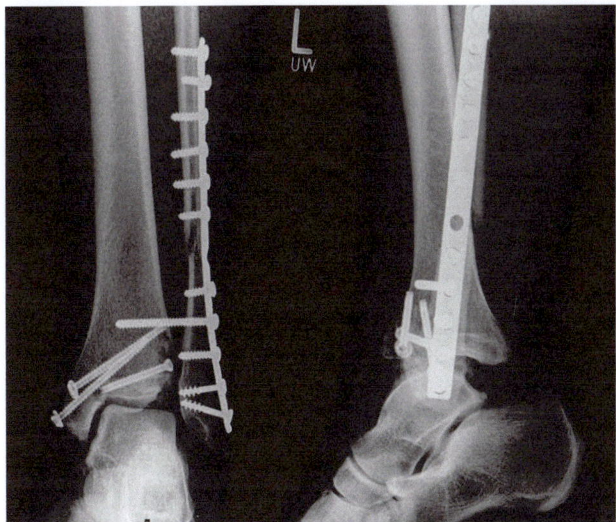
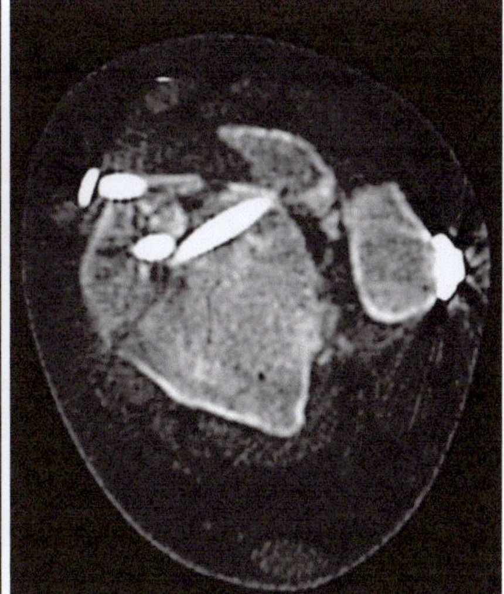

Fig. 10 Obvious incongruity of the ankle mortise following trimalleolar fracture fixation. CT reveals anterior and medial malposition of the anterior distal tibial fragment (anterior malleolar malunion) resulting in fibular malposition due to disintegration of the tibial incisura (fibular notch) and syndesmotic incongruity. In addition, the fibula is shortened. [Adapted from: Rammelt S, Zwipp H. *Korrektur fehlverheilter Fibulafrakturen.* In: Hamel, J, Zwipp H (eds.): Meistertechniken in der operativen Orthopädie und Unfallchirurgie. Sprunggelenk und Rückfuß. Berlin, Springer, 2016, S. 83–92, with permission]

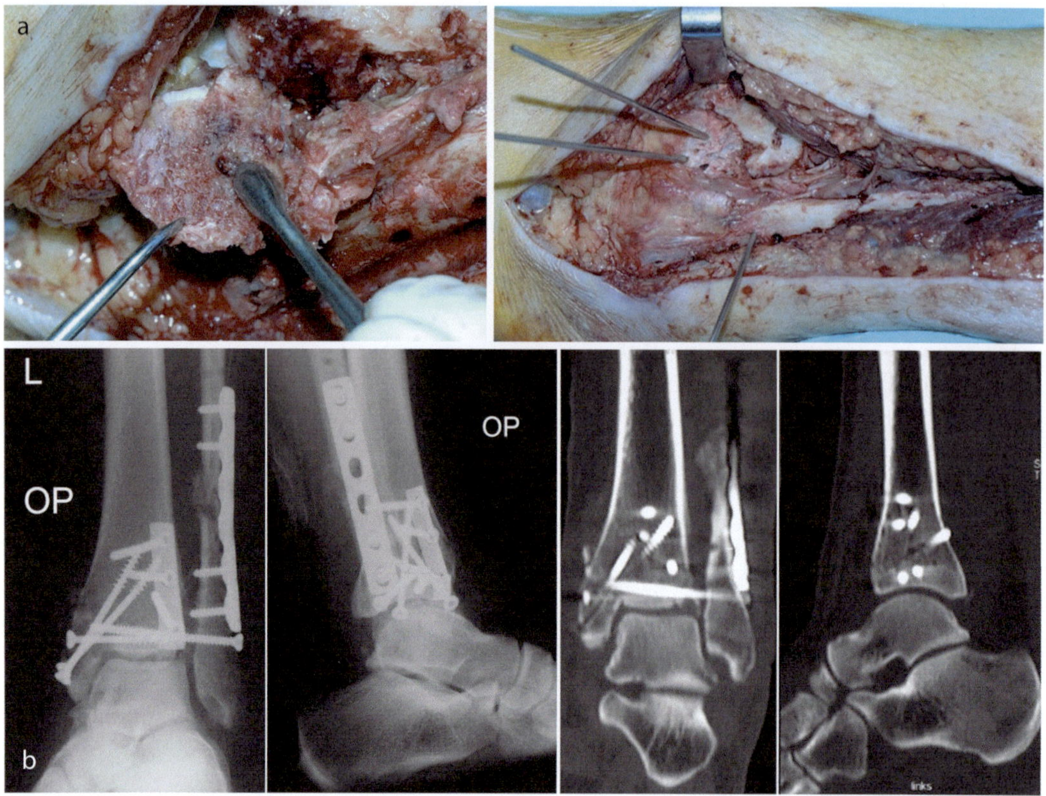

Fig. 11 Early correction of an anterior malleolar malunion (same patient as in Fig. 10). (**a**) Intraoperative images after osteotomy of the anterior malleolar fragment and reduction followed by K-wire fixation. The anterior distal tibia is stabilized with an anterior antiglide plate. A syndesmotic screw is added to enhance syndesmotic healing. The fibula is lengthened and fixed with a locking plate and the distraction site filled with cancellous bone graft. (**b**) Postoperative radiographs and CT scans demonstrate a congruent ankle mortise and joint position. [Adapted from: Rammelt S, Zwipp H. *Korrektur fehlverheilter Fibulafrakturen.* In: Hamel, J, Zwipp H (eds.): Meistertechniken in der operativen Orthopädie und Unfallchirurgie. Sprunggelenk und Rückfuß. Berlin, Springer, 2016, S. 83–92, with permission]

of the ankle joint. The lateral branch of the superficial peroneal nerve and the extensor digitorum longus are gently mobilized medially. The anterior perforating branch of fibular artery consistently penetrates the tibiofibular interosseous membrane at 5 cm above the ankle joint and runs distally across the AiTFL.

The malunited anterior malleolar fragment is mobilized via osteotomy along its former fracture line. In case of nonunion, the fibrous tissue between the fragment and the anterolateral tibia is resected. The fragment is mobilized carefully and left hinging on the AiTFL. In the presence of a plafond impaction (malunited type 3 fracture), a second, incomplete osteotomy is carried out parallel to the joint line and congruity of the plafond is restored under direct vision by mobilizing the articular fragment distally, using the talar dome as a template [41]. In case of AVN, necrotic bone is resected. Bone grafting is performed for resulting subchondral defects, but also after debridement of the fibrous nonunion. Anatomic reduction of the hinged anterior malleolar fragment is then carried out with direct visualization of the articular congruency and held provisionally with K-wire(s). As with acute anterior malleolar fractures, internal fixation may be achieved with an anterolateral distal tibial antiglide plate for malunited type 3 fractures or screws for malunited type 2 fractures. Separate screws may be needed for fragment specific fixation. Malunited syndesmotic avulsions (type 1) are mobilized and reattached to the distal tibia under correct tension with suture anchors [42].

With regards to outcomes, there are only scarce reports on early or late anterior malleolar correction for either isolated Chaput fragment malunion [43], complex correction for failed trimalleolar fracture fixation [42, 44], bony anterior syndesmosis repair [30], or anterior pilon malunions [7, 41], all with good short to mid-term outcomes.

4.6 Supramalleolar Deformities and Malunited Tibial Pilon Fractures

In cases where there are associated supramalleolar deformities, the entire ankle and hindfoot alignment must be assessed properly to look for the primary level of the deformity and any compensatory or additional deformities distally such as talar tilt or anterior shift as well as excessive heel varus or valgus. Furthermore, though coronal plane deformities (varus or valgus) are more frequently encountered, sagittal plane malalignment must also be reviewed and corrected at the same time [4, 45].

Posttraumatic **supramalleolar malunions** mostly result from tibial pilon fractures and may be combined with intra-articular deformities [6, 7, 44, 46]. Partial impaction of the tibial plafond articular surface can occur medially with supination-adduction fractures, laterally with pronation-abduction fractures, or as the result of posterior or anterior malleolar fractures [37, 39, 41]. Supramalleolar malunions can also result from premature closure of the medial physeal plate following (undetected) medial malleolar fractures in childhood [47]. If the joint cartilage is still intact over more than half of the articular surface, a supramalleolar or intra-articular osteotomy can be performed to correct the eccentric loading on the ankle joint [6, 7, 13, 14, 41, 44–49]. The aim is to correct varus, valgus, excessive ante- or recurvatum, and intra-articular malunion of the tibial plafond. The principle applied in this procedure is similar to the high tibial osteotomy which is to transfer the eccentric load away from the eroded cartilage and towards to normal side of the joint. Additionally, one must also consider correction of the ligamentous instability and inframalleolar compensatory deformities (hindfoot and midfoot) due to chronic hindfoot malalignment [4, 14]. Supramalleolar tibial osteotomy has also been added to fibular lengthening osteotomy for malunited pronation-external rotation fractures in order to offload the particularly vulnerable lateral tibial plafond following malleolar malunion [49].

The supramalleolar osteotomy is performed using an opening or closing wedge technique depending on the clinical presentation. The surgeon must take into account the quality of the soft tissue coverage, the presence of bone loss, any shortening of distal tibia, and available technical knowledge. Opening wedge supramalleolar osteotomy is regularly preferred in cases of posttraumatic shortening of the distal tibia due to impaction or bone loss provided the medial soft tissue envelope is not compromised (Fig. 12). A fibular osteotomy is usually added in cases of concomitant fibular deformity or if the distal medial opening wedge is >10° [13]. A disadvantage of opening wedge osteotomy includes the need for bone graft with longer time to healing and the risk of nonunion when compared to closing wedge osteotomy [14]. Alternative techniques including oblique sliding and dome osteotomies have been shown to be able to correct angular deformity and length without the need for bone grafting [50]. A combination of supramalleolar osteotomy and intra-articular osteotomy via medial malleolar osteotomy can also be performed for malunited medial malleolar fractures with impaction [44].

If **inframalleolar deformities** are noted such as talar tilt in a varus ankle deformity, an oblique tibial osteotomy can be performed to address both the supramalleolar varus deformity and reduce (close) the ankle mortise to address ankle instability [51]. Often, excessive heel varus is present and will benefit from a combination of valgus (closing wedge or Dwyer) osteotomy, lateral shift of the calcaneus, and reefing of the

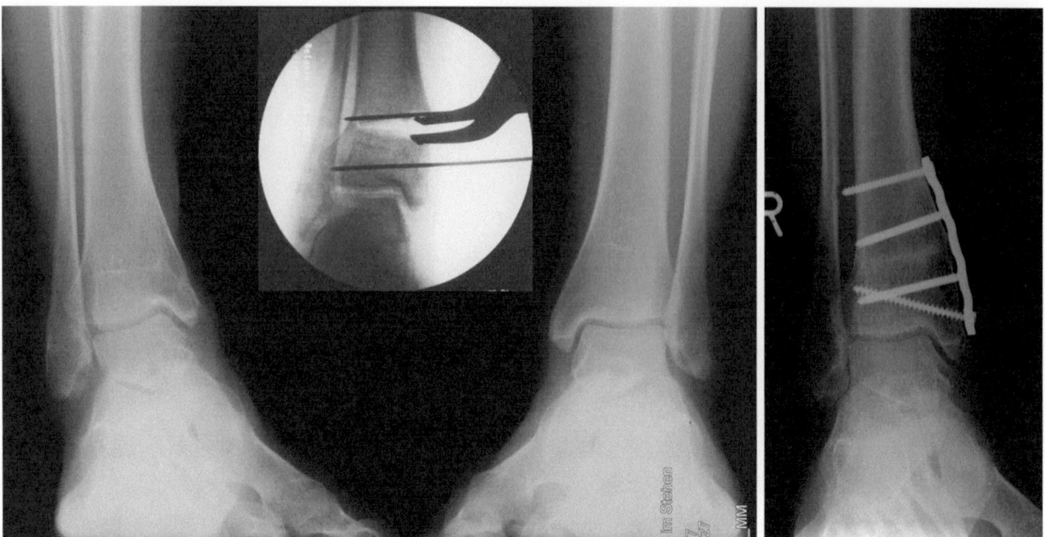

Fig. 12 Opening wedge supramalleolar osteotomy in a 23-year old patient for varus deformity resulting from a medial malleolar fracture 10 years ago with subsequent premature closure of the physeal growth plate. The patient was increasingly symptomatic since 3 years

chronically avulsed or elongated lateral ligaments [4]. In case of erosion or impaction of the medial tibial plafond resulting in an intra-articular deformity, the osteotomy line is directed more obliquely at the apex of intra-articular deformity to correct the deformity right at the center of rotation and angulation (CORA) resulting in a plafond-plasty [48]. Conversely, lateral impaction of the tibial plafond or avascular necrosis of the anterolateral tibial metaphysis resulting from abduction injuries may warrant an intra-articular osteotomy with lateral bone grafting [4, 41].

The surgical approach is typically dictated by pre-existing scars and implants, the apex of the deformity, and the direction of correction. Distal tibia osteotomy is performed via an (antero-) medial approach while osteotomies of the distal fibula warrant a lateral approach. The osteotomy should ideally be performed at the level of the CORA to gain maximal correction. However, in malunited ankle or pilon fractures, the CORA often lies very close to or at the ankle joint. Therefore, if a joint preserving osteotomy is planned, the osteotomy must be performed more proximally [14, 46]. The exact site and angle of the osteotomy should be planned preoperatively and marked intraoperatively with K wires while the amount of correction is confirmed with intraoperative fluoroscopy. For stability reasons, the osteotomy line should be targeted at the proximal 1/3 of the intrasyndesmosis plane. Nha et al. stated that osteotomy performed at the suprasyndesmosis plane has a higher risk of lateral hinge fracture while osteotomy performed at the proximal 1/3 of the intrasyndemosis plane can tolerate an opening wedge of up to 20° without lateral hinge fracture or with stable lateral cortical fracture without the need for fibular osteotomy due the ligamentous support of the syndesmosis [52]. In addition, overcorrection of the deformity by 3° to 5° in the coronal plane is recommended by most authors to achieve a lateral distal tibial angle between 93° and 95° [13, 14].

Once the osteotomy line is marked with a K-wire and confirmed with fluoroscopy, an oscillating saw can be used under continuous water irrigation to reduce thermal damage. One must ensure that the saw blade is perpendicular to the tibia and parallel to the K wire marker. Subsequently, the osteotomy is stopped a few millimetres short of the opposite cortex to prevent hinge fracture and secondary displacement of the distal fragment during deformity correction. An osteotome can be inserted into the osteotomy line initially to spread it open just enough to insert a lamina spreader for further controlled opening of the wedge. Once the amount of correction is acceptable, bone graft is inserted into the opening wedge and fixation is performed typically with a medial locking plate. In case of poor bone quality, a medial or posterior blade plate may provide superior stability (Fig. 13). Care is taken to correct additional sagittal plane deformities (inclination/declination of the distal tibia) [4, 45].

Simple **intra-articular malunions** can be corrected with intra-articular osteotomies along the former fracture line in exceptional cases with still intact cartilage in young, active, and compliant patients with sufficient bone stock [6, 7]. For long-standing deformities, an oblique supramalleolar osteotomy can be guided to the apex of the deformity ("plafond-plasty") [41, 48].

If a fibular osteotomy is needed, an oblique osteotomy increases the bony surface contact area. The fibula can be fixed with a one third tubular plate. In cases where there is concomitant medial malleolar and supramalleolar deformities, a double osteotomy may be needed to first correct the supramalleolar varus deformity followed by medial malleolar osteotomy for

lengthening and narrowing of the ankle mortise [6, 44]. A combination of medial locking plate and screws can be used for fixation of this double osteotomy.

Favorable results have been reported after supramalleolar, intra-articular osteotomy (plafond plasty), and medial malleolar osteotomies to correct eccentric loading [7, 13, 14, 22, 45–51]. In fact, a recent study on second-look arthroscopic evaluation of 29 ankles after supramalleolar osteotomy without marrow stimulation for medial ankle osteoarthritis showed that 26 (89.7%) ankles showed cartilage regeneration at the medial compartment of the ankle joint as a result of load redistribution and none had deterioration of cartilage status at 2.9 years postoperatively [53].

In addition, there are a few published series and reports on corrective intra-articular osteotomy for malunited pilon fractures reporting good outcomes at 2–5 years [6, 7, 41, 54]. Patients have to be counselled that posttraumatic arthritis may progress despite correction, but only a small percentage (14%) will need a secondary fusion [6]. Frequently, medial plates will have to be removed because they are felt through the skin and result in irritation in tight shoewear.

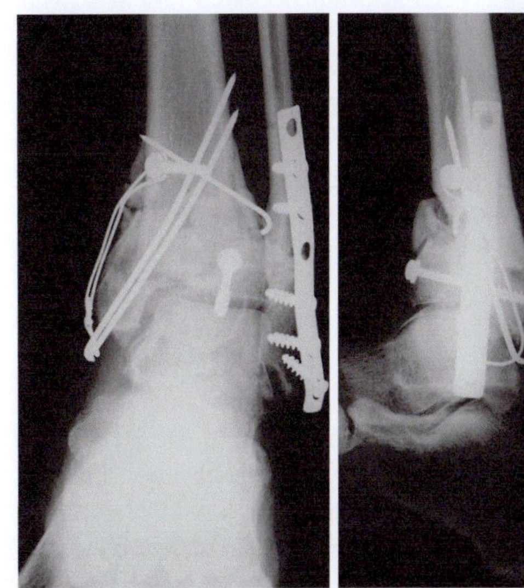
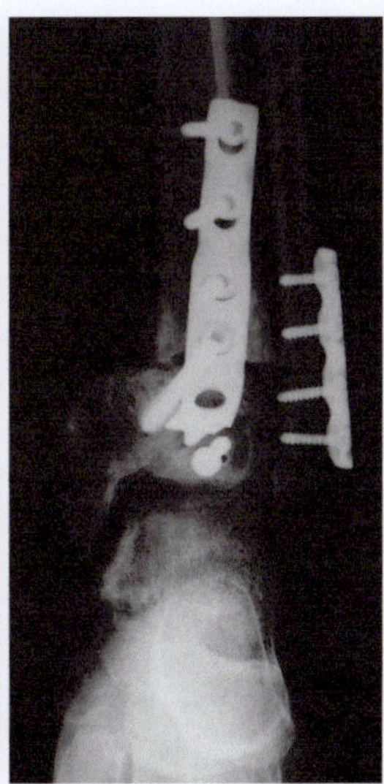
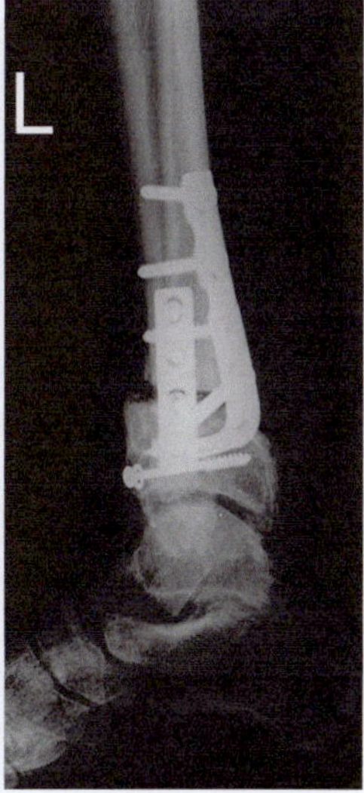

Fig. 13 Closing wedge supramalleolar osteotomy in a 55-year old, poorly compliant patient with varus malalignment and inclination of the distal tibia following trimalleolar fracture fixation with impaction of the plafond. A posterior blade plate is used to achieve correction and stable fixation

5 Late Syndesmosis Injuries of the Ankle

The management of syndesmotic injuries is a key to success in the treatment of malleolar fractures as chronic instability can lead to posttraumatic ankle arthritis [19, 20, 30]. It was reported that 20–45% of all operatively treated ankle fractures involved syndesmosis injuries [55]. In addition, up to 52% of syndesmotic injuries were found to be malreduced after closed reduction and 16% even after open reduction and fixation with postoperative CT scanning [10, 12, 55].

Late or chronic syndesmotic injury is a broad umbrella term encompassing a spectrum of symptoms and functional deficits of variable severity and duration. The 2016 ESSKA-AFAS consensus on syndesmotic injuries have classified syndesmotic injuries based on duration since trauma as **acute** being **<6 weeks**, subacute as between 6 weeks and 6 months, and **chronic** being **>6 months** [56]. Irrespective of the time from injury, syndesmotic instability can be classified as **frank or latent diastasis**, the latter becoming evident on stress examination [57]. In this section, evaluation and reconstructive options for subacute and chronic ligamentous syndesmosis injuries will be discussed as bony syndesmosis instability secondary to malleolar malunions has been addressed earlier. It goes without saying that any **concomitant bony deformities** have to be addressed simultaneously in every case of chronic syndesmotic instability in order to achieve a sufficient correction—and vice-versa [4, 30].

5.1 Specific Preoperative Evaluation and Planning

The presenting complaint can be non-specific ankle pain upon weight-bearing with persistent swelling and limited range of motion following a high ankle sprain, typically an eversion injury [30]. It may also be associated with subjective feeling of instability ("giving way") on uneven grounds masquerading as lateral ligament complex instability. Clinical examination includes palpation of the anterolateral ankle (anterior syndesmosis) where tenderness may be aggravated with dorsiflexion of the foot. Forced external rotation of the foot against a fixed lower leg may also reproduce the pain as the syndesmosis is stressed [19]. Calf or syndesmosis squeeze test can be performed as well although it may not be that specific in chronic injuries. Han et al. reported that palpation of the anterior syndesmosis produced a dull tenderness in 18 out of 20 patients with chronic syndesmotic injuries, only 3 out of 20 had a positive external rotation test and 2 out of 20 had positive calf squeeze test reflecting a 90%, 15%, and 10% specificity respectively [58]. Other recommended tests include a 'fibular translation' test that is performed by drawing the fibula forward and backward while the tibia is fixed with the contralateral hand. A manual 'Cotton' test may be performed by cupping the heel and applying medial and lateral forces to the talus with the ankle in neutral position stabilized by the contralateral hand [56]. Keep in mind that symptoms from posttraumatic ankle arthritis may overlap with those of syndesmotic instability.

Weight-bearing radiographs of both ankles in lateral and mortise views are indispensable for assessing any ankle malalignment including chronic syndesmotic instability [30]. The most relevant radiographic parameter for syndesmotic integrity is the "ligne claire" (tibiofibular clear space [TCS]) as originally described by Chaput (Figs. 3 and 14). It is considered the most reliable indicator as it is not significantly affected by tibial rotation [19, 56]. Other radiographic measures include the tibiofibular overlap (TFO) and the medial clear space (MCS). On weight-bearing mortise views, syndesmosis integrity is maintained if the TCS is less than 6 mm and TFO is greater than 1 mm although this reference is larger in males [10, 30] and may be completely absent as normal variant [59]. Furthermore, the TCS measured in mortise view seems to increase with age [56]. Because of the considerable anatomic variability, bilateral radiographs are essential [59]. A TCS and MCS widening of 2 mm or more compared to the contralateral unaffected ankle is considered to be pathologic [30, 60]. In addition, sagittal instability of the syndesmosis will regularly be present when the fibula migrates posteriorly reinforcing the importance of analysing the lateral view of the ankle radiographs [30]. Schreiber et al. [61] described use of the posterior tibiofibular distance, while Grenier et al. [62] proposed the anteroposterior tibiofibular (APTF) ratio to ensure sagittal instability is not missed.

CT scanning of both ankles is the gold standard for assessment of syndesmosis integrity. The standard view would be the coronal cut located at 10 mm proximal to the tibial plafond (Fig. 14) although more inferior levels closer to

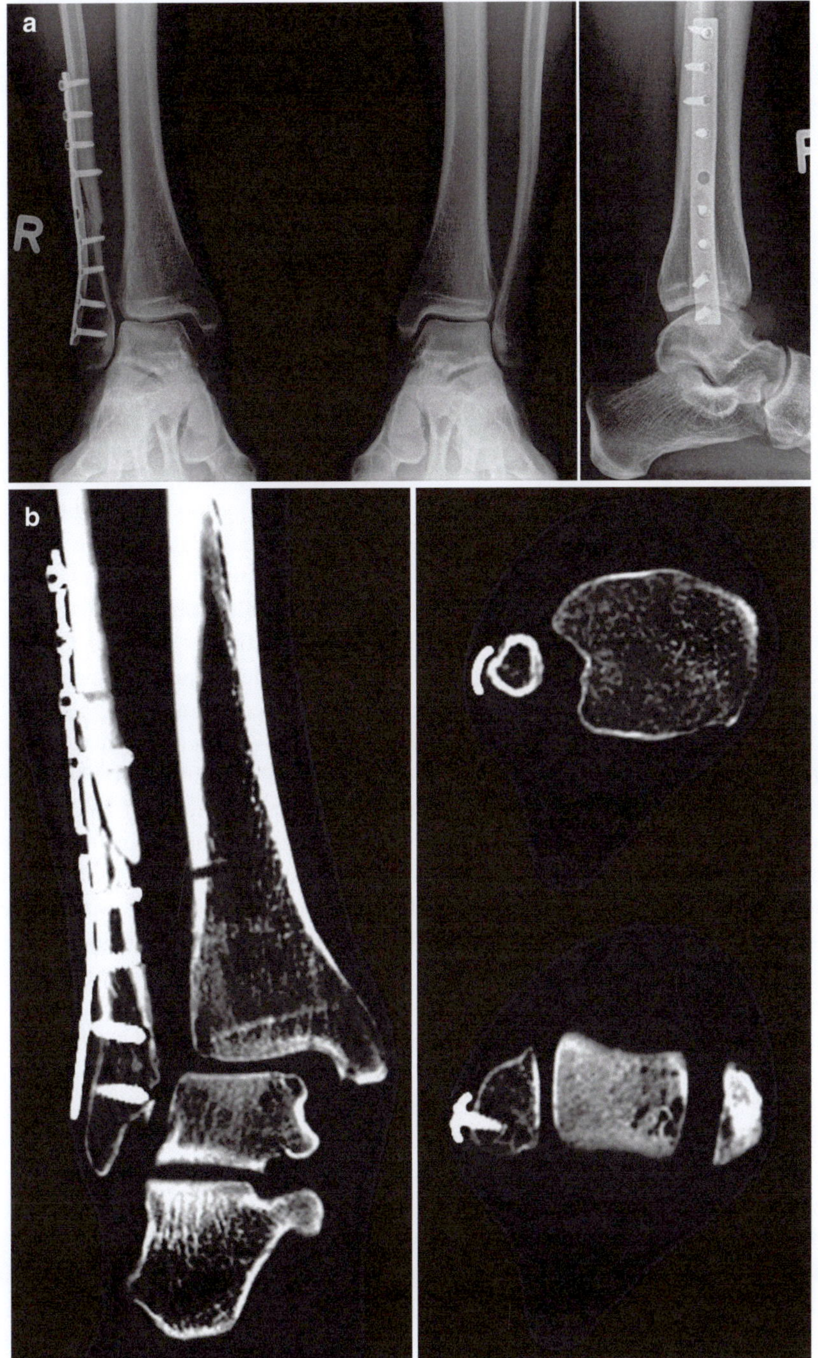

Fig. 14 (**a**) Standing radiographs and (**b**) CT imaging of chronic syndesmotic instability as evidenced by tibiofibular diastasis with marked widening of the MCS. In addition, there is fibular shortening and valgus following a pronation-external rotation injury

the tibial plafond have been reported [10, 30, 59]. As with plain radiographs, there is a high interindividual but low intraindividual variability of the radiographic measurements [59, 62]. Any side-to-side difference in fibular translation or syndesmosis diastasis more than 2 mm is considered pathological [30]. In addition, weight-bearing CT scans have recently gotten a role in the assessment of subtle syndesmosis injuries combining the benefits of physiologic loading and three-dimensional imaging. However, it is still unclear if it is superior to conventional CT scanning in the diagnosis of acute or chronic instability [63].

Ankle arthroscopy, as an invasive procedure, only allows for evaluation of the anterior portion of syndesmosis with the interosseous and posterior part less accessible [56, 60]. Granted, it allows assessment of associated injuries such as cartilage or lateral ligamentous injuries.

5.2 Treatment of Subacute Syndesmosis Injury

This group of patients presents from 6 weeks to 6 months post injury with a variable temporal progression of symptoms. In patients with no diastasis, symptoms are generally due to the impingement of hypertrophic synovium and scar tissue within the tibiofibular space and adjacent anterolateral part of the ankle joint. Treatment consists of **arthroscopic debridement** of the syndesmotic scars with excellent outcomes including improved range of motion and relief of symptoms [30, 58, 64]. Usually, there is no need for additional "prophylactic" syndesmotic stabilization with screws or suture button device as they have been reported to not produce improved outcomes [58, 65]. Syndesmotic stabilization is only needed if it is clinically unstable after debridement upon arthroscopic or fluoroscopic stress examination.

In another group of patients with subacute syndesmosis injury and instability, the patients display diastasis of the ankle mortise in standing radiographs, typically after returning to full weight-bearing with or without removal of the syndesmotic screw or flexible implant. The ankle joint is eccentrically loaded thus having a higher predisposition to arthritis [9, 60]. In this scenario, the aim is to debride any interposed scar tissues and **repair the AiTFL** provided that adequate remnant ligaments are present. It has been reported that anatomical reconstruction or repair of the anterior syndesmosis may be sufficient to produce fibrotic healing with good outcomes [66]. Favourable results have been achieved when debridement or AiTFL repair was followed by **syndesmotic stabilization** with a combination of position screw and/or suture button [30, 66]. If there is dystopic ligament healing or elongation, medial and proximal advancement of a bone block from the anterior tibia (Chaput) tubercle to tighten the stretched out AiTFL coupled with a position screw placement, produced good outcomes as well [67]. Likewise, a malunion or nonunion of a posterior malleolar (PiTFL) avulsion is debrided, advanced, and fixed with a screw followed by reduction of the distal fibula into the incisura and syndesmotic stabilization (Fig. 15).

If the medial clear space remains displaced after syndesmotic reduction, the medial gutter and **deltoid ligament** must be explored and intervening scar tissues removed. Occasionally, a torn and unstable deltoid ligament may necessitate repair or reconstruction especially in the presence of valgus tilt of the talus [30].

If there is insufficient soft tissue or remnant syndesmosis tissue left after debridement for repair or approximation, soft tissue reconstruction of the syndesmosis via **ligamentoplasty** is a viable option [68]. The authors prefer to use a split peroneus longus tendon graft for a near-anatomic reconstruction of the AiTFL, interosseous ligament and PiTFL to recreate the dynamic three-point fixation of the distal fibula. Using a split peroneus longus tendon has minimal functional deficit after transfer as it has minimal contribution to foot eversion and does not result in lateral ankle instability, in particular with half of the tendon remaining in place. The technique involves a direct lateral approach to the distal fibula. The peroneus longus tendon is exposed behind the fibula and separated from the peroneal brevis. Using the same approach, the syndesmosis is exposed and all scar tissues debrided. The

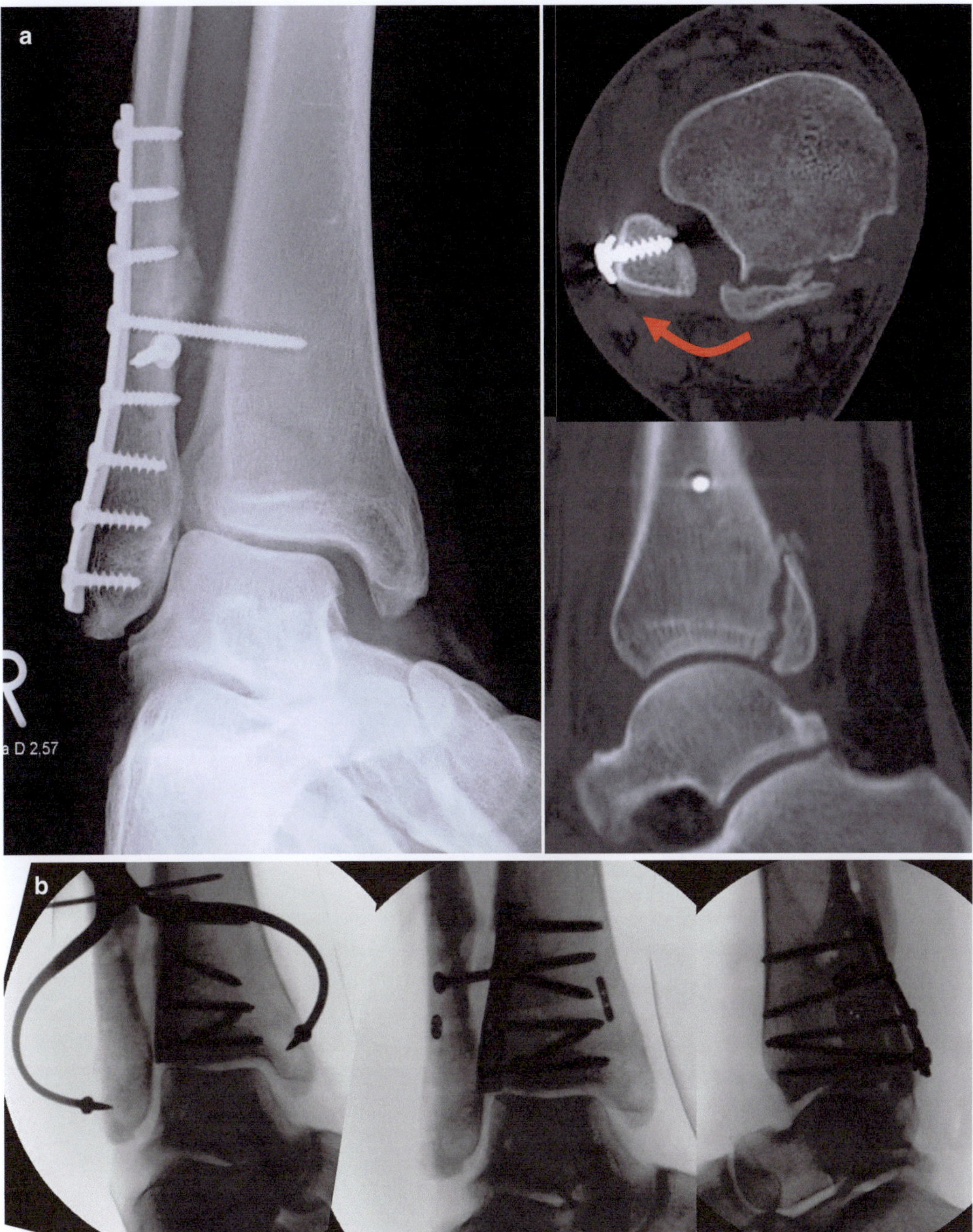

Fig. 15 (**a**) Subacute syndesmotic instability with diastasis following lateral malleolar fixation but neglect of PiTFL avulsion resulting in nonunion of the posterior malleolar fragment and rotational instability of the distal fibula without fibular shortening. (**b**) The posterior malleolar fragment is debrided, reduced, and fixed with an antiglide plate via a posterolateral approach recreating the fibular notch and facilitating fibular reduction. A flexible implant (suture button) is employed to enhance syndesmotic fixation

peroneus longus tendon is divided into equal parts from the tip of the fibula upwards to a 15–18 cm length. The anterior split portion of the tendon is guided through three bone tunnels in the distal tibia and fibula, mimicking the ana-tomic trajectory of the syndesmotic complex (Fig. 16). The fibula is reduced into the tibial incisura with a large pointed reduction forceps, and anatomic reduction is checked with mortise and lateral radiographs. If the medial clear space

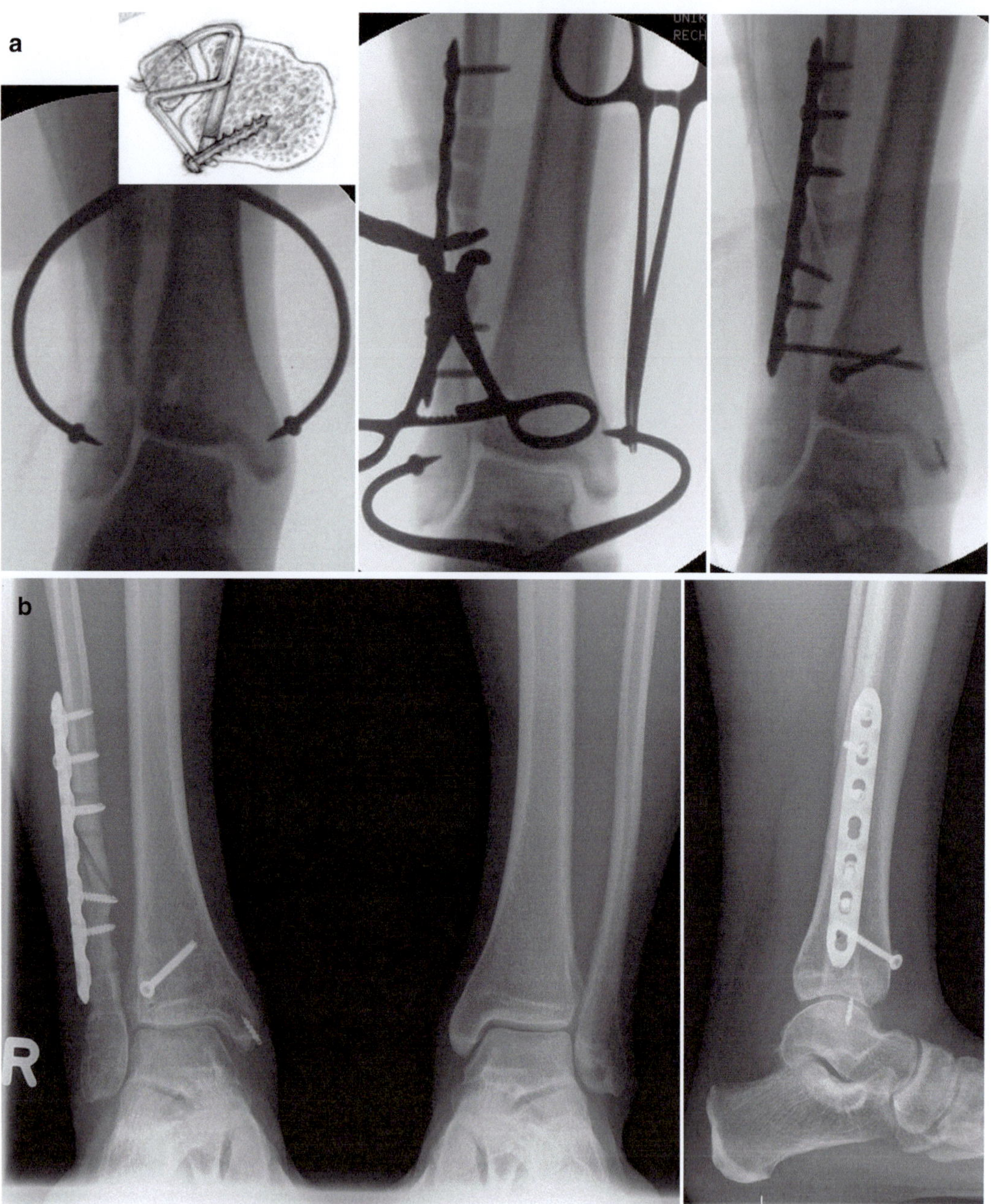

Fig. 16 Peroneus longus ligamentoplasty (same patient as in Fig. 14). (**a**) Following debridement of the syndesmosis and medial gutter, a split peroneus longus tendon is used to restore the three-point-suspension of the syndesmosis [68]. Despite syndesmotic stabilization, there is still talar shift and tilt doe to fibular shortening and valgus which is corrected by an oblique distal fibular osteotomy. The chronically unstable deltoid ligament is reefed to the medial malleolus with a suture anchor. (**b**) At 1 year, weight-bearing radiographs demonstrate a stable ankle mortise. The syndesmotic screw was removed at 8 weeks, alternatively, it may be left in place

is still wide, scar and pannus tissue is debrided via a small anteromedial approach. Once reduction and fixation is satisfactory, a syndesmotic screw is inserted to protect the ligamentoplasty for at least 8 weeks postoperatively. The free end of the tendon graft is secured under correct tension at the anterolateral tibial tubercle with a 3.5 mm cancellous screw and washer. Published results from the first 16 patients followed for an average of 18 months were encouraging with 93.8% reporting significant pain relief and a mean Karlsson score of 88 [68]. Since then, the authors have treated more than 150 patients using similar method with mostly good outcomes. Failures were seen in the presence of symptomatic arthritis or bony defects at the distal tibia or fibula at the time of revision surgery [30].

There are several other types of tenodeses or ligamentoplasties available for reconstruction using multiple types of grafts. Connors and colleagues used a split semitendinosus allograft to reconstruct the AiTFL and interosseous ligament via a tiered double level bone tunnel followed by stabilization with 2 syndesmotic screws which were removed at 6 months [69]. Morris et al. reconstructed the AiTFL and interosseous ligament with a free hamstring autograft [70]. Other options of grafts include peroneus brevis, free gracilis, and plantaris tendons, fascia lata, and free hamstrings tendon allograft [30]. More recently, fixation devices like internal bracing have been employed for replacement or reinforcement of the AiTFL and interosseous portion of the syndesmosis [71]. All of these soft tissue reconstructions of the syndesmosis have been reported to produce good outcomes and pain relief in the short to medium term.

5.3 Treatment of Chronic Syndesmosis Injury

Chronic injuries of the syndesmosis (beyond 6 months) may present with frank or latent diastasis and posttraumatic arthritic changes depending on the time from injury and amount of instability. The syndesmotic space is filled with scar tissue and pannus at the time of presentation. Thorough debridement typically leaves few remnants for direct syndesmotic repair leaving either ligamentoplasty or tibiofibular fusion as treatment options in the absence of advanced posttraumatic ankle arthritis.

With good bone stock at the distal tibia and fibula, many authors advocate dynamic soft tissue reconstruction of the syndesmosis via **ligamentoplasty** as described above [30, 56, 68–70]. This will allow some residual tibiofibular motion and thus a near physiologic action of the ankle joint. Tibiofibular fusion remains a salvage option in cases of failed ligamentoplasty or when soft tissue reconstruction is not feasible due to poor bone quality, avascular necrosis of the lateral tibial plafond or severe scarring of the peroneal tendons.

Tibiofibular fusion with bone grafting for chronic syndesmotic instability has been described by several authors [30, 72]. Following debridement of scars and debris in the syndesmotic region, necrectomy is performed in case of AVN of the anterolateral distal tibia [30, 33]. Syndesmotic fusion is achieved with interposition of a corticocancellous bone block and permanent screw fixation. In case of poor bone stock in the distal fibula, screws may be augmented by a small plate. Only a few small series are reported in the literature and are limited to short-term results. Olson and colleagues, in the largest series of ten patients, reported favourable outcomes of tibiofibular arthrodesis at a follow-up of 2 years [72]. There were three reoperations but no secondary ankle arthrodesis was necessary. Although elimination of the three-dimensional fibular motion also affects tibiotalar motion resulting in unphysiological stiffness, secondary ankle fusion has not been reported in the short-term yet, and long-term results of tibiofibular fusion are still pending. Furthermore, even complete posttraumatic tibiofibular synostosis, although associated with limited plantar- and dorsiflexion at the ankle, does not seem to lead to relevant symptoms or inferior results in the affected patients [73]. It appears therefore that tibiofibular synostosis is relevant only with concomitant malposition of the distal fibula [30].

In the presence of advanced ankle arthritis, joint preserving procedures will ultimately fail. Unfortunately, chronic diastasis and instability of the syndesmosis rapidly progresses to ankle arthritis due to significant reduction in contact area and abnormal loading forces in the ankle joint as outlined above. In a study of 735 tibial plafond fractures, it was reported that the 95% rate of posttraumatic ankle arthritis was significantly associated with failure to diagnose syndesmosis injuries and syndesmotic avulsions at the distal tibia and fibula [74]. Primary cartilage damage at the time of injury coupled with inflammatory cytokines further add to the risk of late posttraumatic ankle arthritis and secondary damage to the cartilage surfaces from eccentric loading [75]. In these scenarios, corrective ankle fusion or total ankle replacement with syndesmotic stabilization is the treatment of choice [4, 25, 30]. These treatment options are dealt with in separate chapters of this book.

References

1. Weber BG. Lengthening osteotomy of the fibula to correct a widened mortice of the ankle after fracture. Int Orthop. 1981;4(4):289–93.
2. Reidsma II, Nolte PA, Marti RK, Raaymakers EL. Treatment of malunited fractures of the ankle: a long-term follow-up of reconstructive surgery. J Bone Joint Surg Br. 2010;92(1):66–70.
3. Rammelt S, Swords M, Dhillon M, Sands A, editors. AO manual of fracture management. Foot & Ankle. Stuttgart: AO Foundation; 2020.
4. Rammelt S, Zwipp H, Hansen ST. Posttraumatic reconstruction of the foot and ankle. In: Browner J, Krettek A, editors. Skeletal trauma: basic science, management and reconstruction. Philadelphia: Elsevier; 2019. p. 2641–90.
5. Capogna BM, Egol KA. Treatment of nonunions after malleolar fractures. Foot Ankle Clin. 2016;21(1):49–62.
6. Rammelt S, Zwipp H. Intra-articular osteotomy for correction of malunions and nonunions of the Tibial Pilon. Foot Ankle Clin. 2016;21(1):63–76.
7. Rammelt S, Marti RK, Zwipp H. Joint-preserving osteotomy of malunited ankle and pilon fractures. Unfallchirurg. 2013;116(9):789–96. German.
8. Ramsey PL, Hamilton W. Changes in tibiotalar area of contact caused by lateral talar shift. J Bone Joint Surg Am. 1976;58(3):356–7.
9. Thordarson DB, Motamed S, Hedman T, Ebramzadeh E, Bakshian S. The effect of fibular malreduction on contact pressures in an ankle fracture malunion model. J Bone Joint Surg Am. 1997;79(12):1809–15.
10. Vasarhelyi A, Lubitz J, Gierer P, et al. Detection of fibular torsional deformities after surgery for ankle fractures with a novel CT method. Foot Ankle Int. 2006;27(12):1115–21.
11. Dujardin F, Abdulmutalib H, Tobenas AC. Total fractures of the tibial pilon. Orthop Traumatol Surg Res. 2014;100(1 Suppl):S65–74.
12. Sagi HC, Shah AR, Sanders RW. The functional consequence of syndesmotic joint malreduction at a minimum 2-year follow-up. J Orthop Trauma. 2012;26(7):439–43.
13. Takakura Y, Tanaka Y, Kumai T, Tamai S. Low tibial osteotomy for osteoarthritis of the ankle. Results of a new operation in 18 patients. J Bone Joint Surg Br. 1995;77(1):50–4.
14. Krause F, Veljkovic A, Schmid T. Supramalleolar osteotomies for posttraumatic malalignment of the distal tibia. Foot Ankle Clin. 2016;21(1):1–14.
15. Moody ML, Koeneman J, Hettinger E, Karpman RR. The effects of fibular and talar displacement on joint contact areas about the ankle. Orthop Rev. 1992;21(6):741–4.
16. Rammelt S, Bartoníček J. Posterior malleolar fractures: a critical analysis review. JBJS Rev. 2020;8(8):e19.00207.
17. Roberts V, Mason LW, Harrison E, Molloy AP, Mangwani J. Does functional outcome depend on the quality of the fracture fixation? Mid to long term outcomes of ankle fractures at two university teaching hospitals. Foot Ankle Surg. 2019;25(4):538–41.
18. Mont MA, Sedlin ED, Weiner LS, Miller AR. Postoperative radiographs as predictors of clinical outcome in unstable ankle fractures. J Orthop Trauma. 1992;6:352–7.
19. Rammelt S, Obruba P. An update on the evaluation and treatment of syndesmotic injuries. Eur J Trauma Emerg Surg. 2015;41(6):601–14.
20. Kaftandziev I, Bakota B, Trpeski S, Arsovski O, Spasov M, Cretnik A. The effect of the ankle syndesmosis reduction quality on the short-term functional outcome following ankle fractures. Injury. 2021;52(Suppl 5):S70–4.
21. Reilingh ML, Beimers L, Tuijthof GJ, Stufkens SA, Maas M, van Dijk CN. Measuring hindfoot alignment radiographically: the long axial view is more reliable than the hindfoot alignment view. Skelet Radiol. 2010;39(11):1103–8.
22. Faict S, Burssens A, Van Oevelen A, Maeckelbergh L, Mertens P, Buedts K. Correction of ankle varus deformity using patient-specific dome-shaped osteotomy guides designed on weight-bearing CT: a pilot study. Arch Orthop Trauma Surg. 2021;143:791. Epub Sep 25.
23. Lockard CA, Chang A, Shin RC, Clanton TO, Ho CP. Regional variation of ankle and hindfoot cartilage T2 mapping values at 3 T: a feasibility study. Eur J Radiol. 2019;113:209–16.
24. Mosca M, Buda R, Ceccarelli F, Fuiano M, Vocale E, Massimi S, Benedetti MG, Grassi A, Caravelli

S, Zaffagnini S. Ankle joint re-balancing in the management of ankle fracture malunion using fibular lengthening: prospective clinical-radiological results at mid-term follow-up. Int Orthop. 2021;45(2):411–7.

25. Manke E, Yeo NEM, Rammelt S. Ankle arthrodesis. A review of current techniques and results. Acta Chir Orthop Traumatol Cechoslov. 2020;87(4):225–36.

26. Rammelt S, Bartoníček J, Kroker L, Neumann AP. Surgical fixation of quadrimalleolar fractures of the ankle. J Orthop Trauma. 2021;35(6):e216–22.

27. Curtis MJ, Michelson JD, Urquhart MW, Byank RP, Jinnah RH. Tibiotalar contact and fibular malunion in ankle fractures. A cadaver study. Acta Orthop Scand. 1992;63(3):326–9.

28. Weber D, Weber M. Corrective osteotomies for malunited malleolar fractures. Foot Ankle Clin. 2016;21(1):37–48.

29. Weber M, Ganz R. Malunion following trimalleolar fracture with posterolateral subluxation of the talus-reconstruction including the posterior malleolus. Foot Ankle Int. 2003;24(4):338–44.

30. Rammelt S, Boszczyk A. Chronic syndesmotic injuries: arthrodesis versus reconstruction. Foot Ankle Clin. 2020;25(4):631–52.

31. Heineck J, Serra A, Haupt C, Rammelt S. Accuracy of corrective osteotomies in fibular malunion: a cadaver model. Foot Ankle Int. 2009;30(8):773–7.

32. Sneppen O. Treatment of pseudarthrosis involving the malleolus. A postoperative follow-up of 34 cases. Acta Orthop Scand. 1971;42(2):201–16.

33. Assal M, Sangeorzan B, Hansen ST. Post traumatic osteonecrosis of the lateral tibial plafond. Foot Ankle Surg. 2007;13(1):24–9.

34. Hoelsbrekken SE, Kaul-Jensen K, Mørch T, Vika H, Clementsen T, Paulsrud Ø, Petursson G, Stiris M, Strømsøe K. Nonoperative treatment of the medial malleolus in bimalleolar and trimalleolar ankle fractures: a randomized controlled trial. J Orthop Trauma. 2013;27(11):633–7.

35. Drijfhout van Hooff CC, Verhage SM, Hoogendoorn JM. Influence of fragment size and postoperative joint congruency on long-term outcome of posterior malleolar fractures. Foot Ankle Int. 2015;36(6):673–8.

36. Li Y, Chen Y, Liu X, Chen J, Gan T, Zhang H. Patient pain and function after correction of posterior malleolar malunion. Foot Ankle Int. 2021;42(12):1536–46.

37. Bartoníček J, Rammelt S, Kostlivý K, Vaněček V, Klika D, Trešl I. Anatomy and classification of the posterior tibial fragment in ankle fractures. Arch Orthop Trauma Surg. 2015;135(4):505–16.

38. Klammer G, Kadakia AR, Joos DA, Seybold JD, Espinosa N. Posterior pilon fractures: a retrospective case series and proposed classification system. Foot Ankle Int. 2013;34(2):189–99.

39. Rammelt S, Bartoníček J, Kroker L. Pathoanatomy of the anterolateral tibial fragment in ankle fractures. J Bone Joint Surg Am. 2022;104:353–63.

40. Lauge-Hansen N. Fractures of the ankle. II. Combined experimental-surgical and experimental-roentgenologic investigations. Arch Surg. 1950;60(5):957–85.

41. Li X, Xu Y, Guo C, Yang C, Zhu Y, Xu X. Anterior distal tibial plafond-plasty for the treatment of post-traumatic ankle osteoarthritis with anterior translation of the talus. Sci Rep. 2021;11(1):4381.

42. Marx C, Schaser KD, Rammelt S. Early corrections after failed ankle fracture fixation. Z Orthop Unfall. 2021;159(3):323–31.

43. Ito K, Tanaka Y, Katsui R, Taniguchi A. Corrective osteotomy for malunion of a tillaux-chaput fracture: a case report. Clin Med Case Rep. 2017;1:103.

44. Guo C, Liu Z, Xu Y, Li X, Zhu Y, Xu X. Supramalleolar osteotomy combined with an intra-articular osteotomy for the reconstruction of malunited medial impacted ankle fractures. Foot Ankle Int. 2018;39(12):1457–63.

45. Wagner E, Wagner P. Correction of sagittal plane deformity of the distal tibia. Foot Ankle Clin. 2022;27(1):129–44.

46. Krähenbühl N, Susdorf R, Barg A, Hintermann B. Supramalleolar osteotomy in post-traumatic valgus ankle osteoarthritis. Int Orthop. 2020;44(3):535–43. An additional fibula or calcaneus osteotomy was necessary for 55% and 23% of all patients, respectively.

47. Rammelt S, Godoy-Santos A, Schneiders W, Fitze G, Zwipp H. Foot and ankle fractures during childhood: review of the literature and scientific evidence for appropriate treatment. Rev Bras Ortop. 2016;51:630–9.

48. Mann HA, Filippi J, Myerson MS. Intra-articular opening medial tibial wedge osteotomy (plafond-plasty) for the treatment of intra-articular varus ankle arthritis and instability. Foot Ankle Int. 2012;33(4):255–61.

49. Hintermann B, Barg A, Knupp M. Corrective supramalleolar osteotomy for malunited pronation-external rotation fractures of the ankle. J Bone Joint Surg Br. 2011;93(10):1367–72.

50. Kim J, Henry JK, Kim JB, Lee WC. Dome supramalleolar osteotomies for the treatment of ankle pain with opposing coronal plane deformities between ankle and the lower limb. Foot Ankle Int. 2021;23:10711007211050639.

51. Lee WC, Moon JS, Lee K, Byun WJ, Lee SH. Indications for supramalleolar osteotomy in patients with ankle osteoarthritis and varus deformity. J Bone Joint Surg Am. 2011;93(13):1243–8.

52. Nha KW, Lee SH, Rhyu IJ, Kim HJ, Song JG, Han JH, Yeo ED, Lee YK. Safe zone for medial open-wedge supramalleolar osteotomy of the ankle: a cadaveric study. Foot Ankle Int. 2016;37(1):102–8.

53. Lim JW, Eom JS, Kang SJ, Lee DO, Kang HJ, Jung HG. The effect of supramalleolar osteotomy without marrow stimulation for medial ankle osteoarthritis: second-look arthroscopic evaluation of 29 ankles. J Bone Joint Surg Am. 2021;103(19):1844–51.

54. Li X, Xu X. Joint preservation for posttraumatic ankle arthritis after tibial plafond fracture. Foot Ankle Clin. 2022;27(1):73–90.

55. Tornetta PIII, Axelrad TW, Sibai TA, et al. Treatment of the stress positive ligamentous ankle fracture: inci-

dence of syndesmotic injury and clinical decision making. J Orthop Trauma. 2012;26(11):659–61.

56. van Dijk CN, Longo UG, Loppini M, Florio P, Maltese L, Ciuffreda M, Denaro V. Classification and diagnosis of acute isolated syndesmotic injuries: ESSKA-AFAS consensus and guidelines. Knee Surg Sports Traumatol Arthrosc. 2016;24(4):1200–16.

57. Edwards GS Jr, DeLee JC. Ankle diastasis without fracture. Foot Ankle. 1984;4(6):305–12.

58. Han SH, Lee JW, Kim S, Suh JS, Choi YR. Chronic tibiofibular syndesmosis injury: the diagnostic efficiency of magnetic resonance imaging and comparative analysis of operative treatment. Foot Ankle Int. 2007;28(3):336–42.

59. Mukhopadhyay S, Metcalfe A, Guha AR, Mohanty K, Hemmadi S, Lyons K, O'Doherty D. Malreduction of syndesmosis—are we considering the anatomical variation? Injury. 2011;42(10):1073–6.

60. Xenos JS, Hopkinson WJ, Mulligan ME, Olson EJ, Popovic NA. The tibiofibular syndesmosis. Evaluation of the ligamentous structures, methods of fixation, and radiographic assessment. J Bone Joint Surg Am. 1995;77(6):847–56.

61. Schreiber JJ, McLawhorn AS, Dy CJ, Goldwyn EM. Intraoperative contralateral view for assessing accurate syndesmosis reduction. Orthopedics. 2013;36(5):360–1.

62. Grenier S, Benoit B, Rouleau DM, Leduc S, Laflamme GY, Liew A. APTF: anteroposterior tibiofibular ratio, a new reliable measure to assess syndesmotic reduction. J Orthop Trauma. 2013;27(4):207–11.

63. Krähenbühl N, Bailey TL, Weinberg MW, Davidson NP, Hintermann B, Presson AP, Allen CM, Henninger HB, Saltzman CL, Barg A. Is load application necessary when using computed tomography scans to diagnose syndesmotic injuries? A cadaver study. Foot Ankle Surg. 2020;26(2):198–204.

64. Ogilvie-Harris DJ, Gilbart MK, Chorney K. Chronic pain following ankle sprains in athletes: the role of arthroscopic surgery. Arthroscopy. 1997;13(5):564–74.

65. Ryan PM, Rodriguez RM. Outcomes and return to activity after operative repair of chronic latent syndesmotic instability. Foot Ankle Int. 2016;37(2):192–7.

66. van den Bekerom MP, de Leeuw PA, van Dijk CN. Delayed operative treatment of syndesmotic instability. Current concepts review. Injury. 2009;40(11):1137–42.

67. Beumer A, Heijboer RP, Fontijne WP, Swierstra BA. Late reconstruction of the anterior distal tibiofibular syndesmosis: good outcome in 9 patients. Acta Orthop Scand. 2000;71(5):519–21.

68. Grass R, Rammelt S, Biewener A, Zwipp H. Peroneus longus ligamentoplasty for chronic instability of the distal tibiofibular syndesmosis. Foot Ankle Int. 2003;24(5):392–7.

69. Connors JC, Grossman JP, Zulauf EE, Coyer MA. Syndesmotic ligament allograft reconstruction for treatment of chronic diastasis. J Foot Ankle Surg. 2020;59(4):835–40.

70. Morris MW, Rice P, Schneider TE. Distal tibiofibular syndesmosis reconstruction using a free hamstring autograft. Foot Ankle Int. 2009;30(6):506–11.

71. Lenz CG, Shepherd D. Dynamic syndesmotic stabilisation and reinforcement of the antero-inferior tibiofibular ligament with internal brace: early results and clinical outcome. Foot Ankle Orthop. 2022;7(1):2473011421S00042.

72. Olson KM, Dairyko GH Jr, Toolan BC. Salvage of chronic instability of the syndesmosis with distal tibiofibular arthrodesis: functional and radiographic results. J Bone Joint Surg Am. 2011;93(1):66–72.

73. Marvan J, Dzupa V, Krbec M, et al. Distal tibiofibular synostosis after surgically resolved ankle fractures: an epidemiological, clinical and morphological evaluation of a patient sample. Injury. 2016;47(11):2570–4.

74. Haller JM, Githens M, Rothberg D, Higgins T, Barei D, Nork S. Syndesmosis and syndesmotic equivalent injuries in tibial plafond fractures. J Orthop Trauma. 2019;33(3):e74–8.

75. Godoy-Santos AL, Ranzoni L, Teodoro WR, Capelozzi V, Giglio P, Fernandes TD, Rammelt S. Increased cytokine levels and histological changes in cartilage, synovial cells and synovial fluid after malleolar fractures. Injury. 2017;48(Suppl 4):S27–33.

Ankle Infections: Postoperative and Septic Arthritis

Joseph D. Galloway, Emily E. Wild, and Michael S. Sirkin

1 Introduction and Epidemiology

Ankle infections encompass a broad spectrum of pathology which can lead to significant morbidity. Careful preparation and adherence to treatment principles, along with a thorough understanding of the epidemiology and risk factors, as well as the diagnostic and treatment options can lead to a successful outcome.

Here, we will focus on native ankle septic arthritis and postoperative ankle infections with particular emphasis on fracture related infections (FRI) and those involving hardware. Postoperative infections can arise in the elective setting or post-traumatic with injuries being categorized as high and low energy, and open versus closed with somewhat different implications. It is helpful to identify the depth of infection as being confined to the skin structures as a cellulitis, or deeper more aggressive infections forming abscesses and necrosis, and those involving the joint space or bone such as osteomyelitis. Additionally, it is useful to stratify infections by duration as either acute (typically less than 4–6 weeks) or chronic.

Soft tissue infections can occur more readily in the ankle due to impaired perfusion and altered sensation that may be preexisting in the patient [1]. One epidemiological study found an incidence of cellulitis of 199 cases in 100,000 person-years, with a 21.6% rate of hospitalization and recurrence [2]. Postsurgical patients most often present acutely with cellulitis. These patients are at a high risk due to preexisting skin insult and lymphatic drainage interruption [1]. While cellulitis is typically treated with antibiotics alone, the presence of deep space infections may require operative intervention [3]. Therefore, determination of the depth of infection and any abscess formation is key and relies both on careful examination and, frequently, advanced imaging.

The incidence of septic arthritis has been reported to be from 2 to 10 cases per 100,000 persons, with approximately 3–7% of the cases involving the foot or ankle [4]. Postoperative ankle joint infections have been reported in 1–5% of cases most commonly through direct inoculation with typical skin flora [3]. Therefore, the best treatment of postoperative infections, is prevention.

Osteomyelitis represents a deep infection that has invaded the bony architecture. An important distinction must be made between an acute osteomyelitis, representing vascularized viable bone, and chronic osteomyelitis with bone necrosis. Whereas the former may often be treated with systemic antibiotics, the later always requires a debridement for eradication.

J. D. Galloway (✉) · M. S. Sirkin
Department of Orthopaedics, Rutgers New Jersey
Medical School, Newark, NJ, USA
e-mail: sirkinms@mac.com

E. E. Wild
Department of Orthopaedics, SUNY Downstate,
Brookdale Hospital, Brooklyn, NY, USA

© The Author(s), under exclusive license to Springer Nature Switzerland AG 2023
D. Herscovici Jr. et al. (eds.), *Evaluation and Surgical Management of the Ankle*,
https://doi.org/10.1007/978-3-031-33537-2_19

2 Risk Factors for Infection

A thorough understanding of the risk factors associated with ankle infection will help tailor the clinician's index of suspicion for diagnosis and prognostication. Recognizing those factors that are modifiable can aid in treatment.

Injury related risk factors are nonmodifiable. Traumatic ankle injuries are at baseline elevated risk for infection compared to elective surgery. Tissue disruption and devascularization from the injury impede the body's native defenses [3]. Specifically, open fractures, high-energy mechanisms, and wound contamination level each confer a statistically significant increased risk of developing a surgical site infection [5]. Higher energy injuries such as tibia plafond fractures have historically had an elevated risk of wound breakdown and infection with historic rates of infection after acute operative treatment from 13 to 50% [6–8]. While the injury itself is not modifiable, the use of a staged treatment protocol with spanning external fixation (Fig. 1), elevation for edema resolution and delayed internal fixation can reduce the rates of wound breakdown and deep infection to about 5% [6].

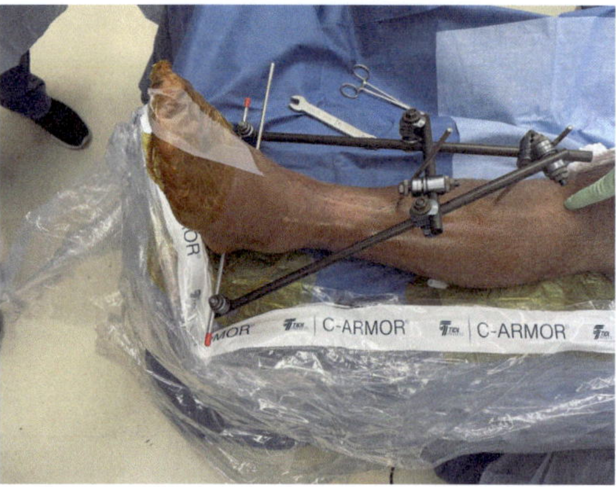

Fig. 1 Shows a patient with a high energy pilon fracture who underwent temporary ankle spanning external fixation in the acute phase to allow for improvement in the swelling and the damaged soft tissue envelope. Careful inspection now reveals transverse extensor surface skin creases at the ankle joint, and the longitudinal stress-relaxation stretch marks in the skin indicative of resolution of the swelling phase

Patient-related risk factors which compromise immune surveillance, metabolism, and vascularity are critical to identify. It is helpful to think of patient risk factors as systemic and local factors. Systemic factors include malnutrition, renal failure, liver failure, diabetes, chronic heart disease, alcohol use, tobacco use, steroids, immunodeficiency, malignancy, obesity, and extreme age [9, 10]. Local factors include lymphedema, venous stasis, peripheral vascular disease, and localized scarring and fibrosis [9]. Patients with any of these factors have been termed a compromised host or "Class B" host, and nearly 80% of osteomyelitis cases are reported in class B hosts [9].

While not all patient factors are modifiable, those which are should be addressed preoperatively in elective surgery cases. Nutritional status should be optimized, with the involvement of a nutritionist in a multidisciplinary team. Patients should be counseled on smoking cessation and reduction of excessive alcohol consumption. Smoking has been identified as an independent risk factor in the failure of treatment in fracture related infections [11]. American Society of Anesthesiologists (ASA) grade ≥ 3 has been found as an independent risk factor for infection, thus for elective procedures patients should be medically optimized by their primary physician [5]. Obesity has been routinely found as an infection risk factor with Body Mass Index (BMI) ≥ 30 carrying a significant increased risk [5, 12]. However, in the acute traumatic setting, modification of these factors is usually not an option. Additionally, for patients with degenerative pain in the lower extremities, often exercise and weight reduction is painful leading to a vicious cycle begetting further comorbidities such as diabetes and heart disease further elevating their risk [13].

Diabetes mellitus is worth a special note ankle infection. The overall risk of any foot and ankle infection in diabetic patients is eight times higher than that of the general population and postoperative infection rates double that of healthy cohorts [14]. Additionally, diabetics have a blunted immune response to infection leading to lower cure rates and as a result a significantly higher risk of amputation after infection [15]. One report found a postoperative infection rate up to 60% and amputation rates up to 42% in diabetic open ankle fractures [16]. There is a clear association between glucose control and postoperative surgical site infections, with Jupiter et al. demonstrating a significant risk of infection development with hemoglobin A1c greater than 7.0% [17]. Hyperglycemia, even without a diagnosis of diabetes, has been identified as an independent risk factor for infection in orthopaedic trauma patients. Blood glucose levels $\geq$200 mg/dL on presentation is a significant risk factor in the development of both 30 and 90 day deep surgical site infection [18, 19]. In situations where surgical delay for improved diabetic management is not feasible, tight perioperative glucose control is a requirement and close follow up with a multidisciplinary team post-op can improve the chances of a good outcome. Finally, special attention must be paid to diabetic patients with ulcers not only for local reasons but also due to the risk of seeding infection at an ankle surgical site. All factors must be addressed when treating diabetic ulcers, including nutritional status and shoe wear modifications.

Age over 65 has been associated with higher infection rates and can be attributed to their higher risk of associated medical comorbidities, such as declining nutritional state, declining mental capabilities, and decreased mobility [13]. One study found that age was an independent risk factor for infection that linearly increased up to age 65, but thereafter paradoxically decreased. The authors proposed the "hardy survivor" effect, as a possible explanation [20]. While many of the factors associated with age are nonmodifiable, these serve to guide index of suspicion as well as prognostication.

2.1 Surgeon and Surgery-Related Risk Factors

Many risk factors for infection are directly under the surgeon's control. These factors include issues such as surgical time, soft tissue handling, antibiotic usage, and post-operative protocols. The Surgical Care Improvement Project (SCIP) guidelines lay out several controlled variables [21]. (1) Prophylactic antibiotics should be received within 1 h prior to incision [21]. Infection rates are significantly higher in cases that are not given preoperative antibiotics compared to those that are [22]. Additionally, for longer procedures, the antibiotics should be redosed after two half-lives (about every 4 h for cefazolin) [23]. (2) Prophylactic antibiotics should be selected for activity against the most probable microbe, in this case *Staphylococcus aureus*. (3) Euglycemia should be maintained, with well-controlled morning blood glucose concentrations on the first two postoperative days. (4) Hair at surgical site should be removed with clippers, not with a blade. (5) Urinary catheters should be discontinued within 2 postoperative days. (6) Normothermia should be maintained perioperatively [21]. Appropriate surgical site preparation can improve infection risks and postoperative outcomes. The foot may contain up to three million microorganisms/cm^2 [13]. Using an alcohol-based skin prep prior to surgical incision is a mandatory step. Studies have shown that chlorohexidine is superior in decreasing bacterial load [24].

Regarding operative time, any increase in time between surgical incision and finished closure allows for more contamination of the surgical wound, increasing the risk for surgical infection [13]. While we are not aware of any set surgical time limit above which infection rates dramatically increase, cases in excess of 90 min of open wound time have a higher odds ratio of infection [5]. The surgeon should aim to be both expedient and thorough. Careful preoperative planning with contingencies will minimize tinkering time in the OR, and a surgical plan will avoid against missed steps keeping the case moving.

The most directly controllable factor is surgical technique and soft tissue handling. Overly aggressive stripping and retraction causes disruption of the microvasculature, leading to ongoing ischemia and impeded local host infection defense. Open fractures and fracture related infections (FRIs) require careful debridement of all necrotic tissue including skin, muscle, fascia, and bone when needed. Focusing on a small exposure may lead to incomplete debridement and persistent nonviable and infected tissue. Additionally, good hemostatic technique should be observed to avoid postoperative hematoma and dead space for bacteria to thrive.

3 Diagnosis

Evaluation of a patient with suspected ankle infection begins with a detailed history and physical examination. Special attention should be given to patient comorbidities and risk factors for infection [25]. History should include any prior injury or surgery, evaluation of onset and duration of symptoms, fever and chills (not always present), malaise, pain, weightbearing tolerance, history of prior infections anywhere, and general medical health [1]. Often patients with ankle infections will exhibit no systemic signs of infection such as fever (only seen in 30–40% cases) [25, 26].

Physical exam should pay attention to the cardinal signs of infection (swelling, redness, tenderness, and warmth), surgical scars, draining sinus, lymphedema, skin health including induration and assessment of vascular status (shiny skin, alopecia, venous insufficiency). Attention should be given to localization of the infection, the most important aspect being the depth of infection. While cellulitis will be tender to touch, marked tenderness along the joint line and extreme pain with minimal joint motion of the ankle may be indicative of a septic arthritis [25].

Necrotizing fasciitis is beyond the scope of this chapter but deserves a brief note. It represents a rare but very aggressive deep necrosing infection, occurring usually in immunosuppressed patients, spreading rapidly along the myofascial planes. The hallmark clinical history and exam are extreme pain out of proportion to exam, often appearing early like a cellulitis with erythema, warmth, tenderness, and tachycardia. Delay in diagnosis contributes to the high reported mortality rate of 50–70% from septic shock [1, 3, 27, 28]. Blisters and bullae can develop but these are usually intermediate to late findings. One of the most consistent findings is progression of erythema and symptoms despite an adequate intrave-

nous antibiotic regimen, highlighting the importance of serial exams, and a high index of suspicion for diagnosis. Classically these patients can deteriorate rapidly with hallmark depletion of their serum sodium and declining renal function. The Laboratory Risk Indicator for Necrotizing Fasciitis (LRINEC) score can aid in diagnosis but should not replace clinical judgement. The treatment for necrotizing fasciitis involves an emergent widely based debridement of all necrotic skin, subcutaneous tissue and fascia, and broad spectrum IV antibiotics [1, 3, 27, 28].

3.1 Labs

Peripheral blood tests in the workup of a suspected ankle infection of any kind include peripheral blood cultures (typically two sets), complete blood count (CBC), erythrocyte sedimentation rate (ESR), and C-reactive protein (CRP) levels. However, these markers only represent inflammation in the body and thus have a poor specificity [25]. In a review of 30 patients with native septic ankles, Holtom et al. reported elevated ESR and CRP in all patients, but only 47% had elevated peripheral WBC [29]. We find it useful to also check a HgA1c in patients, as uncontrolled diabetes is a strong risk factor for infection, but also, we have not infrequently uncovered a new diagnosis of prediabetes or diabetes in a patient. If the suspected infection is postoperative and there are wound healing issues, we recommend also checking metabolic and nutrition labs such as basic metabolic panel (chem-7), thyroid panel, prealbumin, and albumin levels [10]. Total lymphocyte count of <1500 cells/mm^3 and albumin <3.5 mg/dL, and serum transferrin <200 mg/dL are indicative of malnutrition and reduced ability to heal a wound [30]. It is useful to consult a nutrition expert in the case of these patients.

3.2 Aspiration and Tissue Culture

If infection involving the joint is suspected then the gold standard in diagnosis is an aspiration of synovial fluid [25]. This is typically done with an

18G hypodermic needle attempting to avoid apparent cellulitic skin. This may be done either anteromedial, just medial to the palpable tibialis anterior tendon at the level of the joint line aiming into the superomedial joint gutter, or alternatively through an anterolateral approach midway between the anterior border of the fibula and the peroneus tertius at the level of the joint [25]. Traditionally a synovial WBC count >50,000 cells/mm^3 has been used for a diagnostic threshold of septic native arthritis around the body [25, 31]. Data should be interpreted with caution and respect to the pretest clinical suspicion as a cutoff of 50,000 has been shown to have sensitivity of only 64% [31]. Fluid should be sent for culture, gram stain, and crystal analysis. Culture remains the gold standard for diagnosing a septic joint, however up to 20% of patients with septic ankles have been reported to be culture negative [29].

Regarding draining wounds, cultures should be obtained from deep tissue in the operating room (discussed in section below). We do not recommend superficial tissue or fluid samples nor routine culture swabs as these have a low diagnostic yield [32–35].

3.3 Imaging

Imaging can be a substantial aid to appropriate diagnosis and treatment plans. Plain radiographs should routinely be obtained in evaluation. In postoperative settings, radiographs should be scrutinized for maintenance of reduction and alignment, change in implant position or any lucent halo which may indicate loosening. Early in an infection, radiographs may only show soft tissue swelling, but with delayed presentations of septic arthritis there may be evidence of joint destruction. Late changes in bony structure can also be evaluated on plain radiographs, including cortical erosion and periosteal reactions. It is mandatory to examine radiographs for the presence of subcutaneous gas, which in the absence of an open wound, raises concern for an aggressive necrotizing infection [25].

Computed tomography (CT) is more sensitive to bony and joint destructive changes, and if renal function allows, the addition of contrast is very useful in looking for deep soft tissue abscess in postoperative infections [25]. This is instrumental in debridement planning as when extensile measures are needed for identifying skip abscesses. In fracture cases, CT is useful in assessing union. This is important if a question exists about the necessity for hardware retention.

In subacute postop infections, we have found MRI to be useful in looking for bony edema tracking up the marrow space away from the local hardware which might be indicative of intramedullary osteomyelitis which may necessitate reaming of the marrow space. The addition of contrast to MRI enhances evaluation for soft tissue abscess [25, 36]. For native septic arthritis, we do not recommend routine CT or MRI scanning unless something atypical in the history or physical leads to suspicion of soft tissue abscess or bony extension. Tagged WBC bone marrow scintigraphy with technetium-99 m sulfur colloid has been reported with 86–98% accuracy in prosthetic joint infections [25], however we have not found this to be particularly useful in the non-arthroplasty setting.

Vascular studies, such as palpation or doppler of the distal pulses, can provide valuable information about the potential to heal any wounds or infections. Knowledge of any insufficiency is critical in surgical planning of a debridement in assessing whether primary or secondary healing is viable or whether flap coverage will be required. Ankle-Brachial Index (ABI) >0.9 is considered normal, with a value <0.45 concerning for a poor healing response. A toe wave pressure of 0.45 is predictive of good healing while a pressure of 0.2 is indicative of poor healing. Duplex ultrasonography can assess for arterial stenosis and occlusive venous insufficiency, which may warrant referral to vascular surgery for consideration of intervention angiography [1].

4 Treatment

Once a diagnosis of infection has been established the management depends upon the presence or absence of joint involvement, amount of joint degeneration, presence or absence of fracture, instability, presence of hardware, and extent of bony involvement.

Treatment requires an aggressive surgical debridement of all infected and all nonviable tissues. Compromised tissue left in place provides a nidus for persistent infection and bacterial adherence with biofilm formation [33]. Several biopsies of both soft tissue and bone should be taken at the time of the initial debridement as routine swab cultures and aspiration have been shown to not be representative of the chronic infection and adherent bacteria [33].

A brief word about urgency and antibiotics. Lee et al. reported that patients who were treated with antibiotics with or without debridement or aspiration within 5 days of symptom onset had a greater chance to regain ankle function, although most ankles still had residual mild or severe pain at the time of the latest follow-up [37]. Treatment of infections is urgent but should be stepwise with a prioritized goal of a targeted diagnosis. We do not recommend an initial treatment course of antibiotics be started until a deep culture can be obtained, unless based on clinical evaluation you have determined the infection to be superficial cellulitis only. The only other exception to this rule is in the physiologically septic patient, who should be promptly started on empiric broad spectrum antibiotics immediately after obtaining blood cultures [25].

4.1 Native Septic Joint Arthroscopic or Aspiration

The mainstay of management of ankle joint infections is an operative debridement. Serial aspirations have been reported with success in the treatment of native septic ankles [25]. However, this excludes cases with hardware or extra-articular involvement, and it is the author's opinion that aspiration should be reserved for the medically infirm and end-stage arthritic joints.

Arthroscopic debridement has been used in ankle infections and reported favorable outcomes with smaller incisions, shorter hospitalization, and more rapid rehab compared with open arthrotomy [25, 38]. Typical portals are anteromedial and anterolateral (similar to aspiration sites) with one for an inflow with a 4 mm 30° scope and the other as an outflow or working portal for an arthroscopic shaver [25]. An arthroscopic debridement does not allow for addressing extra-articular extension or hardware in FRIs and should be relegated to native septic arthritis.

4.2 Fracture Related/Hardware

Fracture related infections are distinct from native septic arthritis or osteomyelitis as well as from infected periprosthetic joints in the matter of instability. Stability of the tissue not only lessens ongoing damage to surrounding tissue, but also creates an environment favorable to infection resistance [39–41]. However it is well known that metal implants involved in an infection allow for bacteria to form a biofilm, consisting of a glycocalyx which confers significant resistance to both the body's immune response as well as to antibiotics [33, 39, 42].

Thus, in the care of fracture related infections there are two objectives which somewhat oppose one another which are the eradication of infection, impeded by the presence of a foreign body, and the need for stability both for fracture union and a favorable environment for infection clearance.

More specifically, the primary aims of treatment of fracture related infections can be stated as:

1. Fracture consolidation.
2. Eradication of infection at final treatment.
3. Healed soft tissue envelope.
4. Restoration of function.
5. Prevention of chronic osteomyelitis [43].

Rittman and Perren stated that the stabilizing effect of implants outweighed the disadvantage of the foreign body effect [41]. It has thus been recommended that hardware should be retained in the face of infection until fracture healing so long as the hardware is stable and functioning [44]. Therefore, two concepts have been laid out in consideration. Firstly, debridement, antimicrobial therapy, and implant retention, so called "DAIR" protocol. Secondly, debridement, antimicrobial therapy, and implant removal or exchange. The determination of what to do with the hardware is influenced by the time from injury, extent of bony healing and stability, amount of necrotic tissue and dead space, maintenance of acceptable fracture alignment, and implant fixation and contribution to stability [43, 45].

One proposed treatment algorithm is to attempt to maintain hardware in a patient presenting up to 10 weeks out from the time of surgical fixation. Although 10 weeks is a rather arbitrary number, it should serve as a treatment guide depending upon the abovementioned factors. These patients should undergo a debridement and retention of hardware, if stable and still functional, or removal of hardware if it is loose. This is not intended as a definitive treatment, but rather as a temporizing measure to suppress the infection long enough to allow for fracture healing and stability so that the hardware could be removed later. In patients presenting greater than 10 weeks from ORIF, the fracture is presumed to have enough stability and they undergo a debridement and removal of hardware [16].

The final consideration in what to do with hardware regards the alignment of the fracture. In those patients who have lost acceptable alignment and the fracture is not united, we will either remove the hardware, perform a debridement and then revision reduction, and internal fixation. Or if there is purulence at the time of debridement we will remove the implants, perform a debridement, use local antibiotics (described later), and plan for revision fixation later after wound sterilization. In such cases a spanning external fixator is applied to provide bony and soft tissue stability, as an antibiotic intramedullary rod will not function well so distally; rarely a splint may suffice.

When hardware must be retained for the stability of the fracture and to aid in initial treatment of infection, the decision must be made as to whether those implants should be taken out later. In a review of 69 infected fractures managed with hardware in place, Rightmire et al. reported a disappointing 68% union rate, with the remaining requiring hardware removal or exchange ultimately. Furthermore, they reported in those with successful union, the rate of infection recurrence in those with hardware left in place was 32% compared to 16% in those who had hardware removed after union. They recommend strong consideration of hardware removal and debridement after obtaining fracture union [11].

In the case of chronic osteomyelitis, treatment is determined by four factors; the condition of the host, the functional impairment caused by infection, the site of involvement, and the extent of bony necrosis [9]. Concomitant adjacent osteomyelitis has been reported in 30% of patients with septic arthritis, and is most commonly found in compromized hosts with one or more risk factors. In such patients, the clinician should have an elevated index of suspicion, and it may be useful to obtain an MRI of the foot and ankle to evaluate for adjacent osteomyelitis [29].

4.3 Tissue Sampling

Deep tissue samples are recommended to be sent for both microbiological as well as histopathological examination. Multiple samples should be taken, each with a new clean surgical instrument and each in a separate tissue culture bottle for aerobic and anaerobic growth [32, 43, 46]. These should preferentially be taken from suspected areas of fracture related infection, such as periosteum and membrane at implant bone interface and care to avoid the skin and any superficially draining areas. We recommend multiple, at least three to five, deep samples be taken from distinct areas of the wound. Multiple samples growing the same organism avoid confusion over a single sample possibly growing a known skin contaminant. Regardless of number of samples, it is important to be systematic and even develop a protocol in the approach to biopsies as this has been found to have a higher diagnostic yield than random sampling and no protocol for antibiotic management [32]. We do not recommend superficial tissue or fluid samples nor routine culture swabs as these have a low diagnostic yield [32–35]. We do not recommend any additional biopsies or cultures be taken at final debridement as we have not found this to be helpful in changing management. The most accurate biological diagnosis would be the one from the initial biopsy and cultures, and treatment should be based on those.

Novel techniques for diagnostics include genomic sequence identification such as Next-generation sequencing through 16s rRNA gene profiling have been reported to identify organisms in 77% more cases than traditional microbiological identification techniques in fracture nonunion biopsies. These genetic material profiling techniques may provide a way to identify further infections in cases which otherwise would be classified as "culture negative" infections. We have not yet instituted this in our practice, but promising results are coming out of the arthroplasty literature [47].

4.4   Debridement

Irrigation and debridement remain the keystone in the treatment of fracture related infections. Surgical approach will typically proceed through prior surgical incisions, and strict careful soft tissue handling techniques are critical to maintain a viable soft tissue envelope [48]. The purpose of irrigation is reduction of bacterial load and the removal of loose debris. The optimum volume of fluid is unknown but should be sufficient to macroscopically clean the entire wound bed [49].

Debridement should be systematic and thorough with the goal of removing all necrotic bone, necrotic and ischemic soft tissue, and any nonessential or nonfunctioning foreign bodies (e.g., braided suture and loose hardware). When using prior incisions, any local sinus tracts should be excised. It may be beneficial to excise a few millimeters of dense adherent scar tissue not contributing to healing on either side of the incision. Preoperative planning should include a strategy for management of any soft tissue defects if primary closure will be complicated by an adequate debridement. Often inflamed tissue will retract

significantly after debridement, amplifying the apparent tissue loss in the limited realestate about the ankle (Fig. 2). Accessory sinus tracts remote from intended debridement approach may be left as these will typically close secondarily after the infection is treated [48].

If it is determined that further bone exposure beyond the initial surgical bed is needed, this should proceed in an extraperiosteal plane to preserve vascularity to the bone [48]. The extent of debridement of bone requires careful inspection and clinical judgement and will be affected by duration of infection. In general, all bone left behind should have bleeding surfaces, following the theory that bleeding infected bone may heal with systemic antibiotic therapy [43]. Bilgili et al. showed that in the face of infection with hardware, fracture healing proceeds in a histopathologically similar albeit slower manner to uninfected tissue. In a rat model fracture callus was shown to have lower stiffness and torque to failure at 6 weeks compared with uninfected tis-

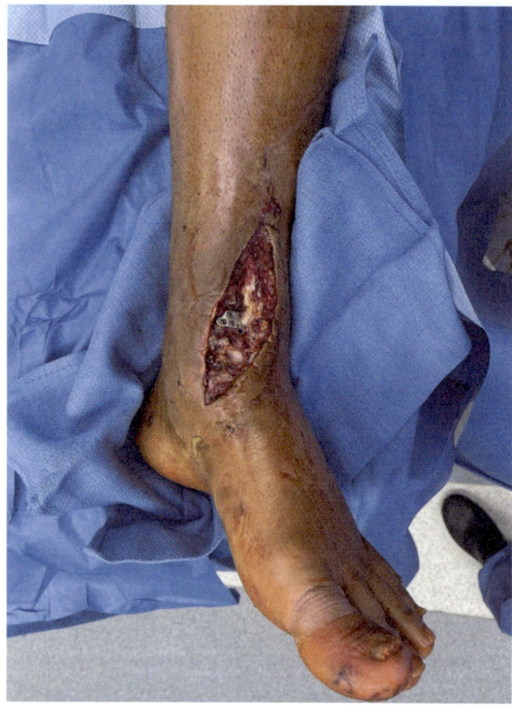

Fig. 2 Shows significant retraction of tissue exacerbating the apparent tissue loss after a debridement of an infected pilon fracture

sue [50]. In chronic infections (>6 to 10 weeks duration), bony debridement should proceed until uniform petechial bleeding bone surfaces are encountered (the so called "paprika sign") [9, 48].

The number of debridements required in fracture related infections has been reported from 1 to 11 with an average number of 3 debridements [11]. In chronic osteomyelitis cases, the average number of debridements has been reported as 3.8 [9]. In FRI requiring hardware retention, if purulence is found on initial debridement, we recommend serial irrigation and debridement until no further purulence is encountered before definitive closure or coverage.

In native septic ankles or in FRI diagnosed early and with no obvious purulence and having viable soft tissue envelope amenable to primary closure, a single irrigation and debridement may be sufficient. In these, careful serial exams and laboratory trend may show improvement on systemic antibiotics. In these we have followed a protocol developed by the senior author for incision management and monitoring. Wounds which are closed have a closed incisional vacuum (ciVAC) dressing applied for 72 h and are then changed to a dry gauze dressing for 12 h to evaluate for persistent drainage. Wounds with drainage, other than wound edge oozing, should have a new ciVAC dressing applied for another 72 h and the protocol is repeated. This is followed for three sequential ciVACs cycles, or about 9–10 days after which if the wound drainage has not noticeably decreased a repeat irrigation and debridement is performed and the protocol is restarted.

We apply these ciVACs with an open cell polyurethane ether sterile foam dressing applied to a broad surface area encompassing the incision and surrounding inflamed skin. We use a layer of nonadherent emollient gauze under the foam sponge to prevent skin irritation. This not only aids in drainage management and monitoring, but also provides a durable sterile dressing for the wound, promotes blood flow to the local area, and reduces edema through the incision. The rationale behind a broad surface is to apply even pressure to decrease shear forces in the wound

bed. However, others have advocated for a strip of polyurethane ether sponge applied directly to the skin in a narrow strip encompassing just the incisional margins, while still others have advocated for use of a polyvinyl alcohol white sponge to decrease skin irritation [51, 52]. We prefer to use −125 mmHg pressure at a low continuous setting. Others have reported use on closed incisions ranging from −50 to −200 mmHg [52, 53].

4.5 Local Antimicrobial Therapy

Local administration of antimicrobials is an effective means of managing 'dead space' and allows for administration of a supra-therapeutic dose of antibiotics not tolerated systemically [43, 49]. This is usually not required in the treatment of native septic ankles. However, in FRIs requiring extensive debridement, the resultant 'dead space' lacks perfusion resulting in a low pH low oxygen tension environment ideal for bacterial proliferation despite systemic antibiotics. Additionally, in chronic infections (>4 to 6 weeks) and those requiring hardware retention with presumed antibiotic resistant biofilms, local supra-therapeutic doses of antibiotics up to 1000 times the minimum inhibitory concentration (MIC) improve sterilization of the wound [49].

We recommend use of high concentration antibiotic loaded PMMA beads or spacer depending on the size and shape of any bone defect. We prefer to make our own beads with high viscosity bone cement. At the first debridement, without organism identification, we will typically add 2 g of vancomycin and 2.4 g tobramycin powder. The powder is homogenously crushed with a blunt instrument such as the butt end of a Cobb elevator and mixed with the cement powder. The monomer is then added and mixed until a medium doughy texture is reached which may be workable into 5–7 mm beads. These are placed on a #1 polypropylene suture. The neutrophilic infiltration and the adhesive inflammatory exudate at the site of an infected wound can be significant complicating bead identification and retrieval. We find use of dyed bone cement or addition of a few drops of methylene blue dye aids in bead identification. Additionally, after cement hardening and determining the number of beads that will fit in the wound, the suture is tied in a knot around the terminal beads to facilitate removal at the next washout (Fig. 3). With local antimicrobial use, consideration must be given to cytotoxic effects of different agents to osteoblasts, fibroblasts, and chondroblasts. Additionally, when used with polymethylmethacrylate (PMMA), the antimicrobial must be heat stable to up to 100 °C. A literature review and consensus paper from the Fracture Related Infections group found aminoglycosides and glycopeptides to both be heat stable with vancomycin, and tobramycin being least cytotoxic [49, 54]. Rifampin, doxycycline, penicillin, ciprofloxacin, and gentamicin produced significantly greater reduction in osteocyte activity, however in later rat in vivo models, gentamicin has not been found to impede fracture healing in infection treatment [54, 55].

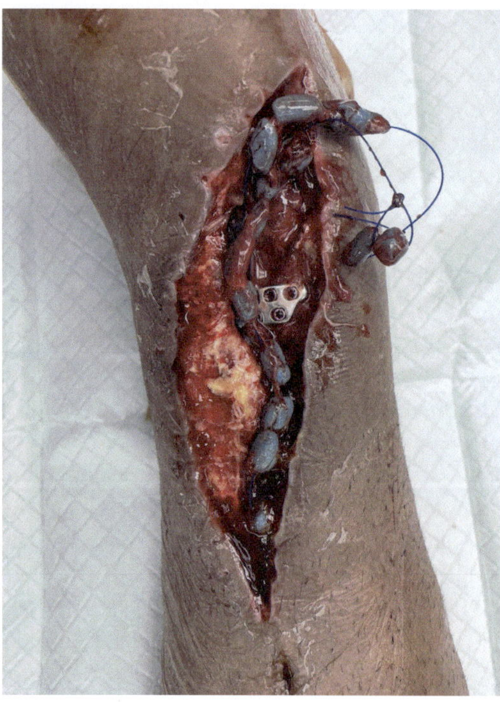

Fig. 3 Antibiotic polymethylmethacrylate beads on a prolene suture. Note the knot tied around the terminal bead, as well as methylene blue dye in the PMMA ensures retrieval of all beads after they have been in an inflamed wound

4.6 Soft Tissue

Preoperative planning should account for soft tissue coverage. Whenever possible, primary closure is preferable, but it must be tension free with the ability to evert skin edges as the inflamed skin will tend to invert. Suprafascial elevation and local flap advancement may be valuable techniques if the skin is healthy enough to tolerate. Avoid braided sutures as these may harbor microorganisms contributing to recurrent infection. Superficially, absorbable sutures should be avoided as they will instigate local inflammation in already compromised skin. Nylon suture is least reactive, and most tension free wounds can be closed with 3–0 vertical mattress sutures [48].

When adequate debridement will result in a soft tissue coverage defect, usually the distal third of the tibia and ankle area there may ultimately a need for a free tissue transfer for coverage [43]. There is limited data on the optimal timing of coverage. Single stage debridement and coverage of chronic osteomyelitis has been described, however this requires advanced coordination with plastic reconstructive surgeons or personal expertise in soft tissue transfers [56]. We typically perform serial debridements every 2–4 days until no further frank purulence is encountered. This is done in coordination with plastic reconstructive surgeons with the aim of definitively covering the wound either at the time of or within 3 days of the last "clean" debridement (Fig. 4). If the wound is going to require tissue transfer for coverage and requires multiple washouts, the wound should be managed with an antibiotic bead pouch. We fashion ours by making and inserting antibiotic cement beads as described above. The surrounding skin is cleaned of any residue with alcohol and then tincture of benzoin is applied to the skin. An occlusive adhesive such as Ioban™ 3M™ is then used to create an airtight seal. Finally, an 18G spinal needle and syringe is inserted from a remote location through the subcutaneous tissue into the wound, and the remaining air is aspirated from the bead pouch.

Some have described using negative pressure wound therapy (NPWT) dressings on wounds

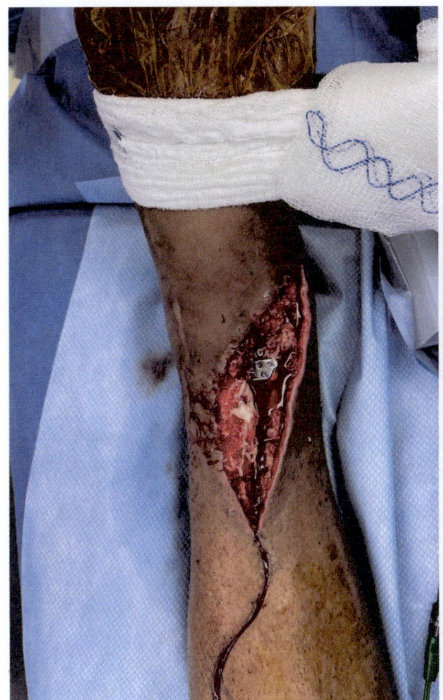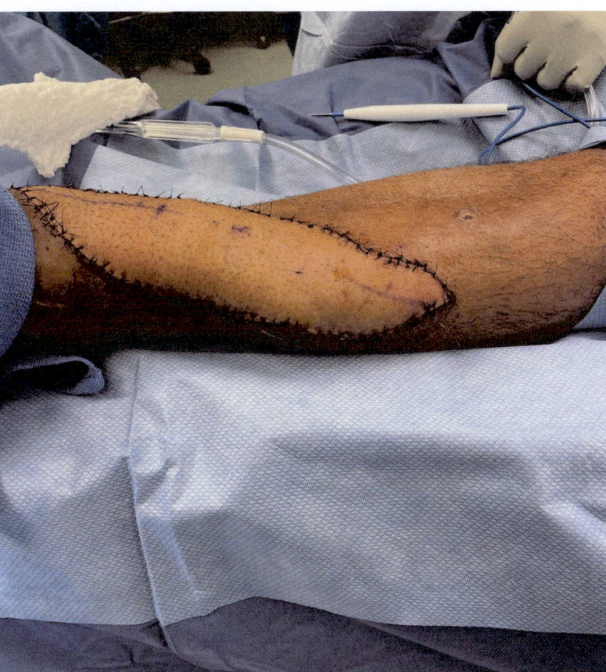

Fig. 4 Note healthy bleeding at all surfaces after two debridements with no further necrosis or purulence noted, at this time, due to the distal third of the tibia location of this soft tissue defect this patient underwent a free tissue transfer with an anterolateral thigh fasciocutaneous flap anastomosed to the anterior tibial artery

pending coverage. These have been shown to stabilize the wound environment, reduce edema, improve tissue perfusion, and stimulate beneficial cells at the wound surface [52]. This is an effective short-term tactic pending definitive coverage. However, in a frankly infected wound bed we prefer a bead pouch as NPWT sponges may lead to colonization with resistant organisms and possibly persistent infections [43, 57]. Some have proposed the use of surgical drains when dead space is present, however we are not aware of any studies evaluating the outcome of debridement with or without a surgical drain [3, 25, 48].

5 Overall Management/ Medical/Antibiotics

Management of antibiotics requires knowledge of the local antibiogram, resistance, patterns, as well as the common infecting organisms. Infecting organisms have been reported as *Staphylococcus aureus* in 54–65% of patients and oxacillin-resistant in 13–23% [16, 29]. Other organisms include staphylococcus epidermidis 23%, and the remainder were *Enterobacter cloacae*, *Propionibacterium acnes*, Acinetobacter, Serratia, *Pseudomonas aeruginosa*, and Vancomycin-resistant Enterococcus [16]. Ultimately, antibiotics should be tissue culture specific. Organism identification should not be based on any superficial or draining sinus tract swabs as these are often colonized and not representative of the underlying infection which may be sessile [42].

For native septic joints, antibiotics should be initially held until a sample is obtained such as through aspiration, but then empiric broad spectrum antibiotics covering both gram-positive and gram-negative organisms should be started expediently to reduce the ongoing damage of the infection in the joint. In postoperative infections, we recommend antibiotics be held prior to obtaining cultures unless the patient is exhibiting systemic signs of sepsis. After organism identification, therapy may be narrowed to lessen side effects and reduce production of resistant organisms. Antibiotics typically are given for at least 6 weeks postoperatively for deep soft tissue and joint infections [25]. If hardware is being maintained for fracture healing, then antibiotics are continued until healing, debridement, and removal of hardware, and then generally continued for 6 weeks post hardware removal.

There is evidence that rifampin can have better penetration of sessile forms of staphylococcus than other antibiotics. In a randomized controlled trial of patients presenting with acute or subacute infections (less than 2 months of symptoms), involving Staphylococcus epidermidis or Staph aureus organisms, had stable implants at debridement, and able to tolerate long-term treatment (3–6 months) with a rifampin-ciprofloxacin protocol experienced a 2-year follow-up cure rate of 100% [58].

Ultimately the duration of antibiotic treatment should be individualized for each patient guided by clinical and laboratory evaluation. We recommend this be determined in conjunction with infectious disease consultants as they can weigh in on local microbial resistance patterns, cost considerations, adverse drug reactions, and interactions [3, 16]. The Fracture Related Infections (FRI) group has recommended patients with FRIs to be managed by a multidisciplinary group. Antibiotic stewardship programs with design for improving appropriate use of medications through the selection of antibiotic regimen, dosing, duration of therapy, and route of administration are recommended. Treatment of FRIs requires expertise in bone and soft tissue reconstruction, microbiology and local antibiograms, antibiotics effects and side effects, as well as advanced diagnostic imaging. Proposed members of such teams include infectious disease physicians, clinical pharmacists, local hospital infection control department, nurses, musculoskeletal radiologists, nuclear medicine specialists, and orthopaedic and plastic reconstructive surgeons [43]. Involvement of each of these may be guided on a case-by-case need. When such multidisciplinary approach is not feasible, consideration should be given to referring the patient to a center with more specialization and multidisciplinary capability for complex cases [43, 46].

6　Outcome

Following their protocol for hardware retention less than 10 weeks or removal after 10 weeks, Zalavras et al. reported complete infection clearance in 13/18 (72%) of patients with the remaining 5 experiencing recurrence. Four of these were in compromised hosts as described by Cierny-Mader [9, 16]. Three were in patients with hardware retention, and two of these were cleared of infection after repeat washout and hardware removal after fracture consolidation. An additional two patients had recurrence with instability due to hardware loosening and malreduction. These patients were in compromised hosts and ultimately underwent amputation to ultimately yield an amputation rate of 3/18 (17%). Two of these were in diabetic patients, however patients should be counselled that peri-implant infections about the ankle are serious infections and failed salvage may result amputation [16]. Additionally, smoking has been found to be an independent predictor of failure of treatment of fracture related infections, with an estimated risk of failure 3.7 times higher than nonsmokers [11].

In late presentations of FRI where bony union has occurred and debridement with hardware removal can be performed, there is a high rate of successful infection clearance. One study reported no recurrences in 14 patients for whom hardware could be removed at the time of debridement [16].

If infection has been going on for a prolonged time and involves the joint, it is unlikely the patient will have a good outcome maintaining the joint as there may be significant breakdown of the articular cartilage. However, reasonable results can be expected with a structured protocol for managing the infection followed by a talocrural fusion. Thordarson et al. reviewed 5 patients with septic arthritis presenting with average 8 months of infection and radiographic evidence of joint destruction and osteomyelitis. They were all treated with aggressive debridement, deep biopsy, and targeted antibiotics, followed by a second debridement 3–5 days later and free flap coverage. After infection clearance and flap maturation, the patients underwent an ankle fusion at average 3.7 months after debridement and all went on to union at average 3.5 months. All patients were ambulatory without aid and satisfied with their outcome [59]. Another series reported 19 patients with chronic infections treated with aggressive I&D, hardware removal, antibiotic bead placement with gentamycin. On average, they underwent 2 washouts before free flap coverage (in 7/19 patients) and external fixator placement. After average 6 months, patients underwent arthrodesis at average 6 months with about a 50% union rate, in those who did not unite on initial treatment, they were repeat debrided and additional stability and bone graft added. Eighteen of 19 patients went on to stable union. The one patient with pseudarthrosis was a heavy smoker [60].

Given the recurrence risk after treatment of any infection, patients should be followed for a minimum 12 months after final therapy conclusion [43].

7   Conclusion

The treatment of infections about the ankle, especially postoperative fracture related infections is complex and requires a thorough and systematic approach for a successful outcome. The key recommendations in evaluation and treatment can be summarized as:

- Establish a diagnosis, with suggestive signs of infection mandating further investigation and prompt treatment. Diagnosis requires deep tissue sampling, not superficial swabs.
- Empiric broad-spectrum antibiotics should be started after obtaining culture samples and should be tailored to culture with a multidisciplinary approach.
- Stability is required in treatment of fracture related infections.
- Careful and thorough debridement is the mainstay of treatment and should not be compromised. When appropriate debridement results in defects, strategies should be employed for dead space management and vascularized soft tissue coverage.

- Low pressure irrigation should be used with enough volume to clean the surgical field and flow clear.
- Local high concentration of antibiotics should strongly be considered.
- Optimize the patients' health status through a multidisciplinary approach. Smoking cessation should be sought, metabolic factors corrected, nutritional deficiencies screened and improved, and weight reduction strategies.
- Multidisciplinary approach is beneficial and should be implemented in complex FRI cases. Consider transfer to a specialized center when a team approach or experience is lacking.
- Patients should be followed for a minimum of 1 year following definitive treatment of these infections.

References

1. Anakwenze OA, Milby AH, Gans I, Stern JJ, Levin LS, Wapner KL. Foot and ankle infections: diagnosis and management. J Am Acad Orthop Surg. 2012;20:684–93. https://doi.org/10.5435/JAAOS-20-11-684.
2. McNamara DR, Tleyjeh IM, Berbari EF, Lahr BD, Martinez JW, Mirzoyev SA, et al. Incidence of lower-extremity cellulitis: a population-based study in Olmsted county, Minnesota. Mayo Clin Proc. 2007;82:817–21. https://doi.org/10.4065/82.7.817.
3. Donley BG, Philbin T, Tomford JW, Sferra JJ. Foot and ankle infections after surgery. Clin Orthop Relat Res. 2001;391:162–70. https://doi.org/10.1097/00003086-200110000-00017.
4. Kaandorp CJE, Van Schaardenburg D, Krijnen P, Habbema JDF, Van De Laar MAFJ. Risk factors for septic arthritis in patients with joint disease. A prospective study. Arthritis Rheum. 1995;38:1819–25. https://doi.org/10.1002/ART.1780381215.
5. Shao J, Zhang H, Yin B, Li J, Zhu Y, Zhang Y. Risk factors for surgical site infection following operative treatment of ankle fractures: a systematic review and meta-analysis. Int J Surg. 2018;56:124–32. https://doi.org/10.1016/J.IJSU.2018.06.018.
6. Sirkin M, Sanders R, DiPasquale T, Herscovici D. A staged protocol for soft tissue management in the treatment of complex pilon fractures. J Orthop Trauma. 2004;18:78–84.

7. Bourne RB, Rorabeck CH, Macnab J. Intra-articular fractures of the distal tibia: the pilon fracture. J Trauma. 1983;23:591–6. https://doi.org/10.1097/00005373-198307000-00008.

8. Kellam JF, Waddell JP. Fractures of the distal tibial metaphysis with intra-articular extension--the distal tibial explosion fracture. J Trauma. 1979;19:593–601. https://doi.org/10.1097/00005373-197908000-00007.

9. Cierny G, Mader JT, Penninck JJ. A clinical staging system for adult osteomyelitis. Clin Orthop Relat Res. 2003;414:7–24. https://doi.org/10.1097/01.blo.0000088564.81746.62.

10. Lee MS, Grossman JP. Complications in foot and ankle surgery: management strategies. Berlin: Springer; 2017. https://doi.org/10.1007/978-3-319-53686-6.

11. Rightmire E, Zurakowski D, Vrahas M. Acute infections after fracture repair: management with hardware in place. Clin Orthop Relat Res. 2008;466:466–72. https://doi.org/10.1007/s11999-007-0053-y.

12. Bamgbade OA, Rutter TW, Nafiu OO, Dorje P. Postoperative complications in obese and nonobese patients. World J Surg. 2007;31:556–60. https://doi.org/10.1007/S00268-006-0305-0.

13. Boyd J, Chmielewski R. Prevention of infection in foot and ankle surgery. Clin Podiatr Med Surg. 2019;36:37–58. https://doi.org/10.1016/J.CPM.2018.08.007.

14. Flynn JM, Rodriguez-Del-Río F, Pizá PA. Closed ankle fractures in the diabetic patient. Foot Ankle Int. 2000;21:311–9. https://doi.org/10.1177/107110070002100407.

15. Game F. Management of osteomyelitis of the foot in diabetes mellitus. Nat Rev Endocrinol. 2010;6:43–7. https://doi.org/10.1038/NRENDO.2009.243.

16. Zalavras CG, Christensen T, Rigopoulos N, Holtom P, Patzakis MJ. Infection following operative treatment of ankle fractures. Clin Orthop Relat Res. 2009;467:1715–20. https://doi.org/10.1007/s11999-009-0743-8.

17. Jupiter DC, Humphers JM, Shibuya N. Trends in postoperative infection rates and their relationship to glycosylated hemoglobin levels in diabetic patients undergoing foot and ankle surgery. J Foot Ankle Surg. 2014;53:307–11. https://doi.org/10.1053/J.JFAS.2013.10.003.

18. Anderson BM, Wise BT, Joshi M, Castillo R, O'Toole RV, Richards JE. Admission hyperglycemia is a risk factor for deep surgical-site infection in orthopaedic trauma patients. J Orthop Trauma. 2021;35:E451–7. https://doi.org/10.1097/BOT.0000000000002101.

19. Richards JE, Kauffmann RM, Zuckerman SL, Obremskey WT, May AK. Relationship of hyperglycemia and surgical-site infection in orthopaedic surgery. J Bone Joint Surg Am. 2012;94:1181–6. https://doi.org/10.2106/JBJS.K.00193.

20. Kaye KS, Schmit K, Pieper C, Sloane R, Caughlan KF, Sexton DJ, et al. The effect of increasing age on the risk of surgical site infection. J Infect Dis. 2005;191:1056.

21. Rosenberger LH, Politano AD, Sawyer RG. The surgical care improvement project and prevention of postoperative infection, including surgical site infection. Surg Infect. 2011;12:163–8. https://doi.org/10.1089/SUR.2010.083.

22. Dayton P, DeVries JG, Landsman A, Meyr A, Schweinberger M. American college of foot and ankle surgeons' clinical consensus statement: perioperative prophylactic antibiotic use in clean elective foot surgery. J Foot Ankle Surg. 2015;54:273–9. https://doi.org/10.1053/J.JFAS.2015.01.004.

23. Modha MRK, Morriss-Roberts C, Smither M, Larholt J, Reilly I. Antibiotic prophylaxis in foot and ankle surgery: a systematic review of the literature. J Foot Ankle Res. 2018;11:61. https://doi.org/10.1186/s13047-018-0303-0.

24. Yammine K, Harvey A. Efficacy of preparation solutions and cleansing techniques on contamination of the skin in foot and ankle surgery: a systematic review and meta-analysis. Bone Joint J. 2013;95-B:498–503. https://doi.org/10.1302/0301-620X.95B4.30893.

25. Movassaghi K, Wakefield C, Bohl DD, Lee S, Lin J, Holmes GB, et al. Septic arthritis of the native ankle. JBJS Rev. 2019;7:1–9. https://doi.org/10.2106/JBJS.RVW.18.00080.

26. Gupta MN, Sturrock RD, Field M. A prospective 2-year study of 75 patients with adult-onset septic arthritis. Rheumatology (Oxford). 2001;40:24–30. https://doi.org/10.1093/RHEUMATOLOGY/40.1.24.

27. Wong CH, Khin LW, Heng KS, Tan KC, Low CO. The LRINEC (laboratory risk indicator for necrotizing fasciitis) score: a tool for distinguishing necrotizing fasciitis from other soft tissue infections. Crit Care Med. 2004;32:1535–41. https://doi.org/10.1097/01.CCM.0000129486.35458.7D.

28. Wong C-H, Chang H-C, Pasupathy S, Khin L-W, Tan J-L, Low C-O. Necrotizing fasciitis: clinical presentation, microbiology, and determinants of mortality. JBJS. 2003;85:1454–60.

29. Holtom PD, Borges L, Zalavras CG. Hematogenous septic ankle arthritis. Clin Orthop Relat Res. 2008;466:1388–91. https://doi.org/10.1007/s11999-008-0229-0.

30. Cross MB, Yi PH, Thomas CF, Garcia J, Della Valle CJ. Evaluation of malnutrition in orthopaedic surgery. J Am Acad Orthop Surg. 2014;22:193–9. https://doi.org/10.5435/JAAOS-22-03-193.

31. Li SF, Henderson J, Dickman E, Darzynkiewicz R. Laboratory tests in adults with monoarticular arthritis: can they rule out a septic joint? Acad Emerg Med. 2004;11:276–80. https://doi.org/10.1111/J.1553-2712.2004.TB02209.X.

32. Hellebrekers P, Rentenaar RJ, Mcnally MA, Hietbrink F, Houwert RM, Leenen LPH, et al. Getting it right first time: the importance of a structured tissue sampling protocol for diagnosing fracture-related infections. Injury. 2019;50:1649–55. https://doi.org/10.1016/j.injury.2019.05.014.

33. Gristina AG, Costerton JW. Bacterial adherence and the glycocalyx and their role in musculoskeletal infection. Orthop Clin North Am. 1984;15:517–35.

34. Aggarwal VK, Higuera C, Deirmengian G, Parvizi J, Austin MS. Swab cultures are not as effective as tissue cultures for diagnosis of periprosthetic joint infection. Clin Orthop Relat Res. 2013;471:3196–203. https://doi.org/10.1007/s11999-013-2974-y.

35. Mackowiak PA, Jones SR, Smith JW. Diagnostic value of sinus-tract cultures in chronic osteomyelitis. JAMA. 1978;239:2772–5. https://doi.org/10.1001/jama.1978.03280530036018.

36. Mathews CJ, Weston VC, Jones A, Field M, Coakley G. Bacterial septic arthritis in adults. Lancet (London, England). 2010;375:846–55. https://doi.org/10.1016/S0140-6736(09)61595-6.

37. Lee CH, Chen YJ, Ueng SW, Hsu RW. Septic arthritis of the ankle joint. Chang Gung Med J. 2000;23:420–6.

38. Mankovecky MR, Roukis TS. Arthroscopic synovectomy, irrigation, and debridement for treatment of septic ankle arthrosis: a systematic review and case series. J Foot Ankle Surg. 2014;53:615–9. https://doi.org/10.1053/j.jfas.2013.10.012.

39. Chang CC, Merritt K. Infection at the site of implanted materials with and without preadhered bacteria. J Orthop Res. 1994;12:526–31. https://doi.org/10.1002/jor.1100120409.

40. Merritt K, Dowd JD. Role of internal fixation in infection of open fractures: studies with Staphylococcus aureus and Proteus mirabilis. J Orthop Res. 1987;5:23–8. https://doi.org/10.1002/jor.1100050105.

41. Rittmann WW, Perren SM. 4. Discussion. In: Rittmann WW, Perren SM, editors. Cortical bone healing after internal fixation and infection: biomechanics and biology. Berlin: Springer; 1974. p. 63–9. https://doi.org/10.1007/978-3-642-65977-5_4.

42. Gristina AG, Costerton JW. Bacterial adherence to biomaterials and tissue. The significance of its role in clinical sepsis. J Bone Joint Surg Am. 1985;67:264–73.

43. Metsemakers W-J, Morgenstern M, Senneville E, Borens O, Govaert GAM, Onsea J, et al. General treatment principles for fracture-related infection: recommendations from an international expert group. Arch Orthop Trauma Surg. 2020;140:1013–27. https://doi.org/10.1007/s00402-019-03287-4.

44. Worlock P, Slack R, Harvey L, Mawhinney R. The prevention of infection in open fractures: an experimental study of the effect of fracture stability. Injury. 1994;25:31–8. https://doi.org/10.1016/0020-1383(94)90181-3.

45. Berkes M, Obremskey WT, Scannell B, Ellington JK, Hymes RA, Bosse M. Maintenance of hardware after early postoperative infection following fracture internal fixation. J Bone Joint Surg Am. 2010;92:823–8. https://doi.org/10.2106/JBJS.I.00470.

46. Govaert GAM, Kuehl R, Atkins BL, Trampuz A, Morgenstern M, Obremskey WT, et al. Diagnosing fracture-related infection: current concepts and recommendations. J Orthop Trauma. 2020;34:8.

47. Goswami K, Tipton C, Clarkson S, Chang G, Tan TL, Fram B, et al. Fracture-associated microbiome and persistent nonunion: next-generation sequencing reveals new findings. J Orthop Trauma. 2022;36:S40–6. https://doi.org/10.1097/BOT.0000000000002305.

48. Tetsworth K, Cierny GIII. Osteomyelitis debridement techniques. Clin Orthop Relat Res. 1999;360:87.

49. Metsemakers W-J, Fragomen AT, Moriarty TF, Morgenstern M, Egol KA, Zalavras C, et al. Evidence-based recommendations for local antimicrobial strategies and dead space management in fracture-related infection. J Orthop Trauma. 2020;34:18.

50. Bilgili F, Balci HI, Karaytug K, Sariyilmaz K, Atalar AC, Bozdag E, et al. Can normal fracture healing be achieved when the implant is retained on the basis of infection? An experimental animal model. Clin Orthop Relat Res. 2015;473:3190–6. https://doi.org/10.1007/s11999-015-4331-9.

51. Stannard JP, Volgas DA, McGwin GIII, Stewart RL, Obremskey W, Moore T, et al. Incisional negative pressure wound therapy after high-risk lower extremity fractures. J Orthop Trauma. 2012;26:37.

52. Streubel PN, Stinner DJ, Obremskey WT. Use of negative-pressure wound therapy in orthopaedic trauma. JAAOS - J Am Acad Orthop Surg. 2012;20:20.

53. Stannard JP, Robinson JT, Anderson ER, McGwin G, Volgas DA, Alonso JE. Negative pressure wound therapy to treat hematomas and surgical incisions following high-energy trauma. J Trauma. 2006;60:1301–6. https://doi.org/10.1097/01.ta.0000195996.73186.2e.

54. Rathbone CR, Cross JD, Brown KV, Murray CK, Wenke JC. Effect of various concentrations of antibiotics on osteogenic cell viability and activity. J Orthop Res. 2011;29:1070–4. https://doi.org/10.1002/jor.21343.

55. Fassbender M, Minkwitz S, Kronbach Z, Strobel C, Kadow-Romacker A, Schmidmaier G, et al. Local gentamicin application does not interfere with bone healing in a rat model. Bone. 2013;55:298–304. https://doi.org/10.1016/J.BONE.2013.04.018.

56. McNally MA, Ferguson JY, Lau ACK, Diefenbeck M, Scarborough M, Ramsden AJ, et al. Single-stage treatment of chronic osteomyelitis with a new absorbable, gentamicin-loaded, calcium sulphate/hydroxyapatite biocomposite: a prospective series of 100 cases. Bone Joint J. 2016;98-B:1289–96. https://doi.org/10.1302/0301-620X.98B9.38057/ASSET/IMAGES/LARGE/38057-GALLEYFIG2F.JPEG.

57. Yusuf E, Jordan X, Clauss M, Borens O, Mäder M, Trampuz A. High bacterial load in negative pressure wound therapy (NPWT) foams used in the treatment of chronic wounds. Wound Repair Regen. 2013;21:677–81. https://doi.org/10.1111/wrr.12088.

58. Zimmerli W, Widmer AF, Blatter M, Frei R, Ochsner PE. Role of rifampin for treatment of orthopedic implant-related staphylococcal infections: a random-

ized controlled trial. J Am Med Assoc. 1998;279:1537–41. https://doi.org/10.1001/jama.279.19.1537.

59. Thordarson DB, Patzakis MJ, Holtom P, Sherman R. Salvage of the septic ankle with concomitant tibial osteomyelitis. Foot Ankle Int. 1997;18:151–6. https://doi.org/10.1177/107110079701800307.

60. Hulscher JBF, Te Velde EA, Schuurman AH, Hoogendoorn JM, Kon M, Van Der Werken C. Arthrodesis after osteosynthesis and infection of the ankle joint. Injury. 2001;32:145–52. https://doi.org/10.1016/S0020-1383(00)00156-X.

Nonoperative Management of Ankle Arthritis

David E. Karges and Philip Shaheen

1 Introduction

Ankle arthrosis is a leading cause of lower extremity chronic disability in North America, well known to affect quality of life to the same level as end-stage hip arthritis [1]. Chronic ankle pain is often associated with both mechanical and nonmechanical sources. Mechanical ankle pain is generally due to static and dynamic forms of axial load activity such as standing and walking. The etiology of mechanical ankle pain is commonly osteoarthritis, post-traumatic arthritis, malalignment conditions to the ankle and hindfoot, ankle instability, and symptomatic tendinopathies. Whereas nonmechanical ankle pain is due to inflammation without repetitive loading or presence of mechanical stresses. The etiology of nonmechanical ankle pain is associated with systemic inflammation due to rheumatoid arthritis, hemophilia, diabetes and neuropathic injury, complex regional pain, and emotional conditions.

Isolating the cause of mechanical ankle pain can be challenging when an individual presents with multiple locations of foot and ankle pain. Subtle weight shifting may occur in an attempt to off-load other possible primary causes of musculoskeletal pain such as hip arthrosis, or calcaneal valgus or varus hindfoot deformity, or even a plantarfascial soft-tissue pain. An initial history and clinical evaluation of a patient's ankle pain is an important step in determining primary and secondary causes of chronic pain. The spectrum of different grades of ankle arthritis and the numerous associated soft-tissue pathologic conditions which may present adjacent to the arthritic joint make the assessment by clinical and radiographic evaluation the minimum necessary to achieve information so the cause of ankle pain is ascertained.

The decision between nonoperative versus surgical management will rely on chronicity and severity of ankle symptoms, daily function, response to medical management, demands required of a painful ankle during active hours of the day, and risk/benefit analysis concerning treatment options. The role and effectiveness of conservative care, however, makes it a wise initial form of care.

2 Nature of Ankle Arthrosis

The condition of ankle arthritis is largely due to three main causes, osteoarthritis (OA), rheumatoid arthritis (RA), and most commonly post-

D. E. Karges (✉)
Department of Orthopaedic Surgery, University of Minnesota/CentraCare, Saint Cloud, MN, USA
e-mail: david.karges@centracare.com

P. Shaheen
Department of Orthopaedic Surgery, Saint Louis University, Saint Louis, MO, USA
e-mail: philip.shaheen@health.slu.edu

traumatic arthritis (PTAA) [2]. Post-traumatic arthritis is a leading cause of ankle arthritis making up 70% of cases with OA reported at 12% and RA being the primary form of inflammatory arthritis [3] (Figs. 1, 2, 3, 4, 5, and 6).

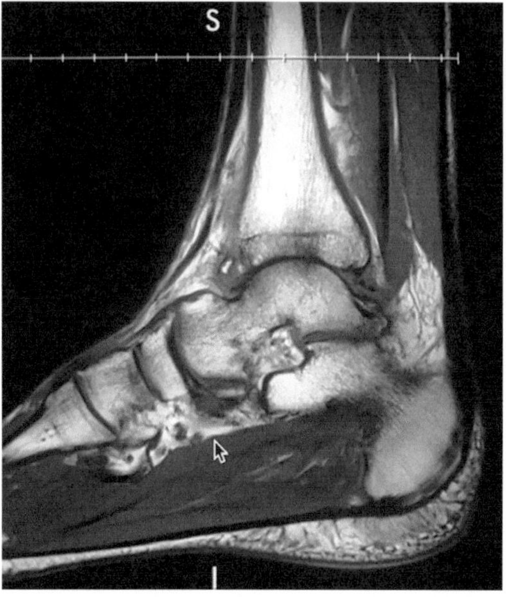

Fig. 1 Osteoarthritic ankle MRI image revealing narrowing of ankle joint cartilage

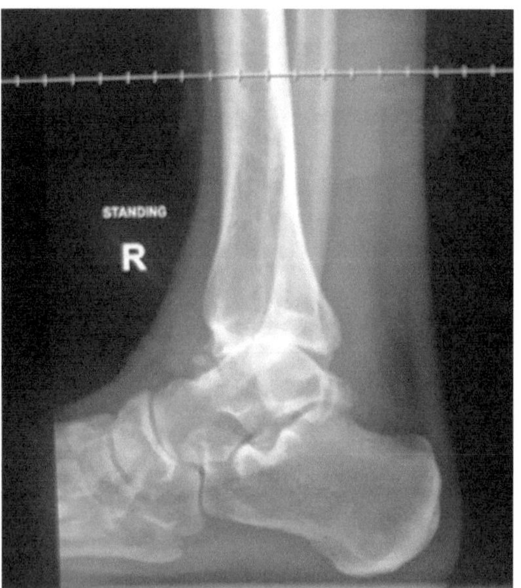

Fig. 2 Plain X ray of same OA ankle

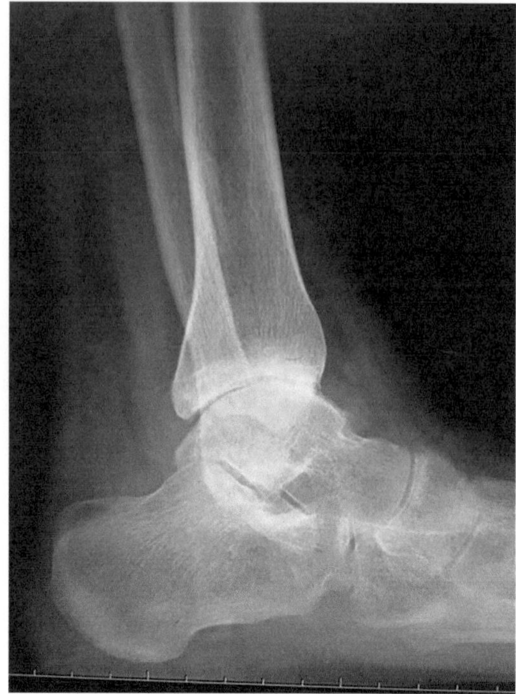

Fig. 3 Rheumatoid arthritic ankle joint image

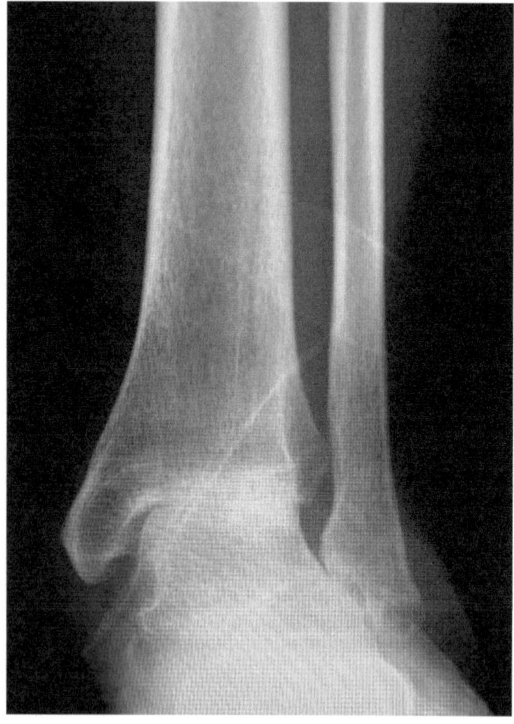

Fig. 4 AP X ray same RA ankle, advanced ankle arthritis with degenerative loss of syndesmotic ligaments

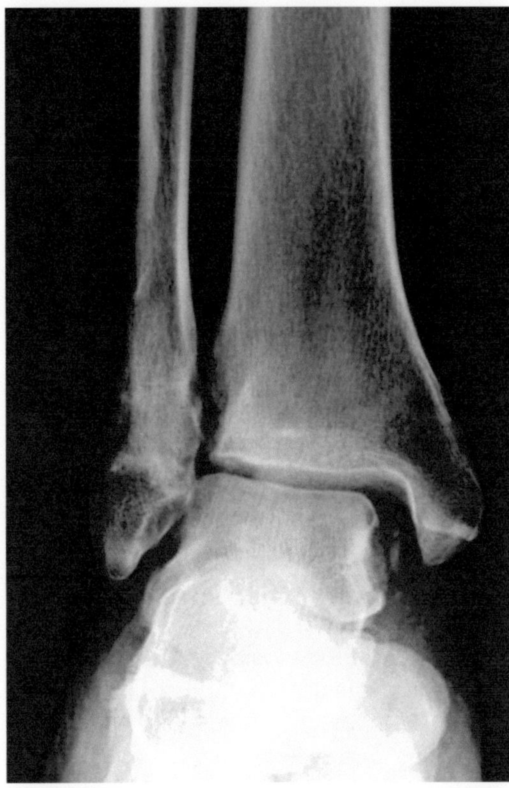

Fig. 5 Plain X-ray of early post-traumatic ankle and deltoid ligament disruption

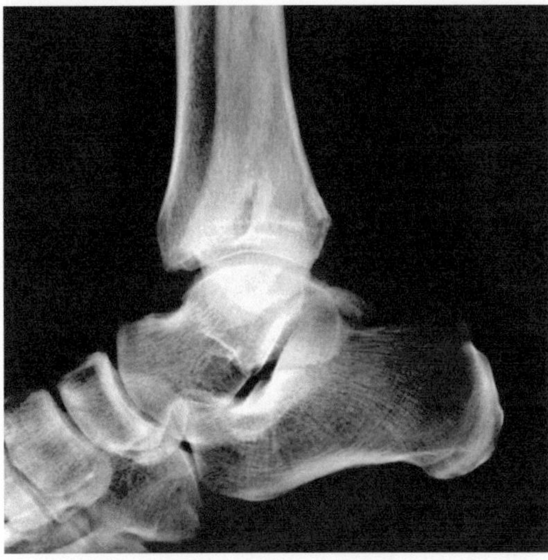

Fig. 6 Early anterior and posterior anterior malleolar spurring

There is no single cause of osteoarthritis of the ankle. Most importantly, repetitive loading and repeated stress to the ankle over an extended period of time presents a major risk factor for ankle osteoarthritis. In addition increased age, obesity, family genetics associated with primary OA and abnormal ankle joint alignment all impact the daily loading of the ankle and are variables leading to OA of the ankle.

Inflammatory arthritis is not caused by daily "wear and tear" to the articular surface of the ankle. Degenerative change of the cartilage surface and subchondral bone scaffolding to the joint is due to auto-immune disorders in which the immune system attacks native healthy cartilage and bone.

Although the cause of rheumatoid arthritis remains unknown, RA is believed to be associated with the Class II type histocompatibility complex human lymphocyte antigen DR4. It is believed a viral infection may be responsible for activating the antigen and triggering the inflammatory synovitis response. Subsequent destruction of an articular joint results from both B and T cells which precipitate synovial inflammation by way of release of degradative proteases [4].

Clinically, the inflammatory course of an ankle RA condition tends to follow one of three main directions. Most commonly, patients experience a polycyclic course (70%) of inflammation with multiple episodes of synovitis and remission. Patients with a single inflammatory episode, monocyclic course (20%), lasting for months are known to experience little chance of permanent ankle degeneration whereas the progressive variant (10%) is the most destructive and does not experience remission [5].

Although osteoarthritis and inflammatory arthritis are well-regarded types of ankle arthritis, post-traumatic arthritis is the most common form of arthritis to impact the ankle joint. The demographic of patients who develop post-traumatic arthritis are often younger and more active sustaining ankle arthritis due to an initial injury and subsequent arthrosis from repetitive load with daily activity.

Few investigations evaluating ankle arthrosis have attempted to reveal precise morphological, biomechanical, and biochemical changes with articular cartilage and subchondral bone following articular degenerative changes with each of the three main causes of ankle arthritis. The presence of pro-inflammatory and anti-inflammatory mediators in OA and RA is well documented [6, 7]. Metabolic profiling of the synovial fluid environment in experimentally tested ankles with OA shows the joints to be more hypoxic and acidotic that normal joints. OA is known to be associated with oxidative conditions in arthritic joints. Fat metabolism is believed to be a source of energy for the degenerative process in arthritic OA joints and these synovial findings are consistent, as well, with studies evaluating RA synovial joints [8, 9].

The ankle is a ligamentous joint with primary stability from the medial deltoid ligament complex. An ankle injury sustaining compromise of the deltoid ligament attachment to the medial talus, if left untreated, will predictably ensue a biomechanical alteration which impairs tibiotalar contact during repetitive loading. Injury of the deep deltoid ligament, directly allows the talus to translate laterally. This lateral translation of the talus has revealed up to a 40% diminished articular contact surface-area between the dome of the talar articulation with the plafond, resulting in increased peak-contact pressures during weightbearing of the ankle joint [10]. Structural changes to the articular surface of the joint, associated with the post-injury attenuation of the deltoid ligament complex have significant effect on the chronic degenerative change of the ankle. The role of mechanical loading in the repair of cartilage and subchondral bone, the metabolic changes in the cartilage, and the role of cytokines and viability of chondrocytes after articular injury may all contribute to the progression of post-traumatic arthrosis. Inflammatory cytokines and elevated levels of metabolite concentrations have also been well documented in human synovial fluid PTAA studies revealing degradation of tissue constituents in arthritis.

3   Pathoanatomy Effects

The mechanics of normal gait, from heel strike to toe-off, is important to understand for the orthopaedic surgeon. The initial phase, known as the "Stance Phase", involves heel-strike to flat-foot.

During this transition, the subtalar joint inverts precipitating lateral heel-strike. As weight transfers forward the subtalar joint everts, unlocking the midtarsal (Chopart's) joints, and the midfoot becomes supple for shock absorption. The Tibialis Anterior muscle contracts eccentrically controlling the initiation of plantarflexion of the foot.

As body weight advances over the foot and the gait-cycle transitions from flat-foot to heel-rise, the gastrosoleus lever contracts to control foot dorsiflexion. The Posterior Tibialis contracts concentrically returning the subtalar joint to inversion, externally rotating the tibia and initiating pelvic and contralateral leg motion which is the "Swing Phase."

Asymmetric arthritis of the ankle, whether OA, inflammatory or post-traumatic arthritis will change the gait of an individual due to three main factors: pain, stiffness, and lower extremity muscle atrophy. Pain due to arthritis will shorten the stance phase which comprises 60% of a gait cycle. Individuals with asymmetric ankle arthritis develop weakness not only in the compartments of the leg but atrophy and deconditioning of the thigh and pelvic gluteal musculature occurs, and balance of the affected lower extremity becomes impaired. Progressive weakness of the pelvic musculature, Gluteus Medius and Minimus, on the stance side will cause the contralateral pelvis to droop when the leg is in swing phase, resulting in a "Trendelenburg Gait." The loss of flexibility to the arthritic ankle joint affects pace, slowing down the gait cycle.

An additional cause precipitating ankle arthritis is malalignment of the ankle and hindfoot leading to early-stage degenerative change of the ankle joint. Varus malalignment of the hindfoot affects increased load across the medial plafond of the ankle and will progress to a degenerative state over time. The primary abnormalities associated with the varus hindfoot are the plantarflexed first metatarsal and loss of eversion with heel-strike creating a lateral overload of the lateral column of the foot. This malalignment leads to subsequent ankle instability following attenuation of lateral ligaments and capsule and hypertrophy of the Peroneus Longus, which progresses the varus deformity of the foot and ankle. Over time, medial arthritic changes to the ankle joint ensue. The literature reveals few publications discussing ankle arthritis in which hindfoot alignment is actually measured [11–13].

In early-stage ankle arthritis, progression of a varus ankle malalignment presents commonly, but the alignment change is considered to be mild. However, with increasing grades of ankle arthritis the varus malalignment is known to increase. This increased grade of varus to the ankle may precipitate a compensatory valgus hindfoot alignment. With this understanding, the treatment for a varus ankle should be carefully considered so as not to disregard the lateral subfibular impingement associated with a valgus hindfoot that may result when aligning the ankle [14].

The underlying impact of end-stage ankle arthritis on objective outcome data such as physiologic health, mental health, employment, and daily activity is not known, however baseline data, focused on subjective scoring of conservative management of advanced ankle arthritic patients is clear. Nonoperative treatment involving medical management, physiotherapy, brace application, and structural shoe design tends to fail in the advanced arthritic individual. When controlled subjective scoring of ankle arthritis patients has been compared to patients with no lower extremity limitations, the functional impact on daily life to patients with severe ankle arthritis has been shown to be pronounced. Data-driven research is believed to be of utmost importance when attempting to understand patient limitations, determining patient needs, and providing treatment recommendations [15].

4 Principles of Nonoperative Care

The correction and treatment of ankle arthritis is a difficult task to accomplish nonoperatively when looking at all-comers presenting with ankle arthritis. Patients with end-stage ankle arthritis, in particular, will require more than medical management to suppress daily inflammatory

symptoms. These advanced conditions benefit from structural bracing which support ankle and hindfoot loading. In addition, orthotics and custom shoe design help to improve comfort with daily activity. Importantly, there are few risks associated with nonoperative care of ankle arthritis.

Early treatment goals focus on prevention and palliative care to restore the foot and ankle to a comfortable and powerful lever. This is generally accomplished by providing immobilization to the ankle, maintaining a plantigrade functional foot that has motion and can endure different terrain.

Foot and ankle arthritis and lower extremity deformity must all be assessed when determining a treatment plan. If nonoperative care cannot be performed effectively, foot and ankle surgery is indicated to maintain the plantigrade foot by way of arthrodesis, resection arthroplasty, or replacement arthroplasty. The goal of all foot and ankle treatment is to provide pain relief while maintaining ambulatory capacity.

5 Imaging

Individuals with post-traumatic and osteoarthritis of the ankle commonly present with isolated ankle pain and stiffness. This is in contrast to the patient with a condition of inflammatory ankle arthritis in which pain symptoms are often present in multiple joints of the foot and ankle including the subtalar, midfoot, and metatarsal phalangeal joints. A thorough evaluation of the ankle and foot including weight bearing three-view X rays of the ankle are required to provide information to confirm an ankle arthritis diagnosis. The ankle X rays series is comprised of an anteroposterior (AP), mortise, and lateral radiograph. The AP view reveals the ankle in the natural anatomic position. The mortise view is an AP view with 10° internal rotation. This view projects the entire tibial plafond and both the medial and lateral malleoli with the entire talar dome. The lateral ankle plain X ray is a 90° projection to the mortise view. The image displays the calcaneus and talus in full profile and the lateral alignment of the hindfoot and ankle with respect to the distal tibia and lateral malleolus of the fibula. This image also shows the midfoot and metatarsal bases in profile.

Objective radiographic information consistent with joint space narrowing across the dome of the talus, subchondral sclerosis, subchondral cyst formation, asymmetric cartilage degeneration of the joint, and osteophyte formation are revealing of ankle arthritis (Figs. 7, 8, and 9). Computerized tomography (CT) and Magnetic Resonance imaging (MRI) help in providing detailed information regarding arthritis, ankle and hindfoot alignment, and associated soft tissue degenerative conditions.

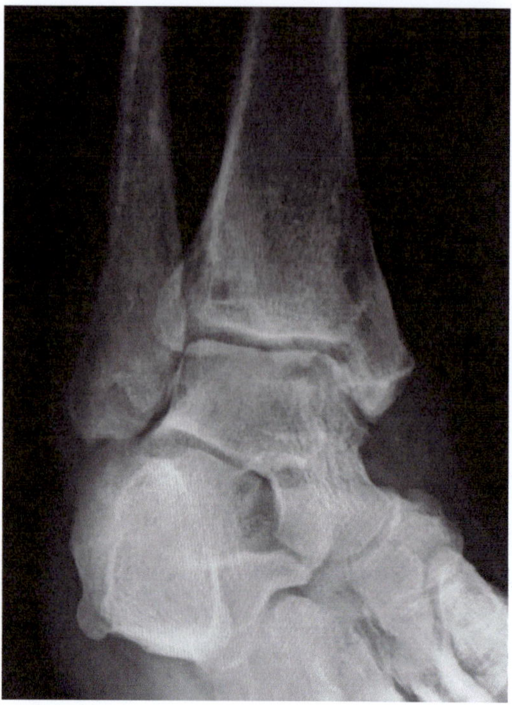

Fig. 8 Mortise X ray of same arthritic ankle with multifocal subchondral cyst formation

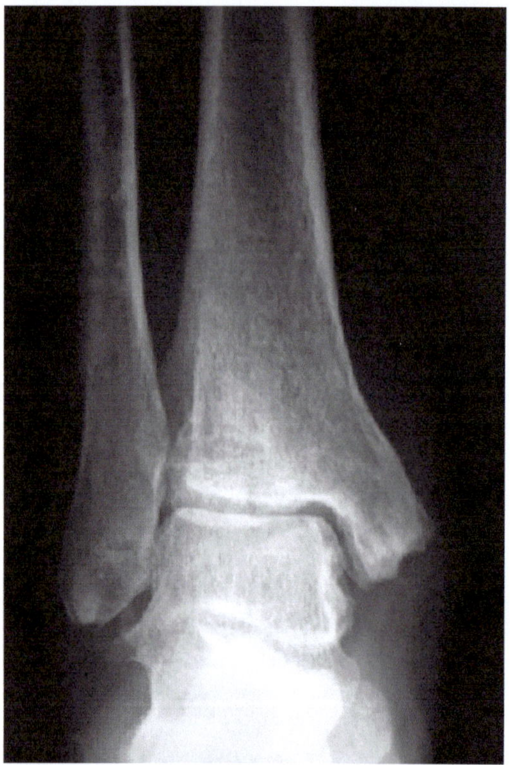

Fig. 7 AP X ray of early post-traumatic ankle arthritis, minimal joint space narrowing

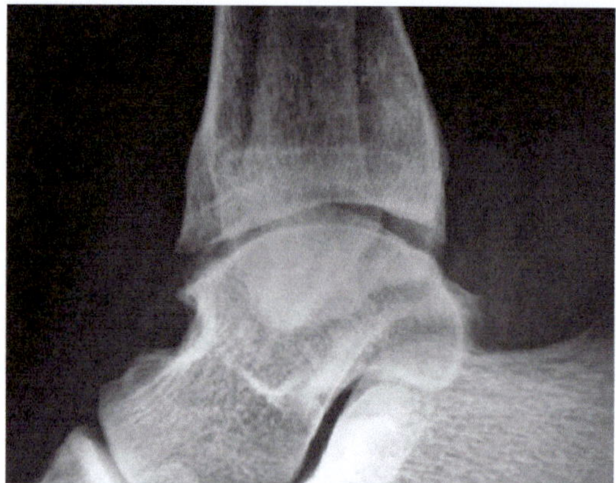

Fig. 9 Lateral plain X ray with anterior spur formation of post-traumatic ankle

6 Clinical Evaluation of the Arthritic Ankle

The process of diagnosing, staging, and rendering appropriate management to the arthritic ankle patient starts with a detailed interview of the arthritic history. While there is research to support nonoperative treatment options for arthritis of the hip and knee, data to support effective nonoperative management of the arthritic ankle is limited. Recommendations such as weight loss, application of an ambulatory assist such as a cane or walker, bracing, modification in shoe design, and anti-inflammatory medical management all play key roles in successful nonoperative care. However, when counseling patients with end-stage ankle arthrosis on benefits and disadvantages of conservative care, the understanding of limitations in repetitive loading on an arthritic ankle even with use of structural products must be revealed.

The younger patients with ankle arthritis, those in their 20s to 40s, routinely present with a history of a traumatic injury to the symptomatic ankle. A reason for the initial evaluation, if not a follow-up visit from a past traumatic ankle injury, can merely be persistent ankle pain, swelling, stiffness, inability to perform work on uneven terrain, ankle instability, or development of deformity to the ankle. The younger ankle arthritis patients may feel they have a normal ankle. They may work as a laborer, attempt to perform exercise activities, and have little understanding of the pathologic change causing the ankle symptoms.

There are no hard and fast rules regarding indications to nonoperative recommendations of ankle arthritis when counseling patients on their treatment. Severity of daily pain, response to anti-inflammatory agents, ankle/hindfoot and knee stiffness, work demands, ankle function with activity, and health comorbidities all provide treatment direction. However, objective lower extremity imaging data associated with ankle alignment such as angulation/tilt, rotation, translation, and length factor into the condition of ankle arthritis. Any chronic altered distribution to weight-bearing stresses will lead to abnormal force concentrations across the ankle. Animal and biomechanical studies and a few retrospective clinical studies have addressed the concern of what amount of malunion is tolerable when recommending nonoperative treatment to the arthritic ankle [16, 17].

Tilt of the ankle joint leads to shear stress, and contact pressure changes to the articular cartilage. Contact surface area can decrease up to 40% with angular malalignment. Distal tibial deformities produce worse contact pressures with sagittal plane deformity when it is greater than 15° whether anterior or posterior. With any subtalar joint stiffness there can be an exacerbation of ankle arthritic symptoms.

Ankle alignment less than 15° varus or 10° valgus and medial shift less than 20 mm to the mechanical axis has been found tolerable to daily function and a strong consideration for nonoperative management. However, what is normal alignment for a mechanical axis of the lower extremity? The mechanical axis of the leg passes from the femoral head to the posterior tuber of the calcaneus. The average mechanical axis crosses the knee 10 mm medial to the anatomic center of the knee on the frontal plane and anterior to the center of rotation of the knee in the sagittal plane. The mechanical axis of the tibia corresponds to its anatomic axis of the tibial spine. When standing, the knee joint is oriented in 3° of valgus relative to the mechanical axis. Despite this, the orientation of the ankle joint is parallel to the floor 90° to the tibial axis.

To best assess deformity, the surgeon must consider all three dimensions comprising leg length, ankle rotation, and angular alignment when considering nonoperative custom structural devices for ankle stabilization. A simple method of determining leg length is standing with a leveling block, of specific measure, until the ASIS level is balanced bilaterally. A patient's input concerning the feel of a level pelvis when standing on a measured block is a valuable subjective way to help correlate an objective measurement. Another technique is measuring tibial leg length in the prone position with knees flexed 90° and determine any discrepancy in sole height. Lastly, CT scanograms of hip, knee, ankle, and hindfoot can precisely determine length discrepancy.

Rotation is determined with patient prone and knees flexed 90° and ankles in neutral position. Compare rotation of foot with the unaffected side. Angular alignment is less precise but can be performed by superimposing, weightbearing X rays intersecting medullary lines of both the proximal and distal segments of the leg and foot.

Isolation of the location of pain in the patient with radiographic findings of an arthritic ankle is a necessary step when counseling someone on a treatment plan. Personal experience has clearly revealed to me that an arthritic ankle is not always the source of pain, even in a patient with a post-traumatic, osteoarthritic, or inflammatory ankle arthritic history. All patients must be evaluated for associated reasons of pain besides ankle arthritis such as pes planus, cavus and, cavovarus hindfoot deformity and well as midfoot arthritis and commonly an acquired Achilles contracture.

A patient must stand to assess hindfoot alignment. Calcaneal-valgus deformity, a common cause of medial and lateral subfibular ankle pain can be more debilitating than low grade ankle arthritic symptoms. A patient presenting with ankle symptoms but has a flat-foot on stance, must be questioned about the location of pain, posteromedial or subfibular, or both. Posteromedial pain, particularly when reproducible with direct focal pressure is diagnostic of Posterior Tibial tendonitis (PTT). Lateral subfibular pain is diagnostic of an impingement process, due to hindfoot valgus malalignment, in which the lateral process of the talus collides with the distal lateral malleolus. This pain can be exquisite and lead patients, and surgeons, to misdiagnose the condition as ankle arthritis. A selective injection of 1% Lidocaine (1.5–2 cc) and cortisone (1 cc triamcinolone) to the PTT tendon sheath or subfibular lateral ankle location is an additional way to determine pain from calcaneal valgus deformity versus ankle arthritis.

The lateral cavus hindfoot deformity which may create medial ankle arthritis is another ankle-hindfoot alignment deformity which must be evaluated as a possible cause of ankle pain in a treatment plan where the patient shows signs of ankle arthritis. A patient with subtle cavus deformity and postero-lateral peroneal tendonitis is wise to be treated with a selective injection into the peroneal tendon sheath and assessed as to whether the pain comes from the ankle, the peroneal tendonitis, or both locations.

Arthritis of the subtalar joint (S-T) is commonly found post-traumatically with calcaneus and talus injuries. However numerous conditions such as osteoarthritis, infection, hindfoot coalitions, posterior tibial tendonitis, and rheumatoid arthritis are other known causes. It is unknown if end-stage ankle arthritis and the associated stiffness may precipitate S-T arthritis due to increased focal pressure over such a small hindfoot surface-area. Symptoms of S-T arthritic pain vary with repetitive motion, static loading of the hindfoot, temporal periods of the day, and vigorous activity. However, the pain can be exquisite and preclude an individual from bearing weight on the foot. Radiographic narrowing of the S-T joint visualized on a weight-bearing plain lateral and mortise X ray is helpful objective information to correlate with the clinical exam. If expected, the selective injection, again, provides valuable diagnostic information which can be used with a treatment plan in addition to treatment for ankle arthritis.

7 Nonoperative Treatment Options

Since it is known that ankle arthritis affects a younger patient's demographic whose etiology is commonly traumatic compared to the demographics for knee and hip arthritis, a goal to avoid early surgical planning is clear. The various conservative treatments available to suppress and control ankle arthritic symptoms include analgesics, articular corticosteroid injections, offloading and immobilization of ankle motion with bracing, physiotherapy, orthotics, shoe modification, ambulatory assistive devices, and weight control. Viscosupplementation, historically a conservative treatment option for knee arthritis, was felt to be a weak injection treatment for ankle arthritis with short lifetime [18]. However, studies researching this treatment now show these joint lubrication agents provide improvement in joint function, stiffness, and analgesia [19].

8 Management

8.1 Oral, Topical, and Intra-articular Anti-arthritic Agents

The medical management of ankle arthritis is well regarded to focus on control of pain with repetitive loading. Oral narcotic analgesics have been a source of pain control for decades and have led to serious dependency and overuse such that opiate prescriptions have increased in number over 500% in the past two decades [20]. Early, yet progressive statewide laws, regulations, and policies nationwide are active in provider practices to diminish prescription of narcotic drugs. These laws are largely modeled after federal guidelines and vary across states [21]. The anticipation is that licensed prescription of narcotics will diminish because of nationwide policies, and generations of new orthopaedic surgeons will continually improve nonnarcotic protocols to manage arthritic pain.

Over 20 anti-inflammatory drugs (NSAIDS) are available on the market for use in common oral treatment of arthritic pain control. The NSAIDS inhibit prostaglandins which are a natural response to tissue stress. Prostaglandins are made at locations of tissue damage such as degenerative articular joints where they cause inflammation and pain. They are generated from arachidonic acid-derived prostaglandins by the action of cyclooxygenase (COX) isoenzymes. Their synthesis is blocked by NSAIDS including those selective for inhibition of COX-2 isoenzymes, which are a dominant source of prostaglandin formation in inflammation [22].

The NSAIDS manufactured for public anti-arthritic consumption make up approximately 40% of all cases. The medicine is available in lower dose over the counter (OTC) and higher dose prescription forms. Oral NSAIDS have been a form of safe, anti-arthritic treatment for decades however their routine use in the treatment of ankle arthritis is wisely to be counseled by a physician. The use of NSAIDS is not without risk. Over 100,000 hospitalizations a year are due to gastrointestinal complications and toxicity related to the use of these agents, but with careful attention to oral management these medicines play a powerful role in nonoperative, mild to severe, pain care [23]. Ibuprofen and Diclofenac are the commonly prescribed drugs to provide relief of pain.

Topical and patch forms of NSAIDS are available. The diclofenac sodium 1.5% topical and the diclofenac hydroxyetheyl pyrrolidine 1.3% patch and the diclofenac sodium gel 1% are useful in treating pain due to arthritis and soft-tissue injuries.

Glucosamine sulfate and chondroitin sulfate are naturally occurring substances found in connective tissues. When taken orally, studies have shown the absorption of glucosamine sulfate can be traced to cartilage surfaces in as early as 4 h. Similar to NSAIDS, these agents have shown a unique anti-inflammatory effect to cartilage surfaces. Studies suggest these agents may inhibit breakdown of cartilage [24]. Chondroitin sulfate is a larger molecule and also is believed to work as an anti-inflammatory agent reducing joint pain. However, these agents have often been disappointing for patients due to the incomplete relief of pain provided [25].

Intra-articular cortisone and hyaluronic acid (HA), platelet-rich plasma (PRP), and mesenchymal stem cell injections have a role in nonoperative care of ankle arthritis. Cortisone injections have been used for decades in the management of ankle arthritis. The majority of studies report varying strength of triamcinolone as a drug of choice over methylprednisolone. Regardless of etiology, studies reporting on corticosteroid injections have shown the treatment to be safe, responsive to symptoms and particularly diagnostic, even more than X ray findings, when attempting to isolate the location of pain in the foot and ankle [26]. Regarding the ankle, a study has shown, however, that therapeutic effects of pain relief do not extend beyond 3 months, and repeated injections have shown reduced benefit [27].

Viscosupplementation is a commonly used injection therapy in the treatment of knee arthritis. More recently, this treatment has been carefully evaluated for its place with ankle arthritis. Both prospective and meta-analysis studies concerning the use of HA in treatment of ankle arthritis has revealed the therapy safe and most effective with three weekly, 1 mL injections to the ankle [28]. Meta-analysis studies have also confirmed that multiple doses be administered for best outcome. Many of the studies recommend a three-injection protocol with the use of fluoroscopy to confirm injection location [29].

The use of intra-articular PRP injections is a fairly new treatment in management of nonoperative ankle arthritis care. PRP is defined as plasma with a minimum concentration of one million platelets/uL. Growth factors are stored in alpha-granules within platelets [30]. These factors have been shown in animal studies to diminish inflammatory effects, indirectly provide analgesic response to soft-tissue and articular surfaces, and possibly show protective properties to articular cartilage. A recent study concluded PRP treatment is safe, showed no adverse side effects and the outcomes of a three- injection protocol was effective in reducing ankle pain [31]. In summary, PRP has been found to be safe and injections can reduce ankle pain due to OA.

Stem cell injections are an uncommon treatment in nonoperative management of ankle arthritis. Stem cells are harvested from patient blood and bone. This process of collecting stem cells is similar to an isolated process of harvesting marrow from the anterior pelvic ileum. These cells are then cultured in a lab setting before injection into a joint. Research is very limited. There is currently no standard dosage of injection, frequency of treatment and outcome data. The purpose of stem cell treatment to an arthritic ankle joint is the belief that stem cells may synthesize cartilage cells, suppress inflammation and diminish ankle pain, and play a role in cytokine protein release that may help avoid cartilage degeneration. However, there is no standard protocol for treatment of stem cell therapy [32].

8.2 Obesity and Ankle Arthritis

The vast majority of orthopaedic and medical literature discussing obesity and ankle arthritis focuses on the different surgical options and outcomes. Obesity is defined as a body mass index (BMI) equal or greater than 30 kg/m². Obesity remains an epidemic in developed countries and is known to affect more than 35% of adults in the United States [33]. Patients are at higher risk for complications and outcomes particularly with surgical management [34]. Obese patients treated nonoperatively for ankle arthritis have been shown to clearly display increased stress on soft-tissues and joints of the foot and complain of associated nonspecific foot pain. However, there is little data to support that weight loss will reduce foot and ankle pain [35].

8.3 Physiotherapy

Physiotherapy is a well-regarded, safe and generally effective nonoperative treatment to manage ankle arthritis. The approach to therapy focuses on improved ankle function, range of motion, balance, stability and strength of the ankle. However, for optimal benefit with physiotherapy, these exercises should take place under the supervision of a licensed physiotherapist [35]. An initial treatment protocol is range of motion, balance, proprioception, and progressive strengthening. Next, functional exercises of the foot and ankle are wise as a form of therapy designed to bridge the gap from standard range of motion and strengthening to a type of rehabilitation tailored to mimic foot and ankle function required for a specific activity or sport. These exercises have shown to be effective in pain desensitization [36]. Additional modalities are thermotherapy (warming tissues), ultrasound and both laser and TENS unit treatment have been used for symptomatic relief [37].

With progression of ankle arthritis there is degeneration of basic life activities. In summary, aerobic exercise and both supervised and self-supervised physical therapy regimens are essential as they improve endurance and conservation of gait and maximize core function and posture during active work.

8.4 Ankle Bracing

Nonoperative bracing of the ankle and hindfoot remains a common initial treatment in the management of early, to end-stage, ankle arthritis. Orthopaedic foot and ankle surgeons are wise to develop an understanding of lower extremity, ankle and foot biomechanics associated with pathologic conditions found with ankle arthritis. This understanding helps to optimize brace, orthotic and shoe designs in conservative management of ankle arthritic. The goals when applying these structural devices should be to off-load axial force to the foot and ankle, diminish shear, provide cushion, and yet stabilize forces during gait in an effort to avoid surgery. In summary, the goal of these modifications in brace and footwear are to comfortably immobilize painful motion and compensate for loss of motion and stiffness by improving the transition from heel-strike to toe-off.

When counseling a patient about conservative management of ankle arthritis, a relatively quick and easy brace design to assess the benefit of brace treatment is the proprietary, removable cast or fracture boot. The design to these braces includes a locked ankle component in neutral position with a rocker-bottom sole design. Studies evaluating the prefabricated adjustable design of these braces have been comparable to custom orthoses, but they preclude the ability to be in normal shoewear which can be a reason for their temporary use [38].

The pain in ankle arthritis is largely due to symptomatic tibiotalar sagittal motion associated with repetitive loading during gait. The types of ankle brace indicated in management of ankle arthritis continues to expand in design. Historically, the ankle-foot orthosis (AFO) was a tall custom, double-upright brace attached to the shoe, whereas the molded AFO (MAFO) is a brace design to fit inside a shoe. With the condition of ankle arthritis, the AFO should be designed without any ankle hinge that will increase sagittal plane motion. Either brace design can be a lace-up or Velcro strap design made of leather, plastic with polypropylene or carbon-fiber to secure ankle immobilization but allow energy transfer from heel-strike to toe-off (Figs. 10, 11, and 12).

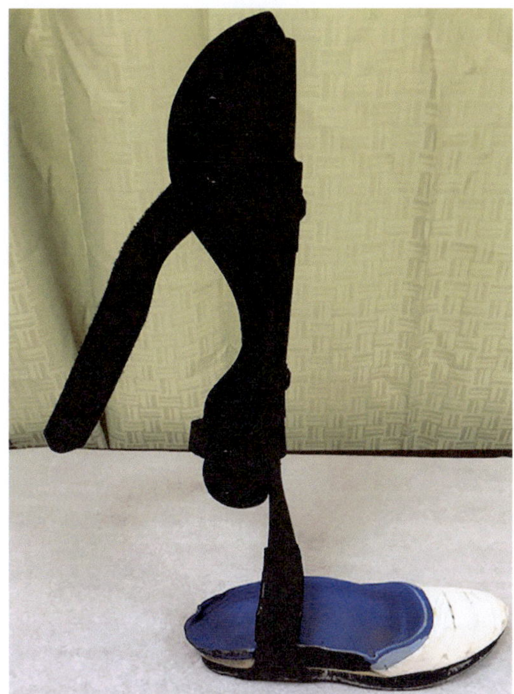

Fig. 10 Dynamic carbon fiber AFO with foot plate and orthotic

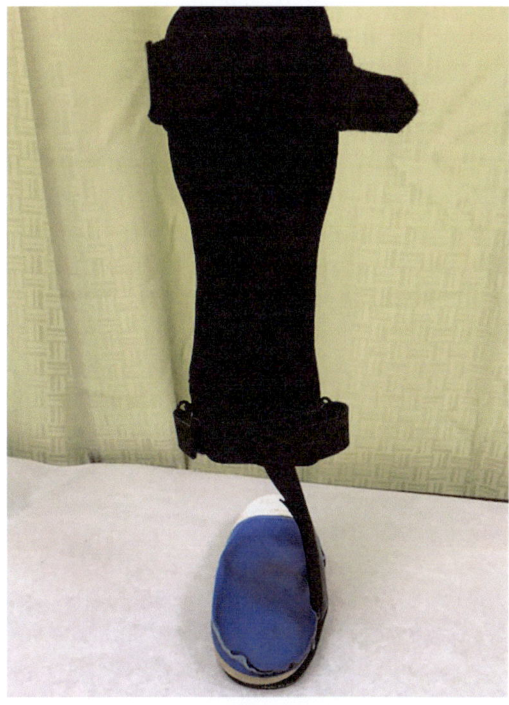

Fig. 11 Dynamic carbon fiber AFO with foot plate and orthotic

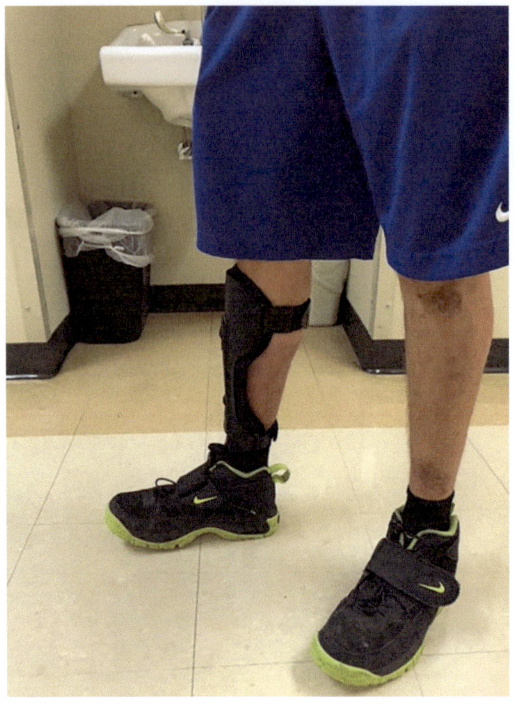

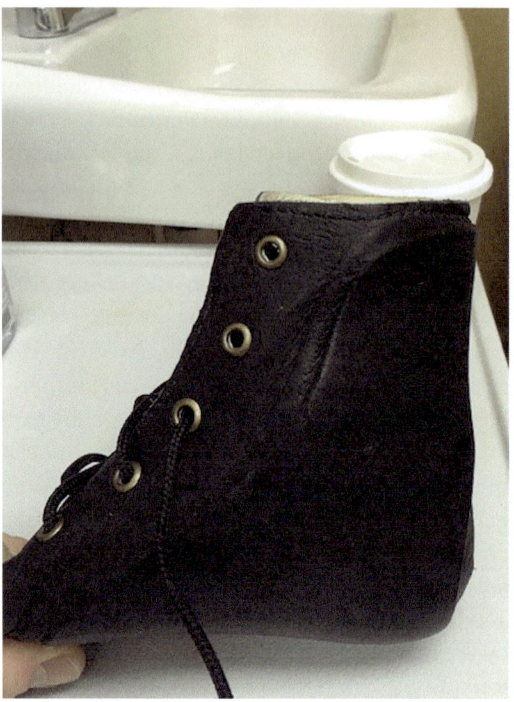

Fig. 12 Low profile carbon fiber AFO allowing for commercial shoewear

Fig. 13 Arizona custom ankle brace

The Arizona brace is another excellent brace designed to immobilize sagittal plane motion of the ankle and hindfoot while allowing to fit in a shoe which can improve patient compliance [39] (Figs. 13 and 14).

Both designs, MAFO and Arizona brace, off-load axial pressure sustained by the ankle during gait at the cost of diminishing sagittal motion to the ankle. However there is little data available to provide an indication of which brace design is best in clinical cases of ankle arthritis [40]. My personal experience with use of these two braces is a preference for the Arizona brace, over the MAFO, due to its shorter height, excellent control of ankle and hindfoot motion, and better patient acceptance. The disadvantage of the Arizona brace is its persistent bulky fit in the counter of any shoe or boot.

The Patellar-Tendon-Bearing brace (PTB) is a custom, ankle off-loading brace that plays a significant role in conservative care with the end-stage ankle arthritic patient. The brace was initially, in the 1960s, a cast-brace for treatment

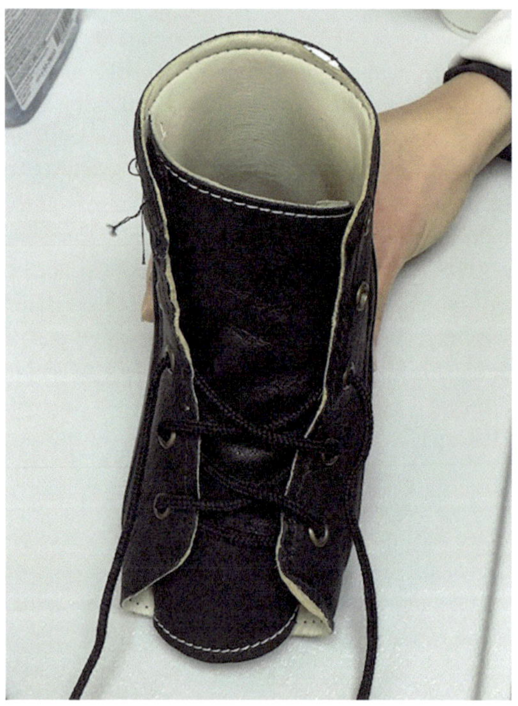

Fig. 14 Arizona custom ankle brace

of tibial fractures and tibial nonunions [41]. The traditional design of this brace is most effective with ankle arthritis (Figs. 15 and 16). Low profile medial and lateral upright bars fix into the heel component of a shoe or boot and the brace extends proximally to an infrapatellar circumferential strap or thermoplastic knee orthosis that tightens. Distally, within the heel component of the shoe and fixed to the brace, the plantar hindfoot is carefully suspended in the shoe so hindfoot pressure is minimized with repetitive loading. The brace has shown repeatedly in studies to reduce peak-plantar pressures effectively reducing ankle and hindfoot forces in gait but transferring this load during gait to the midfoot. The midfoot force is therefore improved by combining the rocker-bottom sole-modified shoe with the PTB brace.

A new custom addition in brace technology is the Intrepid Dynamic Exoskeletal Orthosis, or IDEO brace. Pain which remains a concomitant issue with ankle bracing with arthritis is known to have shown a significant reduction with the

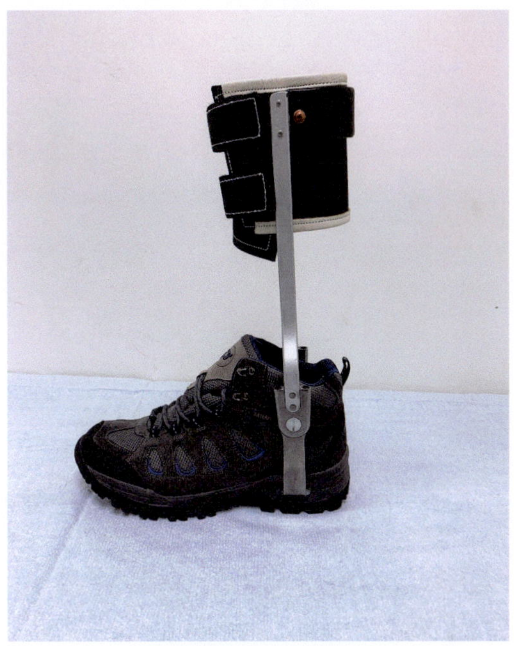

Fig. 16 Classic Patellar-Tendon-Bearing brace

advent of the IDEO brace. The brace was developed at the Center for the Intrepid at the Brooke Army Medical Center in San Antonio, Texas in 2009 [42]. The brace is molded out of lightweight carbon fiber and was initially designed to offer a limb salvage treatment option to soldiers who sustained complex lower extremity foot and ankle injury during military conflicts.

The brace is designed like a spring in which a foot plate is attached to a posterior series of carbon fiber ankle struts which are attached in the back of the calf to a cuff. As the foot plate is loaded with weight bearing, this bends the ankle struts, fixed proximally to the calf; and generates energy to the ankle in plantarflexion. The loading of the ankle struts is designed in a fashion where force and pain are removed from the ankle (Figs. 17 and 18). This orthosis has shown excellent potential in management of civilian post-traumatic arthritis and osteoarthritis of the ankle with numerous contemporary hybrid designs fashioned after the original Intrepid design [43] (Figs. 19, 20, 21, 22, 23, and 24). The only contraindication reported to the IDEO brace was ipsilateral knee range of motion less than 90° [42]. Data reviewing use of the IDEO brace with

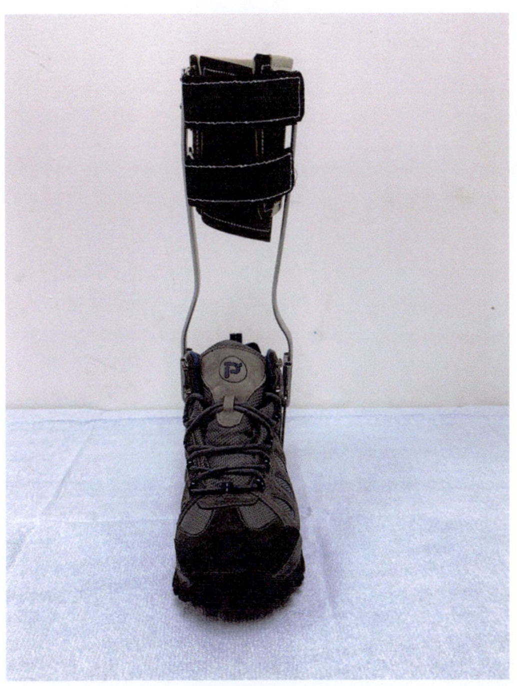

Fig. 15 Classic Patellar-Tendon-Bearing brace with metal uprights attached outside of shoe and leather calf cuff

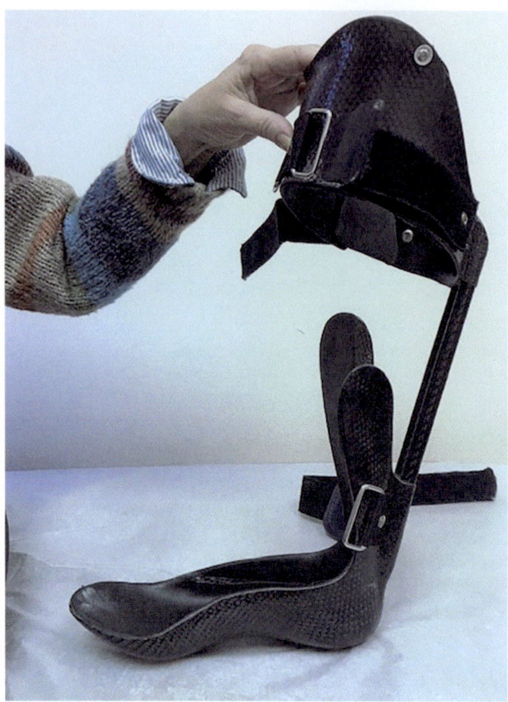

Fig. 17 Original Intrepid lab design of IDEO brace

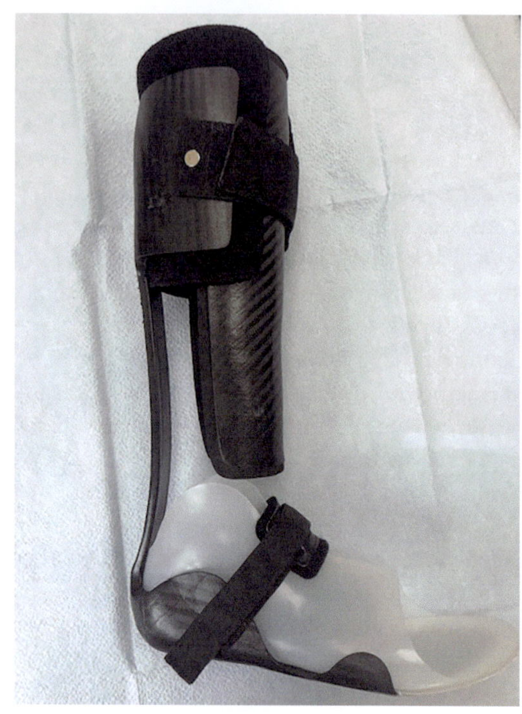

Fig. 19 Hybrid design of IDEO brace

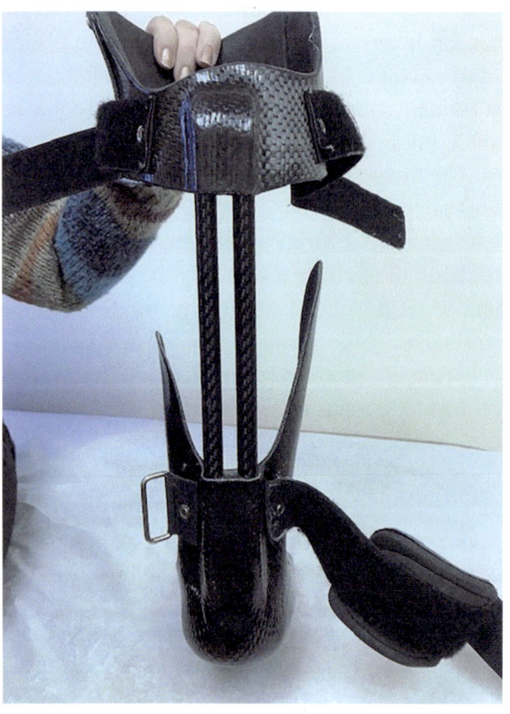

Fig. 18 Original Intrepid lab design of IDEO brace

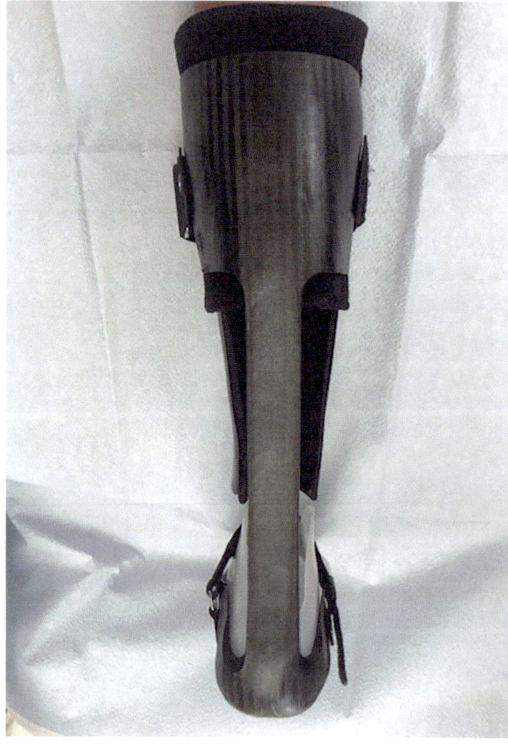

Fig. 20 Hybrid design of IDEO brace

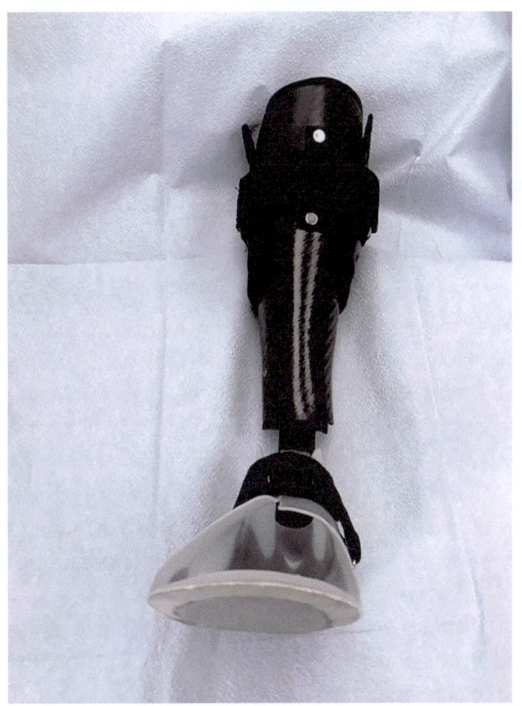

Fig. 21 Hybrid design of IDEO brace

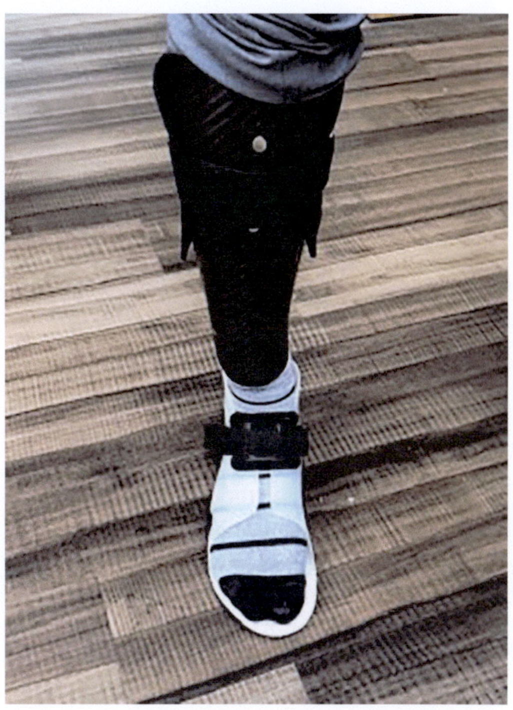

Fig. 23 Low profile design of the IDEO brace

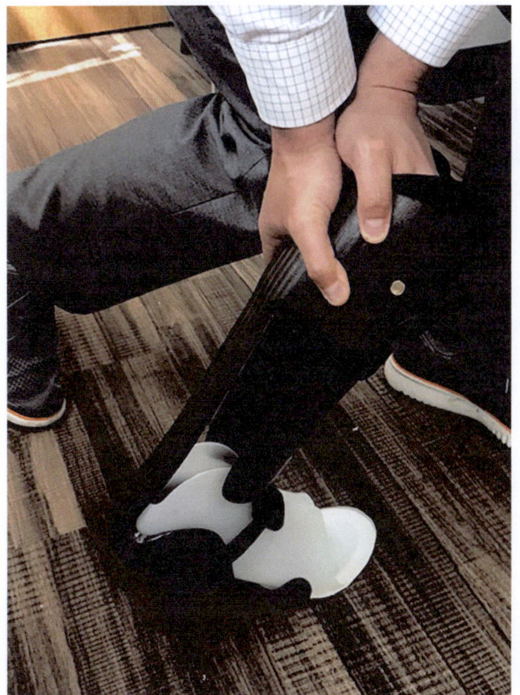

Fig. 22 Energy transmission of posterior strut to foot plate with ankle dorsiflexion

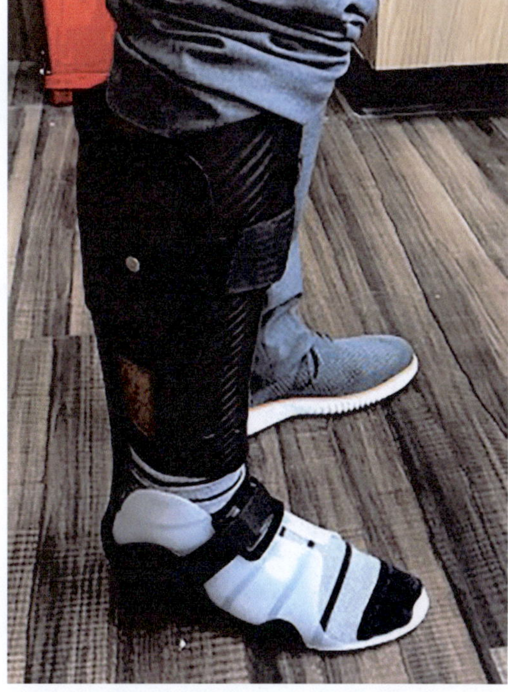

Fig. 24 Low profile design of the IDEO brace

immediate specialized physical therapy training, known as Return to Run (RTR), has shown largely best results with this brace [44]. The practical disadvantage of the IDEO brace is cost and access to a RTR physical therapy program. When both, brace and RTR therapy, are combined even the end-stage ankle arthritic patient may have potential to achieve a more functional outcome than a surgical cohort.

8.5 Orthotics and Shoe Modification

Foot orthoses and shoe modification are important tools in the nonoperative management of ankle arthritis. Orthotics, like braces, are used to decompress pressure sites, decrease shear, provide support, and stabilize or help correct flexible deformities of the foot. The condition of ankle arthritis is commonly associated with different grades of secondary arthritis, stiffness, malalignment, and instability of the foot, requiring structural products to optimize gait when pursuing conservative management of the ankle.

The types of custom orthotics prescribed are the accommodative which cushion and support hindfoot to digits, the semi-rigid which cushion, support, and control a foot morphology, the rigid which focuses on arch support and the partial amputation foot prosthesis which protects a partial foot amputation [45].

The accommodative custom orthotic is an effective, supportive insert for the individual with mild deformity requiring cushion, hindfoot wedging for mild angular malalignment and possibly forefoot metatarsal off-loading. I have routinely used a moderate density sponge rubber material for the contact surface area which distributes forces nicely and is well liked by patients. However, this material is more compressible requiring new orthotics every 1–2 years from experience.

The most common custom orthotic design, in my experience treating the arthritic foot and ankle condition is the semi-rigid orthotic. These orthotics are made of different materials, polyethylene foams, vinyls, and cork composites. The semi-rigid design can be easily modified, in ankle braces, to optimize clinical changes such as off-load pressure points when attempting to avoid ulcer formation in a neuropathic foot or adjust hindfoot alignment. These are excellent, comfortable, strong orthotics which work well particularly in the hindfoot and plantar surface of the foot [46].

The rigid orthotic has not worked well in my practice managing the arthritic ankle. The materials may work supporting the arch and flexible deformities, but they are rigid and don't give way over time often causing focal areas of pain on the plantar foot. They are not adjustable and I have found the semi-rigid orthotic more agreeable with patients. The partial foot prosthesis works well when combining with the semi-rigid orthotic when necessary.

Undermanaging patients diagnosed with ankle arthritis, foot arthritis, and foot deformity with inappropriate footwear is a common cause of persistent patient complaints associated with ankle arthritis. The purpose of shoe and sole modification is to improve locomotion in gait, make gait more efficient, and importantly, less painful.

The rocker-bottom sole modification to a shoe historically presented much value to the patient with a painful midfoot and, or forefoot condition. However clinical data has shown the rocker-bottom shoe to also play a role in management of ankle arthritis [47]. There are six different designs [48]. The two main focal points in design of the rocker-bottom sole modified shoe are the midstance apex location of the sole beginning under the anterior location of the ankle and extending beyond the midtarsal joints assisting the foot as it begins to perform toe-off. The primary apex to a rocker-bottom sole is at the location of the metatarsal-phalangeal joints (Fig. 25).

Commercial rocker-bottom sole modified shoes have clearly advanced in design and technology with a gently beveled heel devoid of imbalancing the patient during heel-strike. The commercial rocker-bottom sole extends from the metatarsals to beyond the metatarsal phalangeal joint providing a smooth transition from heel to forefoot. The rocker-bottom shoe has become a

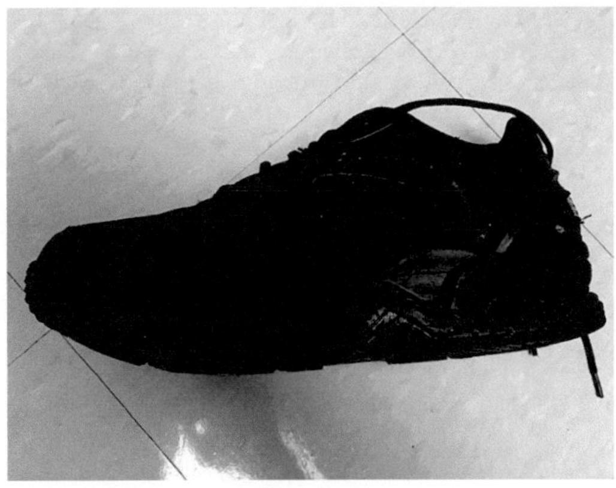

Fig. 25 Rocker- bottom shoe design

popular shoe model for all comers. However, its design plays a therapeutic role in the gait of ankle and midfoot arthritic patients. Patients with ankle and midfoot arthritic conditions that benefit from a rocker-bottom sole are recommended to consider relasting their work shoes, or boots, to achieve the therapeutic function from the sole modification [49].

9 Summary

Ankle arthritis has numerous causes with post-traumatic articular injury of the joint clearly responsible for the vast majority of ankle pathology. When diagnosing early stages of ankle arthritis, the surgeon must evaluate the entire foot and ankle for associated soft-tissue, malalignment, and instability problems which may contribute to the ankle pain. Long term, an early conservative foot and ankle treatment plan may have a better opportunity to help the patient avoid the need of a surgical reconstruction. Research focused on conservative management of end-stage of ankle arthritis is clear. Nonoperative treatment involving medical management, physiotherapy, brace application, and structural shoe design tends to fail with this individual.

However, it is prudent to counsel patients of their conservative care options according to the patients' particular stage of arthritis, functional demands required of the arthritic ankle and possibly any preexisting foot deformity. To be practi-

cal, when discussing the ability to restore function and resolve pain using structural modifications to the foot and ankle, the patient must be clear that when these products are removed from the foot, the painful daily symptoms recur. The benefit of conservative ankle arthritis care, when successful, is largely the minimal risk associated with the management. Yet, when surgical indications of ankle arthritis are clearly present, operative management to ankle arthritis can routinely provide patients with the desired goals of a painless, functional ankle.

References

1. Glazebrook M, Daniels T, Younger A, et al. Comparison of health-related quality of life between patients with end-stage ankle and hip arthrosis. J Bone Joint Surg Am. 2008;90(3):499–505.
2. Martin RL, Stewart GW, Conti SF. Posttraumatic ankle arthritis: an update on conservative and surgical management. J Orthop Sports Phys Ther. 2007;37(5):253–9.
3. Saltzman CL, Salamon ML, Blanchard GM, Huff T, Hayes A, Buckwalter JA, Amendola A. Epidemiology of ankle arthritis: report of a consecutive series of 639 patients from a tertiary orthopaedic center. Iowa Orthop J. 2005;25:44–6.
4. Tenten-Diepenmaat M, Joost Dekker MW, Heymans LD, Roorda T P, Vliet V, Van der Leeden M. Systematic review on the comparative effectiveness of foot orthoses in patients with rheumatoid arthritis. J Foot Ankle Res. 2019;12:1–16.
5. Smyth CJ, Janson RW. Rheumatologic view of the rheumatoid foot. Clin Orthop. 1997;340:7–17.
6. Fleming A, Crown JM, Corbett M. Early rheumatoid disease. Onset. Ann Rheum Dis. 1976;35:357–60.
7. Kapoor M, Martel-Pelletier J, Lajeunesse D, Pelletier JP, Fahmi H. Role of proinflammatory cytokines in the pathophysiology of osteoarthritis. Nat Rev Rheumatol. 2011;7:33–42.
8. Martel-Pelletier J, Alaaeddine N, Pelletier JP. Cytokines and their role in the pathophysiology of osteoarthritis. Front Biosci. 1999;4:D694–703.
9. Mircic M, Kavanaugh A. Inhibition of IL6 in rheumatoid arthritis and juvenile idiopathic arthritis. Exp Cell Res. 2011;317:1286–92.
10. Harrington KD. Degenerative arthritis of the ankle secondary to long-standing lateral ligament instability. J Bone Joint Surg Am. 1979;61:354–61.
11. Hayashi K, Tanaka Y, Kumai T, Sugimoto K, Takakura Y. Correlation of compensatory alignment of the subtalar joint to the progression of primary osteoarthritis of the ankle. Foot Ankle Int. 2008;29(4):400–6.

12. Pagenstert GI, Hintermann B, Barg A, Leumann A, Valderrabano V. Realignment surgery as alternative treatment of varus and valgus ankle osteoarthritis. Clin Orthop Relat Res. 2007;462:156–68.
13. Aminian A, Sangeorzan BJ. The anatomy of cavus foot deformity. Foot Ankle Clin. 2008;13:191–8.
14. Lee WC, Moon JS, Lee HS, Lee K. Alignment of ankle and hindfoot in early stage ankle osteoarthritis. Foot Ankle Int. 2011;32(7):693–9.
15. Agel J, Coetzee JC, Sangeorzan BJ, Roberts MM, Hansen ST Jr. Functional limitations of patients with end-stage ankle arthrosis. Foot Ankle Int. 2005;26:537–9.
16. Wu WL, Su FC, Cheng YM, et al. Gait analysis after ankle arthrodesis. Gait Posture. 2000;11:54–61.
17. Wan L, de Asla R, Rubash HE, Guoan L. In vivo cartilage contact deformation of human ankle joint of full body weight. J Orthop Res. 2008;26:1081–9.
18. Mori S, Naito M, Moriyama S. Highly viscous sodium hyaluranate and joint lubrication. Int Orthop. 2002;26(2):116–21.
19. Kirchner M, Marshall D. A double-blind randomized controlled trial comparing alternate forms of high molecular weight hyaluronan for the treatment of osteoarthritis of the knee. Osteoarthr Cartil. 2006;14(2):154–62.
20. Paulozzi LJ, Budnitz DS, Xi Y. Increasing deaths from opioid analgesics in the United States. Pharmacoepidemiol Drug Saf. 2006;15(9):618–27.
21. Riggs CS, Billups SJ, Flores S, Patel RJ, et al. Opioid use for pain management after implementation of a medicaid short-acting opioid quantity limit. J Manag Care Spec Pharm. 2017;23(3):346–54.
22. Nathan C. Points of control in inflammation. Nature. 2002;420:846–85.
23. Bradley JD, Brandt KD, Katz BP, et al. Treatment of knee osteoarthritis: relationship of clinical features of joint inflammation to the response to a nonsteroidal anti-inflammatory drug or pure analgesic. J Rheumatol. 1992;19:1950.
24. Bassleer C, Henrotin Y, Franchimont P. Invitro evaluation of drugs proposed as chondroprotective agents. Int J Tissue React. 1992;14:231–41.
25. Clegg DO, Reda DJ, Harris CL, et al. Glucosamine, chondroitin sulfate and the two in combination for painful knee osteoarthritis. N Engl J Med. 2006;354(8):795–808.
26. Ward ST, Williams PL, Purkayastha S. Intra-articular cortisone injections in the foot and ankle: a prospective n1-year follow-up investigation. J Foot Ankle Surg. 2008;47:138–44.
27. Khoury NJ, el-Khoury CY, Saltzman CL, Brandser EA. Intraarticular foot and ankle injections to identify source of pain before arthrodesis. Am J Roentgenol. 1996;167:669–73.
28. Chang KV, Hsiao MY, Chen WS, Wang TG, Chien KL. Effectiveness of intra-articular hyaluronic acid for ankle osteoarthritis treatment: a systematic review and metanalysis. Arch Phys Med Rehabil. 2013;94:951–60.
29. Murphy EP, Curtin M, McGoldrick NPO, Thong G, Kearns SR. Prospective evaluation of intra-articular sodium hyaluronate injection in the ankle. J Foot Ankle Surg. 2017;56:327–31.
30. Marx RE. Platelet-rich plasma (PRP): what is PRP and what is not PRP? Implant Dent. 2001;10:225–8.
31. Taisuke F, et al. Safety and efficacy of intra-articular injection of platelet-rich plasma in patients with ankle arthritis. Foot Ankle Int. 2017;6:365–74.
32. Melick G, Hayman N, Landsman AS. Mesenchymal stem cell applications for joints in the foot and ankle. Clin Podiatr Med Surg. 2018;35(3):323–30.
33. Ogden CL, Carroll MD, Kit BK, Flegal KM. Prevalence of obesity in the United States, 2009-2010. NCHS Data Brief. 2012;82:1–8.
34. Bamgbade OA, Rutter TW, Nafiu OO, Dorje P. Postoperative complications in obese and nonobese patients. World J Surg. 2007;31(3):556–60.
35. Saltzman CL, Salamon ML, Blanchard GM, et al. Epidemiology of ankle arthritis. Iowa Orthop J. 2005;25:44–6.
36. Peyron JG. The epidemiology of osteoarthritis diagnosis and treatment. Philadelphia: WB Sanders; 1984. p. 9–27.
37. Valderrabano V, Horisberger M, Russell I, et al. Etilology of ankle arthritis. J Clin Orthop Relat Res. 2009;467:1800–6.
38. Crincoli MG, Trepman E. Immobilization with removable walking brace for treatment of chronic foot and ankle pain. Foot Ankle Int. 2001;32(9):725–30.
39. Wapner KL. Conservative treatment of the foot. In: Surgery of the foot and ankle. St Louis, MO: CV Mosby; 1999. p. 115–30.
40. Thompson JA, Jennings MB, Hodge W, et al. Orthotic therapy in the management of osteoarthritis. J Am Podiatr Med Assoc. 1992;82(3):136–9.
41. Sarmiento A. A functional below-the-knee cast for tibial fractures. J Bone Joint Surg Am. 1967;49:855–75.
42. Patzkowski JC, Blanck RV, Owens JG, Wilken JM, Blair JA, Hsu JR. Can an ankle-foot orthosis change hearts and minds? J Surg Orthop Adv. 2011;20(1):8–18.
43. Patzkowski JC, Owens JG, Blanck RV, Kirk KL, Hsu JR. Skeletal Trauma Research Consortium: management of posttraumatic osteoarthritis with an integrated orthotic and rehabilitation initiative. J Am Acad Orthop Surg. 2012;20(Suppl 1):S48–53.
44. Owens JG, Blair JA, Patzkowski JC, Blanck RV, Hsu JR. Skeletal Trauma Research C: return to running and sports participation after limb salvage. J Trauma. 2011;71(Suppl 1):S120–4.
45. Janisse DJ, Janisse EJ. Pedorthic and orthotic management of the diabetic foot. Foot Ankle Clin. 2006;11:717–34.
46. Carlson JM. Functional limitations from pain caused by repetitive loading on the skin: a review and discussion for practitioners, with new data for limiting friction loads. J Prosthet Orthot. 2006;18:93–103.

47. Brown D, Wertsch JJ, Harris GF, Klein J, Janisse D. Effects of rocker soles on plantar pressures. Arch Phys Med Rehabil. 2004;85:81–6.
48. Marzano R. Fabricating shoe modifications and foot orthoses. In: Janisse DJ, editor. Introduction to pedorthics. Columbia, MD: Pediatric Foot Association; 1998. p. 717–34.
49. Jones DA, Moed BR, Karges DE. Does modified footwear improve gait after ankle arthrodesis? J Foot Ankle Surg. 2015;55:5.

Post-traumatic Ankle Arthritis: Fusions

David J. Ciufo and Paul T. Fortin

1   Introduction

Ankle arthritis occurs much less commonly than arthritis of the hip and knee. Autopsy and cadaveric studies find advanced degenerative changes at the ankle three times less prevalent than the larger joints [1, 2]. While the ankle cartilage is generally thinner and sees greater stress than these other joints, the tensile properties of talar cartilage degrade more slowly over time during aging [3, 4]. Due to these physiologic differences, the development of primary ankle arthritis is fairly uncommon, less than 10% in several longitudinal studies. These cohorts demonstrated 70% or greater of patients presenting with clinical ankle arthritis were secondary to trauma [5, 6]. Within this post-traumatic subset, the most common etiology was rotational malleolar fractures, followed by chronic ankle instability, pilon/tibial shaft/talar fractures, and osteochondral lesions. Despite variable mechanisms of trauma between fracture and instability, there are similar kinematic changes with loss of plantar/dorsiflexion of the tibiotalar joint but also restrictions in surrounding midfoot mobility [7].

End-stage ankle arthritis has been shown to compromise quality of life much like other lower extremity arthritis, and many patients will fail conservative measures. Due to the relationship with trauma, there is also a need to have durable management for younger patients that have developed this debilitating condition. While the use of ankle arthroplasty is gradually increasing, and outcomes are improving, ankle arthrodesis is still the gold standard for end-stage ankle arthritis [8].

Ankle arthrodesis offers a durable answer for the painful arthritic ankle, while allowing for correction of deformity and instability. Like all surgical options, there are known complications associated with this procedure, even when successful fusion occurs. The most problematic outcome of ankle arthrodesis is the alteration in gait mechanics. The fused ankle often demonstrates a shorter stride length, with increased motion of the nearby subtalar and talonavicular articulations [9]. This is felt to be related to the high incidence of adjacent joint arthritis, with some studies identifying up to 100% prevalence of subtalar arthrosis at 10 years post-ankle arthrodesis [10]. Nonetheless, ankle arthrodesis remains an important tool in the armamentarium of the orthopaedic foot and ankle surgeon or traumatologist in the setting of post-traumatic arthritis.

D. J. Ciufo (✉)
University of Rochester, Rochester, NY, USA

P. T. Fortin
Oakland University William Beaumont School of Medicine, Michigan Orthopaedic Surgeons, Royal Oak, MI, USA

© The Author(s), under exclusive license to Springer Nature Switzerland AG 2023
D. Herscovici Jr. et al. (eds.), *Evaluation and Surgical Management of the Ankle*,
https://doi.org/10.1007/978-3-031-33537-2_21

2 Post-traumatic Biochemical Environment

Due to its unique relationship with trauma, the biochemical profile of the arthritic ankle has received research attention. From a composition standpoint, the ankle demonstrates a higher percentage sulfated glycosaminoglycans (GAGs) with a lower water content than the knee, despite a similar collagen content [11]. This leads to a stiffer, more compression-resistant cartilage at the ankle. Baseline levels of protein and proteoglycan synthesis are higher in the ankle as well, suggesting a higher metabolic activity in this joint, which seems to be related to the extracellular environment rather than differences in cell programming. Additionally, the ankle cartilage is more resistant to catabolism in the presence of pro-inflammatory IL-1 [11].

The biochemical environment surrounding intra-articular fracture has also been the focus of investigation. Synovial fluid studies have been performed at the time of fracture demonstrating significant increases in pro-inflammatory markers including TNF-α, IFN-γ, multiple interleukins and matrix metalloproteinases, and hemarthrosis markers in comparison to the uninjured ankle [12]. The same group was able to perform a 6 month follow-up on several of these patients at the time of syndesmotic screw removal, with repeat analysis of injured and control ankle synovial fluid. The authors demonstrated continued elevation of inflammatory markers, even in the setting of complete bone healing [13]. Similar findings occurred when examining the synovium of fractures histologically, suggesting that the tissue of the ankle is also altered and may play a role in the degenerative environment postfracture [14]. These inflammatory changes have not been found to correlate to fracture treatment or quality of reduction, so are likely the natural history of the injury itself rather than a sequela of altered mechanics [15].

Overall, the basic science aspect of post-traumatic arthritis is a growing field and potential target for therapeutics in the future. While fracture reduction and treatment is key for the surgeon, management of the biological milieu within the joint may play an important role in mitigating cartilage damage in the future.

3 Preoperative Evaluation and Surgical Indications

Prior to indicating a patient for ankle arthrodesis, a thorough history and physical examination should be performed. Patient history should include prior fracture or instability events, medical history of inflammatory or other arthropathies, prior surgeries to the ankle, and any pain or dysfunction of other joints, including other joints in the foot, the knee/hip, or upper extremities, that may affect the patient's ability to rehabilitate postoperatively or accommodate the change in biomechanics. Other important aspects of social history include use of cigarettes or other nicotine sources, drug usage, and functional requirements/expectations, both recreational and vocational. A history of prior attempts at conservative management can also be beneficial. Recent studies have found a relative risk of nonunion of 5.8 in active smokers, so discussions about nicotine cessation are an important consideration, as these risks decline to normal in ex-smokers [16].

Physical examination should include the foot and continue upwards. Alignment of the foot itself, deformity at the hindfoot and ankle, and the entire limb alignment are important to evaluate. The skin should be evaluated for prior incisions, including prior soft tissue flap coverage. Vascular exam should be performed, and doppler pulse exam is necessary if pulses are not palpable. Neurologic exam can include Semmes-Weinstein monofilament testing if there is any concern for neuropathy, which may be present in a traumatized foot. Ankle stability and range of motion are important in surgical planning and patient expectations. Manually stabilizing the ankle demonstrating residual motion through the foot can be helpful for patients to understand the biomechanical changes of the arthrodesis and also help alleviate some of the anxiety associated with the term "fusion." Additionally, special attention on assessment of subtalar motion is critical, as limitations of subtalar mobility can significantly compromise gait mechanics and clinical outcomes. Ability to correct any deformity at the ankle should be evaluated, as well as any compensatory deformity at the foot from longstanding ankle malalignment.

Radiographic evaluation should consist, at a minimum, of weightbearing X-rays of the foot and ankle. Hindfoot alignment films and calibrated full length standing films can be helpful when assessing deformity and associated limb length discrepancy. Computed tomography (CT) scans can be helpful to assess bone quality, bone loss, and surrounding joint arthrosis. With the increasing availability of weightbearing CT (WBCT) in many practices, there is growing evidence that this modality provides increased information on hindfoot alignment, as well as compensatory deformity, that could be beneficial to the surgeon in operative planning [17, 18]. Magnetic resonance imaging (MRI) plays less of a role in routine workup of ankle arthritis but may be beneficial in select settings, such as evaluating for osteochondral lesions, or avascular necrosis (AVN) of the talus which may increase nonunion risk.

Based on the data obtained from the surgeon's evaluation, one can then synthesize an appropriate reconstructive plan for the patient. Once the plan for arthrodesis has been confirmed, there are multiple approaches and techniques the surgeon should be aware of to tailor to the specific patient presentation.

4 Surgical Techniques

Regardless of technique, the standard surgical principles of arthrodesis apply. There should be respect of the soft tissues and blood supply, as well as neurologic structures. Joint preparation is paramount, and all cartilage should be removed with feathering and/ or drilling of the subchondral surface of both the tibia and talus to access healthy bleeding bone. Alignment of the hindfoot should be performed with the ankle in neutral dorsiflexion/plantarflexion, five degrees of valgus, similar or slight external rotation to contralateral foot, and centralizing or slight posterior

shift of the talus under the tibia to maximize biomechanical function. To achieve these goals, there are multiple approaches, which can be selected based on surgeon experience and patient presentation.

4.1 Open (and Mini-Open)

Open preparation of the joint is the gold standard procedure. Direct visualization of the joint for debridement and removal of cartilage, removal of prior implants, application of biologics if indicated, and fixation can be performed through various approaches. Each approach is associated with its own risks and benefits. Overall, open ankle arthrodesis has a fusion rate reported in the 90–95% across multiple approaches [19, 20].

4.1.1 Anterior

This has become a workhorse approach for many surgeons. It has benefit of excellent visualization of the entire ankle joint, allows correction of deformity, and supplemental plate fixation can be directly applied through this approach. Anterior plate fixation in addition to crossed screws has demonstrated improvement in rigidity of the fixation construct, and many manufacturers have begun developing arthrodesis specific instrumentation for this approach [21–23]. Usage of an anterior plate has been shown to lead to an increased fusion rate and decreased complication rate in open arthrodesis [19]. Additionally, the same approach can be used for pilon fracture reduction or ankle joint debridement in earlier arthrosis. This approach can be reused for later conversion to arthroplasty if indicated. The anterior approach is also extensile distally if further work such as talonavicular or naviculocuneiform work is planned for hindfoot and/or midfoot stabilization.

Complications associated with this approach are usually soft tissue related. In nearly all cases, the superficial peroneal nerve and its branches will cross the incision. These must be managed carefully to prevent nerve pain or sensory loss, particularly in revision cases. More catastrophic is wound breakdown. There is a limited soft tissue envelope in this region. The tissue experiences significant tension during sagittal plane motion and has the risk of incisional breakdown due to bowstringing of the tibialis anterior and/or extensor hallucis longus tendons. Contraindications to the approach are prior trauma and incisions, prior flap reconstruction, other indications for fibular excision/osteotomy (osteomyelitis/deformity), or the need to access posterior implants.

This technique continues to evolve with surgeon understanding, technique, and implant design. As pre-contoured plates have become more common, so have lower-profile implants with greater rigidity. In uncomplicated cases, this allows for smaller "mini-open" approaches. Studies have demonstrated good access for joint preparation with these smaller incisions, with the benefit of decreased wound size for healing [24, 25]. Early anterior plating techniques included manual contouring of reconstruction plates, often with nonlocking fixation [21]. This progressed to pre-contoured locking plates, which were often thick and placed the at-risk anterior soft tissue envelope under further tension. Newer implants are smaller, using locking technology and larger screws (often 4.5 mm) to increase stability with a smaller footprint (Fig. 1). When placing an anterior plate, the risk of impingement on the talonavicular joint should be noted on lateral fluoroscopy.

Mini-open techniques are attempts at a less invasive modification of open techniques, and are anterior-based. These can include either a single

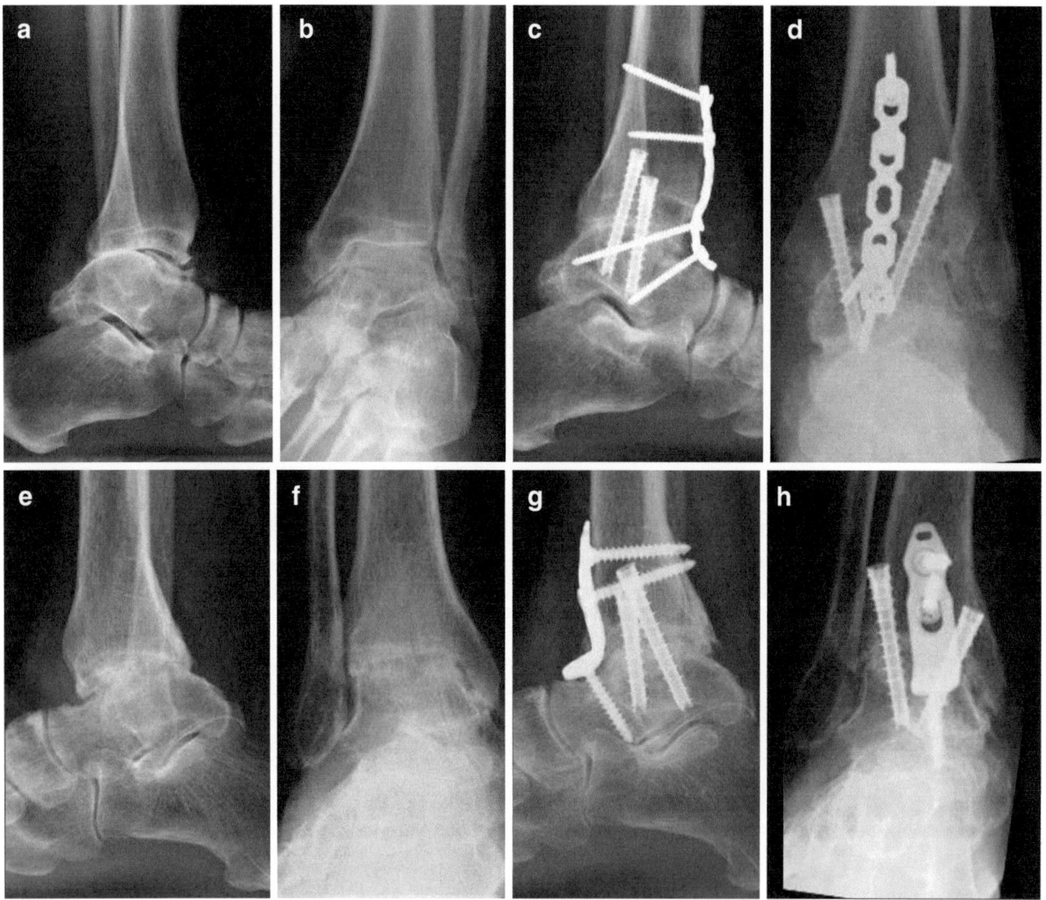

Fig. 1 Comparison of two anterior plating techniques. (**a**, **b**) Lateral and AP preoperative films. (**c**, **d**) Lateral and AP 3 month follow-up films. (**e**, **f**) Lateral and AP preoperative films. (**g**, **h**) Lateral and AP 3 month follow-up films

small anterior approach or multiple smaller incisions [25]. The benefit being that smaller incisions disrupt less blood supply and reduce soft tissue complications. Joint preparation techniques often include burrs in addition to the usual curettes/elevators/osteotomes to help denude cartilage and subchondral bone with less direct visualization. Fixation usually includes cannulated compression screws alone.

Authors' Technique: Tips and Tricks

The anterior approach is our workhorse approach for ankle arthrodesis. The authors prefer to perform the retinacular incision just lateral to the EHL tendon during the approach to maintain the sheath of the tibialis anterior and increase likelihood of a durable repair during closure. The deep approach remains the same, between the TA and EHL tendons, with care to protect the neurovascular bundle. One or two small crossing vessels often delineate the deep approach; these can be coagulated to mobilize the bundle. The retinacular layer should be repaired meticulously during closure with interrupted sutures.

Once the joint capsule is encountered, it is incised, and some tissue redundancy or synovitis can be excised. Anterior osteophytes and loose bodies are excised for visualization. A Gelpi retractor works well for tissue retraction while protecting neurovascular structures. Restoration of alignment may require preferential bone removal from medial or lateral joint. Lamina spreaders of pin distractors can be used to better access the joint surfaces. Curved curettes are helpful in the posterior joint for preparation.

After joint preparation and deformity correction, guide wires for compression screws are placed percutaneously, both medial and lateral, to stabilize the ankle. Additional screws can be place anterior-posterior or posterior-anterior ("home run") as indicated by deformity and bone quality. The wires are drilled and replaced by screws one at a time, to avoid losing fixation during the fixation process. We strive to obtain cannulated screw fixation and compression in the mid-talar body region, both medial and lateral to midline (Fig. 1). If bone quality is poor, or the bone blows out laterally, transfibular fixation is

an option as well. We prefer headless compression screws to avoid implant prominence. The anterior plate will help obtain central compression and stability. Depending on anterior tibial anatomy, an osteotome, or burr may be required to smooth out distal tibial prominence and allow for the plate to seat flush. This also helps reduce anterior soft tissue tension and the chance of talonavicular impingement.

4.1.2 Lateral

The lateral, or transfibular, approach to ankle arthrodesis was initially popularized by Mann [26]. He described an ankle fusion technique that uses a transfibular approach that affords good visualization, avoidance of nerve complications, and rigid fixation without the need for additional bone graft. While an effective technique, there are downfalls to sacrificing the fibula. An intact fibula provides another surface for bony union, a strut against valgus tilt in delayed/nonunion, and importantly, the ability to convert to ankle arthroplasty in the future. Some attempts at modifying the lateral approach have also been used with good success, with attempts to preserve the fibula using this approach [27]. Additionally, it can be challenging to prepare the medial aspect of the joint without a second incision [24].

The early approach described by Mann was a fibular sacrificing approach. This involved a sizeable incision of 15–20 cm along the fibula and aiming distally in the internervous plane between superficial peroneal and sural nerves. Full thickness flaps are developed, and the fibula excised for visualization of the tibiotalar joint. The fibula is osteotomized 3–4 cm proximal to the joint and beveled lateral-medial to avoid soft tissue irritation. This was combined with a 4 cm anteromedial approach to access this portion of the joint. He prepared the joints with flat cuts of the tibia and talus and transfixed the joint with two or three 6.5 mm screws from the lateral talus to the medial tibia for compression. Of note, much like the anterior approach, lateral plate supplementation has also become more common over time. This lateral fibular sacrificing approach is also useful in TTC preparation, as is gives access to both the tibiotalar and subtalar joints, and allows plate fixation across both joints in conjunction with, or substitution for, a TTC nail.

An alternate fibular sparing technique is also available. A similar initial approach is used, but the fibula is left on a posterior soft tissue hinge to maintain vascularity. After ankle or TTC arthrodesis, the inner surface of the fibula can be prepared with a sagittal flat cut, or standard arthrodesis preparation, and fixed back against the tibia at the syndesmosis, and against the talus as well. The lateral aspect of the tibia and talus should be prepared as well. This ideally provides another bony surface for union and maintains a lateral strut which allows later takedown conversion to ankle arthroplasty if indicated. Standard screw placement can still be used, or compression screws from the lateral-medial trajectory afforded by the surgical approach are acceptable. The fibula is fixed with transverse screws (Fig. 2). This can be combined with a mini-open anterior approach if needed for joint preparation, and there has been case series including a combined lateral and anterior approach with plating for TTC arthrodesis [28].

Wound healing is a risk factor, due to the less vascularized nature of the lateral tissues. Additionally, care must be taken to avoid aggressive soft tissue dissection over the talar neck, which may damage the tenuous blood supply to this bone. Peroneal tendons must be identified and protected to maintain function of the subtalar joint as well.

The lateral approach maintains a useful place in the surgeon's toolbox. In the authors' experience, it is more commonly used as a salvage approach at this time, when soft tissue or deformity are limiting factors preventing the anterior approach. In general, outcomes are similar to use of an anterior approach, therefore selection of the correct method falls on the surgeon and the patient presentation [29]. It benefits from avoiding the tenuous anterior skin in the setting of prior trauma, flap coverage, or other soft tissue concerns. This often allows usage of a prior inci-

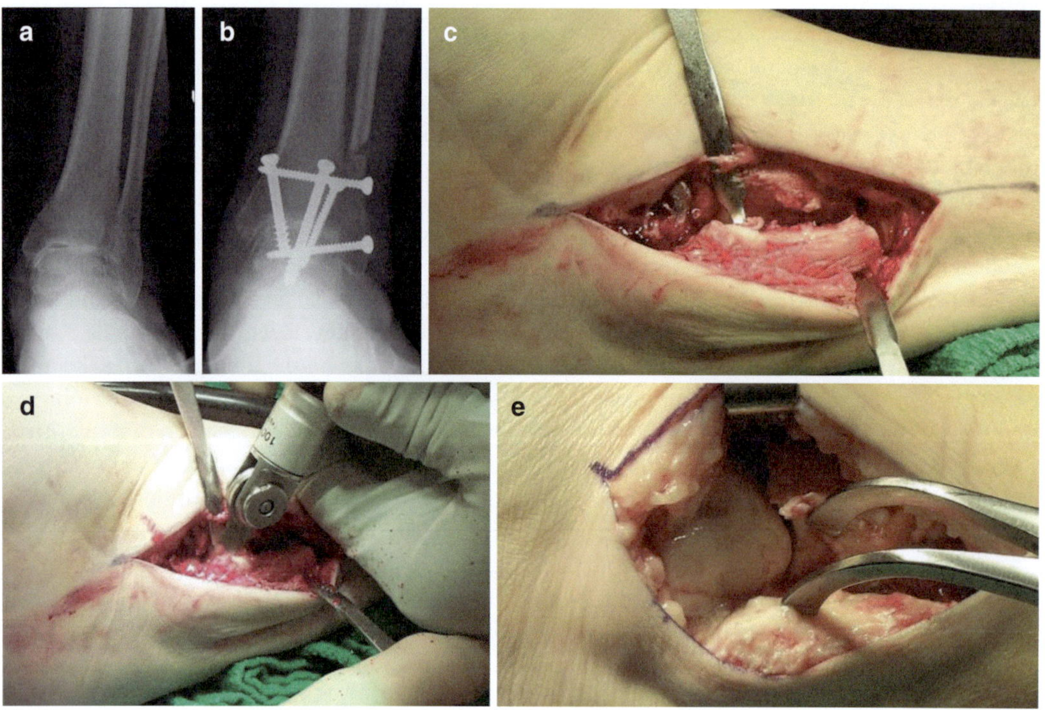

Fig. 2 Lateral approach radiographs and preparation. (**a, b**) Mortise preoperative and postoperative films. (**c**) Intraoperative photo of fibular osteotomy (proximal to right). (**d**) Sagittal cut to prepare internal (medial) surface of fibula. (**e**) Intra-operative view of lateral talus/tibiotalar joint with fibula retracted posteriorly

sion in the setting of post-traumatic arthritis, as prior fibular fracture fixation is common in this cohort. Removal of the fibula decompresses the lateral ankle and often aids in a tension free closure, which can be beneficial in soft tissue compromise or severe deformity. There is greater access to the distal tibia and talar body if bony resection/shortening must be performed for deformity correction. Additionally, the ability to fully access the talar body can be helpful if bulk allograft such as femoral head is needed due to talar collapse or bone loss.

4.1.3 Posterior

A third approach that the surgeon should be aware of is posterior. This can be direct posterior, or through a previously used posterolateral or posteromedial incision that was used in prior fracture fixation. While this approach is less commonly used that the traditional anterior or lateral approaches, it has several valuable indications. As mentioned, if there is failure of posterior implants from prior trauma, this approach can be used to remove these and perform the arthrodesis simultaneously (Fig. 3). In the setting of prior soft tissue reconstruction, or threatened anterior/lateral soft tissue, the posterior approach provides an option with robust soft tissue coverage distant to prior incisions or tissue flaps. Third, the approach can be used to perform a simultaneous tibiotalar and subtalar fusion, while preserving the fibula, in the setting of severe hindfoot post-traumatic arthritis or in the neuropathic patient.

There is limited literature on the isolated posterior tibiotalar arthrodesis, but the approach has been investigated thoroughly in the setting of TTC fusions. It has been described for use in severe deformity, with locked plating or intramedullary nailing. The posterior approach has been compared to the lateral approach and found to be safe and effective [30–34]. These patients are often positioned prone, which also adds some surgical and anesthetic challenges in longer, more complex cases.

4.2 Arthroscopic

As interest in minimally invasive techniques and instrumentation have grown, there has been increasing interest in arthroscopic ankle arthrodesis. The technique was first described in the 1980s, with increasing literature to support it. Smaller incisions and percutaneous fixation offer the benefits of decreased wound healing complications and soft tissue stripping and potentially less disruption of the blood supply to the tibia and talus. This technique can be particularly useful in patients with peripheral vascular disease or soft tissue trauma who have been optimized but remain at increased risk for wound healing complications. Barriers to the technique are the need for arthroscopic equipment and surgeon familiarity with ankle arthroscopy. It can also be more challenging to correct deformity with this approach, but deformity alone is not a contraindication to arthroscopic joint preparation. This is becoming more routine for foot and ankle trained orthopedists, but still not a common skill for traumatologists caring for their own post-traumatic patients. Additionally, no supplemental plating can be performed with this approach.

Longitudinal and comparative studies have demonstrated excellent fusions rates, generally exceeding 90% and approaching 100% in some studies with this technique [35, 36].Some comparative studies have even demonstrated higher fusion success rates with arthroscopic joint preparation compared to open techniques, with shorter time to union [35, 37]. It has also demonstrated some success in AVN of the talus, and this may be a benefit of soft tissue preservation [38]. Deformity correction can be challenging when using arthroscopic techniques. There have, however, been isolated reports of successful arthrodesis despite some larger defomities [39]. The principles of arthrodesis remain the same, and the joint must be fully denuded of all cartilage and sufficient perforation of the subchondral bone performed. Fixation is usually performed with 2–3 cannulated compression screws.

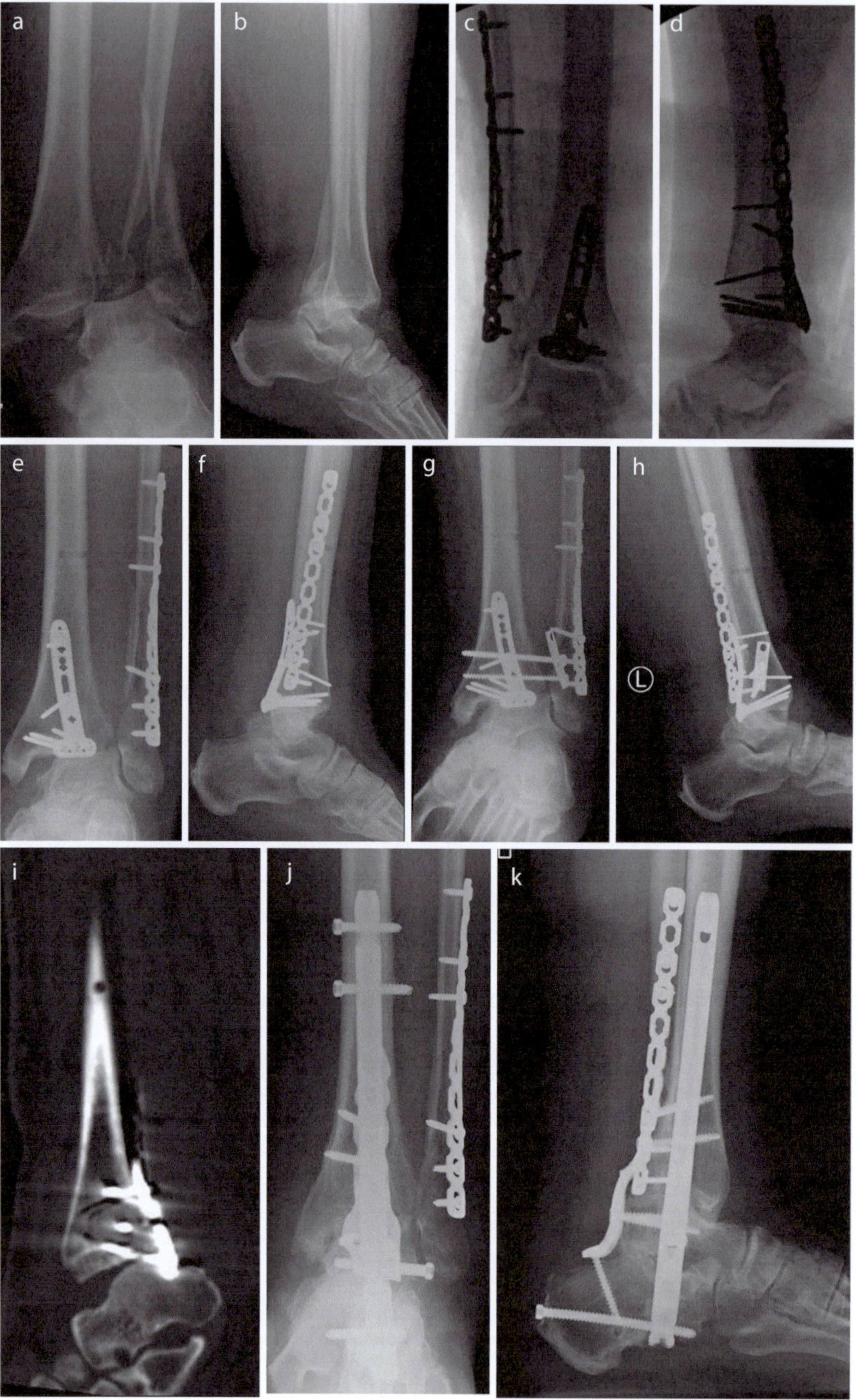

Fig. 3 Patient with BMI of 50, 1 pack per day smoker referred to Foot & Ankle for salvage after failed ORIF and revision ORIF. (**a**, **b**) AP and Lateral injury films. (**c**, **d**) Intraoperative AP and lateral views. (**e**, **f**) Early failure at 6 week follow-up. (**g–i**) Continued loss of reduction after syndesmotic revision. (**j**, **k**) Successful fusion 3 months after posterior approach implant removal and TTC arthrodesis

4.3   External Fixation

External fixation is not a standalone "technique," per se, but an important adjunct to hindfoot salvage and arthrodesis. It plays a particularly important role in the post-traumatic arthritic ankle, especially in the circumstances of infection, poor soft tissue status, and significant tibial axis deformity or malalignment. It has been shown to provide good fusion rates with good maintenance of alignment as well [40]. Like previously discussed techniques, the ankle joint must be prepared (open or arthroscopically) for arthrodesis prior to application of the external ring fixator. Definitive fusion with external fixation is generally performed with a thin wire ring fixator, which provides the greatest stability and options for deformity correction and compression.

Fusion via external fixation provides an excellent salvage opportunity, and the technique fits particularly well with the challenges of the post-traumatic ankle. The simplest of uses can be in a patient with poor soft tissues. By minimizing incisions for implant placement, the soft tissue envelope can be preserved. Additionally, a fixator with adjustable struts can be used in the setting of severe post-traumatic deformity with skin contracture to gradually correct the deformity prior to final arthrodesis, limiting soft tissue complications with acute correction [42–44]. This can be performed entirely with the ring fixator, or a transition to internal fixation after deformity correction, to limit time in the frame. Another valuable, and likely most common, case for ring fixation is the setting of infection. An example may be a pilon fracture that has become infected and failed internal fixation. In such a case, the implants could be removed, the joint prepared for arthrod-esis, and the fixator used to stabilize the fusion site, and soft tissues, primarily while avoiding local instrumentation and allowing antibiotic treatment. These principles carry over from the Charcot literature, demonstrating the benefits of external versus internal fixation in the setting of active infection [45, 46].

Ring fixation is also helpful in the most complex of cases. This is an excellent salvage option in the setting of significant bone loss, or in the need for extensive bony resection for clearance of osteomyelitis [47]. Use of external fixation can allow for simultaneous bony resection and fracture site debridement, excision of necrotic bone, shortening of the tibiotalar region if necessary for soft tissue coverage, and proximal bone transport to salvage the functional length of the limb. While increasingly complex and requiring an experienced surgeon, this option provides for the salvage of a post-traumatic limb in a setting where below-knee amputation may be the only other valid option. Additionally, a fixator can be used to stabilize bone and soft tissue in the setting of multiple debridements or soft tissue reconstruction by the plastic surgery team (Fig. 4).

Ring fixation is a complex task, and both static and dynamic frames have risks to the patient. These devices require expertise not only for application, but for long-term management. It is common to require pin changes for infection and strut changes for dynamic frames. Patients may not tolerate the bulky device for extended periods of time, and it can lead to issues with clothing and ambulation. A severe complication is the potential for fracture through half-pin sites in the tibia [41]. Despite this, this method of fixation confers important and valuable benefits and the option for limb salvage, in select patients.

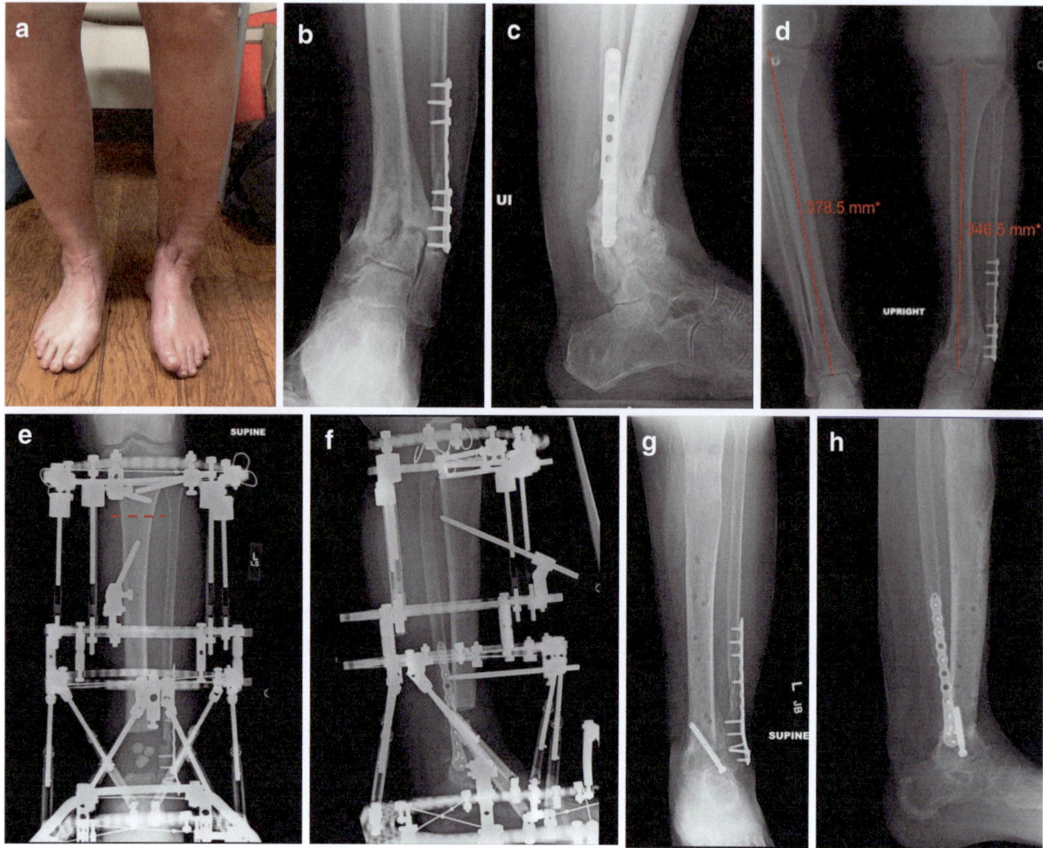

Fig. 4 Reconstruction of infected malunion with bone transport. (**a**) Clinical photo of alignment. (**b**, **c**) AP and lateral views of malunion. (**d**) Limb length view demonstrating loss of length and alignment. (**e**, **f**) AP and lateral in thin-wire frame with proximal osteotomy (red dotted line) and distal excision of necrotic bone and antibiotic spacer. (**g**, **h**) Successful docking and fusion with supplemental hardware distal and well-healed regenerate bone proximal

5 Special Considerations

5.1 The Varus Ankle

Every ankle fusion should involve preoperative planning and consideration of multiple patient specific factors, particularly in the post-traumatic setting. One common deformity requiring special attention is the varus arthritic ankle. Varus deformity can be intra-articular or extra-articular. It can be secondary to the trauma or due to the patient's native anatomy. It can develop from varus malunion of the tibia and or talus, talar neck malunion, compartment syndrome sequelae, or from chronic lateral ankle instability in post-traumatic cases. Varus alignment has been identified as an independent predictor of nonunion in large studies, with greater than double the nonunion rate of a neutral preoperative alignment [20].

The subtalar joint often compensates for malalignment of the ankle, and its flexibility must be evaluated preoperatively, as well as associated foot alignment and compensatory deformity [48]. The compensatory deformities of the foot in general must also be studied during preoperative planning. A host of other foot deformities must be considered when correcting the varus ankle, depending on the associated foot alignment. Most of the concomitant surgical options are those associated with the cavovarus foot in general, including a lateral calcaneal closing wedge/slide, first metatarsal dorsiflexion, claw toe corrections, gastrocnemius recession or Achilles lengthening, plantar fascia release, peroneus longus to brevis transfer, or talonavicular arthrodesis [49, 50]. Of paramount importance is the posteromedial release of the hindfoot. In the setting of significant cavovarus deformity, the soft tissue structures must be aggressively released to allow for deformity correction. This must be patient specific but generally includes the posterior tibial and flexor digitorum longus tendon, talonavicular and subtalar joint capsule, spring and deltoid ligament, plantar fascia, and tarsal tunnel [50]. This will allow for a more balanced plantigrade foot after deformity correction and arthrodesis of the ankle. Many of these soft tissue structures also may contract subsequent to

a lower extremity compartment syndrome and can be seen commonly in post-traumatic foot/ankle deformity. Providing a well-balanced foot for the patient is important to maximize function beneath an ankle arthrodesis.

5.2 Tibial Osteotomy

In the setting of extra-articular fractures, or prior fracture malreduction, the development of post-traumatic arthritis may come from malalignment rather than cartilage and joint trauma. In these unique cases, the ankle joint may be able to be salvaged, at least temporarily, with a corrective osteotomy. In response to injury, ankle cartilage has been shown to produce proteoglycans at an accelerated rate compared to other joints [11]. Therefore, the ankle may be more amenable to joint salvage techniques. At the least, appropriate realignment of the lower extremity axis can improve the outcomes of future ankle arthrodesis or fusion, as well as alignment at the hip and knee. Additionally, these procedures may occur concurrently with the ankle arthrodesis. Attempts at joint preservation with standard supramalleolar osteotomy have been shown to be successful and are worth consideration in patients that are symptomatic with milder radiographic changes and any residual malalignment [51, 52]. Additionally, osteotomies or malunion corrections at other levels along the tibial axis may be required in advance of, or simultaneous with, the planned ankle arthrodesis. These osteotomies can be either intra-articular (Fig. 5) or remote from the tibiotalar joint (Fig. 6), depending on the deformity location. Osteotomy for deformity correction can be accomplished with multiple techniques including open or percutaneous methods and can be stabilized with internal or external fixation [42, 53].

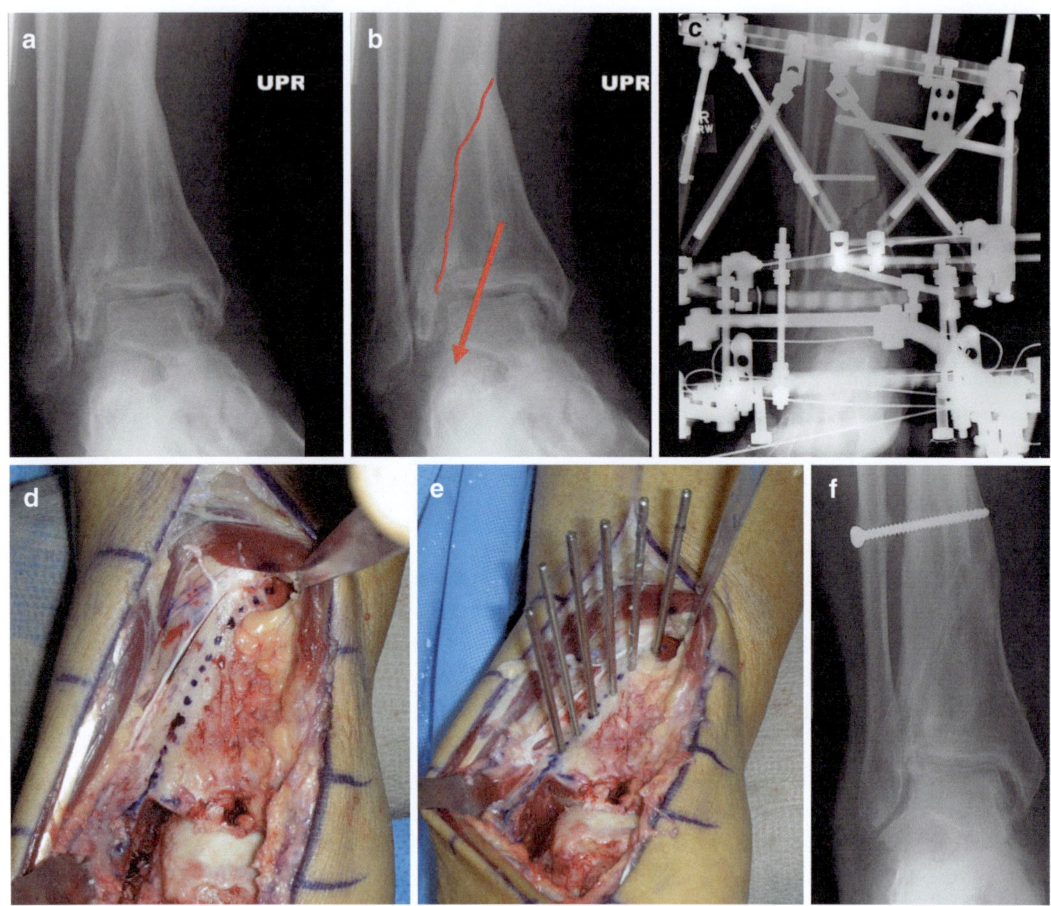

Fig. 5 Joint sparing osteotomy for post-traumatic malunion with early arthrosis. (**a**) AP view demonstrating shortening and varus malalignment. (**b**) Proposed osteotomy site and translation. (**c**) AP image after osteotomy and frame placement. (**d**, **e**) Intraoperative view of osteotomy using multiple drill holes. F: Healed osteotomy with improved alignment

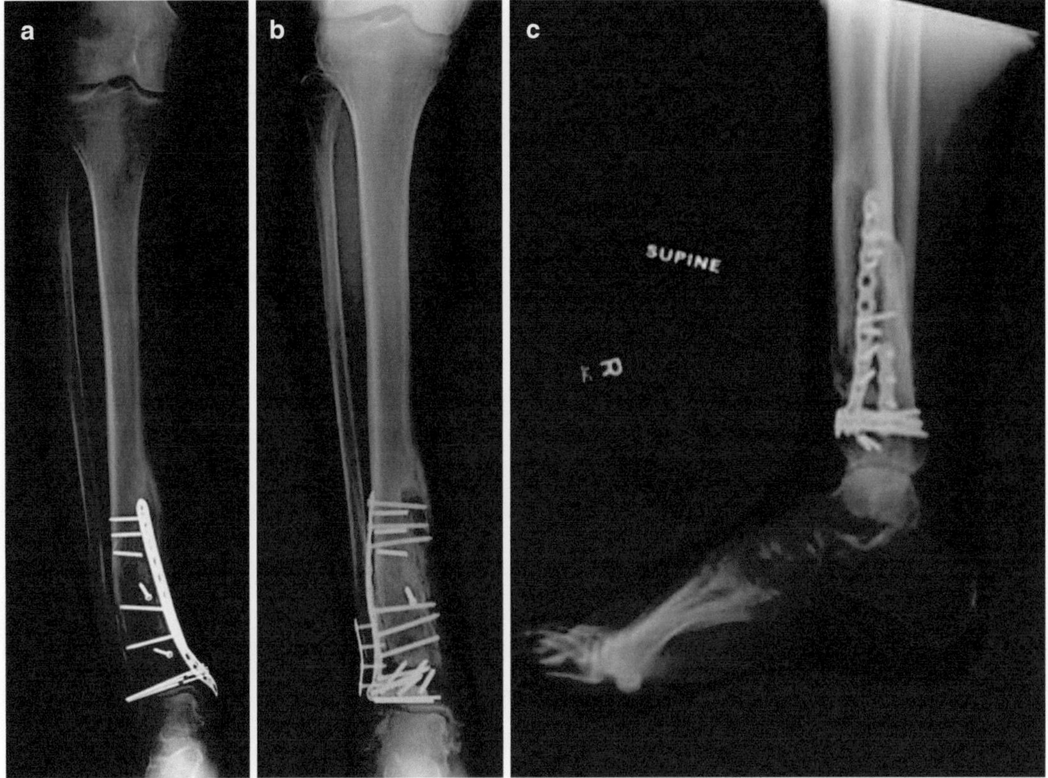

Fig. 6 Salvage of post-traumatic varus malunion with osteotomy and internal fixation. (**a**) AP Tibia demonstrating limb malalignment and implant failure. (**b, c**) AP and lateral views of healed osteotomy with restoration of alignment

5.3 Tibiotalocalcaneal Arthrodesis

Tibiotalocalcaneal (TTC) arthrodesis is a technique useful for revision arthrodesis, severe trauma with concomitant tibiotalar and subtalar arthritis, or for increased stability and fixation in poor bone quality or patients with severe neuropathy. Fusion rates are less favorable than ankle arthrodesis alone, often in the 85–90% range, with complication rates approaching 30%, but this technique should be reserved for complex and salvage situations [54]. This can be performed through multiple approaches, similar to tibiotalar arthrodesis mentioned above. This should be tailored based on soft tissue considerations, prior incisions, direction of deformity and the need for removal of any implants present. In the setting of minimal deformity, a combination of standard anterior tibiotalar and separate sinus tarsi approaches is possible. A single transfibular

incision can be used to address both joints simultaneously, as can the posterior approach (Achilles splitting or posterolateral/posteromedial). Fixation options include TTC nails, plate fixation, external fixation, or some hybrid of these options, as seen in Figs. 3 and 4 [28, 31].

The same techniques of arthrodesis apply, with careful soft tissue handling and respect for the blood supply, meticulous joint preparation, deformity correction, and rigid fixation. This technique can also be beneficial in the setting of talus AVN or significant bone loss, in order to salvage limb length. The classic technique is to use a femoral head allograft to replace excised bone, but this has been shown to have poor arthrodesis rates in some populations [55]. There is developing interest in custom implants to fill a post-traumatic void, with three-dimensional printing of custom mesh implants to incorporate into fusion constructs as a limb salvage option, though long term studies are lacking at this time [56, 57].

5.4 Conclusion

In summary, post-traumatic ankle arthrosis is one of the most common presentations of symptomatic arthritis in the orthopaedic surgeon's patient population. This is a multifactorial process, with many treatment options available in the surgeon's armamentarium, from approach to fixation techniques. The biological basis of these changes remain under investigation, but maintaining appropriate anatomic alignment is key for the surgeon. Techniques for treatment will likely continue to evolve, but arthrodesis currently remains the gold standard for management of post-traumatic tibiotalar arthritis.

References

1. Huch K, Kuettner KE, Dieppe P. Osteoarthritis in ankle and knee joints. Semin Arthritis Rheum. 1997;26:667–74.
2. Muehleman C, Bareither D, Huch K, Cole AA, Kuettner KE. Prevalence of degenerative morphological changes in the joints of the lower extremity. Osteoarthr Cartil. 1997;5:23–37.
3. Kempson GE. Age-related changes in the tensile properties of human articular cartilage: a comparative study between the femoral head of the hip joint and the talus of the ankle joint. Biochim Biophys Acta. 1991;1075:223–30.
4. Athanasiou KA, Niederauer GG, Schenck RC. Biomechanical topography of human ankle cartilage. Ann Biomed Eng. 1995;23:697–704.
5. Saltzman CL, et al. Epidemiology of ankle arthritis: report of a consecutive series of 639 patients from a tertiary orthopaedic center. Iowa Orthop J. 2005;25:44–6.
6. Valderrabano V, Horisberger M, Russell I, Dougall H, Hintermann B. Etiology of ankle osteoarthritis. Clin Orthop Relat Res. 2009;467:1800–6.
7. Deleu PA, et al. Post-sprain versus post-fracture post-traumatic ankle osteoarthritis: impact on foot and ankle kinematics and kinetics. Gait Posture. 2021;86:278–86.
8. Seaworth CM, et al. Epidemiology of total ankle arthroplasty: trends in New York State. Orthopedics. 2016;39:170–6.
9. Sturnick DR, et al. Adjacent joint kinematics after ankle arthrodesis during cadaveric gait simulation. Foot Ankle Int. 2017;38:1249–59.
10. Ling JS, et al. Investigating the relationship between ankle arthrodesis and adjacent-joint arthritis in the hindfoot: a systematic review. J Bone Joint Surg Am. 2015;97:513–9.
11. Kuettner KE, Cole AA. Cartilage degeneration in different human joints. Osteoarthr Cartil. 2005;13:93–103.
12. Adams SB, et al. Inflammatory cytokines and matrix metalloproteinases in the synovial fluid after intra-articular ankle fracture. Foot Ankle Int. 2015;36:1264–71.
13. Adams SB, et al. Inflammatory microenvironment persists after bone healing in intra-articular ankle fractures. Foot Ankle Int. 2017;38:479–84.
14. Furman BD, et al. Articular ankle fracture results in increased synovitis, synovial macrophage infiltration, and synovial fluid concentrations of inflammatory cytokines and chemokines. Arthritis Rheumatol. 2015;67:1234–9.
15. Pham TM, et al. Association of acute inflammatory cytokines, fracture malreduction, and functional outcome 12 months after intra-articular ankle fracture- a prospective cohort study of 46 patients with ankle fractures. J Orthop Surg Res. 2021;16:338.
16. Allport J, Ramaskandhan J, Siddique MS. Nonunion rates in hind- and midfoot arthrodesis in current, ex-, and nonsmokers. Foot Ankle Int. 2021;42:582–8.
17. Barg A, et al. Weightbearing computed tomography of the foot and ankle: emerging technology topical review. Foot Ankle Int. 2018;39:376–86.
18. Richter M, Seidl B, Zech S, Hahn S. PedCAT for 3D-imaging in standing position allows for more accurate bone position (angle) measurement than radiographs or CT. Foot Ankle Surg. 2014;20:201–7.
19. van den Heuvel SBM, Doorgakant A, Birnie MFN, Blundell CM, Schepers T. Open ankle arthrodesis: a systematic review of approaches and fixation methods. Foot Ankle Surg. 2021;27:339–47.
20. Chalayon O, et al. Factors affecting the outcomes of uncomplicated primary open ankle arthrodesis. Foot Ankle Int. 2015;36:1170–9.
21. Tarkin IS, et al. Anterior plate supplementation increases ankle arthrodesis construct rigidity. Foot Ankle Int. 2007;28:219–23.
22. Kestner CJ, Glisson RR, Nunley JA. A biomechanical analysis of two anterior ankle arthrodesis systems. Foot Ankle Int. 2013;34:1006–11.
23. Plaass C, Knupp M, Barg A, Hintermann B. Anterior double plating for rigid fixation of isolated tibiotalar arthrodesis. Foot Ankle Int. 2009;30:631–9.
24. Chinnakkannu K, et al. Mini-open vs. transfibular approach for ankle arthrodesis, which approach is superior in joint preparation: a cadaver study. Indian J Orthop. 2020;55:135–41.
25. Paremain GD, Miller SD, Myerson MS. Ankle arthrodesis: results after the miniarthrotomy technique. Foot Ankle Int. 1996;17:247–52.
26. Mann RA, Van Manen JW, Wapner K, Martin J. Ankle fusion. Clin Orthop Relat Res. 1991;(268):49–55.
27. Smith JT, Chiodo CP, Singh SK, Wilson MG. Open ankle arthrodesis with a fibular-sparing technique. Foot Ankle Int. 2013;34:557–62.

28. Ciufo DJ, Grant AM. Orthogonal locked plating for tibiotalocalcaneal arthrodesis. Tech Foot Ankle Surg. 2022;21(1):40–7. https://doi.org/10.1097/BTF.0000000000000295.

29. Kim JG, et al. Ankle arthrodesis: a comparison of anterior approach and transfibular approach. Clin Orthop Surg. 2018;10:368–73.

30. Mulligan RP, Adams SB, Easley ME, DeOrio JK, Nunley JA. Comparison of posterior approach with intramedullary nailing versus lateral transfibular approach with fixed-angle plating for tibiotalocalcaneal arthrodesis. Foot Ankle Int. 2017;38:1343–51.

31. Kile TA, Donnelly RE, Gehrke JC, Werner ME, Johnson KA. Tibiotalocalcaneal arthrodesis with an intramedullary device. Foot Ankle Int. 1994;15:669–73.

32. Nickisch F, Avilucea FR, Beals T, Saltzman C. Open posterior approach for tibiotalar arthrodesis. Foot Ankle Clin. 2011;16:103–14.

33. Pellegrini MJ, et al. Outcomes of tibiotalocalcaneal arthrodesis through a posterior achilles tendon-splitting approach. Foot Ankle Int. 2016;37:312–9.

34. Fetter NL, DeOrio JK. Posterior approach with fibular preservation for tibiotalocalcaneal arthrodesis with an intramedullary nail. Foot Ankle Int. 2012;33:746–9.

35. Quayle J, et al. Arthroscopic versus open ankle arthrodesis. Foot Ankle Surg. 2018;24:137–42.

36. Ferkel RD, Hewitt M. Long-term results of arthroscopic ankle arthrodesis. Foot Ankle Int. 2005;26:275–80.

37. Myerson MS, Quill G. Ankle arthrodesis: a comparison of an arthroscopic and an open method of treatment. Clin Orthop Relat Res. 1991;(268):84–95.

38. Kendal AR, Cooke P, Sharp R. Arthroscopic ankle fusion for avascular necrosis of the talus. Foot Ankle Int. 2015;36:591–7.

39. Dannawi Z, Nawabi DH, Patel A, Leong JJH, Moore DJ. Arthroscopic ankle arthrodesis: are results reproducible irrespective of pre-operative deformity? Foot Ankle Surg. 2011;17:294–9.

40. Morasiewicz P, et al. Radiological evaluation of ankle arthrodesis with Ilizarov fixation compared to internal fixation. Injury. 2017;48:1678–83.

41. Jones CP, Youngblood SA, Waldrop N, Davis WH, Pinzur MS. Tibial stress fracture secondary to half-pins in circular ring external fixation for charcot foot. Foot Ankle Int. 2014;35:572–7.

42. Paley D, Lamm BM, Katsenis D, Bhave A, Herzenberg JE. Treatment of malunion and nonunion at the site of an ankle fusion with the Ilizarov apparatus. J Bone Joint Surg. 2006;88:119–34.

43. Paley D. Principles of deformity correction. Berlin: Springer; 2002. https://doi.org/10.1007/978-3-642-59,373-4.

44. Paley D, Chaudray M, Pirone AM, Lentz P, Kautz D. Treatment of malunions and mal-nonunions of the femur and tibia by detailed preoperative planning and the Ilizarov techniques. Orthop Clin North Am. 1990;21:667–91.

45. Conway JD. Charcot salvage of the foot and ankle using external fixation. Foot Ankle Clin. 2008;13:157–73.

46. Lee DJ, Schaffer J, Chen T, Oh I. Internal versus external fixation of charcot midfoot deformity realignment. Orthopedics. 2016;39:e595–601.

47. Lovisetti G, Kirienko A, Myerson C, Vulcano E. Ankle salvage following nonunion of distal tibia fractures. Foot Ankle Int. 2018;39:1210–8.

48. Wang B, Saltzman CL, Chalayon O, Barg A. Does the subtalar joint compensate for ankle malalignment in end-stage ankle arthritis? Clin Orthop Relat Res. 2015;473:318–25.

49. AlSayel F, Valderrabano V. Arthrodesis of a varus ankle. Foot Ankle Clin. 2019;24:265–80.

50. Fortin P, Guettler J, Manoli AR, Oak MI. Idiopathic cavovarus and lateral ankle instability: recognition and treatment implications relating to ankle arthritis. Foot Ankle Int. 2002.

51. Krähenbühl N, Susdorf R, Barg A, Hintermann B. Supramalleolar osteotomy in post-traumatic valgus ankle osteoarthritis. Int Orthop. 2020;44:535–43.

52. Choi JY, Kim KW, Suh JS. Low tibial valgization osteotomy for more severe varus ankle arthritis. Foot Ankle Int. 2020;41:1122–32.

53. Goodier WD, Calder PR. External fixation for the correction of adult post-traumatic deformities. Injury. 2019;50:S36–44.

54. Hegeman E, Dowd TC, Huh J. Outcomes following intramedullary nail vs plate fixation for tibiotalocalcaneal arthrodesis: a systematic review. Foot Ankle Orthop. 2022;7:2473011421S00230.

55. Jeng CL, Campbell JT, Tang EY, Cerrato RA, Myerson MS. Tibiotalocalcaneal arthrodesis with bulk femoral head allograft for salvage of large defects in the ankle. Foot Ankle Int. 2013;34:1256–66.

56. Heidari KS, Lalli T. Case report: tibiotalocalcaneal arthrodesis utilizing a titanium mesh implant for limb salvage after failed charcot reconstruction. Foot Ankle Orthop. 2022;7:2473011421S00231.

57. Steele JR, et al. Comparison of 3D printed spherical implants versus femoral head allografts for tibiotalocalcaneal arthrodesis. J Foot Ankle Surg. 2020;59:1167–70.

Total Ankle Arthroplasty for Posttraumatic Arthritis of the Ankle Joint

Albert T. Anastasio, Brandon Haghverdian, Ben Umbel, and Mark E. Easley

1 Introduction

1.1 The Anatomy of the Ankle Joint

The ankle joint is comprised of articulations between the distal tibia, the fibula, and the talus. Multiple ligamentous structures provide static constraint to the ankle, and normal range of motion for the joint is 20 degrees of dorsiflexion and 50 degrees of plantarflexion, with minimal contribution to inversion and eversion [1]. Compared to cartilage found in other joints, the cartilage found in the ankle has greater stiffness and decreased permeability. The chondrocytes found within the ankle can synthesize proteoglycans at an increased rate, contributing to an increased repair capacity of the joint.

The tibial plafond and medial malleolus articulate both dorsally and medially with the talus. The tibial plafond articular surface is 88–92 degrees relative to the lateral tibial shaft axis in the coronal plane, and there is a slight posterior slope to the plafond in the sagittal plane. The articular surface of the talus is comprised of 60% articular cartilage and a central trochlea is present on the talus to allow for tibial articulation and increased stability of the ankle joint [2]. The fibula articulates with the lateral talus and provides a lateral buttress for the ankle joint. The fibula also serves as the attachment point of several important ligamentous structures including those comprising the distal tibiofibular syndesmosis and the lateral ankle ligamentous complex.

1.2 Consideration of Adjacent Joints

The ankle joint acts in close concert with the surrounding joints, particularly the subtalar joint, the talonavicular joint, and the calcaneocuboid joints. The joints of the midfoot also play a crucial role in maintaining normal ankle biomechanics [3]. To function optimally, the ankle joint must rest on a stable platform—degenerative and traumatic conditions which affect the adjacent joints surrounding the ankle can have profound implications on the ankle and tibiotalar joints themselves.

1.3 Pathogenesis of Ankle Arthritis

Posttraumatic arthritis has been implicated as the most common reason by far for the development of severe degenerative change to the ankle joint

A. T. Anastasio · B. Haghverdian · B. Umbel · M. E. Easley (✉)
Division of Foot and Ankle, Department of Orthopaedic Surgery, Duke University, Durham, NC, USA
e-mail: albert.anastasio@duke.edu; brandon.hagverdian@duke.edu; benjamin.umbel@duke.edu; mark.e.easley@duke.edu

© The Author(s), under exclusive license to Springer Nature Switzerland AG 2023
D. Herscovici Jr. et al. (eds.), *Evaluation and Surgical Management of the Ankle*,
https://doi.org/10.1007/978-3-031-33537-2_22

[4]. Intra-articular fractures and ankle fracture-dislocations with malunion both contribute highly to the progression of arthritis in the ankle joint. Even fractures of the ankle which have been anatomically fixed through open reduction and internal fixation show high rates of progression to posttraumatic arthritis, given the presence of a potent inflammatory milieu, with a number of factors having been associated with cartilage degradation [5]. Additionally, trauma without bony injury can cause posttraumatic arthritis to the ankle joint. Many patients will report a history of chronic ankle instability with multiple subluxation or sprain events.

While the majority of cases of end stage ankle arthritis are associated with prior trauma, there are a number of other potential causes for degeneration of the ankle joint. These include inflammatory arthropathies, the most common being rheumatoid arthritis [6]. Additionally, hemochromatosis, Charcot neuroarthropathy, septic arthritis, pigmented villonodular synovitis, and more proximal fractures causing biomechanical alignment aberrancies can contribute to or cause ankle arthritis.

2 Clinical Assessment

2.1 History and Physical Examination

Patients with post-traumatic arthritis of the ankle present either with history of a significant bony injury to the ankle, particularly intra-articular fracture, or with a history of chronic ankle instability with recurrent ankle sprains. Typically, patients report pain that is worse with weight-bearing. They may also complain of ankle swelling, joint stiffness, and progressive limitations in their activity level. Symptoms may be particularly severe while going up-hill due to anterior ankle joint impingement with dorsiflexion.

Physical examination of the patient with post-traumatic ankle joint arthritis may reveal antalgic gait as well as obligatory hip external rotation, as the patient attempts to externally rotate the ankle to avoid a painful push-off. Tenderness to palpation at the anterior ankle joint or the medial and lateral gutters may be present. Decreased range of motion with crepitation is common, and both passive and active ranging of the ankle joint may be painful, especially at the extremes of ankle dorsiflexion, given high rates of anterior tibiotalar impingement accompanying posttraumatic arthritis of the ankle. Variable edema may also be present about the ankle joint. The treating provider should carefully evaluate the alignment of the affected limb for the presence of varus or valgus deformity secondary to chronic instability, as significant deformity may need to be addressed during surgery. The treating physician should also assess the patient from the posterior aspect to determine hindfoot alignment. Lastly, a careful vascular exam should be performed on all patients, including assessment of capillary refill as well as palpation of the dorsalis pedis and posterior tibial pulses. If there is any question regarding a patient's vascular status, a low threshold should be maintained for referral for vascular consultation to assess acceptability for invasive surgical intervention [7].

2.2 Imaging

Imaging evaluation of the patient with posttraumatic ankle arthritis begins with weight-bearing radiographs including the AP, lateral, and mortise views of the ankle. If there is any concern for associated hindfoot or leg deformity, weight-bearing views of the tibia and fibula as well as hindfoot (Salztman) alignment views should be obtained. The Saltzman view will allow for careful delineation of degree of varus or valgus deformity through the heel, which can be very important to address at the time of the TAA procedure [8]. AP, lateral, and oblique radiographs of the foot should be performed to evaluate any associated deformity through the forefoot or midfoot. Furthermore, full length hip-to-knee mechanical axis views can be obtained, in the event that there is a more proximal deformity that needs to be considered and addressed (Fig. 1).

Of emerging importance in the evaluation of the candidate for total ankle arthroplasty (TAA)

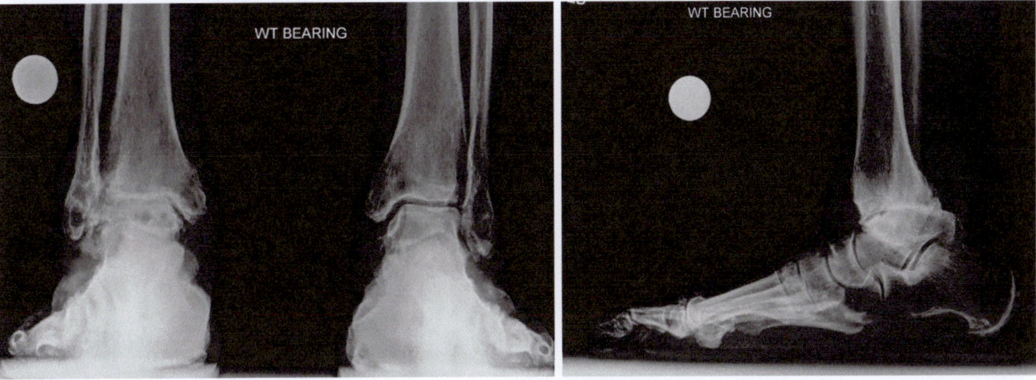

Fig. 1 Imaging evaluation of the patient with posttraumatic ankle arthritis begins with weight-bearing radiographs including the AP and lateral views of the ankle

is the use of weight-bearing computed tomography (CT) scans of the ankle and foot. These scans can provide three-dimensional (3D) visualization of hindfoot alignment and bone stock about the tibia and talus [9]. CT scan can also alert the treating surgeon to the presence of cysts which may need to be addressed at the time of surgery with curettage and bone grafting. CT scan is also used for patient specific instrumentation (PSI) templating, which may confer an advantage in optimizing ideal axial plane rotational alignment [10]. In rare cases where custom or total talus replacements are performed in conjunction with TAA, the contralateral talus may need to be imaged via CT to aid in generation of the talus component. Magnetic resonance imaging (MRI) can be considered in cases where there is concern for pathology present in the surrounding soft tissues, such as peroneal tendon tendinopathy or subluxation. Both CT and MRI can also be useful in identifying avascular necrosis (AVN) of the talus (Fig. 2).

2.3 Indications for TAA

As implantation techniques develop, prosthesis manufacturing technologies advance, and outcomes continue to improve, [11] a higher number of patients presenting with posttraumatic arthritis of the ankle should be considered for TAA as a motion preserving option for end stage ankle joint arthritis. However, careful patient selection

is imperative to ensure proper candidacy for TAA. First, nonoperative management options should be trialed. These include activity and shoewear modification including stiff-soled shoe or rocker bottom alteration. Additionally, an ankle-foot orthosis can be trialed. Pharmaceutical management for posttraumatic ankle arthritis includes nonsteroidal anti-inflammatory medications and topical analgesics as well as viscosupplementation and intra-articular corticosteroid injection.

Once a prolonged period of nonoperative management has failed, patients can be considered for TAA. There are several factors which may influence appropriate patient selection for TAA. Several patient specific comorbidities such as obesity, history of smoking, history of depression, diabetes mellitus, and neuropathy have been linked to failure and poor outcomes after TAA. Neuropathy specifically is a contraindication to TAA. Sensory nerve deficiencies in the affected extremity can cause a patient to lose important protective proprioceptive sensation, thereby precluding TAA. Likewise, if motor deficits are present, the patient will be left without active range of motion of the ankle after TAA. Additional considerations include young age, especially in patients employed in positions where they are on their feet for many hours, given implant longevity limitations. Furthermore, current range of motion and preexisting deformity should be considered in the evaluation of fitness for TAA. Traditionally, cases of severe deformity

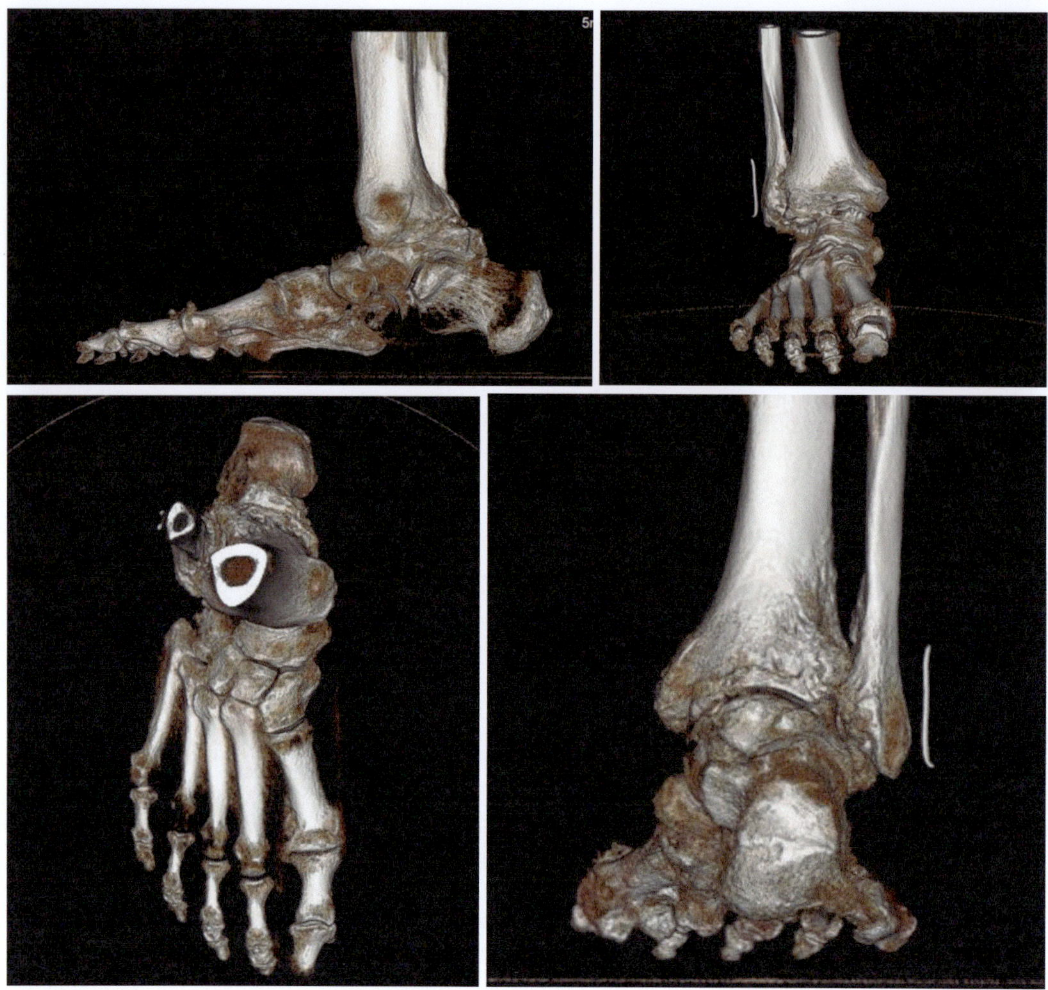

Fig. 2 Weight-bearing CT scans of the ankle can provide 3D visualization of hindfoot alignment and bone stock about the tibia and talus

were thought to be poor candidates for TAA, but more recent literature has indicated that even in cases of severe preoperative deformity, if the deformity through the ankle and surrounding joints is appropriately addressed at the time of TAA, outcomes can mirror those of patients with minor or nonexistent deformity [12–15].

Additional factors to consider in the patient with posttraumatic arthritis who is a potential candidate for TAA include the presence and location of previous surgical scars which may guide surgical approach. If there is concern regarding anterior soft tissues due to prior trauma or surgery, implants which can be placed through a lateral transfibular approach are also available. In

select cases, consultation with a plastic surgeon may be necessary to guide optimal soft tissue management. Plastic surgeons can offer additional procedures such as preoperative flap coverage which may improve candidacy for TAA. Careful neurovascular examination to assess for adequacy of perfusion and for degree of neuropathy is imperative. If dorsiflexion is significantly limited, heel cord lengthening or gastrocnemius recession at the time of TAA can be employed. Additionally, history of previous ipsilateral surgical procedures should be obtained, as the presence of hardware about the leg or ankle may impede placement of either the talar or tibial component of the TAA. A prior ipsilateral total

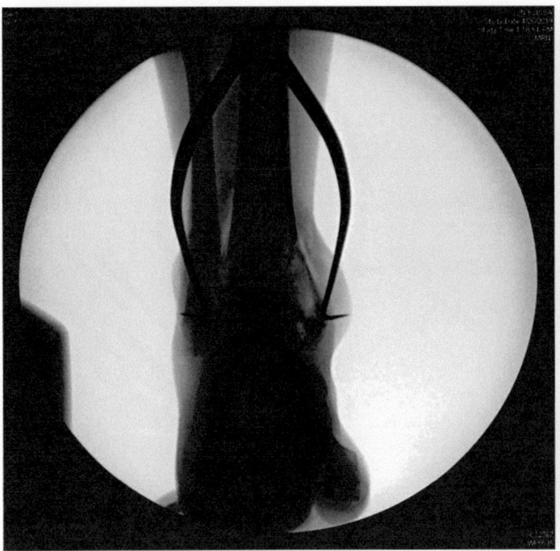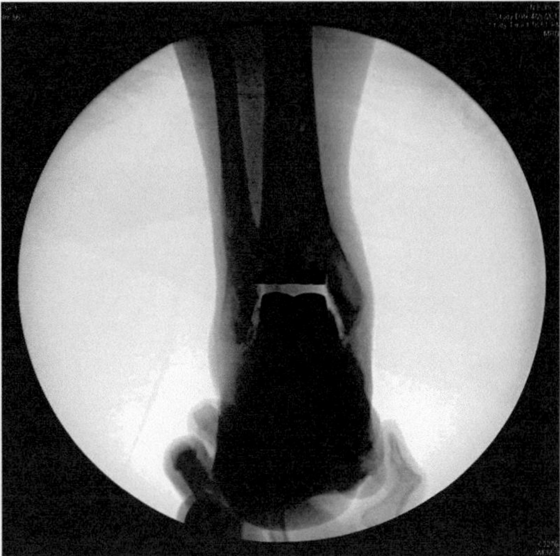

Fig. 3 An example of a conversion from an ankle arthrodesis to a TAA

knee arthroplasty may impede placement of the tibial tubercle pin for the external alignment guide in extramedullary referenced TAA. Lastly, diffuse AVN is often considered a contraindication to TAA. However, if the AVN is isolated to the talar dome, a flat cut talar implant can be utilized in lieu of a resurfacing talar component. In select cases, a total talus may also be considered if there is diffuse AVN. Active infection is an absolute contraindication to TAA.

As an additional use case for TAA, conversion of a painful ankle arthrodesis to TAA is possible, potentially resolving a patient's pain while conferring range of motion to the patient. Several authors have reported favorable outcomes with this procedure, with remarkable preservation of range of motion at early-term follow-up [16]. Conversion of ankle arthrodesis should not be viewed as a panacea, however, as complication rates are substantially higher with this procedure than with primary TAA [17] (Fig. 3).

3 Techniques

Techniques for ankle arthroplasty can be grouped broadly as either variations of distraction arthroplasty or as implant-based TAA. Distraction arthroplasty allows for preservation of the native

ankle joint but is less commonly performed than TAA, given the need for a prolonged period of time in an external fixator frame.

3.1 Distraction Arthroplasty

Ankle distraction arthroplasty is an alternative to ankle arthrodesis or TAA. This technique can be particularly valuable in younger patients, who may be poor candidates for TAA given implant longevity limitations [18]. Distraction arthroplasty involves the use of external fixation to mechanically off-load the ankle joint. The external fixator can be placed for variable amounts of time, with the goal being to allow for stable, congruent range of motion of the joint in the setting of decreased mechanical loading. Ideally, these favorable biomechanical changes would allow for cartilage repair, precluding progression of ankle arthritis and necessity for conversion to TAA or ankle arthrodesis. Adjunctive surgical procedures can be performed in addition to placement of the external fixator to address equinus contracture, anterior tibiotalar impingement, and associated forefoot, midfoot, or hindfoot malalignment [19].

While distraction arthroplasty allows for native joint preservation and may obviate the

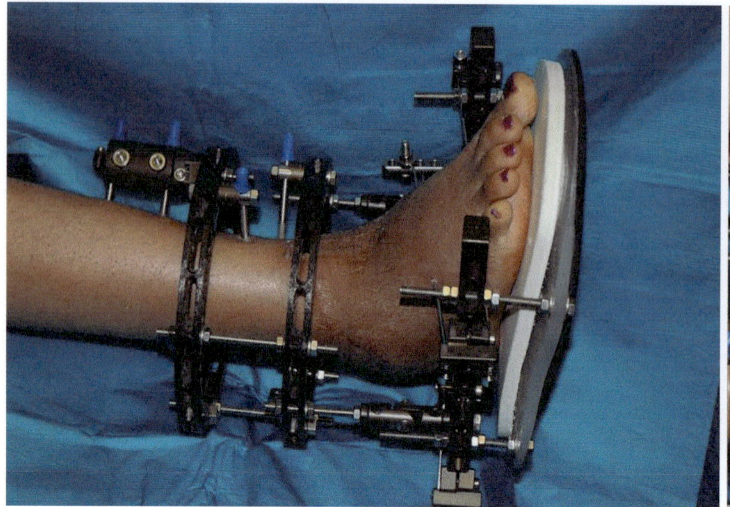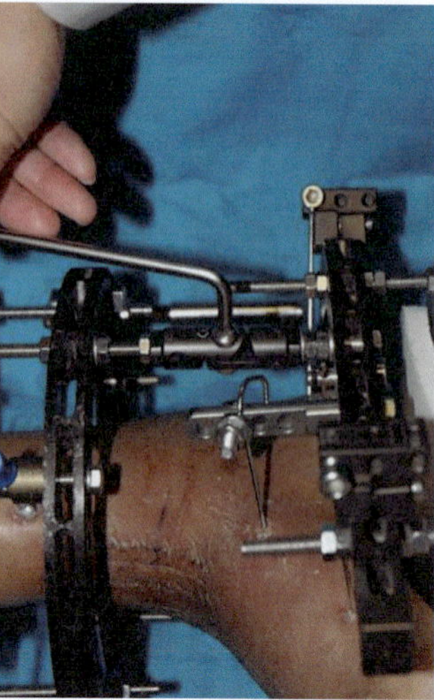

Fig. 4 Ankle distraction arthroplasty, with the external fixator in place. On interval follow up in clinic, the distraction frame can be lengthened to further distract and offload the ankle join

need for conversion to a TAA or ankle arthrodesis, a patient will need to tolerate the external fixator and manage pin care for 2–3 months. Pin site infection rates and other associated complications can be particularly burdensome [20]. Even after a long period of immobilization in the external fixator, progression of ankle arthritis is likely to occur, especially in patients w/ anterior joint space narrowing. Distraction arthroplasty is typically reserved for patients with arthritis with satisfactory alignment and moderate arthritis. Outcomes, while promising short term are generally not as favorable as those for TAA [21]. Distraction arthroplasty is therefore favored in select patients to maximize outcomes after distraction arthroplasty and minimize complications (Fig. 4).

4 Total Ankle Arthroplasty

4.1 History

An alternative to distraction arthroplasty and ankle arthrodesis, TAA is considered by an increasing number of surgeons as the favored surgical treatment of end stage posttraumatic arthritis of the ankle joint. Moreover, patients with end-stage ankle arthritis are aware of the improve-

ments in technology and high patient satisfaction with TAA and now tend to request TAA. Expanding indications for TAA brought on by modern implant designs and improved understanding of correcting coronal plane malalignment as well as addressing other foot and ankle deformities at the time of surgery has led to a more than sixfold increase in utilization of TAA from 1998 to 2010 [22].

Since the first total ankle replacements in the 1970s, implant development, instrumentation, and surgical technique have advanced substantially. As was the case with arthroplasty for other joints, initial implant designs exhibited elevated complication rates, including high incidence of implant failure from excess constraint [23]. Relative success with next generation TAA designs, such as the low-contact stress Buechel-Pappas total ankle replacement (Endotec), were utilized in a trial-only basis in the United States in the 1980s and opened the doors for several pioneers in the field to push the technology forward. Hakan Kofoed developed the mobile-bearing Scandinavian Total Ankle Replacement (STAR; Waldemar Link) and Frank Alvine the fixed-bearing, semi-constrained Agility Total Ankle System (DePuy) [24, 25]. While the Agility ankle is no longer available, the STAR was implanted in the United States on a trial-only basis before garnering FDA approval in the United States in 2009 and continues to be implanted. Between 2000 and 2010, the INBONE (Wright Medical Technology/Stryker) total ankle system, invented by Mark Riley as the TOPAZ ankle, was introduced initially to the US market as the first intramedullary referencing system and is still commonly used today, both in primary and revision TAA. Around the same time, the Salto Talaris total ankle system (developed by Tornier; Integra; now Smith-Nephew) entered the US market after being redesigned from the European-based mobile-bearing Salto total ankle. Since then, numerous other fixed-bearing total ankle system with similar features, have been developed and approved to be implanted in the US, including the Infinity (Stryker), Cadence (Smith-Nephew), Vantage (Exactech), Apex 3D (Paragon28), Quantum (In2Bones/ConMed). The Hintegra total ankle system (Vilex) is unique in that it currently is the only total ankle system available in the United States in both its fixed-bearing and mobile-bearing designs. The Zimmer trabecular metal total ankle system is also unique as it is the only total ankle system implanted through a transfibular lateral approach rather than the anterior approach.

4.2 Approaches

Most TAA systems are designed for implantation via an anterior ankle approach. One system, the Zimmer trabecular metal TAA system features a lateral transfibular approach, necessitating a fibular osteotomy [26]. The anterior approach allows for direct visualization of coronal plane alignment, easy visualization of both the medial and lateral gutters, and supine patient positioning which may reduce anesthesia-related complication risk. Despite advances in TAA including improved soft tissue management, the anterior approach still carries a concerning wound complication rate, even in the absence of peripheral vascular disease or prior anterior ankle surgery. Respecting angiosomes, the recently described anteromedial approach may reduce the anterior wound complication rate [27]. The less frequently utilized lateral approach and Zimmer total ankle system affords direct visualization and an accurate means to identify the ankle's sagittal center of rotation, potentially minimizing bone resection and enhancing TAA biomechanics. Furthermore, when anterior soft tissues are not amenable to TAA, the lateral approach often offers a safe alternative. However, the lateral malleolar osteotomy required to access the ankle from the lateral approach may add morbidity to the procedure (Figs. 5 and 6).

4.3 Implant Design Considerations

There are several factors which implant manufacturers have explored in an attempt to maximize outcomes after TAA. These factors include mobile-bearing versus fixed-bearing prostheses, polyethylene-design considerations, resurfacing versus flat cut talar components, and intramedul-

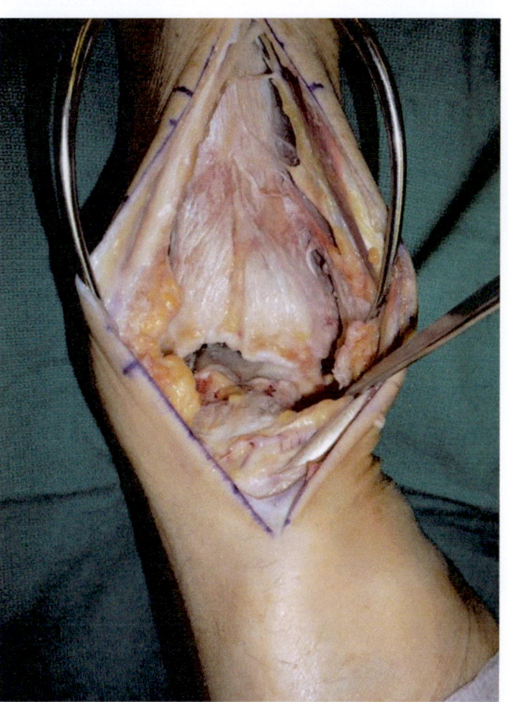

Fig. 5 Excellent exposure to the ankle joint for implantation of TAA can be obtained through use of the anterior approach to the ankle

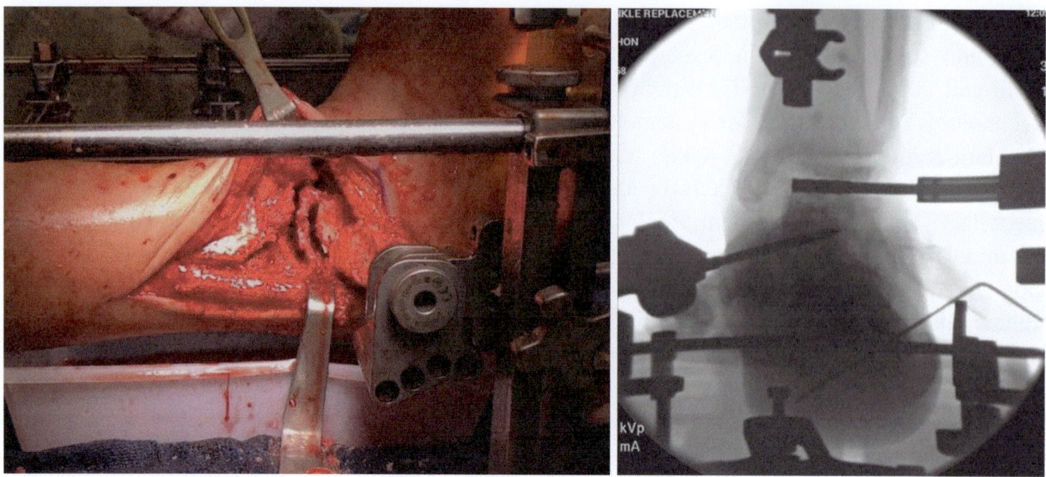

Fig. 6 Lateral approach to the ankle for TAA. (Courtesy of Dr. Lew Schon, MD)

lary versus extramedullary referencing for component alignment. More recently, three-dimensional (3D) printing of PSI and the application of PSI through the use of 3D printed modeling of the cutting guides to improve the accuracy and precision of tibial and talar cuts. With regards to cemented versus uncemented components, the current generation implants largely rely on uncemented bony ongrowth to achieve fixation. In cases where there is advanced osteopenia or question regarding a patient's bone stock or quality of the press fit application of the implant, cementation can be utilized with the majority of the available implants.

Mobile-bearing implants have been designed with the intent to avoid concentrated points of tibiotalar contact and acceleration of polyethylene wear through maintenance of high degrees of conformity at the implant-polyethylene articulation [28]. To achieve this, however, these implants must rely on some degree of constraint to ensure that the ankle remains stable. Thus, the majority of the mobile-bearing prosthesis options available on the market utilize two separate fully conforming articular surfaces. The STAR implant and the HINTEGRA Total Ankle Replacement (Newdeal/Vilex) are examples of mobile-bearing TAA designs. Results of these two mobile-bearing subtypes are generally favorable, [29–31] but long-term studies have reported high rates of polyethylene failure and rates of periprosthetic osteolysis [32]. Importantly, syndesmotic instability is a contra-indication to mobile-bearing TAAs [33]. While mobile-bearing TAA implant options are limited, fixed-bearing implant options, by contrast, are far more abundant in the US market. Generally, fixed-bearing implants exhibit high survival rates, [34, 35] but long term data as well as direct, randomized comparison against mobile-bearing implants is lacking. Polyethylene design considerations also play an important role in the development of TAA systems. Polyethylene manufacturing techniques have improved over recent years, and highly cross-linked polyethylene is favored for TAA over ultrahigh-molecular-weight polyethylene [36]. Vitamin E is often added to TAA polyethylene components to decrease oxidation, and polyethylene sterilization techniques and improved shelf lives are areas of continued evolution. Another area of design innovation involves talar preparation methodology. While the first iteration of many total ankle systems (such as the Salto Talaris) utilized a dome or chamfer cut for the talus, later iterations have included a flat cut talus option, which can be used in the setting of poor talar bone stock.

With regards to extra- and intramedullary referencing to guide tibial preparation and final TAA implant alignment, the vast majority of the available implants utilize a variation of an extramedullary referencing system. Only one implant available today (the INBONE prosthesis) utilizes intramedullary referencing for placement of the tibial component. The intramedullary-referenced design allows for placement of a modular stem, which may aid in tibial component stability in cases where there is marked coronal or sagittal plane malalignment or weak tibial bone support/ structure. Moreover, the Wright/Stryker TAA suite of TAA products is fully modular, ranging in degrees of constraint and stability from the low profile Infinity with a resurfacing talar dome component to the robustly-stabilized INVISION revision system, with all components being compatible. As a distinct disadvantage of the intramedullary referenced TAA, a 6-mm drill hole must be created at the plantar aspect of the foot through the calcaneus, the non-articulating portion of the subtalar joint, and the talus. There is theoretical concern that this technique may threaten the artery of the tarsal canal, thus potentially accelerating rates of postoperative avascular necrosis of the talus [37]. Despite this potential concern, the second generation INBONE II prosthesis has shown excellent short- to mid-term results [38].

As a final implant design consideration, the utilization of PSI for implantation of TAA is increasing. Despite a higher upfront cost, proponents of PSI argue that the accurate, reproducible joint alignment which can be achieved through the utilization of this technology [39] combined with the decreased operative time when compared to extramedullary referenced TAA validate the expense of the implant [40]. Moreover, PSI may address a potentially critical but often overlooked component to total ankle implantation: accuracy of rotational alignment. [good!] While early outcomes and survivorship are favorable, [41] there has yet to be robust data published which demonstrates substantially improved radiographic alignment metrics as well as postoperative outcomes with the utilization of PSI for TAA (Figs. 7 and 8).

4.4 Addressing Concomitant Pathology

As mentioned previously, emerging evidence demonstrates that even in posttraumatic arthritis situations where there is substantial coronal or sagittal plane malalignment with existing deformity through the forefoot, midfoot, and hindfoot, TAA outcomes can be positive if deformity is addressed appropriately. Thus, concomitant procedures will often need to be added to TAA, either in a staged setting or in a single surgical event. Mechanical axis views of the entire limb can assess for the presence of proximal pathology which may need to be addressed prior to TAA. Hindfoot alignment views should be obtained, and special care should be taken to ensure that the patient has been evaluated from behind to further understand heel alignment. In the setting of the varus ankle, a medial release which may consist of release of both the superficial and deep deltoid ligaments is often necessary. More extreme procedures such as medial malleolar osteotomy can also be considered [42]. In the setting of varus ankle deformity, after balancing the ankle with medial release, lateral instability often remains. A lateral ligamentous reconstruction can be undertaken both to tension the lateral ligamentous complex as well as to increase overall joint constraint. We recommend performing the lateral ligament repair with the trial polyethylene component removed to optimize lateral ligamentous tightening. Typically, a smaller polyethylene component can then be placed as the joint space will have decreased (Fig. 9).

In the setting of the valgus ankle, both deltoid and lateral ligamentous instability may require treatment. It may seem paradoxical that lateral ankle instability could coexist with valgus deformity of the ankle, but the valgus deformity is often derived from global ankle instability, and these pathologies are commonly encountered together [43]. Chronic progressive collapsing flat foot deformity frequently accompanies arthritis with valgus through the ankle. Thus, pes planus must be addressed either prior to, at the time of TAA, or subsequently in a staged fashion. With minimizing

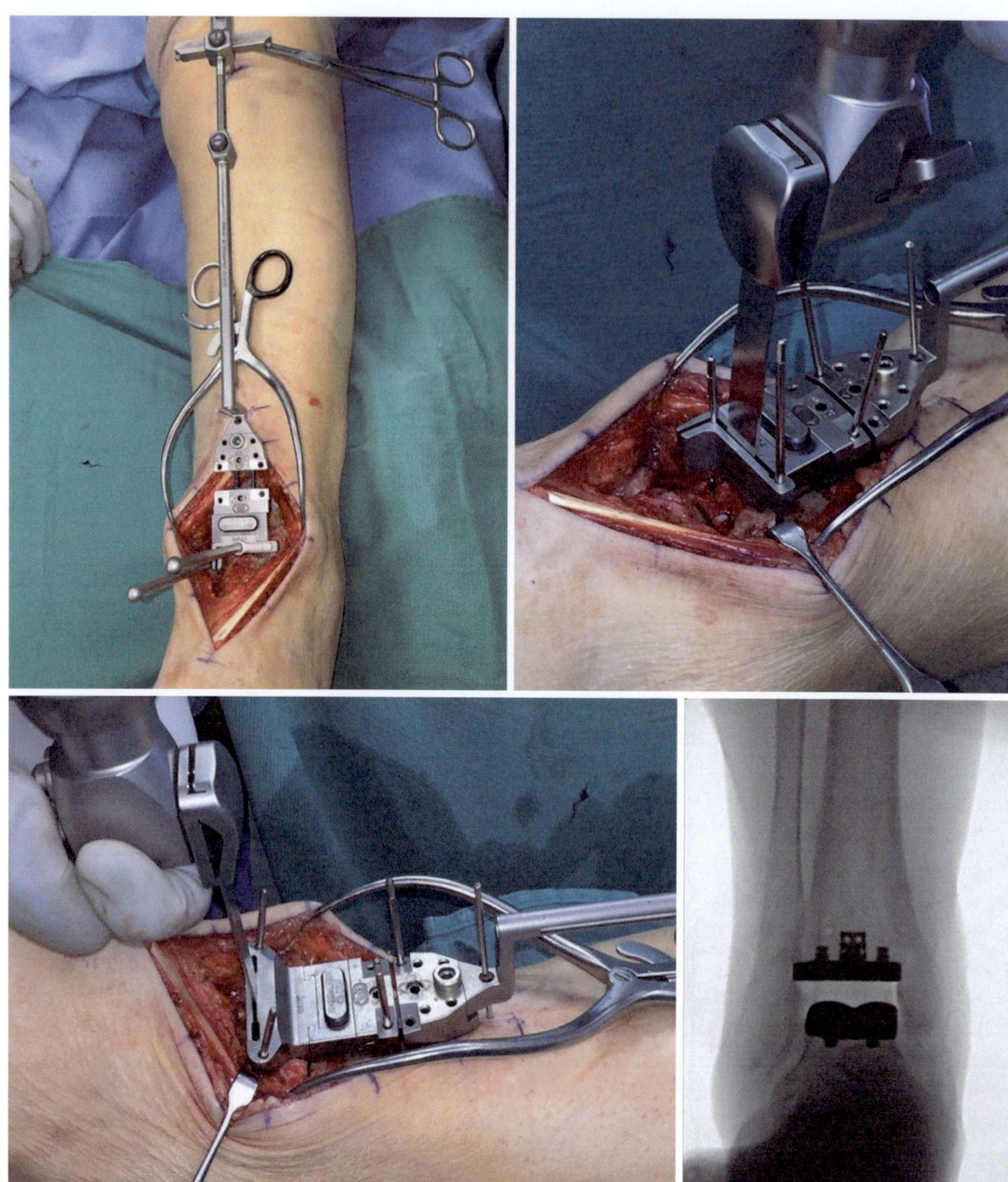

Fig. 7 An example of extramedullary referencing for placement of a TAA. The external alignment guide is placed along the axis of the tibial shaft. The tibial cut is then made through the cut guide, the cut distal tibial bone is removed, and the talar cut guide is then coupled to the extramedullary alignment guide

bony resection and proper repositioning of the platform on which the ankle rests by correcting pes planus, often residual superficial deltoid fibers allow for adequate stability and deltoid reconstruction is not needed. In some instances, even with these techniques, deltoid reconstruction may be necessary, and several techniques have been described [44]. In summation, while addressing concomitant pathology to ensure proper alignment and function of a TAA can be challenging, satisfactory outcomes have been demonstrated when additional procedures have been added to TAA [45] (Fig. 10).

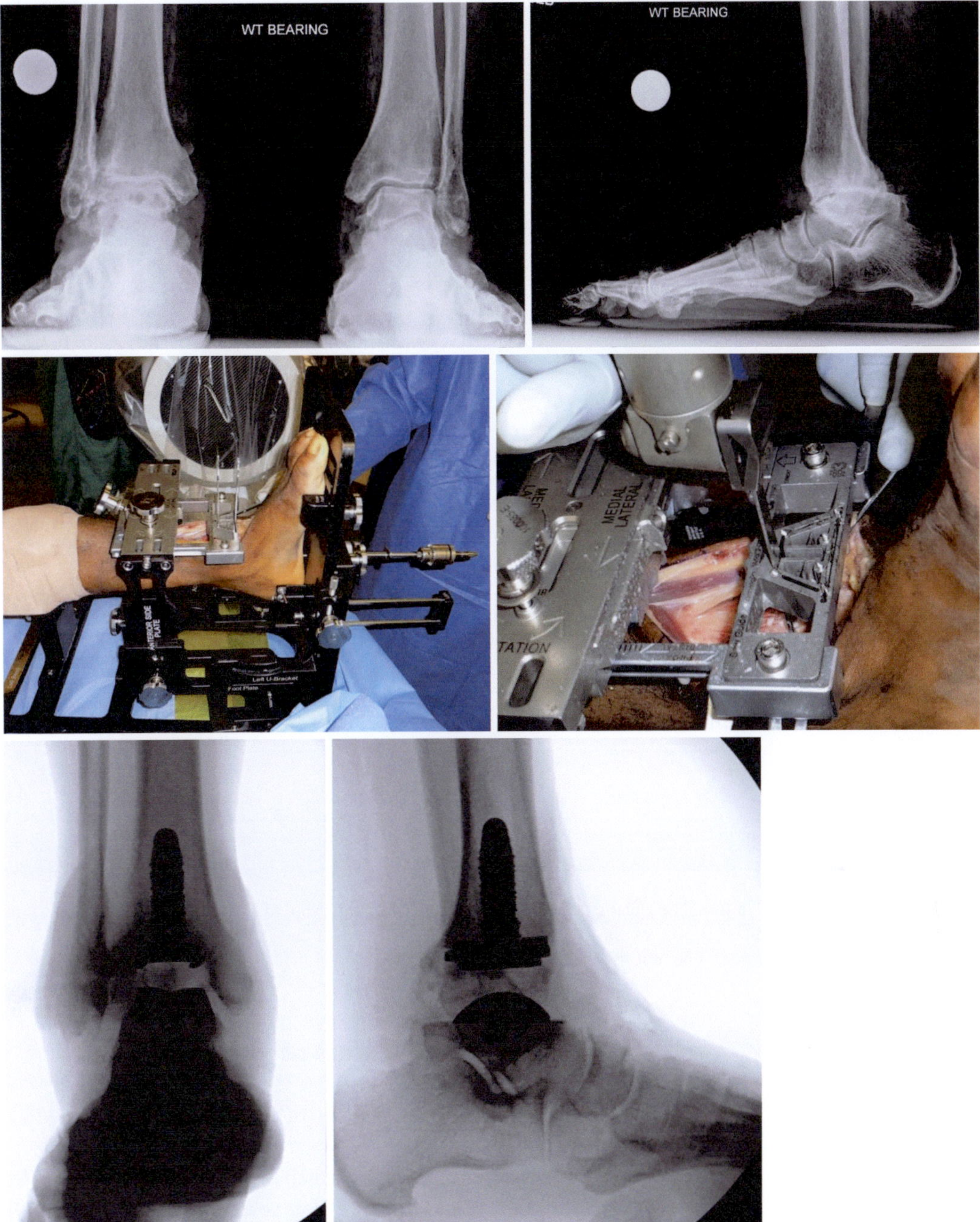

Fig. 8 Preoperative weight-bearing AP and lateral radiographs of the ankle are shown. To carry out intramedullary referencing of a TAA, the foot is placed in a frame, and a 6 mm drill bit is drilled through the calcaneus, nonarticulating portion of the subtalar joint, the talus, and the distal tibia. The cuts are then made through the frame. Final radiographs reveal the modular, stemmed tibial component with the flat cut talus component

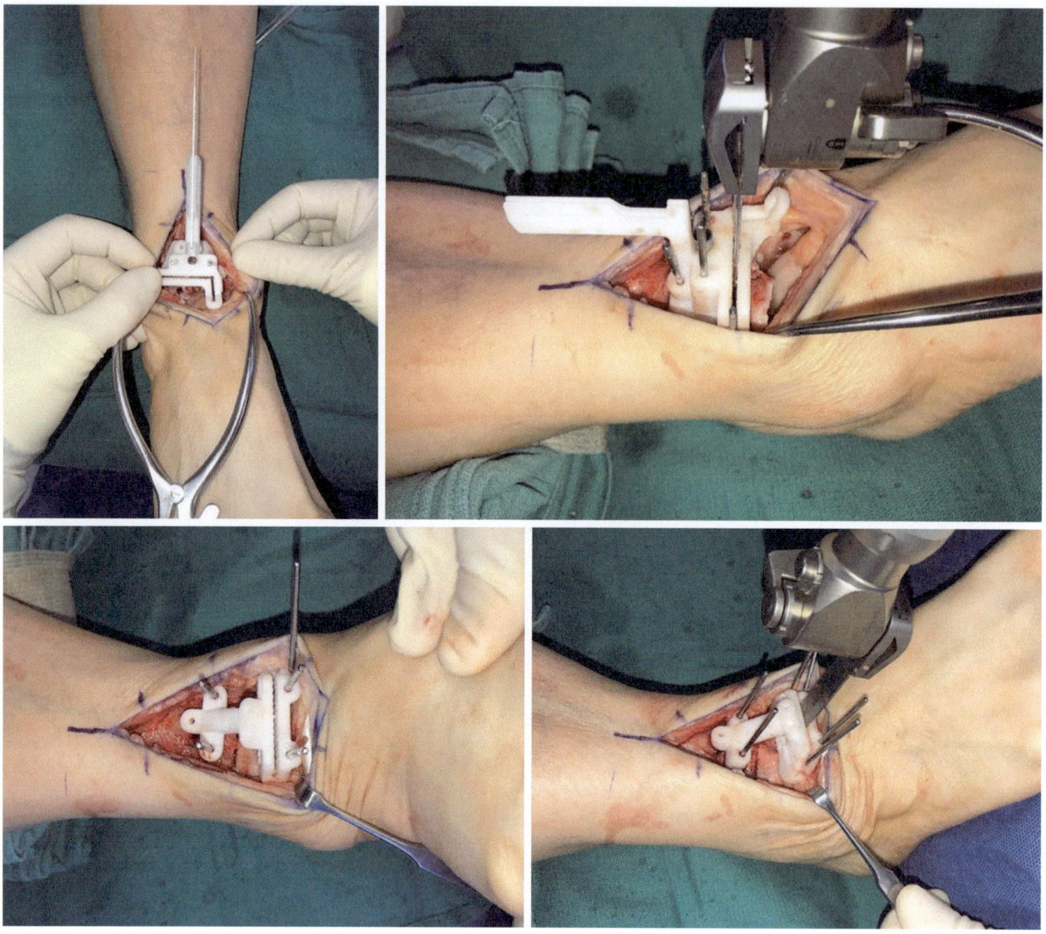

Fig. 9 An example of PSI in use. The tibial cut guide is first placed flush on the distal aspect of the tibia after clearing soft tissue structures. The cut is then made through this guide (top images). The talar cut guide is then placed and the talar cuts are made (bottom images)

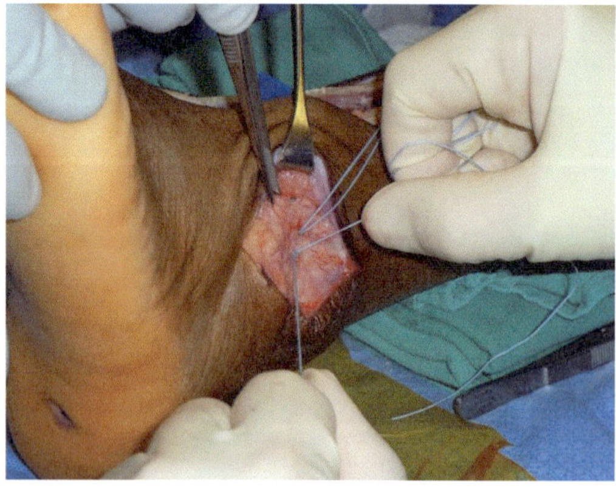

Fig. 10 A Brostrom lateral ligamentous reconstruction after a TAA to stabilize the lateral ligaments. The trial polyethylene component is preferably removed prior to imbrication of the lateral ligaments, and then a smaller polyethylene component is typically placed as the joint space will have decreased

4.5 Future of TAA

With the advent of 3D printing in orthopedics, revolutionary advancements have been made in recent years which expand the indications for TAA. In cases of severe talar bone loss, 3D printing of an entire talus can be utilized in conjunction with the tibial component of a total ankle, to form a total ankle total talus replacement (TATTR). [46] TATTR can also be used in conjunction with talonavicular and subtalar joint arthrodesis to salvage cases exhibiting substantial deformity through the hindfoot as well as severe talar collapse. Furthermore, through the use of 3D printing, the tibial component of a TAA may also be customized to address specific use cases for

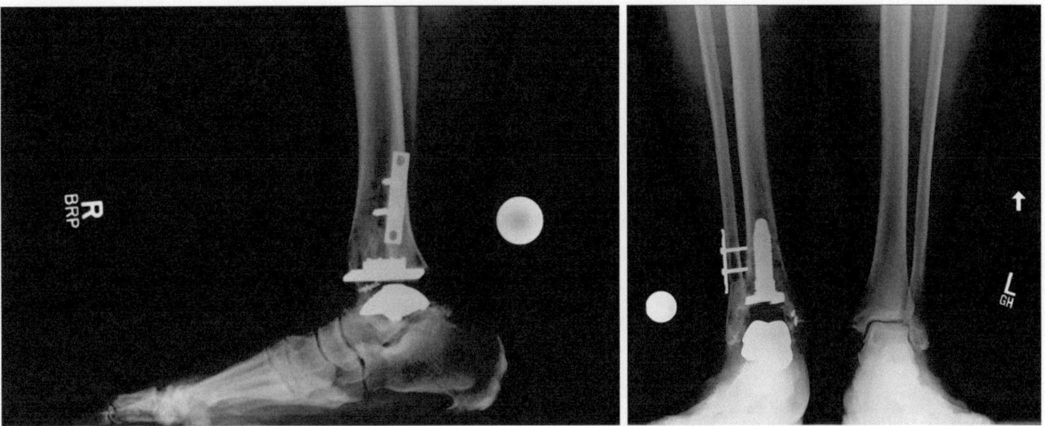

Fig. 11 Example of a failed TAA (left image) with subsequent revision surgery and conversion to a TATTR (right image). The stem for the INBONE prosthesis was utilized in conjunction with the total talus component

tibial bone loss. Additional areas for future development in TAA include dedicated revision systems, improved imaging through the utilization of weight-bearing CT scans from the hip to the foot for full length assessment, and robotic-assisted navigation to guide tibial and talar cuts (Fig. 11).

5 Complications

Even while demonstrating generally favorable outcomes, TAA remains subject to complications which can occur both intraoperatively and postoperatively. Generally, complications which require operative intervention can be addressed through reoperation to address the specific pathology and not require a revision TAA with removal of components. However, in some cases, revision arthroplasty or conversion to ankle arthrodesis is indicated. Revision TAA is associated with lower survivorship rates than primary arthroplasty. Despite a relatively low incidence, especially in the hands of a surgeon with significant experience, [47] the most common intraoperative complication from TAA is medial malleolus fracture. Screw fixation is recommended in the setting of an intraoperative medial malleolus fracture. In the short-term postoperative period, the most common complication encountered are wound-healing problems. Wound issues occurred at a rate of 3.4% in a review of 762 primary TAAs [47].

Outside of the early postoperative window, wound healing issues become less significant. With longer term follow-up, the most common complication encountered after TAA is symptomatic impingement. Operative debridement to clean both the medial and lateral gutters and to debride excessive scar tissue can alleviate symptomology. Importantly, prevention of impingement-related symptoms begins at the index procedure. Surgeons should avoid oversizing the talar component and should ensure that the gutters are clean and without impingement on range of motion of the ankle prior to concluding the surgery. Surgeons should follow their postoperative TAA patients more closely than patients who receive other forms of total joint arthroplasty, as osteolysis can cause cystic formation adjacent to both the tibial and talar components. If these cysts are caught prior to causing implant loosening, several authors have described success with curating and bone grafting of the cysts [48].

If a TAA component is found to be loose or infection is confirmed through joint aspiration, explantation or revision TAA must be considered. In the case of loose components, revision TAA with an intramedullary referenced system can be utilized to achieve enhanced stability. In the case of confirmed infection, we favor a two-stage approach with explantation and placement of antibiotic-impregnated cement spacer, followed by placement of new TAA components once infection has been eradicated. In situations where salvage of range of motion through revision TAA is impossible, ankle or tibio-talo-calcaneal arthrodesis can achieve a stable surface for weight bearing. Unfortunately, fusion success rates following TAA conversion to arthrodesis with structural bone graft or 3D printed spacers are lower than primary arthrodesis scenarios. Thus, the decision to proceed with a revision TAA should be made carefully, and all attempts should be made at salvage prior to consideration of arthrodesis. Below knee amputation remains an option in cases where infection is unable to be eradicated or poor bone stock precludes arthrodesis procedures.

6 Summary

Posttraumatic arthritis is the most common cause for end stage ankle arthritis requiring arthrodesis or arthroplasty procedure. As techniques and implants improve, the indications for TAA over ankle arthrodesis are expanding. Most TAA implants available on the market today utilize uncemented press fit fixation, a fixed-bearing design, and extramedullary referencing to guide tibial and talar cuts. When there is associated pathology with end stage posttraumatic arthritis of the ankle, recent literature suggests that TAA can still be considered, and outcomes can be excellent if proper alignment is achieved and concomitant pathology is addressed. Three-dimensional Printing has an emerging role in TAA, and the utilization of the TATTR in the setting of talar collapse is being reported with more frequency. TAA is not without complications, and wound healing issues in the early stage and implant loosening or subsidence in the midterm to late stage are the most commonly reported complications after this procedure.

References

1. Brockett CL, Chapman GJ. Biomechanics of the ankle. Orthop Trauma. 2016;30(3):232–8.
2. Ledoux WR, Sangeorzan BJ. Clinical biomechanics of the peritalar joint. Foot Ankle Clin. 2004;9(4):663–83. v
3. Niu W, Tang T, Zhang M, Jiang C, Fan Y. An in vitro and finite element study of load redistribution in the midfoot. Sci China Life Sci. 2014;57(12):1191–6.
4. Delco ML, Kennedy JG, Bonassar LJ, Fortier LA. Post-traumatic osteoarthritis of the ankle: a distinct clinical entity requiring new research approaches. J Orthop Res. 2017;35(3):440–53.
5. Punzi L, Galozzi P, Luisetto R, Favero M, Ramonda R, Oliviero F, et al. Post-traumatic arthritis: overview on pathogenic mechanisms and role of inflammation. RMD Open. 2016;2(2):e000279.
6. Jaakkola JI, Mann RA. A review of rheumatoid arthritis affecting the foot and ankle. Foot Ankle Int. 2004;25(12):866–74.
7. Müller AM, Toepfer A, Harrasser N, Haller B, Walther M, von Eisenhart-Rothe R, Gemperlein K, Bergmann K, Bradaric C, Laugwitz KL, Ibrahim T, Dirschinger RJ. Significant prevalence of peripheral artery disease in patients with disturbed wound healing following elective foot and ankle surgery: Results from the ABI-PRIORY (ABI as a PRedictor of Impaired wound healing after ORthopedic surgerY) trial. Vasc Med. 2020;25(2):118–23. https://doi.org/10.1177/13588 63X19883945. Epub 2019 Nov 15. PMID: 32366205.
8. Saltzman CL, el-Khoury GY. The hindfoot alignment view. Foot Ankle Int. 1995;16(9):572–6.
9. Richter M, de Cesar NC, Lintz F, Barg A, Burssens A, Ellis S. The assessment of ankle osteoarthritis with weight-bearing computed tomography. Foot Ankle Clin. 2022;27(1):13–36.
10. Wang Q, Zhang N, Guo W, Wang W, Zhang Q. Patient-specific instrumentation (PSI) in total ankle arthroplasty: a systematic review. Int Orthop. 2021;45(9):2445–52.
11. Shih CL, Chen SJ, Huang PJ. Clinical outcomes of total ankle arthroplasty versus ankle arthrodesis for the treatment of end-stage ankle arthritis in the last decade: a systematic review and meta-analysis. J Foot Ankle Surg. 2020;59(5):1032–9.
12. Reddy SC, Mann JA, Mann RA, Mangold DR. Correction of moderate to severe coronal plane deformity with the STAR™ ankle prosthesis. Foot Ankle Int. 2011;32(7):659–64.
13. Daniels TR. Surgical technique for Total ankle arthroplasty in ankles with preoperative coronal plane Varus deformity of 10° or greater. JBJS Essent Surg Tech. 2013;3(4):e22.
14. Sung KS, Ahn J, Lee KH, Chun TH. Short-term results of total ankle arthroplasty for end-stage ankle arthritis with severe varus deformity. Foot Ankle Int. 2014;35(3):225–31.
15. Lee GW, Lee KB. Outcomes of total ankle arthroplasty in ankles with >20° of coronal plane deformity. J Bone Joint Surg Am. 2019;101(24):2203–11.
16. Hintermann B, Barg A, Knupp M, Valderrabano V. Conversion of painful ankle arthrodesis to total ankle arthroplasty. J Bone Joint Surg Am. 2009;91(4):850–8.
17. Pellegrini MJ, Schiff AP, Adams SB Jr, Queen RM, DeOrio JK, Nunley JA II, et al. Conversion of tibiota-

lar arthrodesis to total ankle arthroplasty. J Bone Joint Surg Am. 2015;97(24):2004–13.

18. Morse KR, Flemister AS, Baumhauer JF, DiGiovanni BF. Distraction arthroplasty. Foot Ankle Clin. 2007;12(1):29–39.

19. Bernstein M, Reidler J, Fragomen A, Rozbruch SR. Ankle distraction arthroplasty: indications, technique, and outcomes. J Am Acad Orthop Surg. 2017;25(2):89.

20. Yang Z, Cui L, Tao S, Zhao J, Wang L, Zhang F, et al. Comparisons between ankle distraction arthroplasty and supramalleolar osteotomy for treatment of post-traumatic varus ankle osteoarthritis. BMC Surg. 2022;22(1):178.

21. Nguyen M, Saltzman C, Amendola A. Outcomes of ankle distraction for the treatment of ankle arthritis. Instr Course Lect. 2016;65:311–9.

22. Singh JA, Ramachandran R. Time trends in total ankle arthroplasty in the USA: a study of the National Inpatient Sample. Clin Rheumatol. 2016;35(1):239–45.

23. Gougoulias N, Maffulli N. History of total ankle replacement. Clin Podiatr Med Surg. 2013;30(1):1–20.

24. Bedard N, Saltzman CL, Den Hartog T, Carlson S, Callaghan J, Alvine G, et al. The agility total ankle arthroplasty: a concise follow-up at a minimum of 20 years. Foot Ankle Int. 2021;42(10):1241–4.

25. Saltzman CL, Mann RA, Ahrens JE, Amendola A, Anderson RB, Berlet GC, et al. Prospective controlled trial of STAR total ankle replacement versus ankle fusion: initial results. Foot Ankle Int. 2009;30(7):579–96.

26. Tan EW, Maccario C, Talusan PG, Schon LC. Early complications and secondary procedures in transfibular total ankle replacement. Foot Ankle Int. 2016;37(8):835–41.

27. Amin A, Mahoney J, Daniels TR. Anteromedial approach for ankle arthoplasty and arthrodesis: technique tip. Foot Ankle Int. 2012;33(11):1011–4.

28. Cracchiolo A III, Deorio JK. Design features of current total ankle replacements: implants and instrumentation. J Am Acad Orthop Surg. 2008;16(9):530–40.

29. Nunley JA, Caputo AM, Easley ME, Cook C. Intermediate to long-term outcomes of the STAR total ankle replacement: the patient perspective. J Bone Joint Surg Am. 2012;94(1):43–8.

30. Mann JA, Mann RA, Horton E. STAR™ ankle: long-term results. Foot Ankle Int. 2011;32(5):S473–84.

31. Brunner S, Barg A, Knupp M, Zwicky L, Kapron AL, Valderrabano V, et al. The Scandinavian total ankle replacement: long-term, eleven to fifteen-year, survivorship analysis of the prosthesis in seventy-two consecutive patients. J Bone Joint Surg Am. 2013;95(8):711–8.

32. Yoon HS, Lee J, Choi WJ, Lee JW. Periprosthetic osteolysis after total ankle arthroplasty. Foot Ankle Int. 2014;35(1):14–21.

33. Hintermann B, Susdorf R, Krähenbühl N, Ruiz R. Axial rotational alignment in mobile-bearing total ankle arthroplasty. Foot Ankle Int. 2020;41(5):521–8.

34. Hofmann KJ, Shabin ZM, Ferkel E, Jockel J, Slovenkai MP. Salto Talaris total ankle arthroplasty:

35. Stewart MG, Green CL, Adams SB Jr, DeOrio JK, Easley ME, Nunley JA 2nd. Midterm results of the Salto Talaris total ankle arthroplasty. Foot Ankle Int. 2017;38(11):1215–21.

36. Schipper ON, Haddad SL, Fullam S, Pourzal R, Wimmer MA. Wear characteristics of conventional ultrahigh-molecular-weight polyethylene versus highly cross-linked polyethylene in total ankle arthroplasty. Foot Ankle Int. 2018;39(11):1335–44.

37. Tennant JN, Rungprai C, Pizzimenti MA, Goetz J, Phisitkul P, Femino J, et al. Risks to the blood supply of the talus with four methods of total ankle arthroplasty: a cadaveric injection study. J Bone Joint Surg Am. 2014;96(5):395–402.

38. Gagne OJ, Day J, Kim J, Caolo K, O'Malley MJ, Deland JT, et al. Midterm survivorship of the INBONE II total ankle arthroplasty. Foot Ankle Int. 2022;43(5):628–36.

39. Hsu AR, Davis WH, Cohen BE, Jones CP, Ellington JK, Anderson RB. Radiographic outcomes of preoperative CT scan-derived patient-specific total ankle arthroplasty. Foot Ankle Int. 2015;36(10):1163–9.

40. Hamid KS, Matson AP, Nwachukwu BU, Scott DJ, Mather RC III, DeOrio JK. Determining the cost-savings threshold and alignment accuracy of patient-specific instrumentation in total ankle replacements. Foot Ankle Int. 2017;38(1):49–57.

41. Rushing CJ, Kibbler K, Hyer CF, Berlet GC. The INFINITY total ankle prosthesis: outcomes at short-term follow-up. Foot Ankle Spec. 2022;15(2):119–26.

42. Doets HC, van der Plaat LW, Klein JP. Medial malleolar osteotomy for the correction of varus deformity during total ankle arthroplasty: results in 15 ankles. Foot Ankle Int. 2008;29(2):171–7.

43. Demetracopoulos CA, Cody EA, Adams SB, DeOrio JK, Nunley JA, Easley ME. Outcomes of total ankle arthroplasty in moderate and severe valgus deformity. Foot Ankle Spec. 2018;12(3):238–45.

44. Haddad SL, Dedhia S, Ren Y, Rotstein J, Zhang LQ. Deltoid ligament reconstruction: a novel technique with biomechanical analysis. Foot Ankle Int. 2010;31(7):639–51.

45. Criswell B, Hunt K, Kim T, Chou L, Haskell A. Association of short-term complications with procedures through separate incisions during total ankle replacement. Foot Ankle Int. 2016;37(10):1060–4.

46. Bejarano-Pineda L, DeOrio JK, Parekh SG. Combined total talus replacement and total ankle arthroplasty. J Surg Orthop Adv. 2020;29(4):244–8.

47. Schimmel JJ, Walschot LH, Louwerens JW. Comparison of the short-term results of the first and last 50 Scandinavian total ankle replacements: assessment of the learning curve in a consecutive series. Foot Ankle Int. 2014;35(4):326–33.

48. Gross CE, Huh J, Green C, Shah S, DeOrio JK, Easley M, et al. Outcomes of bone grafting of bone cysts after total ankle arthroplasty. Foot Ankle Int. 2016;37(2):157–64.

Management of Ankle Wounds

Marten N. Basta, Ari M. Wes,
and Lawrence Scott Levin

1 Wound Assessment

A fundamental aspect of lower extremity reconstruction is the initial wound evaluation. In addition to appropriate knowledge of local anatomy surrounding the wound, a nuanced understanding of the physiology of wound healing and the corresponding morphologic changes is necessary to arrive at a clinically sound treatment plan. The following discussion reviews basic elements of the initial history and exam, which should be explored for each patient.

1.1 Pertinent History

The first step in evaluating patients is to obtain an adequate history. In the setting of a trauma, a careful evaluation, preferably in a trauma center, is recommended. If this has not been performed prior to the authors' initial consultation, it is our responsibility to ensure that an appropriate triage, workup, and treatment has been provided or planned for any concomitant injuries. Critical historical elements to discuss include the mechanism of injury and, if not an immediate consequence of an initial trauma, the etiology of the wound. One should also note what diagnostic studies have been completed, and what if any interventions occurred prior to consultation. If the defect is oncologic in nature, identifying any history of radiation, chemotherapy, or immune-modulating steroid/hormone therapy should also be recorded. Relevant comorbidities, their treatment, and how well they are managed should be noted. For chronic conditions, such as diabetes or COPD, this will give some indication of patient compliance and willingness to cooperate with the reconstructive plan [1]. Other important historical elements should be reviewed as well, examples of which include smoking history, presence of hypercoagulable disorders or use of anticoagulant medications, and baseline functional status..

M. N. Basta (✉)
Reconstructive Oncology, Moffitt Cancer Center,
Tampa, FL, USA
e-mail: Marten.Basta@Pennmedicine.upenn.edu

A. M. Wes
Division of Plastic and Reconstructive Surgery,
Department of Surgery, University of Pennsylvania
Health System, Philadelphia, PA, USA

L. Scott Levin
Department of Orthopaedic Surgery, Perelman
School of Medicine at the University of Pennsylvania,
Philadelphia, PA, USA
e-mail: Scott.levin@pennmedicine.upenn.edu

1.2 Exam

Physical examination should always begin with establishing a baseline vascular and neurologic exam, including sensory and motor components. Sensibility of the plantar foot, dorsum, and distal leg may be tested grossly by touch and areas of

© The Author(s), under exclusive license to Springer Nature Switzerland AG 2023
D. Herscovici Jr. et al. (eds.), *Evaluation and Surgical Management of the Ankle*,
https://doi.org/10.1007/978-3-031-33537-2_23

Table 1 Characterization of favorable and unfavorable wound features [4]

Feature	Favorable	Unfavorable
Depth	Superficial/intermediate: Confined to dermal elements only or into subcutaneous tissue without critical structure exposure	Full thickness skin and subcutaneous tissue loss over critical structure (bone, tendon, neurovascular bundle, hardware)
Complexity	Simple: Single tissue type involved	Complex: Multiple tissues involved
Chronicity	Acute, subacute	Chronic
Etiology	– Sharp traumatic injury – Surgically created wound	– Traumatic crush/contusion or avulsion – Tissue necrosis due to infection – Debridement of infected tissue – Irradiated wound bed – Secondary to systemic disease (i.e., diabetes, PVD) – Idiopathic

Note: *PVD* peripheral vascular disease

hyposensitivity further investigated using a Semmes-Weinstein monofilament. Active knee extension and flexion, as well as foot dorsiflexion, plantar flexion, and eversion should be tested and compared to the unaffected limb. Any focal neurologic deficit, either sensory or motor, should be noted as part of baseline neurologic examination. Vascular assessment includes palpation of femoral, popliteal, posterior tibial and dorsalis pedis pulses, with handheld Doppler exam of any nonpalpable vessels [2]. Additionally, obtaining bilateral ankle-brachial index values may assist in identifying significant vascular compromise if present. Wound evaluation should be systematic and requires characterization of several features of favorable and unfavorable findings, as described below in Table 1 [3]. Basic wound assessment should include location and estimated size of the wound, what tissue types appear to be affected or exposed, gross contamination, whether or not an immediate intervention is needed (i.e. control of bleeding, bedside washout of grossly contaminated tissue, tourniquet removal), and an estimate of the amount of soft tissue defect if any appears missing. These characteristics all contribute to anticipating the optimal reconstruction during initial evaluation..

1.3 Wound Classification

The authors' preference is to classify wounds as stable or unstable based upon an algorithm previously described by the senior author [3]. Stable wounds are characterized by primarily favorable features. These include a typically clean and healthy appearance with a well-vascularized wound bed or are surgically created shallow wounds with no critical structure exposure. For these wounds, the authors have found that soft tissue reconstruction is successfully achieved through one or more of the following modalities: primary closure, delayed primary closure, healing by secondary intent, or application of a skin substitute or skin graft.

Unstable wounds are characterized by presence of any of the following:

- Soft tissue deficit overlying critical structures or comminuted open fractures (i.e. high grade Gustilo injury) [5].
- Devitalized soft tissue with evolving necrosis, particularly if overlying critical structures or hardware.
- Prior surgery with scarring near the wound, indicating decreased vascular supply to the wound and possible further tissue loss [6].
- Oncologic wounds involving radiated tissue or in a vascularly challenged extremity.
- Heavily contaminated/infected wounds involving bone or hardware.

Options for definitive reconstruction are discussed in the last two sections of this chapter.

2 Preoperative Planning

Fundamental aspects of preoperative planning include open communication and coordination of operative management across all the teams that will provide definitive treatment. This should also include any additional workup and specialist consultation if indicated. For example, patients with chronic vascular disease may benefit from a vascular surgery consultation to improve inflow to the affected extremity via angioplasty, focal thrombectomy, or vascular bypass prior to or concurrently with reconstruction. Infectious disease consultation should be considered in the setting of contamination or potential deep space infection, particularly in patients with a history of resistant infections or significant antibiotic allergies [7]. Additionally, patients with significant medical history should have preoperative risk stratification, typically through an internal medicine consult, prior to nonemergent major surgery..

2.1 Diagnostic Evaluation

In addition to adequate plain films, advanced imaging should also be considered to evaluate the involved extremity's vascular anatomy. When vascular impairment is suspected, based on an abnormal physical exam or Doppler examination, adjunctive imaging is recommended. Specifically, the authors recommend advanced vascular imaging studies in all patients with nonpalpable or diminished dorsalis pedis or posterior tibial arterial pulses and in patients with complex soft tissue trauma with underlying comminuted or displaced long bone fractures. Computed tomography angiography (CTA), or in the absence of hardware, magnetic resonance angiography (MRA) are excellent noninvasive imaging modalities that can characterize overall flow and identify focal lesions for potential vascular intervention. Once vascular inflow is optimized, knowledge of a patient's foot and ankle vascular anatomy should guide reconstructive management, including the selection of recipient vessels for flap anastomosis [8]. When possible, healthy vessels outside of the zone of injury are preferred. However, our experience with lower extremity trauma demonstrates successful reconstructive outcomes can be achieved utilizing diseased recipient vessels, assuming proper clinical judg-

ment and proficient microsurgical technique [9]. Thus, diseased vessels are not an absolute contraindication to free tissue transfer.

3 Debridement and Wound Bed Preparation

The most important principle of wound management is wound bed preparation through an adequate debridement. Only after debridement can the true size of the wound be determined and a decision made for the type of coverage that will be needed. Sharp excision of the crushed and contaminated skin should be performed to obtain clear, vertical skin edges. Subcutaneous tissue, fascia, and muscle that are compromised should be excised back to healthy tissue. Structurally relevant bone fragments are preserved. However, if a bone segment is crushed, contaminated, and considered nonsalvageable, it should be excised. In addition, bone that is devoid of soft tissue attachments, usually considered an avascular fragment, should be excised. In most instances, this will result in additional loss of tissue volume, but marginally viable tissue left behind can subsequently desiccate, infarct, and become infected, adding further delay in healing and become a potential source of infection [10].

A critical concept in the treatment of open wounds is to avoid desiccation (drying out) of the tissues. Tissue desiccation results in cell death, tissue necrosis, infection, edema, and further destruction of soft tissue [2]. Continuous wet-to-wet dressings or, preferentially, an antibiotic bead pouch, can be placed to allow exposed structures to be bathed in a physiologic medium [11, 12]. When the adequacy of the initial debridement is uncertain, second- or possibly third-look procedures at 2– or 3–day intervals may be necessary [13]. Specifically, returning for interval serial debridement allows one to evaluate the effectiveness of prior debridement/washout and current antibiotic regimen in the setting of infection, while decreasing the chances of overly aggressive or inadequate one-time debridement. Once the wound has a clean base with bleeding edges and no necrotic tissue or purulence, it has been adequately debrided. Lastly, the use of negative pressure wound vacuum therapy has become an important modality in local wound care. Specific benefits of wound vacuum therapy include decreasing local edema and inflammatory processes, bioburden reduction, promotion of wound bed vascularity and granulation formation [14]. These processes temporize wounds until definitive coverage is possible, and anecdotally, may assist in the conversion of a wound from subacute to acute. Typically, wound vacuum therapy can be used if immediate coverage is not possible and when multiple debridements are anticipated. Reasons to discontinue wound vac therapy include inability to maintain therapeutic seal due to anatomy or defect location or if the sealing tape causes substantial damage to the skin surrounding the wound. Otherwise, wound vac therapy requires less frequent dressing changes, prevents tension from causing wounds to grow in size over time, are generally well-tolerated by patients, and can be continued until definitive coverage in the inpatient or outpatient setting.

4 Limb Salvage vs. Amputation

The decision to offer a patient reconstruction vs. primary amputation is often highly controversial and a potential source for medicolegal claims. With advances in surgical technique, fewer situations are encountered in which salvage is not feasible; however, whether salvage *should* be attempted is now the more imperative question to ask. With no gold standard criteria for decision-making, multiple scoring systems have been developed to try to answer whether a salvage *should* be attempted. As no scoring system considers functionality of a salvaged limb, they should never be used as the sole deciding criteria [10, 15]. However, injury factors with the poorest outcomes for limb salvage include severe muscle injury and absence of plantar sensation secondary to posterior tibial nerve disruption [5]. If limb salvage is attempted, there must be an appropriate conversation with the patient and the family

regarding possible failure. Part of that conversation should include an understanding that even with proper planning and execution, limb salvage may not be possible due to the development of chronic sepsis, intractable pain, or lack of patient desire to continue limb salvage.

After adequate debridement has been obtained, and in conjunction with the patient's or family's request, opinions should be obtained from both orthopedic and reconstructive surgeons regarding salvageability of the extremity. In the acute setting, it is advised to wait at least until after the first debridement to make any decisions [16]. When dealing with pediatric patient populations, every attempt at limb salvage should be made unless such attempts would sacrifice important function elsewhere or put the patient's life at risk [17].

One of the principles of orthoplastic surgery, when dealing with traumatic lower extremity lesions, is to establish parameters and guidelines for treatment of bone and soft tissue early in the patient's course, preferably the night of injury [18]. Once an extremity is deemed salvageable, the choice of stabilization—provisional or definitive (usually chosen by orthopedic surgeons)—and the choice of coverage (usually chosen by plastic surgeons) should all be coordinated by the "orthoplastic" team.

Once salvage is planned, knowledge of which patient and perioperative factors increase the risk for reconstructive failure (and consequent secondary amputation) may improve consent discussions and aid in perioperative planning. A review of the authors' institutional experience with attempted lower extremity salvage identified diabetes, multiple arterial injuries, recipient artery pathology, free flap failure, and residual osteomyelitis as risk factors associated with secondary amputation [19].

5 Soft Tissue Reconstruction of Unstable Ankle Wounds

After a limb is deemed salvageable, a functional reconstruction must be planned, providing stable soft tissue coverage, and if necessary, vascularized bone graft for structural support. This section will focus on options for soft tissue reconstruction..

Soft tissue reconstructive options are best determined by "wound stability" or the relative likelihood of healing any given wound. Clear understanding of this concept is fundamental to management of lower extremity wounds, and decision-making is based upon initial wound assessment (see section "Wound Assessment" and Table 1) and individual patient circumstance. Stable wounds are adequately treated by options lower on the reconstructive ladder; in contrast, reconstructive techniques are required for unstable wounds [20].

Historical experience with lower extremity reconstruction dictates that wounds located in the distal third of the lower leg are best reconstructed with vascularized free flaps utilizing microvascular techniques. This is defined by transfer of tissue from one part of the body to another and re-establishing blood supply via arterial and venous anastomoses, which require tools that magnify one's view (i.e., operating microscope or loupes) [21]. Free flaps may be classified in a variety of ways that are outside the scope of this text; the most clinically relevant classification scheme is based upon the tissue type(s) that is transferred (i.e., muscle, skin, bone, fascia). The flap name reflects this scheme, examples of which include but are not limited to musculocutaneous (muscle and skin), fasciocutaneous (fascia and skin), and osteocutaneous (bone and skin). This section focuses on workhorse fasciocutaneous and musculocutaneous free flaps for ankle soft tissue reconstruction. Fasciocutaneous flaps are typically preferred over muscle flaps for resurfacing foot and ankle wounds due to the concept of *replacing like with like*. Specifically, the thin skin and absence of subcutaneous fat overlying the ankle should be reconstructed by a soft tissue flap that not only includes skin, but has similarly thin skin and minimal to no fat included in the flap. Workhorse flaps include the anterolateral thigh (ALT), lateral arm, scapular/parascapular, radial forearm, and the medial sural artery perforator (MSAP). Muscle flaps (with immediate skin grafts) are often chosen to obliterate dead

space or if fasciocutaneous options are either unavailable or unfavorable (morbidly obese patients). Commonly used muscle flaps include the latissimus dorsi, vastus lateralis, gracilis, or rectus abdominis flaps.

6 Choice of Flap

The free flap donor site is chosen based on the demands of the specific subunit that has been injured [22]. Dorsal foot and ankle wounds have similar soft tissue characteristics and require thin, pliable tissues for proper shoe fitting. As such, these defects are ideally reconstructed using the lateral arm, MSAP, radial forearm, ALT, and scapular fasciocutaneous flaps [23]. These wounds have the highest aesthetic demand, and thus replacement of tissue along subunit intervals with flaps that include skin will improve overall appearance as compared to muscle flaps with a skin graft (Fig. 1).

6.1 ALT Flap Surgical Technique

Compared to other fasciocutaneous flaps, the ALT flap typically allows for a larger skin flap with a longer vascular pedicle and relatively easy dissection, all of which make it among the most reliable free flaps available. The technique of ALT flap harvest has been previously described in detail [24, 25]. The patient is placed into a supine position. A line is drawn from the anterior superior iliac spine (ASIS) to the lateral border of the patella (Fig. 2). Using a hand-held Doppler, the descending branch of the lateral circumflex femoral artery is identified and marked out starting at the midpoint of the line. Perforators, which generally cluster within 3–4 cm inferolateral to the midpoint, are also mapped using the Doppler. After all perforators have been marked, the size of the flap needed should then be determined. The flap skin paddle, which is the skin and fascia supplied by the flap pedicle, must then be designed to be centered over the perforator(s) used. The long axis of the flap should be parallel to the thigh, to decrease tension on closure of

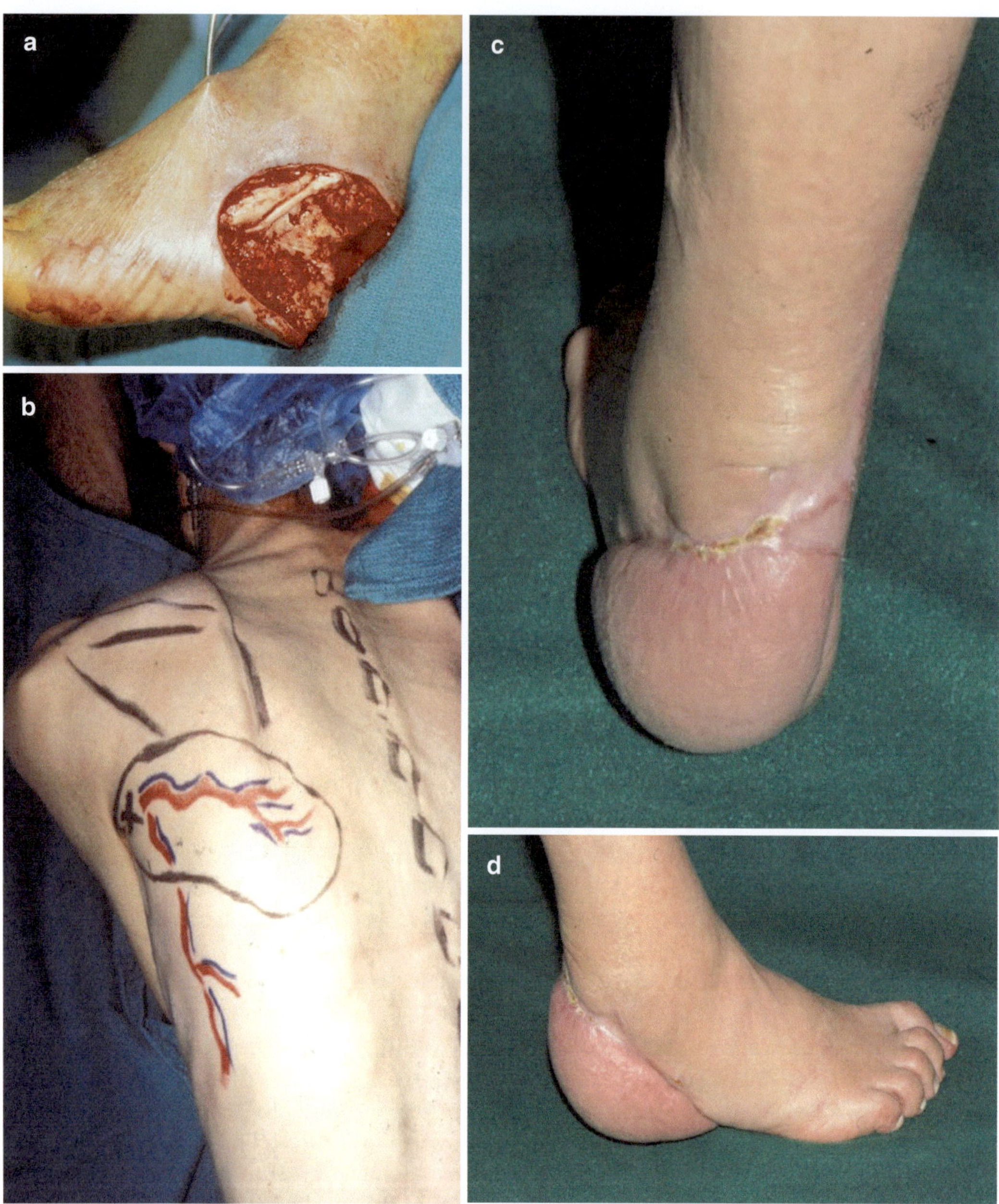

Fig. 1 (**a**) Pictured is a posterior heel soft tissue defect with exposed tendon and loss of weight-bearing plantar subunit. (**b**) A free fasciocutaneous left scapular flap was designed based upon cutaneous branches of the circum-flex scapular system. (**c**, **d**) Lateral and posterior views of postoperative result with re-established padding of the heel without overly bulky flap

donor site. The length of the vascular pedicle can be upwards of 15–16 cm in length if dissected to its most proximal extent (takeoff from the profunda artery), making it among the most versatile flaps for reconstructing defects throughout the body..

Dissection begins with skin incision down to the fascia overlying the rectus femoris muscle.

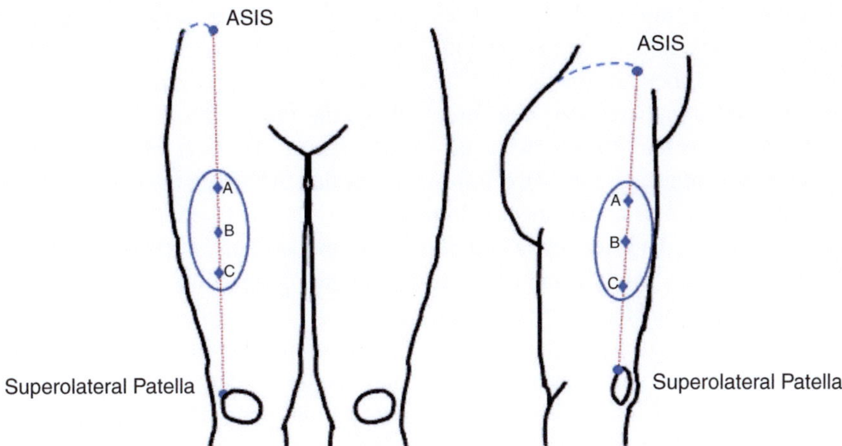

Fig. 2 Schematic diagram of ALT flap design. The anatomic landmarks that guide flap design are the ASIS proximally and the superolateral aspect of the patella distally. The long axis of the flap is centered on this line. Perforators are localized by Doppler exam and marked on the skin (x) and the skin paddle designed with the perforator(s) as centrally located as possible. A general rule of thumb is that a cluster of perforators is located half-way between the ASIS and patella, typically up to three perforators (named according to P. Yu et al. A–B–C perforator system) are identified along the axis approximately 5 cm apart [26]. It is important to mark the flap with the feet in a neutral or slightly internally rotated position to avoid aberrant markings. *ASIS* anterior superior iliac spine, *ALT* anterolateral thigh flap

The medial side of the flap is dissected first. If one is taking this as a fasciocutaneous flap, the fascia is incised and taken off with the skin and subcutaneous tissue. The fascia may be left adherent to the underlying muscles if only skin and subcutaneous tissue is needed (suprafascial dissection). The dissection proceeds laterally until the skin perforators are identified. Once all the perforators have been identified, dissection continues by isolating the perforator(s) along its course from surrounding muscle to the pedicle. Although the ALT flap is consistently well perfused with a single perforator, up to three perforators of appreciable size (>1 mm diameter) may be identified during the dissection. The decision of which perforators to use depends on their anatomic course, relation to one another, and size of the skin paddle needed. Any perforators deemed unnecessary will be ligated or temporarily clamped while isolating the flap on the remaining perforator(s). If perforators were temporarily clamped, the skin paddle perfusion is confirmed after dissection is complete and unused perforators definitively ligated. Once the main pedicle (descending branch of the lateral circumflex femoral artery) is identified, the flap is then dissected from its lateral border towards the pedicle. The pedicle is then dissected proximally, in the intermuscular septum, between the rectus femoris and the vastus lateralis to its origin as the descending branch of the lateral circumflex femoral vessels. A combination of sharp scissor dissection and fine bipolar cautery is used to isolate the pedicle from the surrounding muscle. Some bleeding may occur, but delicate handling of tissue is necessary to avoid damage to terminal vessels that supply the flap's undersurface. Prior to division of the pedicle, heparin is given to anticoagulate the patient. At this location the artery diameter in the pedicle can be upwards of 2 mm..

Closure of the donor site is done in layers with absorbable sutures deep and nonabsorbable sutures or staples for the skin over a closed suction drain. A donor site that is up to 9 cm in size can usually be closed primarily. Larger defects may require the use of a skin graft.

Variations in flap composition include harvesting a musculocutaneous flap by preserving the branches of the main pedicle to the vastus lateralis. When taking the muscle, there is no need to follow the pedicle through the vastus lateralis. Instead, the muscle is dissected along with the overlying skin and subcutaneous tissue. This avoids any unnecessary dissection that may injure the perforator. The harvest otherwise mirrors that of the fasciocutaneous flap. Two infrequent situations when a musculocutaneous flap may be preferred include the presence of a large amount of dead space that would benefit from a thicker flap, or when no suitable single perforator is present and the muscle has not been separated from the fasciocutaneous component above. Prior to final flap pedicle division, the recipient site vessels are exposed and prepared for anastomosis. Recipient vessels are selected based upon the defect location with anterior defects typically utilizing the anterior tibial vessels while medial or posterior defects often anastomosed to the posterior tibial vessels. Once the recipient site is ready, the flap blood supply is divided and the flap oriented to the defect and temporarily secured with staples to allow for vessel anastomosis. After flap reperfusion, a drain is placed deep to the flap, and not in proximity to the anastomosis, and the skin paddle secured with interrupted buried dermal sutures and interrupted nylon skin closure. The authors' preference for dressings includes bacitracin ointment over incisions and a plaster splint without any circumferential compression to prevent pedicle compression. Additionally, no dressings are placed covering the skin of the flap so that it may be visually inspected at any time..

7 Latissimus Dorsi Muscle Flap Surgical Technique

Prior to the popularization of fasciocutaneous and perforator flaps, muscle flaps were the primary reconstructive free flap option. The latissimus dorsi muscle flap is an attractive flap for several reasons, including the relative ease of harvest and the consistent vascular anatomy, which the flap is based upon. The flap demonstrates a dual blood supply (axial—thoracodorsal artery, segmental—lumbar artery perforators), each of which may adequately perfuse the flap

when the other is divided, classifying it as a Mathes-Nahai Type V Muscle Flap [27]. While either blood supply can be used for pedicled flaps, the thoracodorsal artery arising from the subscapular system is the basis for the free latissimus flap. Although the flap may be designed to include one or multiple skin paddles centered along the axis of the thoracodorsal pedicle; the following description is for a muscle-only flap [28].

Patient positioning for latissimus flap harvest may be in either the prone (posterior ankle defects) or lateral decubitus position (anterior or medial/lateral ankle defects), with an ipsilateral flap chosen for lateral defects and contralateral flap for medial defects. Important landmarks for flap design include the anterior border of the latissimus muscle and the tip of the scapula superiorly. The thoracodorsal pedicle runs parallel to the anterior latissimus border and approximately 2–3 cm posterior to it along the underside of the muscle. The incision is designed over the pedicle and may be linear or curvilinear. Harvest begins with sharp dissection down to the superficial surface of the muscle along the length of the incision, followed by elevation of skin and fat flaps over the muscle to the extent needed to cover the defect. Dissection may proceed superiorly until the scapula tip is encountered, anteriorly to the serratus muscle, inferiorly to the posterior superior iliac crest, and medially to the midline of the back. Next, the harvest proceeds with an elevation of the latissimus off the posterior chest wall. The correct plane of elevation may be difficult to identify if beginning inferiorly or anteriorly but is readily apparent along the superior border of the muscle, where an areolar plane is more easily identified. Once this plane is entered, a combination of blunt and bovie dissection is performed to elevate the muscle, taking care to ligate any lumbar perforators medially. The inferior attachments of the muscle must be divided with electrocautery, and muscle elevation continues towards the axilla. The pedicle of the flap will typically be visible along the underside of the muscle, which is followed proximally to the pedicle length required. If dissected proximally to the subscapular origin, up to 10–15 cm of pedicle length may be harvested. Care must be taken to avoid elevating the serratus muscle during the proximal dissection. Pedicle division proceeds with the same principles as described above for the ALT harvest, and either prior to or after pedicle division, the humeral insertion of the muscle must be divided to complete the harvest.

Closure of the donor site is done in layers with absorbable sutures to approximate the superficial fascial layer and the deep dermal layer, followed by standard epidermal closure. Due to wide subcutaneous dissection, seroma formation is the most common donor site complication, and as such two closed suction drains are typically required.

7.1 Postoperative Management

While a large body of literature has demonstrated microvascular flap success rates of 92–98%, reoperation for clinical flap compromise is necessary in about 10% of patients [29]. Therefore, patients are monitored in an intensive care unit or specially designed flap unit with nursing performing flap checks every hour for the first 48 h, and subsequently every 2 h while admitted. These flap checks consist of visual inspection for color of the skin/exposed muscle, palpation for warmth of the flap and capillary refill, and Doppler ultrasound of skin paddle or pedicle signals. Any abnormal findings are indicative of flap vascular compromise and mandate emergent operative exploration and treatment. The patients are typically discharged on postoperative day 7. The lower extremity is maintained in an elevated or flat position for 3 weeks. At that point, a dangling protocol is initiated, which aims to challenge flap venous drainage for incrementally longer periods of time with a clinical endpoint of no congestion in flap skin paddle (mottling, bluish hue or darker discoloration, brisk capillary refill) and minimal increase in swelling with prolonged dangling [30]. For example, the first week of the dangling protocol may call for dangling the extremity off the side of the bed for 15 min once or twice daily, followed by 30 min two or three times daily the next week, and so on until no significant venous congestion is noted with dangling.

8 Vascularized Bone Free Flap Reconstruction

In the foot in ankle, there are few alternative options for ankle arthrodesis, in the setting of large bone gaps. For moderate gaps or ankle arthrodesis in the setting of talus avascular necrosis (AVN), a sliding vascularized tibia flap is an option. Bone transport using an Ilizarov procedure is an additional option; however, it is thought that vascularized bone flaps, as described here, are more resistant to infection and faster to heal then bone transport.

The use of a fibula flap has a long history of success in extremity reconstruction [31]. However, since its origin in 1991, the use of a medial femoral condyle (MFC) flap has quickly gained popularity for smaller complex bone defects [32]. These vascularized bone flaps offer an additional alternative option in bone defects that require vascularized tissue. Other vascularized bone flaps that are used less commonly include the lateral arm flap with humerus cortical component, radial forearm flap, scapular or parascapular flap, and the deep circumflex iliac artery flap with iliac crest [33].

8.1 Indications

In the foot and ankle, vascularized bone flaps have been used successfully in tibiotalar and pantalar arthrodeses, talar avascular necrosis (AVN) and nonunions, navicular AVN, osteomyelitis resulting in significant bone loss and calcaneus nonunions [34]. Conventional bone grafts and/or allografts are typically used as a primary treatment option, but vascularized bone flaps are associated with better outcomes than nonvascularized grafts in segmental defects greater than 6 cm in length and demonstrate faster time to union with less hardware complications in patients undergoing salvage spinal fusion, especially in the setting of chronic osteomyelitis [31, 34]. These vascularized flaps can augment ankle arthrodesis in the setting of large distal tibia defects and tibiotalar degenerative joint disease with significant talar AVN. After failure of primary ankle arthrodesis with conventional techniques, vascularized bone flaps should be considered an option for any secondary surgery. The indications for a MFC flap are for defects of <4 cm when structural support is not required. The fibula flap is used when defects are >4 cm and/or structural support is required [30].

8.2 MFC Surgical Technique

The technique of MFC flap harvest has been previously described in detail [30]. The patient is positioned supine with both legs prepped to the groin. A medial longitudinal incision is made over the posterior border of the vastus medialis beginning at the distal aspect of the medial femoral condyle, which extends proximally for approximately 20 cm. The dissection continues through the subcutaneous tissue until the muscular fascia of the vastus medialis is encountered. This fascia is then incised longitudinally and the vastus medialis muscle retracted anteriorly, revealing the descending geniculate artery. During this approach care should be taken to preserve any substantial perforators to the skin, which could support a cutaneous paddle in addition to the corticocancellous bone flap. Once the feeding vessels are isolated, a rectangular segment of bone, up to 2–3 cm in length and width, may be safely harvested without risking donor site instability. When planning the bone cuts, one should aim to include as many of the plexus branches as possible in the flap and avoid injury to the medial collateral ligament or articular surface of the joint. Next, the periosteum is scored approximately 1 cm beyond the planned bone cuts circumferentially and periosteal elevator used to expose the medial

femoral condyle at sites of osteotomy. The osteotomies are then made with a sagittal saw and a curved osteotome used to carefully free the deep surface of the flap incorporating approximately 1–1.5 cm of cancellous bone. If a skin paddle is to be also included, the authors also identify skin perforators that are traced to the superficial fascia and to the skin island that will be harvested.

The technique of flap inset is tailored to the individual nature of the case. Following temporary ankle stabilization, a bone slot large enough for the bone flap and accompanying pedicle are created and the flap is impacted into the defect. The vascular anastomosis is then performed using the operating microscope. Recipient vessels are selected based upon the defect location with anterior defects typically utilizing the anterior tibial vessels while medial defects often anastomosed to the posterior tibial vessels. The bone flap may be stabilized to adjacent bone using a small k-wire if fixation is deemed necessary by the specific situation [35]. The authors' preference is to admit all patients postoperatively for a period of 2–4 days for flap monitoring accomplished by external Doppler exam and clinical assessment of the skin paddle if one is included (Fig. 3).

8.3 Fibula Surgical Technique

The technique of harvesting a free fibula flap has been described in detail in prior reports [36]. Harvest of the fibula flap can be performed under tourniquet control. The fibula is palpated and marked. The incision is positioned over the posterior border of the fibula. General guidelines regarding the amount of fibula that can be har-

Fig. 3 (**a, b**) Plain radiographs of a patient presenting for lower extremity salvage with navicular nonunion after multiple failed attempts at nonvascularized bone grafting and hardware stabilization. (**c**) Lateral foot demonstrating multiple prior incisions and significantly edematous dorsal foot. This indicated a soft tissue component to vascularized reconstruction would be necessary to provide skin closure. (**d**) Medial femoral condyle bony flap after osteotomies, descending genicular artery pedicle is isolated to the right. (**e**) MFC accompanying skin paddle with perforator arising from MFC vascular pedicle. (**f**) Dorsal view of navicular defect after hardware removal and bony debridement (**g, h**) In situ and fluoroscopy view of navicular defect with compression screw prepared for MFC graft. (**i, j**) View of MFC skin paddle after MFC graft impaction and flap inset

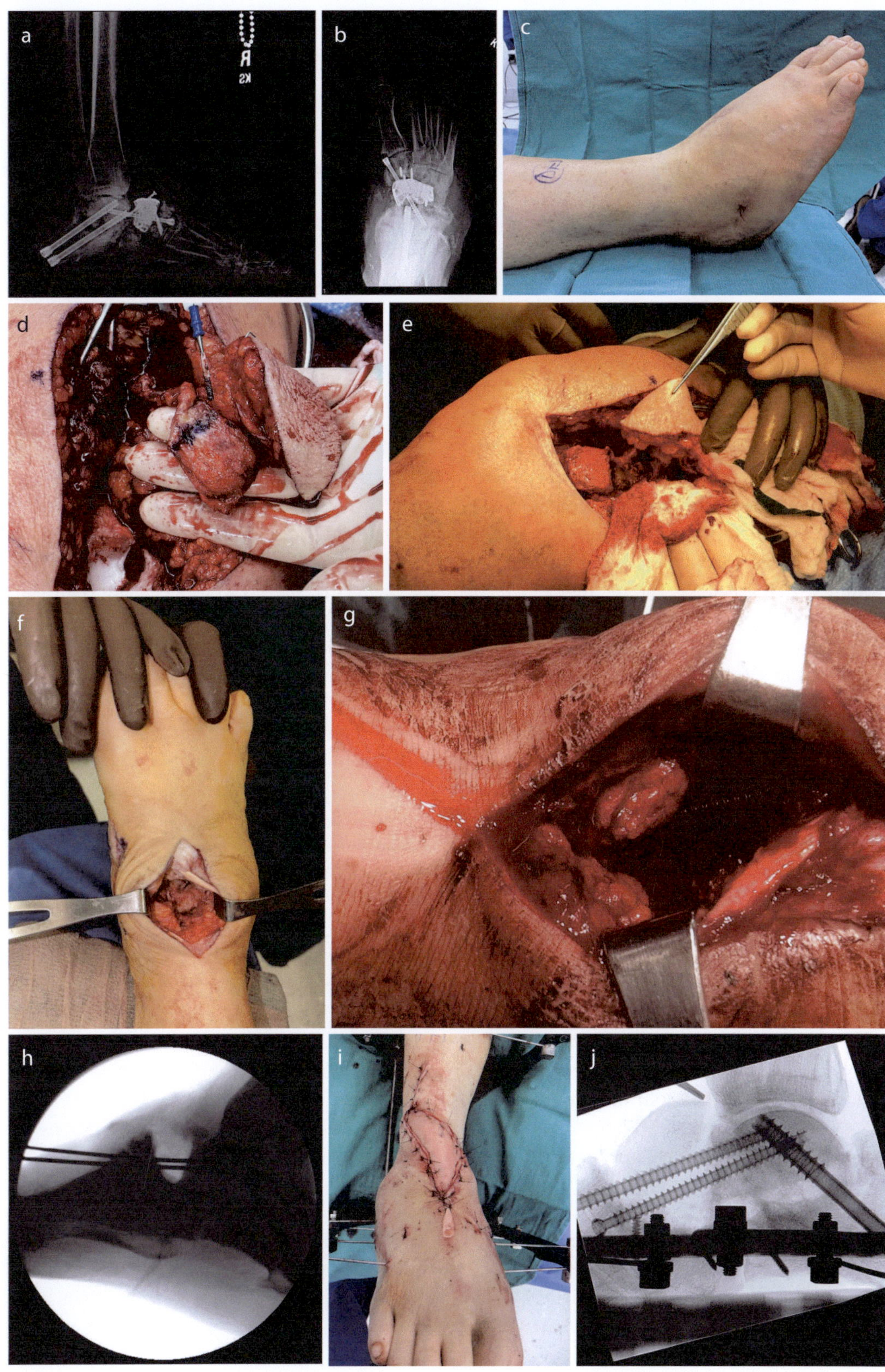

vested safely without disrupting ankle stability while avoiding injury to the peroneal nerve recommend leaving approximately 6–8 cm of fibula intact proximally and distally [37, 38]. The incision usually extends the full length of the fibula or slightly less so to allow for adequate exposure and access to the bony osteotomies and vascular structures proximally. If a skin paddle is harvested, it is centered over the posterior intermuscular septum located at the posterior border of the fibula. Anteriorly, the investing fascia is identified and incised to expose the lateral compartment (peroneal) muscles. The superficial peroneal nerve should be identified and protected. The peroneus longus and brevis are retracted anteriorly, and dissection proceeds to the fibula and the anterior intermuscular septum. The anterior intermuscular septum is incised longitudinally entering the anterior compartment. The anterior tibial vessels and deep peroneal nerve should be identified and protected. The interosseous membrane is identified and incised. When a skin paddle is harvested, the posterior approach is then performed in effort to maintain the skin paddle on the posterior intermuscular septum between the superficial posterior compartment and the lateral compartment. In most situations, skin perforators are visible within the septum. The fibula is carefully freed circumferentially of all attachments along its length, as well as at the planned osteotomy sites (approximately 6 cm inferior to the fibular head and 6 cm superior to the lateral malleolus). Osteotomies at these levels are performed with a sagittal saw or giggly saw. The fibula is retracted laterally, and the distal peroneal vessels are identified and clipped. The fibula and peroneal vessels are then dissected together from distal to proximal in the deep posterior compartment until they join the posterior tibial vessels at the tibioperoneal trunk. The vessels and osseous flap (or osteocutaneous flap) are harvested together [39, 40]. Flap inset is dependent upon the defect characteristics as well as the composition of the flap. The bone may be stabilized using k-wire techniques or a semi-rigid fixation with mini-plates, secured unicortically to surrounding bone, whereas the skin paddle is sutured to provide soft tissue coverage. In all instances, care must be taken to avoid injuring the vascular pedicle running along the medial border of the fibula. Additionally, the authors often secure the perivascular tissue of the pedicle to the periosteum of the bone with chromic suture to prevent sheering or avulsion when placing the bone into the defect. Recipient vessels are selected based upon the defect location and availability of the posterior tibial or anterior tibial vessels..

8.4 Postoperative Management

Principals of postoperative management for soft tissue free flaps also applies here (see previous section). Unique considerations specific to bony free tissue reconstruction include duration of immobilization and weight-bearing status. Typically, partial weight bearing is allowed at 1 month based on overlying soft tissue healing and serial X-rays demonstrating stable bony alignment and evidence of healing and full weight bearing permitted at 2 months if healing continues to progress, and all patients undergo follow up CT scan to confirm union [35].

9 Conclusions

Ankle defects are often challenging to reconstruct; however, successful reconstruction is achieved through a thoughtfully planned multidisciplinary approach to evaluation and management. This chapter serves as a guide to ankle reconstruction involving soft tissue defects, beginning with how to assess a wound on initial consultation. Also discussed are indications for additional work-up or specialist consultation and the importance of adequate debridement. Lastly, free flap reconstructive options are summarized with technical descriptions included for the more common free tissue transfer options for soft tissue-only flaps as well as osteocutaneous free flaps.

References

1. Baumeister SP, Spierer R, Erdmann D, Sweis R, Levin LS, Germann GK. A realistic complication analysis of 70 sural artery flaps in a multimorbid patient group. Plast Reconstr Surg. 2003;112:129–40; discussion 141–142.
2. Levin LS. Soft tissue coverage options for ankle wounds. Foot Ankle Clin. 2001;6:853–66.
3. Cho EH, Garcia R, Pien I, Thomas S, Levin LS, Hollenbeck ST. An algorithmic approach for managing orthopaedic surgical wounds of the foot and ankle. Clin Orthop Relat Res. 2014;472:1921–9.
4. Patrulea V, Ostafe V, Borchard G, Jordan O. Chitosan as a starting material for wound healing applications. Eur J Pharm Biopharm. 2015;97:417–26.
5. Abdou SA, Stranix JT, Daar DA, et al. Free tissue transfer with distraction osteogenesis and Masquelet technique is effective for limb salvage in patients with Gustilo type IIIB open fractures. Plast Reconstr Surg. 2020;145:1071–6.
6. Bibbo C, Ehrlich DA, Nguyen HM, Levin LS, Kovach SJ. Low wound complication rates for the lateral extensile approach for calcaneal ORIF when the lateral calcaneal artery is patent. Foot Ankle Int. 2014;35:650–6.
7. Levin LS. Debridement of soft tissue infections of the lower leg. In: Lee GK, editor. Operative techniques: lower limb reconstruction and amputation, vol. 3. Philadelphia: Wolters Kluwer.
8. Rajan M, Joy M, Levin LS, Kovacs SJ. Recipient vessels: tibia reconstruction. In: Gurunian R, Djohan R, editors. Recipient vessels in reconstructive microsurgery: anatomy and technical considerations. Cham: Springer; 2021. p. 245–50.
9. Cho EH, Garcia RM, Pien I, et al. Vascular considerations in foot and ankle free tissue transfer: analysis of 231 free flaps. Microsurgery. 2016;36:276–83.
10. Heitmann C, Levin LS. The orthoplastic approach for management of the severely traumatized foot and ankle. J Trauma. 2003;54:379–90.
11. Kulkarni GS, Kulkarni S, Babhulkar S. Cement beads and cement spacers: indications, techniques, and clinical results. OTA Int J Orthop Trauma. 2021;4:e118.
12. Thai DQ, Jung YK, Hahn HM, Lee IJ. Factors affecting the outcome of lower extremity osteomyelitis treated with microvascular free flaps: an analysis of 65 patients. J Orthop Surg Res. 2021;16:535.
13. Anakwenze OA, Milby AH, Gans I, Stern JJ, Levin LS, Wapner KL. Foot and ankle infections: diagnosis and management. J Am Acad Orthop Surg. 2012;20:684–93.
14. Reddy V, Stevenson TR. MOC-PS(SM) CME article: lower extremity reconstruction. Plast Reconstr Surg. 2008;121:1–7.
15. Schiro GR, Sessa S, Piccioli A, Maccauro G. Primary amputation vs limb salvage in mangled extremity: a systematic review of the current scoring system. BMC Musculoskelet Disord. 2015;16:372.
16. Lerman OZ, Kovach SJ, Levin LS. The respective roles of plastic and orthopedic surgery in limb salvage. Plast Reconstr Surg. 2011;127(Suppl 1):215S–27S.
17. Momeni A, Lanni M, Levin LS, Kovach SJ. Microsurgical reconstruction of traumatic lower extremity defects in the pediatric population. Plast Reconstr Surg. 2017;139:998–1004.
18. Azoury SC, Stranix JT, Othman S, et al. Outcomes following soft-tissue reconstruction for traumatic lower extremity defects at an orthoplastic limb salvage center: the need for lower extremity guidelines for salvage (L.E.G.S.). Orthoplast Surg. 2021;3:1–7.
19. Piwnica-Worms W, Stranix JT, Othman S, et al. Risk factors for lower extremity amputation following attempted free flap limb salvage. J Reconstr Microsurg. 2020;36:528–33.
20. Levin LS. Foot and ankle soft-tissue deficiencies: who needs a flap? Am J Orthop (Belle Mead NJ). 2006;35:11–9.
21. Heller L, Levin LS. Lower extremity microsurgical reconstruction. Plast Reconstr Surg. 2001;108:1029–41. quiz 1042
22. Hollenbeck ST, Woo S, Komatsu I, Erdmann D, Zenn MR, Levin LS. Longitudinal outcomes and application of the subunit principle to 165 foot and ankle free tissue transfers. Plast Reconstr Surg. 2010;125:924–34.
23. Yu P. Reinnervated anterolateral thigh flap for tongue reconstruction. Head Neck. 2004;26:1038–44.
24. Wang HT, Erdmann D, Fletcher JW, Levin LS. Anterolateral thigh flap technique in hand and upper extremity reconstruction. Tech Hand Up Extrem Surg. 2004;8:257–61.
25. Heitmann C, Guerra A, Metzinger SW, Levin LS, Allen RJ. The thoracodorsal artery perforator flap: anatomic basis and clinical application. Ann Plast Surg. 2003;51:23–9.
26. Yu P, Youssef A. Efficacy of the handheld Doppler in preoperative identification of the cutaneous perforators in the anterolateral thigh flap. Plast Reconstr Surg. 2006;118:928–33; discussion 934–5.
27. Mathes SJ, Nahai F. Classification of the vascular anatomy of muscles: experimental and clinical correlation. Plast Reconstr Surg. 1981;67:177–87.
28. Zhang YX, Messmer C, Pang FK, et al. A novel design of the multilobed latissimus dorsi myocutaneous flap to achieve primary donor-site closure in the reconstruction of large defects. Plast Reconstr Surg. 2013;131:752e–8e.
29. Lese I, Biedermann R, Constantinescu M, Grobbelaar AO, Olariu R. Predicting risk factors that lead to free flap failure and vascular compromise: a single unit experience with 565 free tissue transfers. J Plast Reconstr Aesthet Surg. 2021;74:512–22.
30. Fischer JP, Wink JD, Nelson JA, et al. A retrospective review of outcomes and flap selection in free tissue transfers for complex lower extremity reconstruction. J Reconstr Microsurg. 2013;29:407–16.
31. Levin LS. Vascularized fibula graft for the traumatically induced long-bone defect. J Am Acad Orthop Surg. 2006;14:S175–6.

32. Kazmers NH, Rozell JC, Rumball KM, Kozin SH, Zlotolow DA, Levin LS. Medial femoral condyle microvascular bone transfer as a treatment for capitate avascular necrosis: surgical technique and case report. J Hand Surg Am. 2017;42:841.e1–6.

33. Haddock NT, Wapner K, Levin LS. Vascular bone transfer options in the foot and ankle: a retrospective review and update on strategies. Plast Reconstr Surg. 2013;132:685–93.

34. Erdmann D, Meade RA, Lins RE, McCann RL, Richardson WJ, Levin LS. Use of the microvascular free fibula transfer as a salvage reconstruction for failed anterior spine surgery due to chronic osteomyelitis. Plast Reconstr Surg. 2006;117:2438–45; discussion 2446–7.

35. Haddock NT, Alosh H, Easley ME, Levin LS, Wapner KL. Applications of the medial femoral condyle free flap for foot and ankle reconstruction. Foot Ankle Int. 2013;34:1395–402.

36. Bibbo C, Bauder AR, Nelson J, et al. Reconstruction of traumatic defects of the tibia with free fibula flap and external fixation. Ann Plast Surg. 2020;85:516–21.

37. Baumann DP, Yu P, Hanasono MM, Skoracki RJ. Free flap reconstruction of osteoradionecrosis of the mandible: a 10-year review and defect classification. Head Neck. 2011;33:800–7.

38. Hanasono MM, Zevallos JP, Skoracki RJ, Yu P. A prospective analysis of bony versus soft-tissue reconstruction for posterior mandibular defects. Plast Reconstr Surg. 2010;125:1413–21.

39. Haddock NT, Wapner KL, Scott Levin L. Pedicle and free vascularized bone transfers to the foot and ankle. Tech Foot Ankle Surg. 2013;12:74–8.

40. Piccolo PP, Ben-Amotz O, Ashley B, Wapner KL, Levin LS. Ankle arthrodesis with free vascularized fibula autograft using saphenous vein grafts: a case series. Plast Reconstr Surg. 2018;142:806–9.

Management of Osteochondral Disorders of the Ankle

Alastair Younger

1 Introduction

Osteochondral lesions of the talus (OLT) are common lesions. They can be found in isolation or in combination with other ankle pathology such as ankle instability [1]. The majority are thought to be post traumatic in nature in older patients [2], while in younger patients, these lesions may have a bone developmental origin [3]. They may also be vascular in nature and may have a genetic predisposition to occur. If they remain symptomatic and do not resolve with non-operative treatment, then surgery can be performed. However, many patients are younger compared to the average patient in a foot and ankle practice and have an expectation to return to sport. This occurs in 88% of surgical cases but sometimes at a reduced level [4].

Some patients may fail to get adequate function despite following the guidelines outlined by ICRA [5].

Patients therefore need to be aware of the potential for not being able to return to the sport of their choice or to the level that they wish to achieve.

Patients with malalignment that is overloading the osteochondral defect may require realignment surgery [5], and associated ankle instability needs to be both diagnosed and treated [6]. If both instability and malalignment are treated, then outcomes can be optimized [7]. The incidence of osteochondral lesions occurring in patients with ankle instability treated surgically was approximately 30% in one series [8].

The international consensus group on cartilage repair of the ankle meeting in Pittsburgh in 2017 has assisted the medical community in trying to standardize care with regards to investigation, non-operative treatment, operative intervention, and the use of cartilage or bone graft into the defect [9]. This has been very helpful in trying to codify the treatment of these challenging lesions.

The resources available to treat osteochondral ankle lesions in different centers may determine the treatment. Allograft may or may not be available. Bone graft substitute, cartilage products, and cell products may or may not be affordable.

Arthroscopic procedures are more likely to result in a shorter recovery and maintenance of range of motion [10]. As a result, primary procedures are often arthroscopic, and open procedures are reserved for revision procedures or large initial defects. Some of these procedures are maximally invasive requiring iliac crest or knee harvest sites and tibial osteotomies to gain vertical access to the defect site.

A. Younger (✉)
Department of Orthopaedics, University of British Columbia, Vancouver, BC, Canada

Foot & Ankle Research, St. Paul's Hospital, Vancouver, BC, Canada

© The Author(s), under exclusive license to Springer Nature Switzerland AG 2023
D. Herscovici Jr. et al. (eds.), *Evaluation and Surgical Management of the Ankle*,
https://doi.org/10.1007/978-3-031-33537-2_24

2 Pathology

Failed debridement of OLT results in increased levels of inflammatory mediators in the synovial fluid [11]. Histological analysis of the cartilage in the osteochondral defects show changes suggestive of cartilage degeneration, compared to no degeneration in normal cartilage from allograft donors. Similarly there were raised levels of tumour necrosis factor (TNF) alpha, Interleukin (IL)-2, 6, 10, 13, Matrix Metalloproteinases (MMP) 1, 2, 3, 9 and 10. Medial lesions are more likely to occur than lateral lesions as reported in most papers, and were 60% of all lesions in one systematic review [12]. The location of lesions are mapped out using a grid system as outlined by Elias et al. for the talus [13] and tibia [14]. The grid consists of nine zones of the tibia and talus, with division into each plane into thirds. Zone 1 is anterior and medial, zone 3 anterior and lateral, zone 7 posterior and medial, and zone 9 posterior and lateral.

On the talus the lesions are most commonly on the medial central location [13], and these lesions are deeper and longer than the lateral lesions. The lesions located on the tibia more often medial, with posterior medial being slightly less common than the Centro medial location [14]. The inter and intra observer reliability of this system was reviewed and shown to be reproducible and reliable [15].

The formation of the cyst through a breakdown of the subchondral bone and the subchondral oedema remains debatable. Access of joint fluid may be a precipitating event [16].

Bruns, Maier and Fraissler in separate studies have shown that the OLT lesions are associated with vitamin D deficiency.

3 Terminology

The international cartilage society published their recommendations for terminology in discussing osteochondral lesions [17]. This assists surgeons in understanding the literature with regards to outcomes. They recommended using the term subchondral bone lesion (SBL) if only the bone is affected. This is a rare occasion.

An isolated cartilage lesion has no bone involvement. There was no acronym recommended for classifying this lesion.

A combined cartilage and bone lesion is an osteochondral lesion of the talus, abbreviated to OLT.

Bone marrow stimulation was considered the correct term to cover all procedures in which the defect was debrided, and the bone stimulated via an awl or drill.

Bulk grafts were termed autologous osteochondral transplant (AuOT) or allograft transplant (AlOT).

Subchondral oedema is an increase in fluid in the subchondral bone diagnosed by MRI. The size is also measured by MRI in three planes to calculate a volume of involvement.

Cysts are defined as a lesion under the subchondral bone and characterized by consistency (loculation), communication with the joint, depth, and size, walled or not, and location.

Oedema is classified by size, depth, location, total volume and whether there was communication with the joint.

Acute is defined as under 1 month, sub-acute 1–6 months, and chronic over 6 months since the onset of symptoms [17].

4 Clinical Assessment

Clinical assessment should focus on the key elements of disability. The international consensus group on cartilage repair of the ankle identified assessment of deficit in ADL's and sporting activities, duration of symptoms, history of trauma, mechanism of injury, localization of the pain, mechanical symptoms such as locking and instability, previous treatment and swelling as the core information to obtain in determining treatment options [18].

For physical examination, the physician should inspect for weight bearing alignment, ankle range of motion (compared to the normal side), stability of the lateral and medial collateral ligaments, swelling, and tenderness to palpation [18]. Location of tenderness can be determined by clinical examination, which studies have shown correlates well with the radiotracer uptake on SPECT [19].

If a cartilage lesion is present, deep ankle pain aggravated by activity may be the hallmark symptoms [18].

5 Investigations

Standing AP, lateral and mortise views of the ankle are required for the initial investigation [18] (Fig. 1). Often the defect can be visualized, and the alignment of the ankle can be appreciated. Additional views including a calcaneal axial view, long leg alignment view, as well as AP and lateral views of the foot can be obtained to fully appreciate the associated weight-bearing pathology. Standing radiographs allow for the assessment of alignment and associated lesions such as osteophytes, cystic changes, degenerative change, and size of the OLT plus location. CT allows better estimation of cyst location and size, as well as osteophyte formation and bony impingement (Fig. 2), while MRI allows assessment of cartilage delamination,

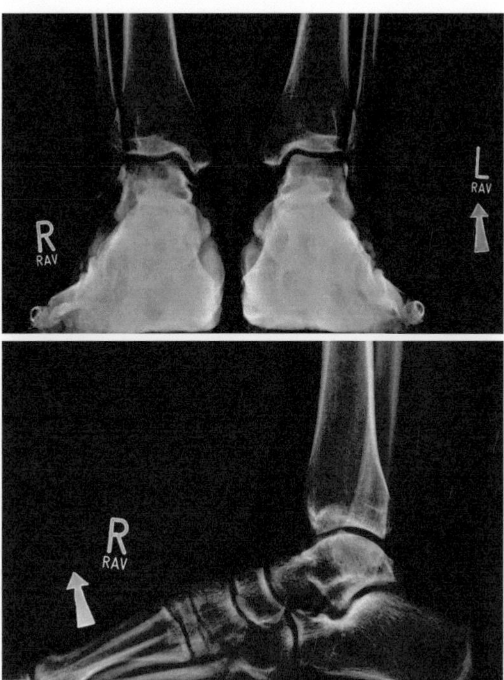

Fig. 1 Standing AP and lateral views showing an osteochondral injury. Long leg alignment views and a calcaneal axial view can also be of value

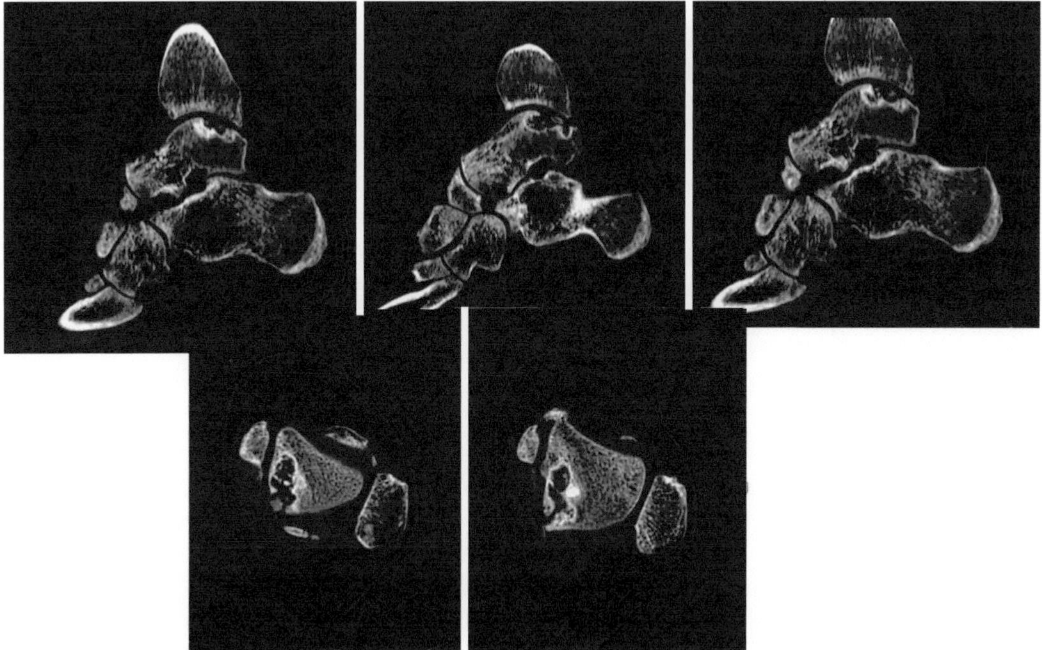

Fig. 2 Assessment of a large cystic defect on the medial talar dome using CT. This lesion was asymptomatic until the subchondral bone fractured (not the same patient as Fig. 1)

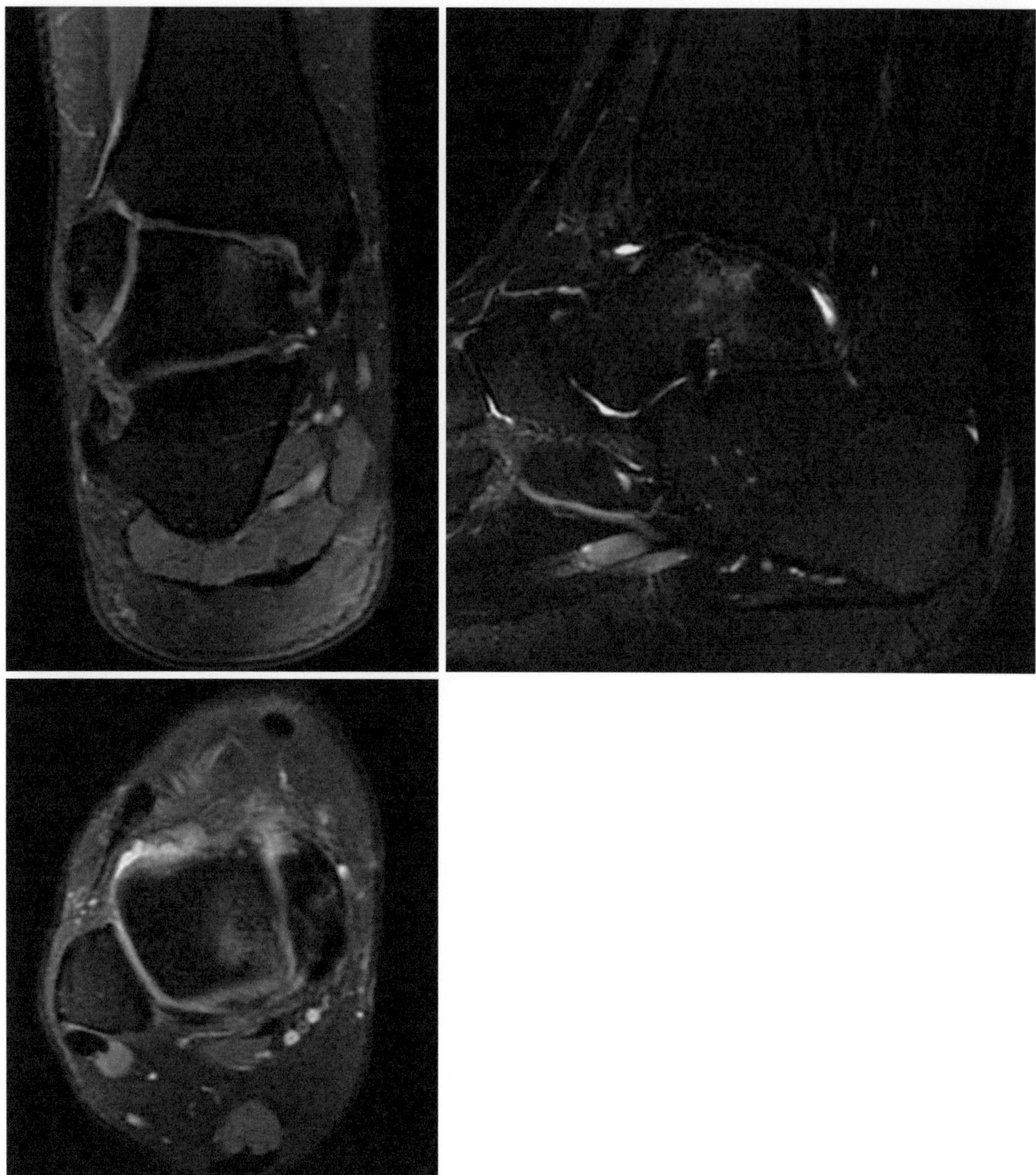

Fig. 3 MRI of the same lesion in Fig. 1

bone marrow oedema, and soft tissue impingement [18] (Fig. 3).

Assessment of sensitivity and specificity shows that plain X-ray is specific (0.91) but not sensitive (0.59) (i.e., it may fail to diagnose an osteochondral defect that is present). The CT scan is more sensitive (0.99) and specific (0.81) than radiographs for OLT identification but not as good as MRI which is reported to be sensitive and specific with a value of 0.96. [20]

As a result, three-dimensional imaging is usually required to understand the full size and location of the defect. MRI remains the principal tool for advanced investigation because it is more sensitive and specific and gives a better estimation on cartilage damage. The bone marrow oedema

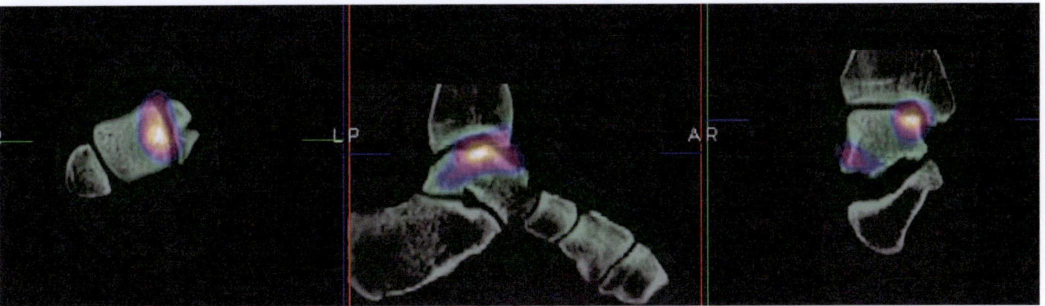

Fig. 4 SPECT of the same patient in Fig. 1 showing bone activity in the osteochondral lesion

indicates the extent of the soft cartilage. Finally, deficiency of the lateral and medial collateral ligaments, the presence of peroneal tendon pathology, and other cartilage lesions or impingement lesions can often be present and assessed via MRI.

The combination of bone scan and CT scan (SPECT) allows visualization of the defect with determination of bone scan uptake superimposed on the CT scan views. Activity of the lesion and other areas of radiotracer uptake such as anterior impingement can also be seen (Fig. 4).

6 Treatment

6.1 Conservative Treatment

Conservative treatment is recommended initially in all patients with asymptomatic lesions, such as incidental findings, non-displaced acute bone and cartilage injuries, older age with lower functional status, adjacent joint arthritis, or a skeletally immature patient [21].

The response to non-operative treatment is affected by patient age, body mass index (higher is worse), acuity of the lesion, size of the lesion (larger is worse), location of the lesion, presence of cystic change (cysts are worse), ankle instability, loose bodies, functional status, associated cartilage injury, medical comorbidities, and progression on imaging [21].

If the patient has an acute non-displaced OLT, ankle immobilization with touch down weight bearing is recommended for 6 weeks. Bone stimulators are unlikely to be beneficial [21].

The goal of non-operative treatment is for a full return to function with occasional pain. Low impact sports are recommended. An MRI should be obtained if there is no improvement in symptoms or radiographs by 3 months. Follow up should be every 6 months until resolution of symptoms. Deterioration may indicate the need for surgery. Concentrated bone marrow aspirate or platelet rich plasma (PRP) may be considered as an adjunct treatment, but there is little evidence to support the use of PRP in this setting [21].

Non-operative treatment can result in symptom resolution in some patients. Bracing, physiotherapy, NSAID medication are the initial treatments. Night splints may be helpful in patients with tight heel cords [21].

6.2 Operative Treatment

Operative treatment is directed at the bone defect and associated pathology.

6.3 Treatment of the Osteochondral Defect

The goal of treatment of the osteochondral defect is to try and get the bone and cartilage void to heal. Appropriate treatment of the primary lesion depends on the location, the residual cartilage condition, and size of the defect [22].

Treatment of the bone defect can be through marrow stimulation, bone graft substitute, autograft, or allograft (Fig. 5). The graft may be can-

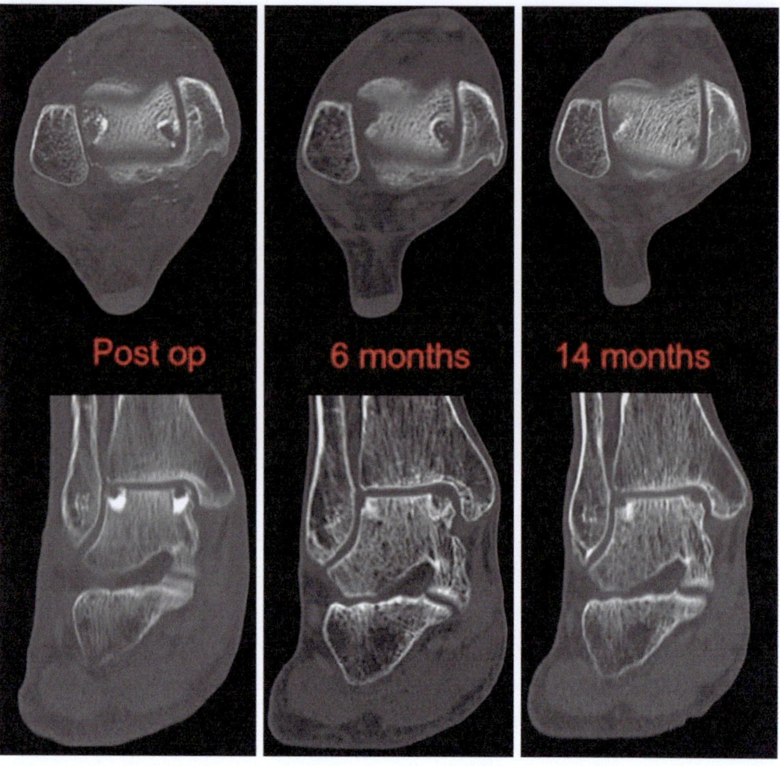

Fig. 5 Treatment of recurrent osteochondral defect on the medial and lateral side of the talus with PDGF and tricalcium sulphate. Gradual healing over time is seen

cellous or bulk such as an OATS. Grafting can be done through the defect by way of joint access or retrograde through the extra-articular bone.

Retrograde grafting can be performed for talar and tibial defects if the cartilage surface is intact. This is a rare case.

If bone is placed in a subchondral defect, it is helpful to seal it from the joint to prevent egress of bone growth factors that may negatively impact the cartilage or the synovium. Fibrin glue over the exposed bone can be used to achieve this seal.

7 Debridement, Curettage, and Bone Marrow Stimulation

Debridement of the osteochondral lesion is routinely performed arthroscopically. For lesions anterior to the 12 o'clock apex of the talus, the lesion can be approached anteriorly. A plantar flexion X-ray can assist in determining if the lesion can be reached [23]. Plantar flexion and occasional limited tibial osteotomy can allow the access to the lesion. Calf tourniquets used during surgery will result in compression of the calf muscles and can limit access to the talus by restricting muscle movement.

Anterior arthroscopy is performed using anterior medial and anterior lateral portals. Care is taken to avoid the superficial branch and deep branch of the peroneal nerve, using blunt dissection and superficial skin incisions.

The author also uses the posterior portals in the supine position as described by Acevedo [24]. This allows access posteriorly to posterior pathology as well as synovitis, loose bodies, or visualization in a tight ankle.

The portal is made just posterior to the medial malleolus and passing behind the tibialis posterior tendon. Because the neurovascular bundle is in this region the deep dissection is blunt, and any shaver should be visualized in the joint before being used. Alternatively, a posterior lateral portal can be made behind the peroneal tendons, a blunt obturator passed through the joint and a switching stick technique used.

Debridement of the osteochondral defect requires removal of all unstable cartilage, and removal of any loose bone. The bone in regions of bone marrow oedema is usually soft secondary to the biologic effects of synovial fluid and needs to be removed. After debridement, the defect should be free of loose cartilage and curetted back to solid bone [25].

Lesions amenable to debridement as a definitive procedure include partial thickness chondral lesions, acute lesions such as those found after ankle fractures, and lesions secondary other disease such as PVNS [22].

Size guidelines exist for the success of debridement. Based on the studies of Choi and Kennedy, smaller lesions do well with debridement, while larger lesions fail [26]. The threshold is debatable, but lesions classified as small should be under 10 mm in diameter, under 100 mm^2 in area, and under 5 mm in depth [27] (Fig. 6). Bone marrow stimulation alone is unlikely to work for lesions greater than 15 mm in diameter [27].

Other factors affecting the success of debridement include the presence of ankle instability, bone marrow oedema, joint malalignment in addition to lesion size, lesion location, cysts, revision procedures, and uncontained lesions [22].

After debridement, an awl or 2 mm drill can be used to penetrate the base of the lesion to allow egress of bone marrow cells to create a new bone base [22]. Releasing the tourniquet can confirm successful penetration by bone bleeding. Two to 3 penetrations should suffice.

The addition of biologics may assist in the healing of the bone and cartilage in the defect. Adjuncts include concentrated bone marrow aspirate, mesenchymal stem cells, platelet rich plasma, and hyaluronic acid [28].

For acute unstable lesions bone marrow stimulation is appropriate, and if the unstable lesion is saucer shaped and large enough that it can be preserved and reattached [29]. Fixation can be achieved using poly-L-lactide pins as described by Nakaska et al. [30, 31], who also showed that fixation was superior to excision and BMS for lesions under 100 mm^2. Alternatives include bone plugs or 2 mm screws. A lesion smaller than 10 mm length or 3 mm depth is better excised than transfixed [32].

Repeat bone marrow stimulation for failed debridement can be considered for cases where the debridement may be incomplete, or when the patient is unwilling to undergo a more invasive open procedure.

BMS has been reported to result in osteoarthritis in 33–34% of patients.

7.1 Post-operative Protocol

Historically non-weightbearing was advocated for 6 weeks. However more recently outcomes have been demonstrated to be similar with 2 weeks non-weightbearing. Range of motion is initiated at 2 weeks with avoidance of shear loading. Various protocols can be used. MRI can be

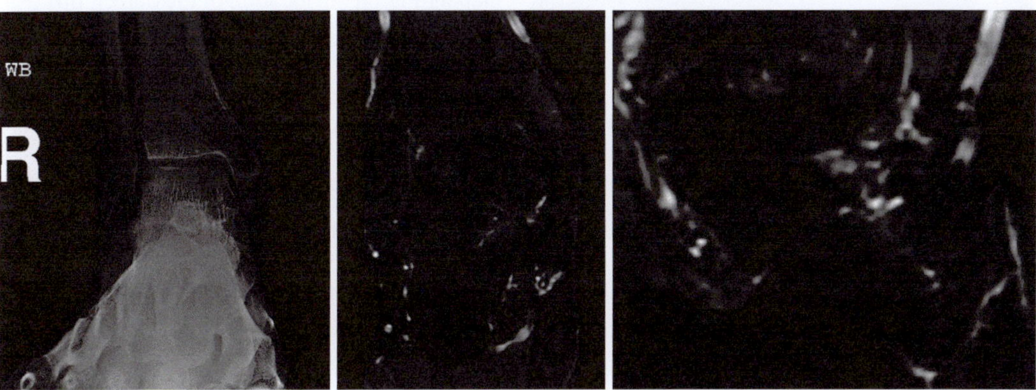

Fig. 6 A lesion of appropriate size and location for bone marrow stimulation (BMS)

used to determine if increased activity can be tolerated. The concomitant procedures can determine the recovery protocol such as lateral ligament reconstruction or calcaneal osteotomy.

After remobilization it is usual to contain shear by using a walker boot or brace.

8 The Cartilage Defect

The cartilage defect is managed by removal of all loose fragments and the filling the defect. In many cases the cartilage defect can be left unfilled, particularly in smaller lesions (Fig. 6). Typically, the defect becomes filled with hyaline cartilage which works well for small defects but may shear with larger defects (Figs. 7 and 8). Cartilage substitutes can be used of various descriptions and various costs; however they may not provide any better graft than marrow stimulation [33]. Cartilage graft can include extracellular cartilage matrix [34–36], juvenile cartilage [37, 38], scaffold [39] or amplified cartilage cells [40] in a single stage [41, 42] procedure, or a two stage procedure.

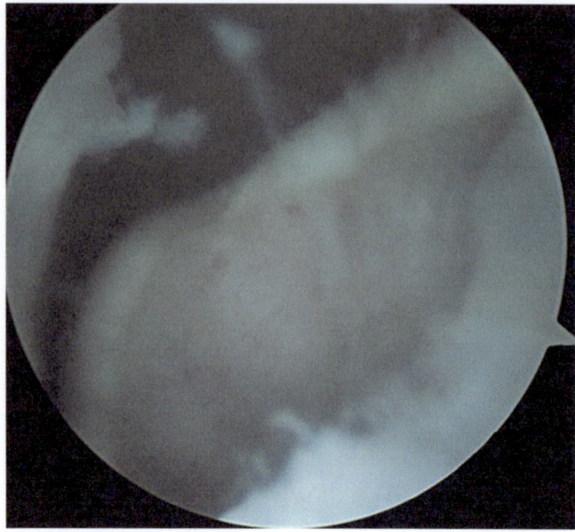

Fig. 8 The same lesion after debridement of loose cartilage and loose bone

9 Larger Defects: Bulk Grafts and Oats

Larger defects may require a bulk graft which can be a fresh frozen graft OATS, a packaged allograft Osteochondral Allograft Transfer (OATS), or an autograft OATS [43]. Mosaicplasty is a little different in technique as the grafts are smaller and defects exist in the cartilage surface [44].

9.1 Procedure

To perform an OATS procedure on the talus, a vertical approach should be obtained through the tibia to gain access to the cartilage surface. Depending on the location of the defect, this usually requires an osteotomy.

9.2 Medial Defects

Medial defects of the talus usually require a medial malleolar osteotomy. They are approached via a high oblique medial malleolar osteotomy [45, 46]. A longitudinal incision is made, and the

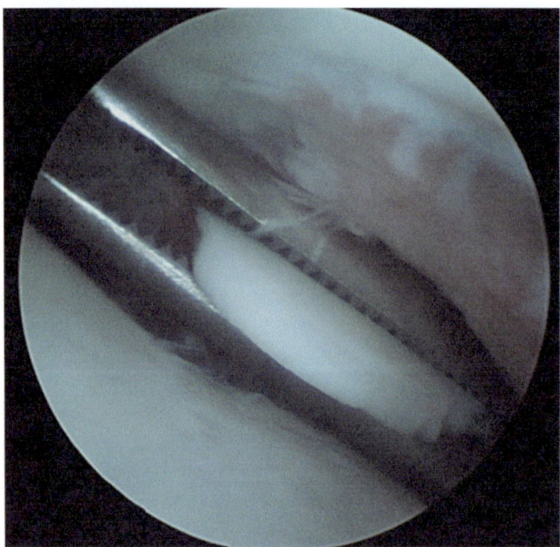

Fig. 7 The same lesion with the cartilage and subchondral bone defect removed

anterior and posterior joint line are outlined. This needs to be performed carefully as an incorrect osteotomy will compromise the approach. The usual error is to enter the joint too medially. To ensure a correct approach a k wire is placed, and its position confirmed on c arm. Predrilling the screw holes for fixation prior to the osteotomy is helpful to maintain articular joint surface congruity. Sometimes full plantar flexion and limited palatoplasty can allow access to the lesion [47].

Before starting the saw cut, retractors are placed anteriorly and posteriorly. The posterior retractor should be placed under the posterior tibial tendon to ensure it does not get cut.

Once performed the anterior and posterior capsule may have to be released to allow the talus to be pulled into valgus hinged on the deep deltoid ligament to improve the visualization. The lesion can then be sized. Because the lesion is usually over 10 mm in size one or two 10 mm grafts are required (Fig. 7).

The guide wire should be carefully placed over the defect. The wire has to be vertically oriented over the joint surface. The wire should end up pointing at the lateral corner of the lateral process of the talus, which is the central axis of rotation of the talus on the lateral view. On the AP view the wire should be perpendicular to the top surface of the talus.

Reaming is performed carefully to avoid heat and irrigation used. A depth of 15 mm should be achieved. The harvested graft should also be planned to match the talar defect as this will often have a shoulder area and may be still a little eccentric in position.

After harvesting the autograft or allograft, the end of the graft is trimmed to be bullet shaped and at the depth of the defect. If desired, platelet rich plasma (PRP) can be placed into the depth of the defect [48, 49].

The graft is carefully placed onto the defect and rotated to best match the defect. It should push in and be flush.

Nested grafts are two or more grafts that are used to fill a defect. They should overlap the adjacent graft by a quarter of the diameter. After one is placed, the second drill hole is prepared, and the second graft placed.

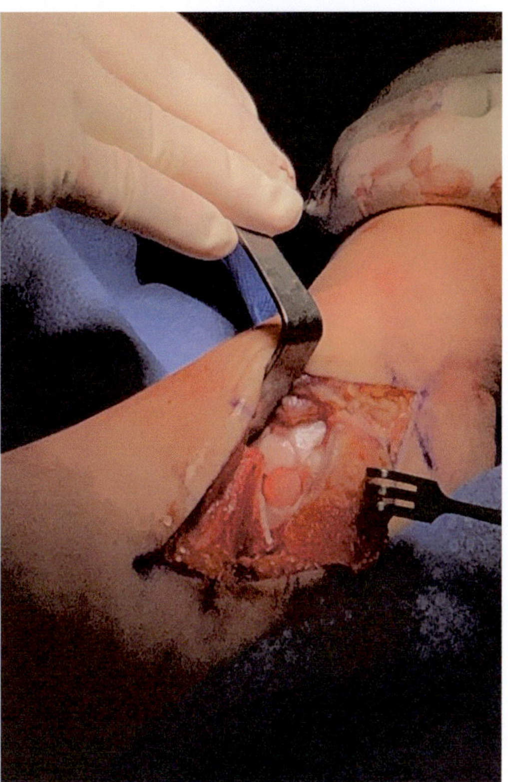

Fig. 9 A medial malleolar osteotomy and double 10 mm OATS autograft for a failed prior debridement of a larger posterior medial lesion

The tibial osteotomy site is reduced and held with screws and or a plate and screws in a stable position (Figs. 9 and 10).

9.3 Lateral Defect

The lateral defect can be approached by an extensile lateral approach. This is performed by sectioning the lateral collateral ligaments. Anterior translation of the talus will often allow vertical access to the defect. If this cannot be achieved after release of the capsule, then a lateral malleolar osteotomy will need to be performed (Fig. 11). This will need to be proximal enough to allow vertical access (Figs. 12, 13, and 14). A transverse osteotomy can be used with external rotation of the fibula, oblique osteotomy with external rotation, or distal rotation similar to the Zimmer ankle approach. Fixation is either with plates or a

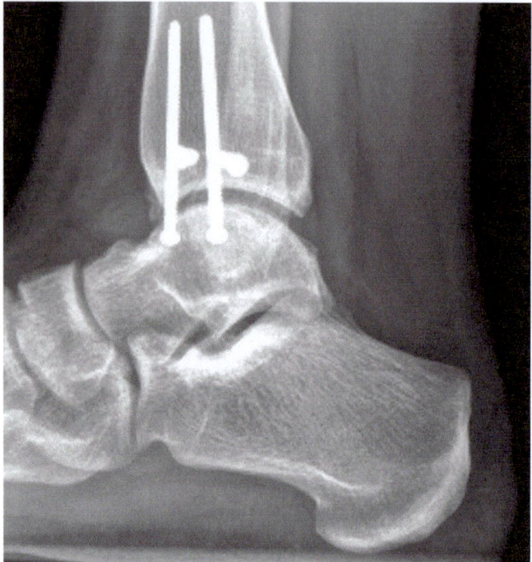

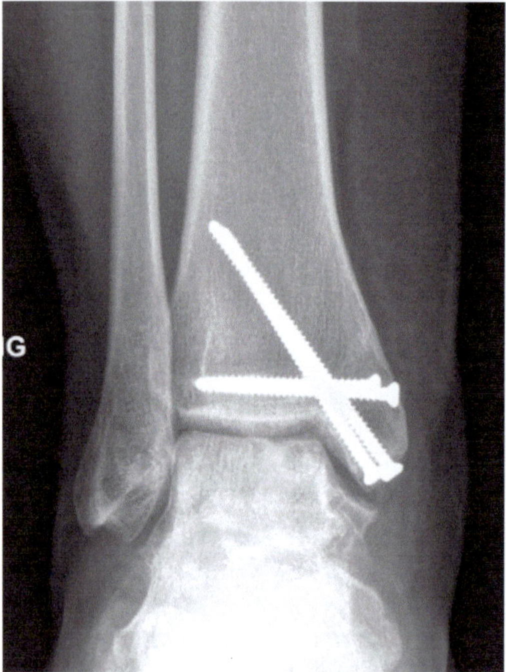

Fig. 10 The postoperative X-ray of the case in Fig. 9 showing screw configuration and osteotomy site

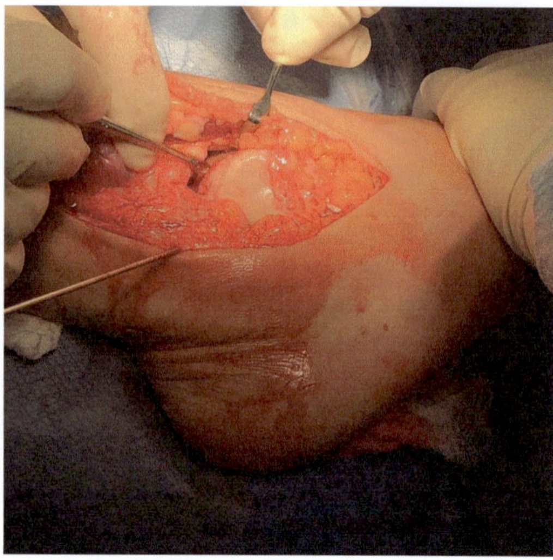

Fig. 11 A lateral malleolar osteotomy to expose a lateral osteochondral defect

Similar prognostic factors exist to bone marrow stimulation, such as size and location. Unconstrained lesions can be treated by OATS. The graft should be congruent and a depth of 12–15 mm used. Two or less grafts have a similar outcome, and three grafts or more may result in a poor outcome.

Cysts may occur after OATS and can be prevented by careful drilling, to avoid thermal injury to bone, a press fit construct, and the use of biologic. The relevance of the cysts are debated [50] (Fig. 15).

The preferred donor site for autograft is the lateral femoral condyle [51]. Donor site morbidity can be reduced by reducing damage to the cartilage, avoiding a tight lateral closure, reducing the soft tissue manipulation, and perform early mobilization of the donor site [52]. Ideally the defect should be backfilled by a plug.

fibular nail. A Chaput osteotomy can also improve access and may allow vertical access to the defect.

The consensus meeting reviewed the role of osteochondral autografts. The recommended indications include cystic lesions more than 1 cm in diameter and revision of failed bone marrow stimulation procedures over 1 cm in size.

9.4 Postoperative Protocol OATS Procedure

Because of the extensive incision and either the lateral ligament repair, or the medial malleolar osteotomy the ankle is splinted for 2 weeks postoperatively. The medial malleolar osteotomy should be stable when fixed, and therefore mobi-

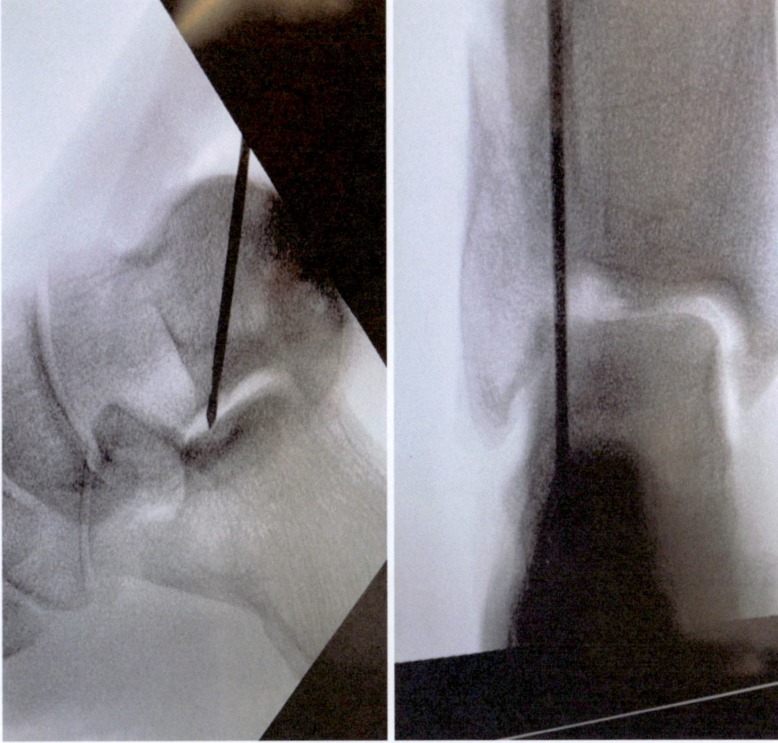

Fig. 12 The correct angle for the OATS drill. The guide wire should be vertical to the joint surface on all planes. On the lateral view the tip of the guide wire should point down to the tip of the lateral process of the talus

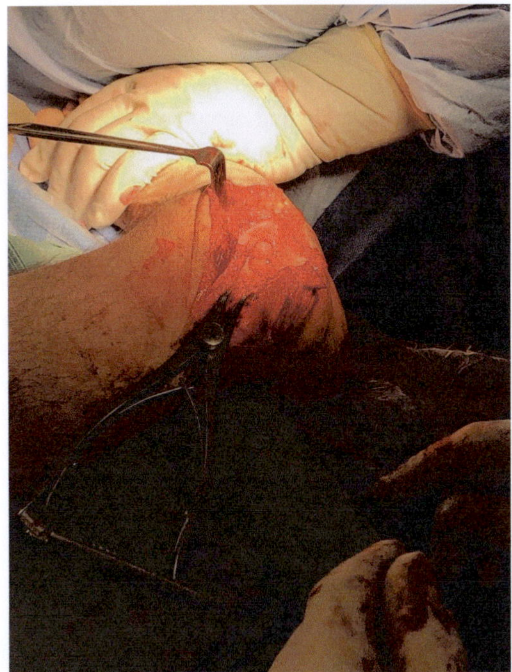

Fig. 13 The final grafts in place

lization can be faster. After suture removal and assuming wound healing, the ankle is mobilized with range of motion. Weight-bearing can be initiated depending on stability of the osteotomy at 2–6 weeks postoperative. Range of motion can be initiated using a stationary bicycle. At 12 weeks proprioception can be initiated.

9.5 Revision Treatment of the Osteochondral Defect

Revision of an osteochondral defect follows the principles of the primary lesion. A thoughtful history and physical is required to ensure that the cause of ongoing pain is correctly identified.

Factors considered important in choice of revision procedure include imaging appearance, mechanical factors such as stability, patient age, presence of other cartilage pathology, presence of a cyst, lesion progression, size of lesion, and type of initial procedure [32].

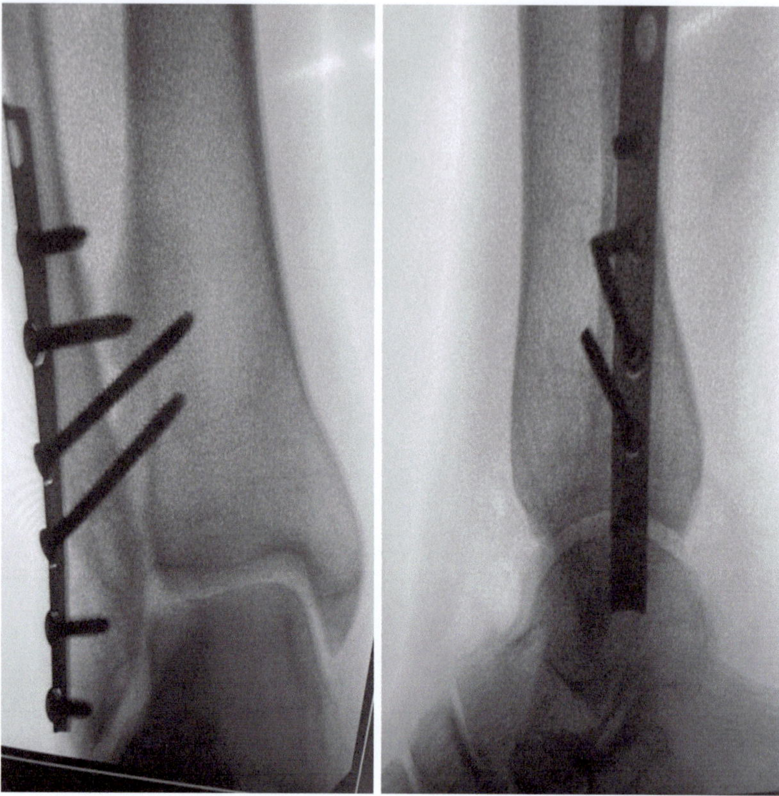

Fig. 14 Fixation of the fibular osteotomy

Revision of the cartilage procedure is contra indicated if the patient has infection, extensive degenerative disease, inflammatory arthropathy, severe stiffness, discrepancy between clinical symptoms and imaging findings, unrealistic expectations for the outcome of the revision procedure, and patient non-compliance [32].

If the primary procedure was a BMS procedure, then an OATS procedure may be the best salvage [53].

A systematic review of five papers showed a success rate for revision BMS at 61%, so revision BMS may not achieve a desirable result and should be considered carefully [54].

Revision may be more successful with an OATS or bulk graft. Park et al. compared primary OATS procedures against revisions and found similar survivorship and outcome scores. Larger lesions were the cause of failure in both groups (over 225 mm^2 on preoperative MRI) [55]. This is not the case of BMS [54]. Yoon et al. also outlined that OATS was a better treatment compared to BMS for failed debridement [53].

Ettinger and Maiorano have advocated a titanium hemicap as a revision device [56, 57].. However only ten lesions were treated in 7 patients in Ettinger's study and 12 patients in the other study. Ettinger observed high body mass index (BMI) as a risk factor for failure. This is unlike Koh et al. that found similar results if longer procedure times for patients over a BMI of 25 [58]. A BMI of 25 is a low threshold for many patient populations.

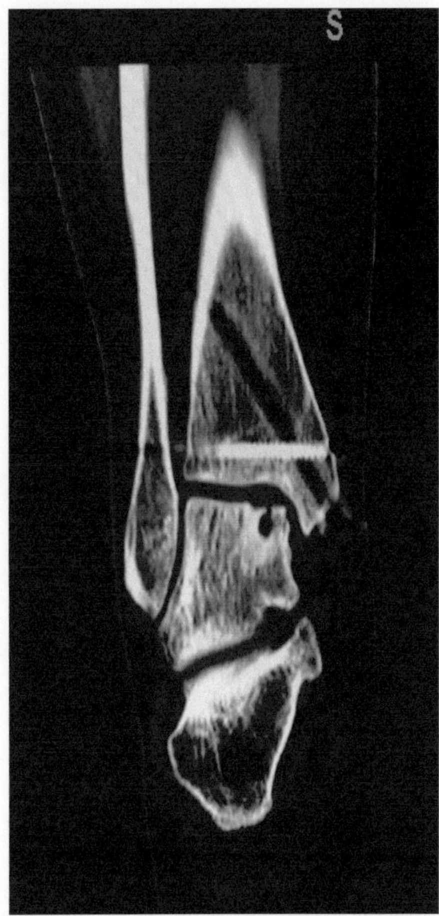

Fig. 15 Cyst defect in an OATS graft

10 Treatment of Bone Marrow Oedema Alone

Subchondroplasty, the injection of Calcium Phosphate into the bone, has been advocated as a treatment for symptomatic subchondral oedema if the overlying cartilage is intact. Concern has been raised about the risk of AVN of the talus from the injection due to over pressurization at the time of injection so caution should be used, and currently the recommendation is to use a low volume of graft (1.5 cc's) [59].

11 Treatment of Lesions of the Tibia

Tibial lesions have a slightly different pathology: The defect is often smaller and the marrow signal greater. The treatment is also challenging as accessing the lesion through the joint is technically challenging. The defect is therefore best addressed retrograde.

Smaller tibial lesions can be treated with debridement and BMS as described by Ferkel and the German registry [60, 61].

Our preferred treatment is to use a tibial targeting device from the knee or biotenodesis set. The lesion is targeted and a k wire from the biotenodesis screw set used (Figs. 16 and 17). The appropriately sized reamer is then used to ream up to but not through the subchondral bone (Fig. 18). The bone is then reamed to a size to allow bone healing. Typically, a 6–10 mm reamer is used. Care is taken not to create heat during the reaming, and so irrigation or reaming with the tourniquet down will achieve this.

Cancellous autograft or allograft is then packed into the defect (Figs. 19 and 20), and platelet derived growth factor at the discretion of the surgeon can be added to stimulate bone healing.

An alternative is to place an OATS graft. However, matching the graft to the defect is difficult to do, and a vertical approach to the joint line is difficult to achieve. An osteotomy can be used to access the tibia to perform the graft [62].

The German registry had a total of 15 cases with over 1 year follow up in a registry of 844 OLT's with a total of 47 being tibial lesions (the majority not having over 1 year follow up). This amounts to 6% of all ankle osteochondral lesions. The majority were treated with BMS [60].

Ferkel reported on arthroscopic treatment of tibial lesions in 17 patients with 14 of 17 doing well with arthroscopic debridement. If there was

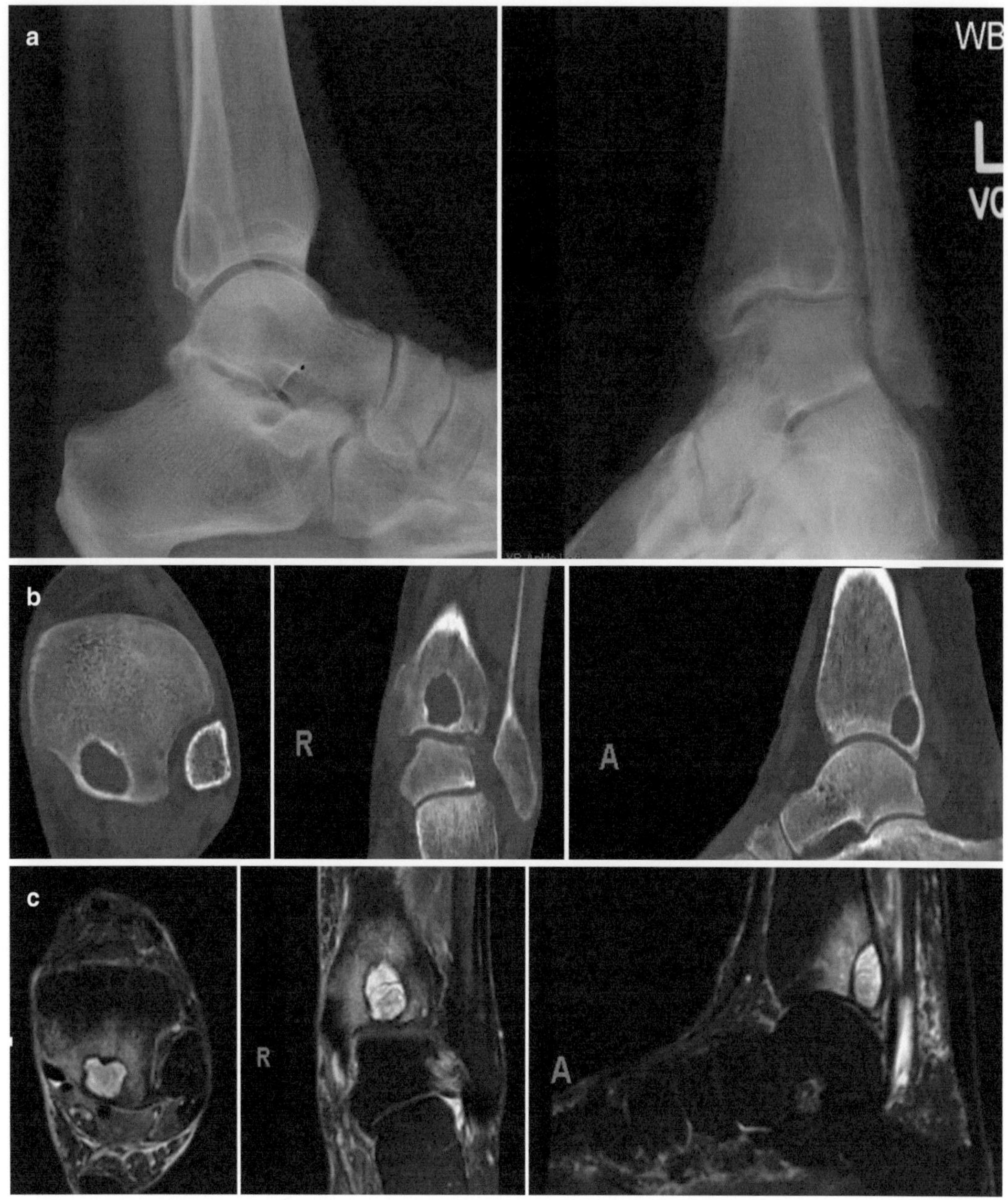

Fig. 16 A large posterior medial cystic defect in the tibia. (**a**) Plain X-rays (**b**) ct appearance (**c**) MRI preop

a cystic component or bone defect, iliac crest graft was added to the defect [61].

Another alternative has been to use injected bone graft made from Calcium phosphate in a subchondroplasty procedure. Some concern has been raised about the risk of AVN. This may however represent a radiographic artefact. As a result, a small amount of graft may be placed and can be of use in isolated bone marrow oedema.

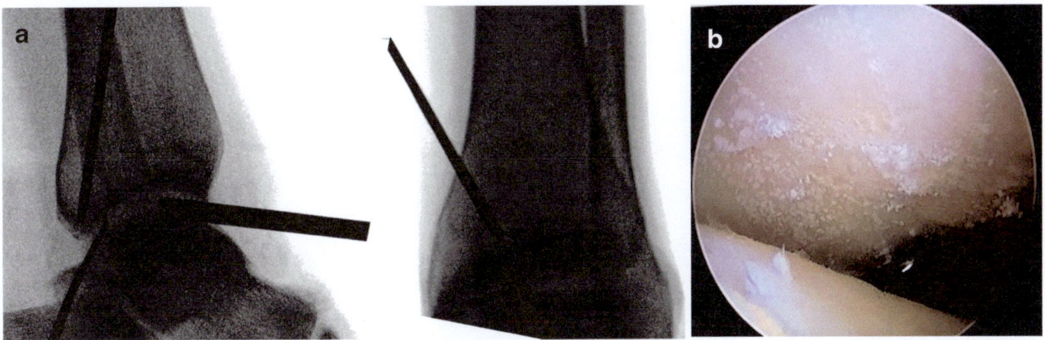

Fig. 17 (**a**) Targeting the lesion using an anterior medial, posterior medial portal, and incision over the distal tibia. The reamer for the biotenodesis screw set was used to access the defect and debridement of the cyst wall was performed arthroscopically. (**b**) Intra-articular view

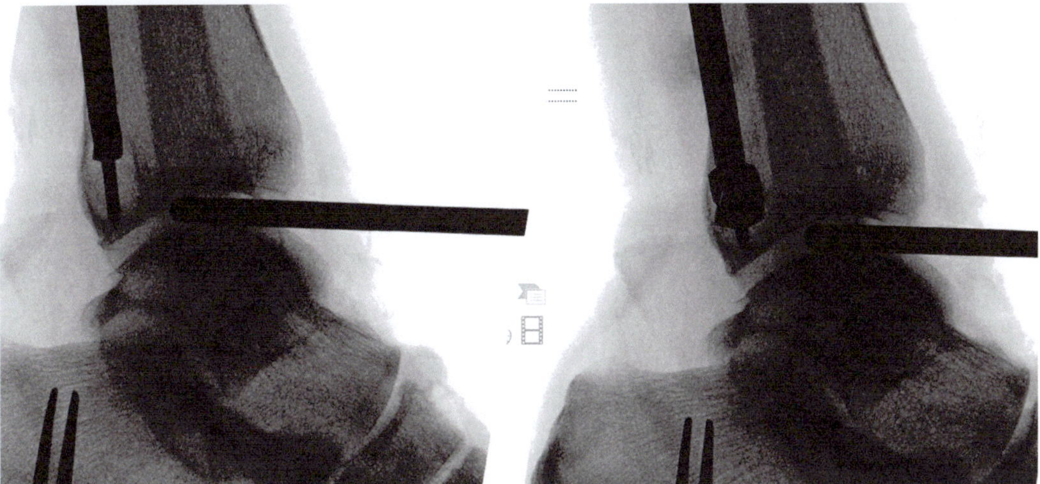

Fig. 18 Reaming to the cyst and staying outside the subchondral bone

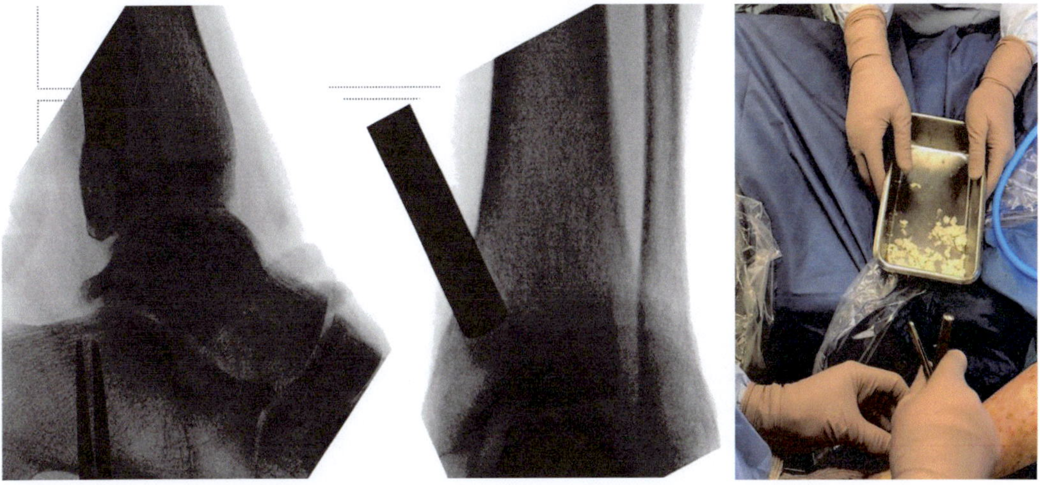

Fig. 19 Grafting the defect with allograft with a 10 mm tamp

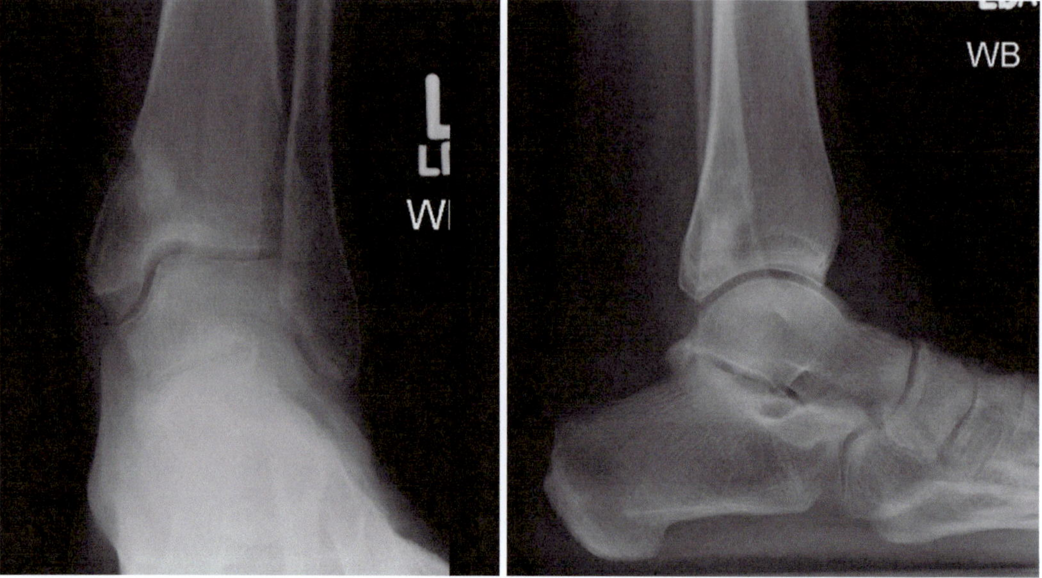

Fig. 20 Postoperative X-rays at 6 months. The patient is symptom free and has unrestricted activity

11.1 Postoperative Recovery After Subchondral Graft Procedures

If bone graft is used, remobilization can be achieved with weight bearing at 2 weeks. If there is concern about shear on a more unstable grafted OCD, delay may be considered.

Return to sport should be delayed until there is clear healing on X-ray and if required CT and MRI. Impact activity should be avoided if there is a residual bone marrow oedema signal.

11.2 Salvage: Fusion or Replacement

In some cases, the treatment of the osteochondral defect is unsuccessful despite a number of strategies and surgeries. In these cases, it may be better to consider fusion of the ankle joint to ensure return of weight bearing function for the patient.

The Consensus meeting recommended fusion or replacement if the failed cartilage procedure cannot be reasonably addressed by a revision procedure, or if there is progressive arthritis in the joint [32].

11.3 Outcomes

In a systematic review by Zengerink et al. in KSST in 2010, they quoted a success rate of 84% for transplantation procedures, 82% if the fragment could be transfixed, 76% for BMS and MFX, and 71% for debridement alone.

However, may factors can change the outcome including lesion size, patient weight, gender, location, vitamin d deficiency [63–65].

Outcomes are hard to interpret because of the scientific quality of the papers. Few are high quality, and the enrolment criteria, surgical procedures, documentation of demographics, outcomes used are all variable [66].

Toal et al. did a systematic review of BMS in 2019 and demonstrated reasonable short-term results [67]. Imaging findings continued to be present potentially indicating deterioration in time.

For OATs, a systematic review showed good to excellent results in 87.4%, 3.6% had donor site morbidity [68] [68]. Mosaicplasty is different than OATS so results should be considered separately.

Return to sport remains a critical outcome measure [69]. With microfracture all ten national basketball players returned to play [69]. In a systematic review 86% of patients returned to play at an average of 4.5 months [70]. However lesion size is critical in this reporting [71].

11.4 Associated Pathology

Osteochondral defects are associated with a number of pathologies. These include lateral ankle instability, hindfoot varus [72], tibial varus [73], anterior medial osteophytes, and peroneal tendinopathy.

Some may require treatment for the success of the osteochondral defect management. In the case of ligamentous instability in the presence of an osteochondral defect, the surgeon may consider performing a lateral ligament reconstruction at the same time of the OLT treatment [74]. This will help treat the osteochondral defect as it prevents shear of the joint surface. It is recommended by the author that any ankle instability present should be managed at the same time as the OLT.

The surgeon may also consider treatment of the hindfoot varus or tibial varus at the same time. This may involve a tibial osteotomy, a calcaneal osteotomy or a combination of both.

Anterior medial impingement and synovitis should also be treated at the time of arthroscopy.

Arthroscopy also allows the assessment of the remaining cartilage. This may assist in future management should the joint remain symptomatic.

11.5 Authors Preferred Technique/ Algorithm

Based on the current research and information the author of this chapter prefers to perform an arthroscopic debridement if there is any uncertainty about the pathology before performing an open or osteotomy procedure. If the lesion is small, no bone graft or cartilage substitute is used. If the lesion is over 5 mm deep or 10 mm long bone grafting using cancellous graft ± platelet derived growth factor is used. This is sealed with fibrin glue, and lyophilized cartilage placed on top.

If the lesion is larger, cystic, or is a revision of a known well debrided and well visualized defect then an OATS autograft is performed.

All associated pathology is treated at the time of the primary procedure with a low threshold to perform a lateral ligament reconstruction, a calcaneal osteotomy (90% of the time lateralizing and done percutaneously), or a tibial osteotomy if needed.

If the OATS procedure fails then I will perform a second look arthroscopy and if there is more diffuse cartilage damage offer an ankle fusion in younger patients or a replacement in older patients.

Bibliography

1. Kerkhoffs GM, Kennedy JG, Calder JD, Karlsson J. There is no simple lateral ankle sprain. Knee Surg Sports Traumatol Arthrosc. 2016;24(4):941–3.
2. Hintermann B, Regazzoni P, Lampert C, Stutz G, Gachter A. Arthroscopic findings in acute fractures of the ankle. J Bone Joint Surg Br. 2000;82(3):345–51.
3. Hannon CP, Smyth NA, Murawski CD, et al. Osteochondral lesions of the talus: aspects of current management. Bone Joint J. 2014;96-B(2):164–71.
4. Steman JAH, Dahmen J, Lambers KTA, Kerkhoffs G. Return to sports after surgical treatment of osteochondral defects of the talus: a systematic review of 2347 cases. Orthop J Sports Med. 2019;7(10):2325967119876238.
5. Wiewiorski M, Werner L, Paul J, Anderson AE, Barg A, Valderrabano V. Sports activity after reconstruction of osteochondral lesions of the talus with autologous spongiosa grafts and autologous matrix-induced chondrogenesis. Am J Sports Med. 2016;44(10):2651–8.
6. Korner D, Ateschrang A, Schroter S, et al. Concomitant ankle instability has a negative impact on the quality of life in patients with osteochondral lesions of the talus: data from the German Cartilage Registry (KnorpelRegister DGOU). Knee Surg Sports Traumatol Arthrosc. 2020;28(10):3339–46.
7. Ahrend MD, Aurich M, Becher C, et al. Preexisting and treated concomitant ankle instability does not compromise patient-reported outcomes of solitary osteochondral lesions of the talus treated with matrix-induced bone marrow stimulation in the first postoperative year: data from the German Cartilage Registry (KnorpelRegister DGOU). Knee Surg Sports Traumatol Arthrosc. 2022;30(4):1187–96.
8. Hadeed MM, Dempscy IJ, Tyrrell Burrus M, et al. Predictors of osteochondral lesions of the talus in

patients undergoing Brostrom-Gould ankle ligament reconstruction. J Foot Ankle Surg. 2020;59(1):21–6.

9. Murawski CD, Hogan MV, Thordarson DB, Stone JW, Ferkel RD, Kennedy JG. Editorial. Foot Ankle Int. 2018;39(1_Suppl):1S–2S.

10. Medda S, Al'Khafaji IM, Scott AT. Ankle arthroscopy with microfracture for osteochondral defects of the talus. Arthrosc Tech. 2017;6(1):e167–74.

11. Danilkowicz RM, Allen NB, Grimm N, et al. Histological and inflammatory cytokine analysis of osteochondral lesions of the talus after failed microfracture: comparison with fresh allograft controls. Orthop J Sports Med. 2021;9(10):23259671211040535.

12. van Diepen PR, Dahmen J, Altink JN, Stufkens SAS, Kerkhoffs G. Location distribution of 2,087 osteochondral lesions of the talus. Cartilage. 2021;13(1_Suppl):1344S–53S.

13. Elias I, Zoga AC, Morrison WB, Besser MP, Schweitzer ME, Raikin SM. Osteochondral lesions of the talus: localization and morphologic data from 424 patients using a novel anatomical grid scheme. Foot Ankle Int. 2007;28(2):154–61.

14. Elias I, Raikin SM, Schweitzer ME, Besser MP, Morrison WB, Zoga AC. Osteochondral lesions of the distal tibial plafond: localization and morphologic characteristics with an anatomical grid. Foot Ankle Int. 2009;30(6):524–9.

15. Martin KD, McBride TJ, Horan DP, et al. Validation of 9-grid scheme for localizing osteochondral lesions of the talus. Foot Ankle Orthop. 2020;5(3):2473011420944925.

16. Shimozono Y, Brown AJ, Batista JP, et al. Subchondral pathology: proceedings of the international consensus meeting on cartilage repair of the ankle. Foot Ankle Int. 2018;39(1_Suppl):48S–53S.

17. Murawski CD, Jamal MS, Hurley ET, et al. Terminology for osteochondral lesions of the ankle: proceedings of the international consensus meeting on cartilage repair of the ankle. J ISAKOS. 2022;7(2):62–6.

18. van Bergen CJA, Baur OL, Murawski CD, et al. Diagnosis: history, physical examination, imaging, and arthroscopy: proceedings of the international consensus meeting on cartilage repair of the ankle. Foot Ankle Int. 2018;39(1_Suppl):3S–8S.

19. Agrawal K, Swaroop S, Patro PSS, Tripathy SK, Naik S, Velagada S. Comparison of bone SPECT/CT and MRI in detection of pain generator in ankle and foot pain: a retrospective diagnostic study. Nucl Med Commun. 2021;42(10):1085–96.

20. van Bergen CJ, Gerards RM, Opdam KT, Terra MP, Kerkhoffs GM. Diagnosing, planning and evaluating osteochondral ankle defects with imaging modalities. World J Orthop. 2015;6(11):944–53.

21. Dombrowski ME, Yasui Y, Murawski CD, et al. Conservative management and biological treatment strategies: proceedings of the international consensus

meeting on cartilage repair of the ankle. Foot Ankle Int. 2018;39(1_Suppl):9S–15S.

22. Hannon CP, Bayer S, Murawski CD, et al. Debridement, curettage, and bone marrow stimulation: proceedings of the international consensus meeting on cartilage repair of the ankle. Foot Ankle Int. 2018;39(1_Suppl):16S–22S.

23. Brohard J, Chin KM. Maximum plantarflexion lateral ankle radiograph for preoperative planning for the arthroscopic treatment of osteochondral lesions of the talus. Foot Ankle Orthop. 2022;7(2):24730114221102453.

24. Acevedo JI, Busch MT, Ganey TM, Hutton WC, Ogden JA. Coaxial portals for posterior ankle arthroscopy: an anatomic study with clinical correlation on 29 patients. Arthroscopy. 2000;16(8):836–42.

25. Murawski CD, Foo LF, Kennedy JG. A review of arthroscopic bone marrow stimulation techniques of the talus: the good, the bad, and the causes for concern. Cartilage. 2010;1(2):137–44.

26. Hunt KJ, Lee AT, Lindsey DP, Slikker W 3rd, Chou LB. Osteochondral lesions of the talus: effect of defect size and plantarflexion angle on ankle joint stresses. Am J Sports Med. 2012;40(4):895–901.

27. Ramponi L, Yasui Y, Murawski CD, et al. Lesion size is a predictor of clinical outcomes after bone marrow stimulation for osteochondral lesions of the talus: a systematic review. Am J Sports Med. 2017;45(7):1698–705.

28. Hwang YG, Lee JW, Park KH, Hsienhao C, Han SH. Intra-articular injections of hyaluronic acid on osteochondral lesions of the talus after failed arthroscopic bone marrow stimulation. Foot Ankle Int. 2020;41(11):1376–82.

29. Reilingh ML, Murawski CD, DiGiovanni CW, et al. Fixation techniques: proceedings of the international consensus meeting on cartilage repair of the ankle. Foot Ankle Int. 2018;39(1_Suppl):23S–7S.

30. Nakasa T, Ikuta Y, Ota Y, Kanemitsu M, Adachi N. Clinical results of bioabsorbable pin fixation relative to the bone condition for osteochondral lesion of the talus. Foot Ankle Int. 2019;40(12):1388–96.

31. Nakasa T, Ikuta Y, Sumii J, Nekomoto A, Kawabata S, Adachi N. Clinical outcomes of osteochondral fragment fixation versus microfracture even for small osteochondral lesions of the talus. Am J Sports Med. 2022;11:3019.

32. Mittwede PN, Murawski CD, Ackermann J, et al. Revision and salvage management: proceedings of the international consensus meeting on cartilage repair of the ankle. Foot Ankle Int. 2018;39(1_Suppl):54S–60S.

33. Ettinger S, Gottschalk O, Kostretzis L, et al. One-year follow-up data from the German Cartilage Registry (KnorpelRegister DGOU) in the treatment of chondral and osteochondral defects of the talus. Arch Orthop Trauma Surg. 2022;142(2):205–10.

34. Shieh AK, Singh SG, Nathe C, et al. Effects of micronized cartilage matrix on cartilage repair

in osteochondral lesions of the talus. Cartilage. 2020;11(3):316–22.

35. Hansen OB, Eble SK, Patel K, et al. Comparison of clinical and radiographic outcomes following arthroscopic debridement with extracellular matrix augmentation and osteochondral autograft transplantation for medium-size osteochondral lesions of the talus. Foot Ankle Int. 2021;42(6):689–98.

36. Ahmad J, Maltenfort M. Arthroscopic treatment of osteochondral lesions of the talus with allograft cartilage matrix. Foot Ankle Int. 2017;38(8):855–62.

37. Manzi J, Arzani A, Hamula MJ, Manchanda K, Dhanaraj D, Chapman CB. Long-term patient-reported outcome measures following particulated juvenile allograft cartilage implantation for treatment of difficult osteochondral lesions of the talus. Foot Ankle Int. 2021;42(11):1399–409.

38. Giza E, Delman C, Coetzee JC, Schon LC. Arthroscopic treatment of talus osteochondral lesions with particulated juvenile allograft cartilage. Foot Ankle Int. 2014;35(10):1087–94.

39. Albano D, Martinelli N, Bianchi A, Messina C, Malerba F, Sconfienza LM. Clinical and imaging outcome of osteochondral lesions of the talus treated using autologous matrix-induced chondrogenesis technique with a biomimetic scaffold. BMC Musculoskelet Disord. 2017;18(1):306.

40. Buda R, Vannini F, Castagnini F, et al. Regenerative treatment in osteochondral lesions of the talus: autologous chondrocyte implantation versus one-step bone marrow derived cells transplantation. Int Orthop. 2015;39(5):893–900.

41. Bai L, Guan S, Liu S, et al. Clinical outcomes of osteochondral lesions of the talus with large subchondral cysts treated with osteotomy and autologous chondral grafts: minimum 2-year follow-up and second-look evaluation. Orthop J Sports Med. 2020;8(7):2325967120937798.

42. Lee KT, Kim JS, Young KW, et al. The use of fibrin matrix-mixed gel-type autologous chondrocyte implantation in the treatment for osteochondral lesions of the talus. Knee Surg Sports Traumatol Arthrosc. 2013;21(6):1251–60.

43. Hannon CP, Baksh N, Newman H, Murawski CD, Smyth NA, Kennedy JG. A systematic review on the reporting of outcome data in studies on autologous osteochondral transplantation for the treatment of osteochondral lesions of the talus. Foot Ankle Spec. 2013;6(3):226–31.

44. Emre TY, Ege T, Cift HT, Demircioglu DT, Seyhan B, Uzun M. Open mosaicplasty in osteochondral lesions of the talus: a prospective study. J Foot Ankle Surg. 2012;51(5):556–60.

45. Hu Y, Yue C, Li X, et al. A novel medial malleolar osteotomy technique for the treatment of osteochondral lesions of the talus. Orthop J Sports Med. 2021;9(3):2325967121989988.

46. Padiolleau G, Amouyel T, Barbier O, et al. Safety of malleolar osteotomies in surgery for osteochondral lesions of the talus. Orthop Traumatol Surg Res. 2021;107(8S):103070.

47. Murawski CD, Kennedy JG. Operative treatment of osteochondral lesions of the talus. J Bone Joint Surg Am. 2013;95(11):1045–54.

48. Yasui Y, Ross AW, Kennedy JG. Platelet-rich plasma and concentrated bone marrow aspirate in surgical treatment for osteochondral lesions of the talus. Foot Ankle Clin. 2016;21(4):869–84.

49. Shimozono Y, Yasui Y, Hurley ET, Paugh RA, Deyer TW, Kennedy JG. Concentrated bone marrow aspirate may decrease postoperative cyst occurrence rate in autologous osteochondral transplantation for osteochondral lesions of the talus. Arthroscopy. 2019;35(1):99–105.

50. Savage-Elliott I, Smyth NA, Deyer TW, et al. Magnetic resonance imaging evidence of postoperative cyst formation does not appear to affect clinical outcomes after autologous osteochondral transplantation of the talus. Arthroscopy. 2016;32(9):1846–54.

51. Hurley ET, Stewart SK, Kennedy JG, Strauss EJ, Calder J, Ramasamy A. Current management strategies for osteochondral lesions of the talus. Bone Joint J. 2021;103-B(2):207–12.

52. Shimozono Y, Seow D, Yasui Y, Fields K, Kennedy JG. Knee-to-talus donor-site morbidity following autologous osteochondral transplantation: a meta-analysis with best-case and worst-case analysis. Clin Orthop Relat Res. 2019;477(8):1915–31.

53. Yoon HS, Park YJ, Lee M, Choi WJ, Lee JW. Osteochondral autologous transplantation is superior to repeat arthroscopy for the treatment of osteochondral lesions of the talus after failed primary arthroscopic treatment. Am J Sports Med. 2014;42(8):1896–903.

54. Dahmen J, Hurley ET, Shimozono Y, et al. Evidence-based treatment of failed primary osteochondral lesions of the talus: a systematic review on clinical outcomes of bone marrow stimulation. Cartilage. 2021;13(1_Suppl):1411S–21S.

55. Park KH, Hwang Y, Han SH, et al. Primary versus secondary osteochondral autograft transplantation for the treatment of large osteochondral lesions of the talus. Am J Sports Med. 2018;46(6):1389–96.

56. Ettinger S, Stukenborg-Colsman C, Waizy H, et al. Results of HemiCAP((R)) implantation as a salvage procedure for osteochondral lesions of the talus. J Foot Ankle Surg. 2017;56(4):788–92.

57. Maiorano E, Bianchi A, Hosseinzadeh MK, Malerba F, Martinelli N, Sansone V. HemiCAP(R) implantation after failed previous surgery for osteochondral lesions of the talus. Foot Ankle Surg. 2021;27(1):77–81.

58. Koh DTS, Tan MWP, Zhan X, et al. Association of elevated body mass index and outcomes of arthroscopic treatment for osteochondral lesions of the talus. Foot Ankle Orthop. 2022;7(2):24730114221103263.

59. Hanselman AE, Cody EA, Easley ME, Adams SB, Parekh SG. Avascular necrosis of the talus after subchondroplasty. Foot Ankle Int. 2021;42(9):1138–43.

60. Gottschalk O, Korner D, Aurich M, et al. Descriptive analysis and short-term follow-up clinical results of osteochondral lesions of the distal tibia based on data of the German Cartilage Register (Knorpelregister((R)) DGOU). Arch Orthop Trauma Surg. 2021;143:809.

61. Mologne TS, Ferkel RD. Arthroscopic treatment of osteochondral lesions of the distal tibia. Foot Ankle Int. 2007;28(8):865–72.

62. Chen W, Tang K, Yuan C, Zhou Y, Tao X. Intermediate results of large cystic medial osteochondral lesions of the talus treated with Osteoperiosteal cylinder autografts from the medial tibia. Arthroscopy. 2015;31(8):1557–64.

63. Malhotra K, Baggott PJ, Livingstone J. Vitamin D in the foot and ankle: a review of the literature. J Am Podiatr Med Assoc. 2020;110(3):Article_10.

64. Oberti V, Sanchez Ortiz M, Allende V, Masquijo J. Prevalence of hypovitaminosis D in patients with juvenile osteochondritis dissecans. Rev Esp Cir Ortop Traumatol (Engl Ed). 2021;65(2):132–7.

65. Telleria JJM, Ready LV, Bluman EM, Chiodo CP, Smith JT. Prevalence of vitamin D deficiency in patients with Talar osteochondral lesions. Foot Ankle Int. 2018;39(4):471–8.

66. Yasui Y, Ramponi L, Seow D, et al. Systematic review of bone marrow stimulation for osteochondral lesion of talus - evaluation for level and quality of clinical studies. World J Orthop. 2017;8(12):956–63.

67. Toale J, Shimozono Y, Mulvin C, Dahmen J, Kerkhoffs G, Kennedy JG. Midterm outcomes of bone marrow stimulation for primary osteochondral lesions of the talus: a systematic review. Orthop J Sports Med. 2019;7(10):2325967119879127.

68. Shimozono Y, Hurley ET, Myerson CL, Kennedy JG. Good clinical and functional outcomes at midterm following autologous osteochondral transplantation for osteochondral lesions of the talus. Knee Surg Sports Traumatol Arthrosc. 2018;26(10):3055–62.

69. Sheu C, Ferkel RD. Athletic performance in the National Basketball Association after arthroscopic debridement of osteochondral lesions of the talus. Orthop J Sports Med. 2021;9(1):2325967120970205.

70. Hurley ET, Shimozono Y, McGoldrick NP, Myerson CL, Yasui Y, Kennedy JG. High reported rate of return to play following bone marrow stimulation for osteochondral lesions of the talus. Knee Surg Sports Traumatol Arthrosc. 2019;27(9):2721–30.

71. Lee KT, Song SY, Hyuk J, Kim SJ. Lesion size may predict return to play in young elite athletes undergoing microfracture for osteochondral lesions of the talus. Arthroscopy. 2021;37(5):1612–9.

72. Easley ME, Vineyard JC. Varus ankle and osteochondral lesions of the talus. Foot Ankle Clin. 2012;17(1):21–38.

73. Li X, Zhu Y, Xu Y, Wang B, Liu J, Xu X. Osteochondral autograft transplantation with biplanar distal tibial osteotomy for patients with concomitant large osteochondral lesion of the talus and varus ankle malalignment. BMC Musculoskelet Disord. 2017;18(1):23.

74. Ackermann J, Casari FA, Germann C, Weigelt L, Wirth SH, Viehofer AF. Autologous matrix-induced chondrogenesis with lateral ligament stabilization for osteochondral lesions of the talus in patients with ankle instability. Orthop J Sports Med. 2021;9(5):23259671211007439.

Index

MIX
Papier aus verantwortungsvollen Quellen
Paper from responsible sources
FSC® C105338

If you have any concerns about our products,
you can contact us on
ProductSafety@springernature.com

In case Publisher is established outside the EU,
the EU authorized representative is:
**Springer Nature Customer Service Center GmbH
Europaplatz 3, 69115 Heidelberg, Germany**

Printed by Libri Plureos GmbH
in Hamburg, Germany